1993

Making Managed Healthcare Work

A Practical Guide to Strategies and Solutions

Making Managed Healthcare Work

A Practical Guide to Strategies and Solutions

Edited by

Peter Boland, PhD
BOLAND
Berkeley, California

AN ASPEN PUBLICATION®
Aspen Publishers, Inc.
Gaithersburg, Maryland
1993

This publication is designed to provide accurate and authoritative information in regard to the Subject Matter covered. It is sold with the understanding that the publisher is not engaged in rendering legal, accounting, or other professional service. If legal advice or other expert assistance is required, the service of a competent professional person should be sought. (*From a Declaration of Principles jointly adopted by a Committee of the American Bar Association and a Committee of Publishers and Associations.*)

Library of Congress Cataloging-in-Publication Data

Making managed healthcare work : a practical guide to strategies and solutions / edited by Peter Boland.

p. cm.
Originally published: McGraw-Hill, Health Professions Division, © 1991.
Includes bibliographical references and index.
ISBN: 0-8342-0391-X
1. Managed care plans (Medical care)—United States. 2. Managed care plans (Medical care)
I. Boland, Peter. II. Title: Making managed healthcare work.
[DNLM: 1. Managed Care Programs—organization & administration—United States.
W 84 AA1 M23 1991a (P)j
RA413.5.U5M35   1993
362.1'068—dc20
DNLM/DLC
for Library of Congress
92-49532
CIP

Editorial Resources: Ruth Bloom

Library of Congress Catalog Card Number: 92-49532
ISBN: 0-8342-0391-X

Printed in the United States of America

2 3 4 5

To
Jane R. Boland
and
Edward W. Boland, M.D.

CONTENTS

CONTRIBUTORS

Kenneth S. Abramowitz, Healthcare Analyst, Sanford C. Bernstein Company, New York, New York

Eric E. Anderson, Ph.D., Chief Operating Officer, Lifelink, Laguna Hills, California

David V. Axene, Principal and Consulting Actuary, Milliman & Robertson Inc., Seattle, Washington

Jerome Beloff, M.D., Vice President and Chief Medical Officer, AV-Med Health Plan of Florida, Miami, Florida

Linda Bergthold, Ph.D., Senior Consultant, National Medical Audit, William M. Mercer, Inc., San Francisco, California

Howard R. Berry, Principal Associate, McManis Associates, Washington, D.C.

Peter Boland, Ph.D., President, Boland Healthcare Consultants, Berkeley, California

Frank M. Brocato, Executive Director, Florida Gulf Coast Health Coalition, Tampa, Florida

Charles R. Buck, Jr., Sc.D., Staff Executive, Health Care Management Programs, General Electric Company, Fairfield, Connecticut

John Burns, M.D., Vice President, Health Management, Honeywell, Inc., Minneapolis, Minnesota

Philip Caper, M.D., Chairman, Codman Research Group, Inc., Lyme, New Hampshire

Joseph G. Charles, Group Director, Employee Benefits, Ryder System, Inc., Miami, Florida

Roberta N. Clarke, Associate Professor, Department Chair, Boston University, School of Management, Boston, Massachusetts

Russell C. Coile, Jr., President, Health Forecasting Group, Alameda, California

Charlotte K. Corcoran, Vice President, Interqual, Inc., North Hampton, New Hampshire

Thomas Davies, Cleremont Business Group, Oakland, California

Hamilton E. Davis, Chairman, Vermont Hospital Data Council, Waterbury, Vermont

Joseph W. Duva, Corporate Director, Employee Benefits, Allied-Signal, Morristown, New Jersey

Lynne J. Eickholt, Director of Managed Care, New England Medical Center Hospitals, Boston, Massachusetts

Carol B. Emmott, Ph.D., Executive Director, California Association of Public Hospitals, San Mateo, California

John C. Erb, Managing Consultant, A. Foster Higgins & Co., Inc., Princeton, New Jersey

Clara Jean Ersoz, M.D., M.S.H.A., Vice President, Medical Affairs, St. Clair Hospital, Pittsburgh, Pennsylvania

Richard H. Eskow, Vice President, American International Healthcare, Rockville, Maryland

Nancy Forney, R.N., MBA, Clinical Director of Surgical Services, St. Clair Hospital, Pittsburgh, Pennsylvania

Peter Fox, Ph.D., Vice President, Lewin/ICF, Washington, D.C.

Jack A. Friedman, Ph.D., Executive Director, Vantage PPO, Sisters of Providence, Portland, Oregon

Mark Gibson, Executive Assistant to the Senate President, Oregon State Senate, Salem, Oregon

Thomas R. Gillem, Director of Quality Education and Communications, Hospital Corporation of America, Nashville, Tennessee

Paul B. Ginsburg, Ph.D., Executive Director, Physician Payment Review Commission, Washington, D.C.

John D. Golenski, S.J., Principal, Bioethics Consultation Group, Berkeley, California

Marika Gordon, M.A., Healthcare Consultant, Los Angeles, California

Robert F. Griffith, Managing Consultant, A. Foster Higgins & Co., Inc., Los Angeles, California

George C. Halvorson, President and Chief Executive Officer, Group Health, Inc., Minneapolis, Minnesota

G. Michael Hammes, President, Heritage National Healthplan, Davenport, Iowa

Marti Harrington, Second Vice President, Planning and Resource Development, Lincoln National Life Insurance Company, Fort Wayne, Indiana

Linda J. Havlin, Flexible and Groups Benefits Consultant, Hewitt Associates, Lincolnshire, Illinois

Douglas A. Hastings, J.D., Epstein, Becker and Green, Washington, D.C.

Randall P. Herman, Principal, Deloite & Touche, Minneapolis, Minnesota

Lisa I. Iezzoni, M.D., Director of Health Services Research, Health Policy Institute, Boston, University

W. Mark Jasper, President, Benefit Panel Services, Los Angeles, California

Kathleen Jennison, M.D., Chief, Quality-of-Care Measurement, Harvard Community Health Plan, Brookline, Massachusetts

Joyce Jensen, Senior Vice President, National Research Corporation, Lincoln, Nebraska

Paul M. Katz, Senior Management Consultant, Milliman & Robertson, San Francisco, California

Paul H. Keckley, Ph.D., President, The Keckley Group, Nashville, Tennessee

John Kitzhaber, M.D., President, Oregon State Senate, Salem, Oregon

Joanne Lamprey, Senior Vice President, InterQual, Inc., North Hampton, New Hampshire

W. Bryan Latham, M.D., President, MedFacts, Miami, Florida

Barbara D. Levine, Assistant Vice President, Health Strategies Group, The Alexander & Alexander Consulting Group, Westport, Connecticut

Kenneth J. Linde, President, Principal Health Care, Inc., Rockville, Maryland

Philip M. Lohman, Ph.D., Research Director, First Consulting Group, Long Beach, California

Mark E. Lutes, J.D., Epstein, Becker and Green, Washington, D.C.

Angelo Masciantonio, Principal, Vantage Health Partners, Inc., Philadelphia, Pennsylvania

Joseph A. Miller, Senior Vice President, Private Healthcare System, Ltd., Lexington, Massachusetts

Joanne Miller, Health Systems Management, Minneapolis, Minnesota

Karen E. Miller, Dr.P.H., Health Care Administrator, Tenneco, Inc., Houston, Texas

Laird Miller, Health Systems Management, Minneapolis, Minnesota

Arnold Milstein, M.D., President, National Medical Audit, William M. Mercer, Inc., San Francisco, California

J. Ian Morrison, Director, Healthcare Program, Institute for the Future, Menlo Park, California

Philip Nathanson, Vice President, Quality and Outcomes Management, Uni-Health America, Burbank, California

Patricia M. Nazemetz, Director, Corporate Benefits, Xerox Corporation, Stamford, Connecticut

Edward Neuschler, Director of Policy Studies, Health Insurance Association of America, Washington, D.C.

Kevin F. O'Grady, M.D., M.S.P.H., Executive Director, Center for Consumer Healthcare Information, Santa Ana, California

Robert E. Patricelli, President and Chief Executive, Value Health, Inc., Avon, Connecticut

Lou Pavia, Senior Vice President, McManis Associates, Washington, D.C.

Jerry Payne, Director of Marketing, Preferred Health Network, Monterey Park, California

James Reep, Chairman, First Consulting Group, Long Beach, California

J. Peter Rich, Partner, McDermott, Will & Emery, Los Angeles, California

Nigel Roberts, M.D., Project Director, Medicare Demonstration, CAPP CARE, Fountain Valley, California

Louis F. Rossiter, Director of Williamson Institute, Medical College of Virginia, Richmond, Virginia

Nancy Rubini, Vice President, Health Care Finance Group, Standard & Poor's Corporation, New York, New York

Charles L. Scalia, Project Manager, Florida Gulf Coast Health Coalition, Tampa, Florida

Mary F. Schmitz, Ph.D., Manager, Corporate Health Services, Southern California Edison Company, Rosemead, California

Leslie Selbovitz, M.D., Principal, National Medical Audit, William M. Mercer, Inc., San Francisco, California

Conrad Sobczak, MBA, Chief Executive Officer, Family Health Plan, Milwaukee, Wisconsin

Manon Spitzer, Director of Marketing and Educational Programs, Codman Research Group, Inc., Lyme, New Hampshire

Gordon M. Sprenger, President and Chief Executive Officer, Lifespan, Inc., Minneapolis, Minnesota

Humphrey Taylor, President, Louis Harris and Associates, Inc., New York, New York

Richard G. Trapp, Florida Gulf Coast Health Coalition, Tampa, Florida

Larry J. Tucker, Flexible and Groups Benefits Consultant, Hewitt Associates, Lincolnshire, Illinois

Henry M. Tufo, M.D., President, Given Health Care Center, Burlington, Vermont

Peter Van Etten, Executive Vice President, New England Medical Center Hospitals, Boston, Massachusetts

Eric R. Wagner, Senior Manager, Price Waterhouse, Washington, D.C.

Gary S. Whitted, Ph.D., Director, Health Cost Management, Employee Benefits Department, Travelers Insurance Companies, Hartford, Connecticut

Ronald H. Wohl, President, In Plain English, Gaithersburg, Maryland

Ed Zalta, M.D., Chief Executive Officer, CAPP CARE, Fountain Valley, California

William D. Zieverink, M.D., Chief of Psychiatry, Executive Director, Emilie Gamelen Institute, Providence Medical Center, Portland, Oregon

The term *managed care* means different things to different people. It defies easy definitions or commonly accepted yardsticks of success and failure. Basically, it involves an unusually dynamic process which fosters organizational change and diversity.

Managed care has become one of the leading forces in the healthcare industry and, as such, is redefining the traditional roles of healthcare buyers and sellers. It is forcing major stakeholders to reassess what works and what does not.

Managed care is not a panacea for rising healthcare costs, over-utilization, cost shifting, excess capacity, and all the other ills which plague the healthcare industry. Rather, it is an approach that brings together different services and technologies to affect price, volume, quality, and accountability simultaneously.

So far, managed care has not lived up to early expectations about its ability to control unnecessary costs and inappropriate medical care. In the process, though, it has greatly increased awareness about the limitations of adversarial relationships and doing "business as usual" regardless of whether the particular delivery system is an HMO, a PPO, or some new hybrid organization.

The technical knowledge is available to make managed care work. What is too often missing is the judgment and political will of key decision makers—providers, purchasers, and payers—to reach a consensus on how to pursue common business objectives. If the essential "building blocks" of managed care (such as effective utilization management, integrated information systems, and quality improvement processes) are correctly assembled and implemented, delivery systems can produce better healthcare at competitive prices.

This requires key players to commit to long-term strategies and to commit the necessary resources to achieve what should be a fundamental goal—the provision of cost-effective healthcare.

Making Managed Healthcare Work examines many of the most important factors that will influence the direction of managed care in the 1990s. A wide range of critical analyses, expert points of view, and case studies on managed care innovation is organized into five broad categories: market dynamics, product characteristics, management information systems, third-generation delivery system capability, and future trends and government initiatives.

The underlying theme of this book is that managed care *can* work if providers, payers, and purchasers are willing to structure new types of business relationships within a partnership approach to delivering healthcare. This entails embracing risk and uncertainty, although far less long-term risk than remaining static in today's rapidly changing environment.

Making Managed Healthcare Work underscores the premise that managed care is most successful when two basic guidelines are followed. An infrastructure of core resources must be present, and each side must recognize that trade-offs are required to establish a partnership approach to managing care and costs in the future.

Peter Boland, Ph.D.
Boland Healthcare Consultants
Berkeley, CA

MAKING
MANAGED HEALTHCARE
WORK

PART ONE

MARKET DYNAMICS

CHAPTER ONE

Delivery Systems

MARKET OVERVIEW AND DELIVERY SYSTEM DYNAMICS

PETER BOLAND, Ph.D., President
Boland Healthcare Consultants, Berkeley, California

Managed care is now the dominant force in the healthcare industry. However, it defies a commonly accepted definition because managed care means different things to different people, depending on their professional affiliation, type of business, and experience in the field.

In essence, managed care is a broad prescription for American healthcare in the 1990s. It entails different financial incentives and management controls intended to direct patients to efficient providers who are responsible for giving appropriate medical care in cost-effective treatment settings. It seeks to maximize value to healthcare purchasers by channeling volume to high quality providers participating in health maintenance organizations (HMOs), preferred provider organizations (PPOs), or other "point-of-purchase" arrangements.

Managed care alters the decision-making of physicians and hospitals by interjecting a complex system of financial incentives, penalties, and administrative procedures into the doctor-patient relationship. Managed care often attempts to redefine what is best for the patient and how to achieve it most economically. It is most successful when physicians, hospitals, financial incentives, and administrative services are fully integrated.

Effective managed care delivery systems control quality and use of services as well as clinical cost and operational expenses. However, the term "managed care" is not necessarily synonymous with either HMOs or PPOs. It depends on the extent to which essential building blocks of managed care (for example, benefit design incentives, utilization management procedures, quality assurance protocols, and information system capability) are integrated into program operations and on whether negotiated performance standards are achieved.

This chapter focuses on seven leading delivery system issues:

1. Trade-offs among major healthcare industry players
2. Different dimensions of quality in relation to performance
3. Managed care negotiations between health plans and providers
4. Purchaser priorities
5. Payer expectations
6. Utilization management trends
7. Managed care results

HEALTHCARE INDUSTRY TRADE-OFFS

One of the most troublesome questions for the healthcare industry to answer is whether managed care is working, or, put another way, to what extent can it be made to work better. The answer depends on a number of factors:

- Expectations
- Points of view
- Time frames
- Interpretation of results

It is working at the conceptual level. The entire field is advancing at a rapid rate, and there is no going back to uncontrolled fee-for-service medicine or reimbursement.

But it is not necessarily working well as an effective strategy for influencing aggregate healthcare spending, improving quality vis-à-vis delivery systems, or laying the groundwork for closer cooperation between healthcare buyers and sellers.

In general, there is a growing consensus that managed care is not working in two key areas:

1. Reduction of overall costs
2. Instability of healthcare premiums

This is exacerbated by the projection that healthcare will continue to consume an increasing portion of the nation's income as measured against the gross national product (GNP) through the 1990s.

For many companies, healthcare is the highest cost category after salaries and raw materials. It directly affects the bottom line, representing up to half of corporate pretax profits, and now threatens the competitiveness of American products in both domestic and foreign markets.

Multiple forces, many of which are related, drive healthcare costs. These include:

- Inflation, both general and healthcare-related
- Rising expectations of consumers (that is, consumer demand), providers, and suppliers about what managed care can do
- Focus on acute care rather than on illness prevention
- Care that is medically unnecessary and inappropriate or services that are ineffective
- Excess capacity of hospitals and other providers
- Inefficient management of healthcare resources
- High-priced technology
- Malpractice insurance rates (and "defensive" medical practices)
- Antitrust regulations
- Aging of the population (and associated severity of illness)

While these factors often seem overwhelming to purchasers, they represent a conflicting dilemma for providers. National trends indicate that aggregate patient days have stopped declining and length of stay is climbing, largely as a result of increased severity of illness and morbidity of hospitalized patients. However, reimbursement has not kept pace with costs because of the growing mix of patients covered by Medicare, Medicaid, HMOs, and PPOs.

The initial focus of employee cost containment strategies was on cost-sharing and price negotiation, neither of which appreciably slowed demand for services. However, demand for expensive care was stimulated both by patients who lacked awareness of treatment alternatives or how to interact with the medical care system and by providers who favored elective procedures and ancillary services from among a growing array of new and established interventions. The unit price of care was modestly controlled through discounts and capitation, but aggregate spending was not held back because frequency of service remained uncontrolled. There were few standards for appropriateness of care.

The market momentum toward managed care is being driven by, more than anything else, employer demands for slowing down the growth rate of employee medical expenses. To control costs, managed care delivery systems attempt to link patients' and providers' healthcare use directly to their associated costs. This connection is absent in traditional fee-for-service medical plans. Managed care plans can achieve this control by giving patients incentives to consider treatment alternatives and by giving providers incentives to use healthcare resources more economically and to practice a "conservative" style of medicine.

In the future, the main focus of healthcare cost management will shift from across-the-board cost containment to management of appropriate utilization, effectiveness, and efficiency—thus reducing the cost of provider inefficiency. The central issue in controlling utilization, particularly in fee-for-service–based plans, is encouraging the use of cost-effective doctors and hospitals.

Delivery system hybrids like open-ended HMOs and exclusive provider organizations (EPOs) are being offered in response to payer demands for more cost control (for example, the HMO model) and consumer resistance to restrictive delivery systems in some areas. Point-of-service HMO plans offer more flexibility than traditional HMOs, while EPOs restrict consumer choice more than traditional PPOs do.

After a decade of healthcare cost containment initiatives, what is clear is that no one vehicle—including managed care—will be effective without the active cooperation and long-term commitment of consumers, employers, payers, and providers working toward long-range solutions. This must include a fair approach to risk-sharing and gain-sharing.

Managed care is not a panacea for rising medical expenses. There are no easy answers, and it will take a comprehensive strategy to cope with rising healthcare costs during the 1990s. Managed care will be no more effective than other "magic bullet" approaches like capitation, data collection and analysis, utilization review (UR), quality assurance (QA), and discounts unless the industry's predominant orientation shifts from short-term risk avoidance to long-term partnerships that change delivery system incentives.

Major players in the field—government, insurers, health plans, hospitals, physicians, suppliers, employers, and health and welfare trust funds—must reassess their willingness to compromise and make different trade-offs in order to frame a unified approach to dampening cost escalation while preserving "controlled access" and quality care. This will require participating in rigorous program evaluation audits and quality assurance reviews—and then acting on the findings in a meaningful way.

Under the current payment system (that is, federal and state governments and insurers), many managed care reimbursement policies are harmful, in the short run, to efficient providers. Efficient, high quality physicians are paid the same as inefficient, poorly motivated doctors. In essence, the best physicians (and hospitals) subsidize the worst ones.

Hospitals will keep raising rates for private patients in relation to the amount of Medicare cutbacks, the amount of discounts to HMOs and PPOs, the effects of HMO capitation, and the impact of utilization review on admissions and resource consumption. However, they will not be able to raise rates enough to offset the 20 to 40 percent discounts and to shift costs to other payers when 85 to 90 percent of their business is HMOs, PPOs, Medicare, and Medicaid. There simply will not be enough "others" to shift costs to in the future. This points toward a new equilibrium in contract care arrangements. There will necessarily be less emphasis on front-end discounts or capitation and more emphasis on risk-based contracts that blend both risk- and gain-sharing features and then distribute them more equitably among payers and participating providers.

In a competitive healthcare environment, physicians will continue to have the last word on costs because they control medical resources—not employers or insurers. While payers and purchasers can strongly influence resource consumption through various incentives and payment controls, as well as directing enrollees to certain providers, they cannot effectively restrain unnecessary care or inappropriate treatment nearly as well as physicians because doctors make the key decisions about how to spend healthcare dollars.

In other words, once a patient seeks care, physicians have a great deal to say about:

- When care is given
- Where it is provided
- How much is rendered and under what conditions
- Whether it is effective
- How long treatment continues (within parameters of acceptable medical standards)

However, hospitals are the location where over half these dollar decisions are implemented. Thus, physicians face a critical choice as managed care stakeholders. Either they must assume an out-front leadership role in implementing cost-effective care or they will become scapegoats for many of the inadequacies of the current system.

Everyone cannot win in managed care. By definition, when some providers are designated as preferred or given exclusive contracts for patient care, others are excluded and therefore lose. HMOs and PPOs want physicians with the necessary clinical skills and motivation to practice cost-effective medicine.

Self-perceived quality providers must decide with whom to align themselves before choice is no longer an option. Managed care organizations need hospitals which strongly support such physicians and are willing to work with selected purchasers and payers for long-term business gain.

It remains to be seen whether selected providers and purchasers (and payers) can make the necessary compromises and trade-offs with each other to develop "win-win" scenarios for the healthcare industry as a whole—which is the only way managed care will work to balance out competing interests in cost management, quality care, and freedom of choice. The "rules of the game" will need to be redrafted by payers, purchasers, and providers so that both risk-sharing and gain-sharing are more equitably spread among the major players.

The alternative is a "survival of the fittest" approach where each stakeholder acts in his or her own "rational self-interest," at least in an economic sense. This would certainly have a positive effect in driving a number of inefficient providers and payers from the market. But it would also cause serious harm to many outstanding community hospitals, academic teaching centers, and county medical facilities which do not have the necessary capital and tools to compete effectively in a profit-oriented managed care marketplace. In the long run, everyone loses if these facilities can no longer maintain adequate levels of care as a result of the adverse effects of cost-shifting.

Cost-shifting and risk transfer alone have not worked to contain aggregate healthcare spending. Cost-shifting has benefited some employers who have transferred an increasing amount of risk to employees and providers. Managed care cannot avoid cost-shifting bencause it inevitably causes a market response, which produces winners and losers. One of the worst effects of this market dynamic is that small businesses and individuals—for whom managed care plans are often out of reach—often bear the brunt of cost-shifting, and they can least afford it.

QUALITY AND PERFORMANCE

Both healthcare providers and purchasers are concerned about the impact of cost containment on quality care. Various managed care features—such as discounts, utilization management, restricted professional autonomy, risk contracts, capitation, and restricted access—are designed to reduce unnecessary utilization and cost. But the inherent danger with these procedures is undertreatment and unduly limited access to necessary care.

As a result, purchasers and payers are increasingly demanding that providers develop policies and procedures for assuring adequate quality. They want to know more about how competing health plans define quality, monitor it, and evaluate it after the fact. In short, they want providers to explain their quality assurance process, to document treatment outcomes, and to justify expenditures.

This new-found focus on quality, however, raises two perennial questions: What will employees and dependents be getting in terms of quality, and how will they know they have it? To satisfy this demand, the market needs indices of quality (before paying for it) and a measurement system for evaluating the process of care, assessing the outcomes of treatment, and monitoring patient satisfaction.

Without such tools, how else will customers really know whether their care was indeed high quality?

There is an assumption in the industry that "quality sells" and that "quality is free." It does sell, particularly among knowledgeable purchasers looking for genuine cost management programs which incorporate quality improvement principles. But defining, measuring, and communicating it is far from free. Measurement systems which document both inpatient and ambulatory care are expensive to implement, costly to maintain, and difficult to translate into plain English for purchasers, who have yet to demonstrate a willingness to pay for them. However, the costs and resources invested may be returned in the form of improved outcomes and increased efficiency. Vague marketing phrases and sales jargon about quality care are no substitute for credible information which documents that medical intervention has had a positive impact on the quality of people's lives.

One of the information challenges of the 1990s will be translating the impact of quality assurance systems on cost management and reporting it to customers in a digestible format. Employers are looking for new reporting techniques which combine inpatient and ambulatory care databases with normative standards and which make operational sense to them. Benefit managers and trust fund administrators need easy-to-read summary data which help them make better decisions about redesigning employee benefits and allocating resources. This means collecting different types of data (for example, data on utilization, cost, and quality) and integrating it in standard reporting formats.

While high quality care provided by an outstanding physician may be free in comparison to second-rate care given by a mediocre physician, there is the cost of validating that care. In order to compete on the basis of quality, health plans must invest heavily in medical software, data processing, and administrative support systems in order to track and measure quality.

This scenario raises a strategic dilemma for providers who want to validate quality care and to pass on the added cost. Managed care plans may be going out on a limb by making the assumption that purchasers are willing to pay the added cost of validating quality care.

Employers and trust funds are certainly "talking quality," but it remains to be seen whether they are ready to buy based on quality or implement quality standards once they are established. So far, there has been little evidence that they are selecting managed care plans based on factors other than capitation or discounts and network size.

Because healthcare prices continue to rise and because employers remain skeptical of health plan assertions about quality, purchasers may be unwilling (that is, large employers) or unable (that is, small employers) to pay the added cost of documenting quality care. It may well become another cost of doing business and competing successfully in the managed care marketplace for providers. If this is the case, then health plans will be forced to absorb such costs until their performance data on quality is powerful enough to be used as a strategic marketing tool—thus justifying the risk of investing in quality assurance technology today. On the other hand, if a working partnership is developed between healthcare buyers and sellers—on a selective basis—the costs of such data systems could be shared.

Unfortunately, most quality assurance systems were developed to allow hospitals to aggregate large amounts of data and to develop defensive strategies to deal with accreditation and outside regulators. They were not devised to give employers the quality-related information they need. Nor were they designed to help balance costs versus outcomes. Furthermore, they were not intended to provide a competitive edge for hospitals and medical groups in addition to more traditional marketing features like discounts and fixed-price contracts. Most providers lacked the marketing knowledge and ability to use quality as a indicator of health plan effectiveness and as a sales technique.

Incentive systems for providers can result in higher quality healthcare if quality indicators are developed as part of performance standards. These indicators can include the following:

- Process of care through review of medical records
- Provider's conformance with appropriateness standards
- Impact of medical encounters on the well-being of patients
- Efficiency of diagnostic and other therapeutic settings
- Intensity of services adjusted for type of patient or case
- Patient satisfaction, based on survey results

Although it is difficult, each of these factors can be translated into incentive-based reimbursement and bonus formulas. However, adequate data management and monitoring resources are required to link compensation to performance.

It should be clear to health plans that the cost of such data acquisition, analysis, interpretation, formatting, and reporting may be greater than the dollars saved in managing the care. However, treatment outcomes will be improved, and this adds significant "value" to the product.

In order for payers, providers, and purchasers to take each other seriously about quality, they will each have to develop standards for acceptable performance and indicators of program effectiveness. This can be developed through a partnership or independently as a market strategy. In either case, it means that quality should be judged according to at least six dimensions: assessment, control, assurance, improvement, treatment outcomes, and treatment analysis. These are briefly summarized in Figure 1.

The first four (that is, control, assessment, assurance, and improvement) relate to the quality measurement and management process. There is a growing consensus among many experts about what constitutes measurable attributes of quality in terms of treatment outcomes, the fifth dimension. The sixth quality category, treatment analysis, links treatment outcomes to each of the other dimensions.

There is a related concern of healthcare payers and purchasers about what happens to the patients after hospital discharge or leaving the physician's care. Payers want to monitor hospital readmission rates, disability periods, lost work time, and return-to-work problems due to poor quality care. While these factors are not usually tracked by providers on behalf of employers, they may be called on to do so in the future.

Each of these quality concepts are valid and necessary for improving care. No one approach is the answer because the issue is multidimensional in nature and technically complex. But the most important fact is that performance data relating to quality is the very substance of what managed care is supposed to be.

Figure 1 *Dimensions of quality.*

Quality Control:	Inspects the production process which delivers care in order to detect possible defects and trouble spots.
Quality Assessment:	Identifies outliers based on selected clinical indicators and targets them for more intensive review.
Quality Assurance:	Informs low quality providers about their performance in relation to good clinical practice standards.
Quality Improvement:	Translates quality into on-the-job expectations for individual work functions (that is, administrative and clinical) and instills greater interdependence through team building within an organization.
Treatment Outcomes:	Measures the effect of medical interventions on patient status in terms of clinical indicators, functional status, access, appropriateness, and satisfaction.
Treatment Analysis:	Focuses on instances of care to determine whether poor outcomes were due to patient, physician (and other caregiver), or system problems.

The overriding problem is that most providers are very reluctant to look at the outcomes of their treatment and how they compare with the outcomes of other providers. For managed care to succeed, there must be a willingness to look at quality-related data and take the necessary actions if the results are poor. In this respect, managed care organizations should have to justify *not* investing in quality monitoring and quality management.

As delivery systems define what they mean by quality, they will be so judged and held accountable for how they manage it. Quality could thus be viewed as a double-edged sword by some providers in the 1990s. Hospitals and physicians will not be able to market quality if they have no practical indices and information on how they measure up.

At this stage in managed care, it is important for hospitals and physicians to support UR and QA procedures which influence overall norms of practice rather than looking primarily for "outliers." They identify "the bad apples," but outlier criteria are not clinically sensitive and will not affect most physicians.

Managed care organizations should get hospitals and physicians as well as purchasers to focus on the results providers achieve on clinical indicators, health status, and patient satisfaction. The techniques which providers use to manage and monitor their results are secondary; the results are what count most.

Nevertheless, providers must reach some general agreement about what quality is and how it should be measured in relation to practice patterns, appropriateness of care, clinical outcomes, functional outcomes, patient satisfaction, and user-defined quality. This requires a level of education, communication, cooperation, and commitment which is difficult to achieve among competing providers, medical institutions, and delivery systems.

Different provider definitions of quality may well arise as a point of strategic product differentiation. But unless hospitals and physicians take the initiative to define and operationalize quality, others, with their own definitions and standards, will develop proprietary products to fill the vacuum.

In essence, quality must incorporate both customer requirements and professional medical standards in order to provide managed care organizations with a competitive edge in the future. Quality will be used more and more as a positioning strategy by providers and as a scorecard by customers.

In managed care, consumer perceptions of quality care are just as valid as those of providers because purchaser and payer expectations drive the market. Consumers view quality in healthcare in a way that is similar to how they recognize it in other products. It depends on service (for example, how quickly appointments can be scheduled, whether the staff was friendly), convenience (for example, how accessible the services are, whether the system is "user friendly"), content (for example, what providers and services are included), price (for example, amount of out-of-pocket expenses), and results (for example, extent and speed of recovery).

Genuine quality requires a meaningful accord between healthcare consumers, buyers, and sellers. Consumer notions about quality are often one-sided and fueled by medical-legal dogma. Unsatisfactory outcomes are frequently viewed as the fault of providers when they may also be due to unrealistic patient expectations or lack of patient compliance with treatment regimens.

Unless users and medical providers develop a common understanding about quality, they will continue to be adversaries rather than partners. Adversarial relationships among hospitals, physicians, and patients can thwart cooperation and communication—thus undermining quality. Focusing on quality can also be a starting point for consumers and providers to bridge the gap between "perceived value" about quality and clinical indications of superior quality care.

In short, quality cannot be wrapped in a "black box" whose technical specifications are beyond the reach of consumers and payers. It must be defined in understandable terms to be credible.

When provider-defined quality is translated into operational terms, practical benchmarks can be developed and performance standards can be established. This enables each side to appreciate their respective roles in achieving different ingredients of quality: patient compliance, administrative procedures, treatment outcomes, and patient health status.

MANAGED CARE NEGOTIATIONS

Managed care plans and providers are becoming far more sophisticated and realistic about negotiating agreements with one another. Although negotiating styles still run the gamut from confrontational to collegial, there is growing consensus that traditional adversarial approaches do not work in managed healthcare. An "us versus them" method does not provide a basis for establishing business trust, consensus, and long-term partnerships. The last-mentioned is needed to deal effectively with persistent cost problems which are multiyear in nature. Likewise, efforts to enhance quality require ongoing commitments of substantial resources over a number of years.

As a result, healthcare buyers and sellers usually focus on at least four broad contract negotiation categories: provider network, reimbursement, cooperation, and contract agreement. Some of the leading issues are briefly listed below.

Provider Network

- Reflect high quality physicians, hospitals, and allied caregivers
- Include full primary and specialty care coverage
- Limit size in order to guarantee volume to network providers versus enrollee access to larger provider panels
- Convenient hours and locations throughout the service area

Reimbursement

- Negotiate competitive rates which give each side a stake in improving the process of care
- Guarantee rates for 1 year or longer
- Provide prompt payment to providers in return for a modest discount
- Show a willingness to implement risk arrangements (for example, per diem, package pricing, DRG, capitation, and pricing by percent of claims) and gain-sharing mechanisms in the near future.

Cooperation

- Establish a framework for an ongoing partnership
- Support utilization management and quality assurance protocols
- Follow claims submission and reimbursement procedures

Contract Agreement

- Adhere to all contract specifications and performance standards
- Continue to serve enrollees for a designated period of time after plan termination, according to a negotiated rate
- Prohibit participating providers from balance billing (other than deductibles and coinsurance)
- Terminate inefficient hospitals (and other vendors), as well as physicians (and other caregivers), that provide medically unnecessary or inappropriate care
- Use binding arbitration to resolve disputes between the health plan, providers, patients, payers, and purchasers

The purpose of managed care negotiations is not to "win," but to establish a viable framework for future relationships. Each side must be able to live with the terms of the agreement and not feel taken advantage of because of inexperience, misrepresentation, or intimidation.

"Risk transfer" can only go so far; then it adversely affects each party in the managed care arrangement, even the side that initially evaded much, if not all, of the risk. It is a mistake to saddle any party with risk they are not in a position to control; it makes for a poor business deal. Accordingly, managed care plans must adjust reimbursement schemes to protect themselves against the impact of particular demographic characteristics and severity-of-illness factors in risk arrangements.

To some extent, however, risk-sharing is a poor substitute for being able to review physician services on an aggregate basis. If accurate data were available for physician practice patterns and overall network performance, there would be less rationale for purchasers and payers to transfer as much risk as possible to providers. Each side would know, based on performance data, who was responsible for inappropriate or unnecessary care and how much it cost. Such providers would be removed from the panel, thus lessening the risk exposure to employers, insurers, managed care organizations, and even hospitals and physicians in the networks.

Likewise, many risk-sharing arrangements also do not address the problem of creative provider billing practices. For example, physicians who unbundle office charges and lab tests (which can result in a 400 to 700 percent markup) would readily agree to a 20 percent withhold in order to collect 80 percent of the charges for unbundled items or for unnecessary procedures.

Hospitals can contract themselves out of business by accepting fixed reimbursement rates without having as much control over costs and utilization as the payer has over revenue. Moreover, hospitals should limit managed care contracts to those that fit into their particular strategy for reimbursement mix, market share, and administrative expense.

Unfortunately, many hospitals jumped into managed care arrangements prematurely and were harmed financially in the process. In some cases, hospitals experienced downgradings on debt and credit ratings as a result of too many unprofitable HMO and PPO contracts. This situation was exacerbated by declining admissions and further cuts in reimbursement for Medicare and Medicaid patients.

Many hospitals are now reassessing the value of each HMO and PPO contract. Some facilities are reducing such contracts by 30 to 50 percent in order to concentrate resources on building better relationships with selected payers (and direct care purchasers) who will likely emerge from the industry shakeout as "winners." These companies are committed to managed care as an on-going line of business and will be more likely to supply significant patient volume as a result.

Contracts which have not produced enough volume or revenue are not being renewed or are being renewed under very different terms. Follow-up agreements are being based on actual experience (that is, track record to date) rather than on financial promises or enrollment projections.

Hospital and physician frustration with "poorly performing contracts" is based not just on a perception of inadequate payment rates and unrealized volume but also on a two- to threefold increase in support staff and the administrative expenses required to service managed care agreements (compared to fee-for-service business).

Providers are becoming more cautious because a managed care plan cannot always deliver what it promises even when it tries to do so. For example, marketing activities generally target a broad area rather than a particular provider's locale. Many patients may be unwilling to switch doctors, and those that do may have different illnesses and severity levels than originally expected, thereby eroding profit margins. In fact, the plan's utilization management system may divert patients to other in-network facilities and caregivers whose charges and fees are lower than another network hospital. Thus, the provider network should be carefully examined. Each of these factors should be negotiated at contract renewal time.

Hospitals no longer take assertions about "eligibles" at face value. They want volume-related rates based on actual new business, not just rollover patients who were shifted from full reimbursement to per diem or discount arrangements.

Each side must put more emphasis on being direct with the other and explicitly state their legitimate business needs. This establishes a concrete frame of reference within which to deal with priorities, trade-offs, performance standards (on all sides), resources, and time tables. Ambiguity and hidden agendas undermine managed care negotiations and end up souring business relationships.

PURCHASER PRIORITIES

Employers vary greatly in their approach to employee benefits and managed healthcare. Most businesses are small to medium-sized and do not have the resources to evaluate managed care options carefully and negotiate aggressive purchasing arrangements with healthcare vendors. Many rely on advice from brokers, third party administrators, insurance company sales representatives, and word-of-mouth. They are essentially carrier-driven, while larger companies often are self-insured and have "administrative service only" (ASO) contracts with insurers. Large corporations and the bigger mid-size firms also depend on employee benefit consultants.

The majority of these companies have access to numerous medical plans—HMOs, PPOs, managed indemnity—but do not set the managed care agenda in each region because their purchasing power is limited by size and inexperience in dealing with the managed care industry.

Some large employers, however, do have the necessary size, internal resources, and know-how to affect the design and delivery of managed care products. Vendors listen when flagship corporations and Fortune 500 companies speak and exert their purchasing clout.

Even though large employers drive the market on cost-containment strategies, they do not speak with one voice. There is considerable debate, for example, about the relative value of HMOs versus PPOs or how to incorporate quality into buying decisions. Employers tend to fall into at least four major categories in their approach to managed care, as shown in Table 1.

Purchasers are still in tremendous flux about what to buy, how to negotiate health plan arrangements to maximize corporate resources, and how to assess vendor performance.

Quality is starting to enter into buying decisions because it is beginning to be defined in terms of industry standards (that is, conformance to customer requirements), professional norms (that is, peer review procedures), and clinical criteria (that is, treatment outcome measures).

However, many businesses are reluctant to use quality as a criteria in selecting health plans or providers because it is difficult to quantify and requires expert staff assistance. It also puts an employer in the

TABLE 1   Employer Purchasing Typology

ROLE	STATUS	ACTION
Passive	Fully insured	Accept products and recommendations from insurer, and offer managed fee-for-service in addition to traditional indemnity coverage.
Reactive	Fully or partially insured	Distinguish between different types of plans and safest "best bet" options to reduce costs and minimize potential employee backlash.
Active	Partially insured or self-insured	Seek out managed care options with cost management features which place providers at risk and correspond with company priorities and employee health characteristics.
Aggressive	Self-insured	Transfer increasing amounts of risk to vendors, define contract specifications, and negotiate performance goals (including quality) with providers; establish direct care relationships with physicians and hospitals; develop company-sponsored preferred provider networks.

position of "crossing over the line" into making medical judgments, that is, questioning practice patterns of local physicians and scrutinizing hospital operations. This is an uncomfortable role for most corporations to adopt, but one that will become increasingly familiar and necessary as employers begin to manage more and more of their managed care activities. Thus, all but a few employers are currently deferring questions about network quality to HMOs and PPOs.

Although their philosophy is often stronger than their actions, larger employers are gradually moving away from buying healthcare based on price alone. They are incorporating different factors into the process of making decisions about what to buy and on what terms. These factors include:

- Management experience
- Financial solvency
- Administrative flexibility
- Operational "bells and whistles" to control unnecessary utilization by plan members and providers and to assure quality
- Ability to generate meaningful utilization, cost, and quality data as well as client reports
- Capacity to meet the service needs of local company managers
- Ease of implementation and claims administration
- Willingness to stand behind their product with rate and performance guarantees

Employers are also starting to reduce the number of healthcare plans and "suppliers" in order to cut administrative costs, gain efficiencies in procurement, and increase control over vendor performance. By reducing the number of suppliers, employers can leverage their purchasing power and increase market share for selected providers.

This means developing a closer working relationship with truly "preferred" providers and basing it on clearly defined performance specifications. That is the new quid pro quo for concentrating blocks of business with fewer suppliers. Large businesses are refining this strategy as the best way to regain control over the quality and cost of medical services they buy.

This approach reflects a broad corporate trend toward developing overall purchasing guidelines and centralizing key administrative functions, like maintaining a medical claims information system, while leaving individual purchasing decisions to local management.

Employers recognize, more and more, that healthcare is local or, at best, regional in nature and that area-specific performance targets are necessary to optimize corporate resources and take advantage of unique health plan arrangements. A number of companies want to increase the value of their healthcare spending, not necessarily reduce how much they spend. This approach tries to maximize the impact of the overall investment rather than limit expenditures to the lowest possible level, since the latter may be "penny wise and pound foolish."

PAYER EXPECTATIONS

Like most other industry players, insurers failed to deliver on early promises about managed care because they did not sufficiently understand the field and misjudged the market. Their assumptions and business expectations were often out of sync with marketplace dynamics and delivery system requirements. Their historical focus was claims payment (that is, accuracy, timeliness, and efficiency) rather than delivery system management. To make matters worse, many states initially prohibited them from negotiating preferred arrangements with providers. As a result, carriers paid a high price to learn what employers are willing to buy and what it takes to develop and manage such products. In short, many carriers were unrealistic about:

- Implementing a national strategy involving 50 to 75 major markets, often due more to internal corporate demands than client needs
- Forming provider networks that were as large as possible without sufficient regard for the associated cost management requirements
- Ascertaining the degree of coordination between benefit design and utilization controls required to manage inappropriate inpatient and ambulatory services
- Providing administrative resources (that is, breadth and depth) needed to support managed care activities successfully
- Estimating the price of competing in saturated HMO markets and competitive PPO markets
- Evaluating the ability of traditional cost-containment approaches, such as employee cost-sharing, to affect price factors and utilization simultaneously
- Identifying the data requirements and data system limitations for underwriting and claims analysis
- Gauging the capacity of actuaries to adequately take cost management features into account so as to price products competitively
- Projecting the financial investment necessary to cover staff recruitment and training, product development, and initial sales cycles
- Relying on hospitals to select network physicians and influence their behavior
- Judging employer commitment to managed care in terms of effective benefit design incentives and limiting choice of providers

In general, carriers did not understand the inherent trade-offs involved in developing a managed care product line. Large insurers tried to implement a poorly defined market-entry strategy with unrealistic expectations about employee penetration levels. In addition, many tried to buy their way into the market through hasty acquisitions and joint ventures which were always costly but not always successful. These financial transactions often dictated an insurer's entire managed care strategy rather than vice versa.

While these lessons learned were expensive, they set the stage for more modest expectations on the part of insurers—but not on the part of purchasers. Even though many payers gradually cut back, their early rhetoric and assertions about cost management resulted in over-stimulating market expectations. Employers and trust fund administrators are now questioning why cost savings generated by utilization management, capitation, and discounts have not been translated into significantly reduced rates or stable premium levels.

A credibility problem on cost savings is developing. The healthcare industry's promises about managed care savings have outpaced performance so far. And purchasers are beginning to ask: "Where are the savings?"

Flagship corporations turned their ire on HMOs initially and are beginning to hold PPOs to the same level of oversight and performance expectations. HMOs too often engaged in "shadow pricing" by setting premiums just below prevailing market rates for insurance premiums. This denied expected cost savings to employers and other payers.

Unless these delivery systems and their carrier sponsors are able to deliver on promised savings, a number of large purchasers may begin bypassing health plans in the early 1990s and start dealing directly with physician groups, hospitals, and other providers of medical services.

UTILIZATION MANAGEMENT

Utilization review grew so quickly during the 1980s that it spawned a whole new industry and a new "medical mystique." Business too often expects UR to control escalating costs even though only modest savings have been generated on an industrywide basis to date. The principal reason is that purchasers do not fully appreciate the illogical or "perverse" nature of healthcare economics. Just as the presence of more physicians results in higher charges (contrary to economic laws of supply and demand), physician constraints such as UR often cause utilization to increase.

In the UR process, it is important to find out three major things:

1. Whether care is medically necessary and appropriate (including frequency of service and duration)
2. Whether lower-cost forms of care are available and efficacious
3. Whether patients improve as a result of treatment

Instead, most UR in the past focused on where treatment was rendered and cost of treatment. These factors are important, but they are not the key to quality assurance or cost management.

A vicious cycle is created by the introduction of increasingly sophisticated UR controls. While utilization review is necessary, a different perspective must be adopted in order to generate real cost savings. Instead of being a mechanism to deny payment, UR systems should build in financial incentives that encourage caregivers to use the most cost-effective levels of care. This would bring providers, purchasers, and regulators into closer alignment about appropriateness of care—where significant cost savings are possible.

Utilization review should not be treated as an end in itself but as a stepping stone to utilization management through individual case management. This will be an integral part of the transition from "managed cost" to "managed care."

This is more likely to occur in the next 5 years as the managed care market shifts more and more risk onto providers and away from payers. Providers will be forced to embrace—and, indeed, control—UR and develop effective utilization management systems as a risk management strategy.

Utilization review procedures should be the basis for managing resource use. The primary focus of UR is identifying bad habits that many physicians have and, secondarily, to "catch the few bad guys" (that is, physician outliers). This is done after the fact through retrospective review or prospectively through precertification or preadmission reviews.

This has led to an "us versus them" mentality with hospitals (and physician offices) under siege from countless utilization review organizations, all demanding immediate data and full cooperation. Provider reaction has often been to maximize reimbursement by second-guessing and outmaneuvering payers of all types—insurers, third party administrators, Medicare, and Medicaid. Tremendous resources are being spent by both sides to fight a battle which neither can win.

It would be far more productive for hospitals to focus on case management, for physicians to concentrate on quality outcomes, and for payers to change their payment schedules so that providers can be rewarded for cost-effective care rather than being tied to lowest common denominator care. However, this will be difficult for inpatient medical facilities because case management usually decreases hospital occupancy. Case management should also be employed by knowledgeable physicians who want to improve cost-efficiency and demonstrate concern for patient comfort by treating them at home whenever possible.

Sophisticated medical software is now widely available and promises to differentiate among hospitals, physicians, and allied health providers based on treatment outcomes and appropriate resource use.

Reliable provider profiles can now give payers, health plans, and hospitals an objective basis for making better decisions about channeling large blocks of managed care business. This has been made possible by the development of protocols and practice guidelines based on independent analyses of what constitutes effective medical care and superior outcomes.

Today, utilization management is expanding rapidly in both scope of services and depth of analytical capability. The UR field is in the process of developing and implementing at least five important innovations, which include the following:

1. Expansion of review and case management programs. This implies development of "medical necessity" criteria and price control databases for:

   - Hospital outpatient services
   - Ambulatory care facilities and settings, including ambulatory surgery
   - Physician office care
   - Long-term care
   - Home-based services
   - Allied health practitioners

2. Targeted case management programs with complete ancillary services at negotiated reimbursement for a variety of health-care services. Included will be such features as:

   - Durable medical equipment
   - Home health services and infusion therapy
   - Psychiatric residential treatment
   - Physical and occupational therapy
   - Rehabilitative services
   - Prescription drugs

3. Quality assurance as a stand-alone product line offered by vendors as well as hospitals and physicians. This means:

   - Defining quality of care in operational terms and then managing it

- Redefining hospital and physician data collection and analysis mechanisms
- Identifying both underutilization and overutilization of services
- Incorporating indices for intensity of services and severity of illness
- Developing inpatient and ambulatory care outcome measures

4. Integration of claims data and utilization review information. This will lead to expanded analytical capability and reporting capacity, resulting in:

- Reports which indicate savings by different types of UR procedures and by case management
- Targeting "high incidence" illnesses by diagnosis and procedure
- In-depth provider profiling
- On-line modification of fee schedules
- Far more sophisticated price and fee negotiation

5. Program specialization and specification. Typical examples could include:

- Increased use of clinical expertise in case management
- Use of UR conducted by medical and nursing specialists trained in treating a patient's particular illness
- Use of review resources designed to focus on particular problem areas
- Identification of tertiary-level DRGs by specific institutions
- Identification of "centers of excellence" based on superior surgical or treatment results

In short, meaningful data will become the number one priority of sophisticated healthcare purchasers.

These five advances will lead to more accurate monitoring of provider performance, thus setting new standards and expectations for cost-effective medical care.

MANAGED CARE RESULTS

Each of the delivery system issues discussed above will have a pronounced impact on the development and direction of managed care in the 1990s. To date, managed care has produced mixed results in relation to three early assertions:

1. Reduce costs
2. Maintain reasonable access to services
3. Assure adequate quality

It has failed on one count (costs) and generally succeeded on another (access), but the data are inconclusive or not available about the third (quality). In short, managed care is suffering from an acute case of unmet expectations on the part of many consumers, employers, physicians, hospitals, and insurers.

Most industry analysts concede that managed care has not succeeded as expected, but it can work if the major stakeholders choose to share healthcare risks and rewards more equitably.

The technical know-how is available to make managed care work effectively. What is missing is the political resolve to move from sporadic ad hoc agreements to on-going multiparty relationships.

The answer to the nagging question "Can managed care work?" lies in forging strategic healthcare alliances based on four broad principles:

1. Long-term partnerships
2. Interdependent business needs
3. Explicitly agreed-upon objectives
4. Performance guarantees which indicate each party's unique responsibilities

Accountability is the glue that will hold managed care partnerships together. It will become increasingly important for each party to know where it stands at each step along the way in making managed care work in the future.

Changing Trends in Healthcare Delivery

KENNETH S. ABRAMOWITZ, Healthcare Analyst

Sanford C. Bernstein Company, New York, New York

COST GROWTH REMAINS OUT OF CONTROL

After 5 years of 8 percent growth in the gross national product (GNP), during which time healthcare costs seemed to be under control, the cost of healthcare should increase sharply by at least 12 percent during the next 5 years, assuming that the general inflation rate remains close to 5 percent. If the nominal GNP grows 7 to 8 percent during 1988–1993 while healthcare costs grow 12 percent, healthcare spending would rise from 11 percent of the GNP in 1989 to 13 to 14 percent by 1993. Leading this surge will be an acceleration in both hospital and physician expenses, which represent 40 percent and 20 percent of aggregate spending, respectively. The decline in hospital utilization that allowed a slowing of inflation is largely finished. The four major forces that continue to drive expenses are (1) more sophisticated and high-priced technology, (2) the aging of the population, (3) massive excess capacity of providers, and (4) inflated demand caused by patient insensitivity to price.

Although healthcare spending is accelerating, the government, which finances close to 40 percent of such expenses, is restraining reimbursement for its beneficiaries through both the Medicare and Medicaid programs. As a consequence, hospital and physician providers are rapidly raising prices so as to shift cost growth to corporate America through the health insurance system. This indirect taxation will cause health insurance payments for hospital costs, for example, to rise from 7 percent to at least 16 percent. As corporations shift more of the burden onto employees, direct patient payments should accelerate from 13 to 19 percent. Ironically, corporate America and its employees will be forced to shoulder the rising costs of treating an aging Medicare population that the federal government will not tax sufficiently to cover its direct costs.

148, 145

HOSPITAL MANAGEMENT COMPANIES RESTRUCTURING, BUT STILL STRUGGLING

National hospital occupancy fell from 75 percent in 1983 to 64 percent in 1989, and massive excess capacity still burdens the hospital system. Clearly, 15 percent of the nation's hospitals should be closed, with the patients moved to the remaining higher quality and higher occupancy hospitals. In reality, perhaps only 5 percent of the hospitals will close by 1993 because neither politicians nor corporate health benefits managers are willing to undergo the short-term pain involved, even though closing the lowest quality hospitals in the country would improve patient care. In addition, another 10 percent of beds are projected to be cut as hospitals close excess floors or wings, even though that does not eliminate hospital overhead expense, which may become less well absorbed. Nevertheless, industry profitability should continue to decline as long as the excess bed supply persists.

Within this pressured market, the market share of proprietary hospitals should rise slightly from 11 to 12 percent for acute care beds and from 13 to 16 percent for psychiatric beds.

The major hospital management companies have restructured their operations during the past 3 years and are now positioned to accelerate their current growth rates of 5 to 10 percent to 10 to 15 percent during the next 5 years. In contrast, the smaller hospital companies are almost all contracting or floundering. The major hospital companies have a more secure base of larger, superior quality hospitals, better cash flows, and higher levels of excess corporate overhead that can be pruned back.

REIMBURSEMENT TRENDS REMAIN NEGATIVE

The reimbursement environment continues to be hostile for hospital management companies as a consequence of the high costs and high inflation rate inherent in these services. However, the negative utilization trends are clearly moderating, as Medicare hospital days per 1000 population are no longer falling and private pay utilization is now falling at a more modest rate of 2 to 3 percent. With the Medicare population growing at 2 percent and the private population growing at 1 percent, actual aggregate patient days have stopped declining, and are now growing at a rate of less than 1 percent; the growing length of stay of an increasingly sick patient base has contributed to this growth.

A far larger negative trend continues to be the deteriorating reimbursement mix of the patients because Medicare, HMO, and PPO admissions have risen as a percentage of the total. Although a typical insurance-reimbursed daily rate might average $1000 to $1200 in 1989, Medicare pays closer to $500 to $600, HMOs pay $700 to $800, and PPOs pay closer to $800 to $900. Moreover, the discounts are rising. Consequently the differential between buyers is growing. By 1993, Medicare may well be paying 35 percent of fee-for-service rates, HMOs 60 percent, and PPOs 70 percent, thereby further encouraging people to join HMOs and PPOs.

FEE-FOR-SERVICE REMAINS UNDER ATTACK

Traditional fee-for-service medicine will continue to decline because it is essentially an unaffordable luxury that encourages demand and inflated charges. However, it represents a very popular system that corporate America has no intention of jettisoning. Consequently, American business, through its insurance carriers, will seek in vain to reform fee-for-service medicine. Managed fee-for-service is growing rapidly as corporations increasingly accept the principle that preadmission hospital certification programs can cut the number of hospital patients by 10 to 15 percent. Unfortunately, hospitals will very quickly raise rates an additional 10 to 15 percent in order to offset the denied hospital utilization.

In the current phase, 1989–1990, corporations have become increasingly involved in setting up formal or informal preferred provider organizations (PPOs), which will not only conduct preadmission certification but will also extract 15 to 25 percent discounts. Unfortunately, by 1991–1992, corporations will discover that while PPOs may modestly reduce hospital cost growth, they will hardly affect physician costs because physicians will quickly unbundle patient charges and increase demand by searching for new pathology.

Corporations and their employees will finally begin to cap what they are willing to pay for healthcare and realize that budgeted care through HMOs is the only cost-effective solution to containing healthcare costs. By 1992–1993, this will occur following 5 years of 20 to 30 percent healthcare cost growth and further cost shifting to employees; after HMOs achieve an estimated 60 percent value advantage, some 2 years after theoretically being forced by the Financial Accounting Standards Board to begin recognizing their liability for retiree healthcare costs; and during a margin squeeze caused by the next recession. In other words, no matter how it is modified, fee-for-service medicine can never contain cost growth as long as patients are free to spend employers' funds on their care and physicians are free to determine utilization and set charges as high as they deem necessary. When the public and private sectors finally realize this, healthcare costs will begin to be contained.

CHAPTER TWO

Legal and Regulatory Environment

REGULATORY AND LEGAL INFLUENCES ON MANAGED CARE

MARK E. LUTES, J.D.
DOUGLAS A. HASTINGS, J.D.
Epstein, Becker & Green, P.C., Washington, D.C.

The growth of managed care systems has always been influenced by regulation.[1] Passage of the HMO Act of 1973 (the "HMO Act"), P.L. 93-222, was the initial stimulus for the HMO sector of the managed care industry's growth spurt. The HMO Act made available feasibility grants, planning grants, and other development funds. The HMO Act amendments of 1976, P.L. 94-460, fostered growth by easing federal qualification requirements in the open enrollment, community rating, and medical staffing areas, thus encouraging additional focus on federal qualification.

Legislative influences continued in the 1980s. The Omnibus Budget Reconciliation Act (OBRA) of 1981 was the impetus behind HMO contracts with state Medicaid programs. The passage of the Tax Equity and Fiscal Responsibility Act (TEFRA) of 1982 made Medicare risk-contracting available to HMOs and competitive medical plans (CMPs). From June 1985 to November 1988, Medicare risk enrollment in HMOs increased from 262,000 to 1,062,000 members. By 1986, Congress had abolished HMO grant and loan requirements. Partly in consequence, a number of plans sought equity capital and a public market in HMO stock was born.

At the same time, the managed care industry's growth and change has itself produced regulatory change. In the 1970s, state legislatures responded to HMO growth by freeing HMOs from the constraints of the service benefit plan (Blue Cross–type) statutes and the insurance laws. The 1980s have seen the passage of statutes that enabled preferred provider arrangements (PPA); this was a response to the trend toward this managed care product. By easing obstacles to PPA growth, such as state "freedom of choice" and "nondiscrimination" rules, these statutes have allowed regulation to catch up with the industry and pushed the development of PPAs ahead.[2]

Regulatory and legal developments are certain to continue to be strong influences on the direction of the managed care industry. This chapter provides an overview of significant legal and regulatory developments that managed care "players" need to be cognizant of and factor into their plans. For convenience they are grouped as federal regulatory developments, state regulatory developments, and general legal influences.

FEDERAL REGULATORY DEVELOPMENTS

Federal HMO Amendments

The 1988 amendments to the federal HMO Act can be expected to facilitate changes in the HMO product by making it more adaptable and competitive in several ways. First, the Amendments acknowledge a need to enhance HMO price competitiveness by modifying the community-rating requirement. HMOs have been required to determine rates using federally prescribed community rating formulas, by community rating and community rating by class. They have not been permitted to establish rates solely on the utilization experience of a group during its previous contract year. The Amendments, with one caveat, will permit federally qualified plans to fix rates on the basis of the plan's "revenue requirements for providing services to the group." The caveat is that, for small groups (less than 100 persons), the modified rates cannot exceed by more than 10 percent the group's rate when calculated by a community-rated formula. This limitation was imposed to protect small groups against the dramatic rate increases that theoretically could result from the new "adjusted community rating" system.

Second, the Amendments bring the federal regulatory structure in line with the wave of "open-ended HMOs" or HMOs with "choice." These are HMOs that allow enrollees to obtain care from nonparticipating providers, although in such cases coinsurance is a prerequisite to the enrollee's reimbursement. The old rule was that federally qualified plans must provide the physician services required by the law only through contracting physicians except for emergency, out-of-area, and infrequently used physician services. The rule has been modified to permit plans to offer up to 10 percent of basic health services through out-of-plan physicians. Moreover, plans can charge their enrollees "reasonable" deductibles for out-of-plan physician services. If the Amendments' implementing regulations do not require plans to calculate the 10 percent as a percentage of each enrollee's benefit package, theoretically the HMO might aggregate its out-of-plan allotment so as to offer a PPA product to several groups.

Third, the Amendments will facilitate HMO sponsorship of other products by eliminating the separate "legal entity" requirement. Federally qualified plans will no longer need to create tandem corporations from which to operate nonfederally qualified plans but will be permitted to offer such products, including single service and indemnity products, through the same corporation. Moreover, by repealing the requirement that one-third of the federally qualified plan's policy-making body be drawn from the membership, the Amendments have eliminated an organizational stumbling block facing plans that seek to organize in such a way as to offer several managed care products.

In another bow to industry trends, the Amendments recognize the development of multistate HMO products. Specifically, the Amendments require the Secretary of Health and Human Services to take into consideration the resources of an organization that owns or controls a plan in determining that plan's fiscal solvency. The controlling organization must, however, offer assurances that it will assume the financial obligations of the plan. While this Amendment will not automatically alleviate the strain that the maintenance of reserves and deposits in numerous states places on multistate HMOs, the federal "example" may encourage state insurance departments to recognize this need of the HMO chains.

While promoting HMO plan flexibility and competitiveness in these ways, the Amendments also spell the end of two aspects of the special status enjoyed by federally qualified HMOs. This could influence a plan's decision to seek federal qualification.

First, the Amendments substantially modify the current regulatory interpretation which has required that an employer's contribution to a federally qualified HMO plan be equal to the largest contribution paid on behalf of an employee to any non-HMO plan offered, up to but not exceeding the HMO premium. Segments of the business community had alleged that HMOs were taking advantage of this equal contribution requirement to "shadow price" — that is, to inflate their premiums to the level of their competitors' prices irrespective of the HMO's actual costs. The Amendments will allow employers to make any contribution that does not "financially discriminate" against an HMO enrollee. The elimination of equal contribution rules can be expected to place new pressures on plans to discount their prices where employers believe the plans are enrolling the employer group's healthiest members.

Second, the Amendments immediately modify the Section 1310 "dual choice mandate" and allow employers to offer HMOs that use the choice option to satisfy their dual choice obligations. Section 1310 requires an employer with 25 or more employees which has been mandated by (received a request from) a federally qualified HMO to offer its employees an HMO option. More important, the Amendments phase out the dual choice mandate as of October 1995. Though many plans rarely use the mandate, the removal of the threat of the dual choice mandate could have some effect on the successful entrance of the HMO product into immature managed care markets.

Government as Payer

Over the past few years the managed care industry has been increasingly involved with the government as a payer. As of 1988, 356 managed care plans participated in the Federal Employees Health Benefits Program (FEHBP). FEHBP enrollment in these plans has grown to over 2 million members. The opportunity for managed care plans to contract with the government under the Medicare program were significantly enhanced by the addition of the risk-contracting option under TEFRA. Previously, managed care plans were confined to arrangements with Medicare under which they were compensated on the basis of what the Health Care Financing Administration (HCFA) deemed to be the reasonable cost of providing Medicare-covered services.

Risk-contracting organizations receive a monthly per capita payment for each enrollee that is equal to 95 percent of what HCFA calculates to be HCFA's adjusted average per capita cost (AAPCC) for Medicare beneficiaries who are in the demographic class to which that enrollee is assigned and who remain in the regular fee-for-service sector. Cost and risk contractors must be federally qualified HMOs or CMPs. CMPs are state-licensed organizations that meet federal requirements in such areas as insolvency protection, provision of Medicare-covered services, and, with respect to open enrollment, grievance and quality assurance procedures. By 1988, the TEFRA risk-contract alternative had attracted 153 new plans to the Medicare program with an aggregate enrollment of around 1 million members.

The industry's involvement with the Medicaid program was boosted in 1981 by the Omnibus Budget Reconciliation Act (OBRA). OBRA granted states the option of establishing their own qualification standards for HMOs contracting with state Medicaid programs. It also amended the requirement that participating HMOs have an enrollment mix of no more than 50 percent Medicare and Medicaid beneficiaries. HMOs contracting with state programs were now permitted to have up to 75 percent of their enrollment be Medicare and Medicaid beneficiaries. By January 1987, the number of Medicaid beneficiaries enrolled in HMOs, health insuring organizations, or under the care of partially capitated primary care physicians had grown to over 2 million.

The managed care industry's dealings with the federal government are likely to continue to escalate. The Civilian Health and Medical Program of the Uniformed Services (CHAMPUS) which provides healthcare to dependents of military personnel, is seeking to increase private sector involvement. One dramatic 1988 development was the implementation of a 4½-year demonstration program giving CHAMPUS beneficiaries the freedom to choose among a CHAMPUS HMO, a CHAMPUS PPA, and the traditional CHAMPUS indemnity system. Three private sector HMOs are cooperating to provide a new CHAMPUS HMO system throughout northern California and Hawaii.

CHAMPUS has a demonstration project in the Norfolk, Virginia, area designed to reduce mental health costs and has home healthcare demonstration projects in the Washington, D.C., area, the state of Washington, and a region encompassing eight western and plains states. In addition, each of the military services has implemented or developed plans for contracts with primary care clinics to provide care for military retirees and dependents of active duty personnel. A variety of managed care organizations may well benefit from the patient or premium stream that CHAMPUS projects might engender, provided that the organizations' agreements with the government are carefully structured to limit the contractors' risk for higher than anticipated utilization by CHAMPUS beneficiaries.

Moreover, HCFA officials continue to tout managed care as the long-term solution to escalating Medicare expenditures. HCFA is implementing demonstration projects for Medicare (Part B only) preferred provider arrangements. HCFA also will test the Medicare insured group concept under which an employer group would be capitated to provide Medicare services to its retired workers. Contracting organizations must meet many of the same requirements that HMOs and CMPs holding cost- or risk-based Medicare contracts must satisfy.

In order for governmental business to remain attractive to managed care organizations, a number of problems will require special legislative and regulatory attention. Moreover, several efforts to "reform" programs will need to take into consideration the needs of managed care companies. For example, a recent study called for a reduction in the number of plans participating in the FEHBP.[3] The report also raised the possibility of bidding for FEHBP business and adjusting premiums to reflect the alleged lower risk of HMO enrollees.

The Medicare risk-contracting program is also receiving attention. HMOs and CMPs which have elected not to renew their risk contracts have alleged that the current AAPCC methodology produces inappropriate payment amounts and is a poor predictor of actual costs and utilization. Congress has directed the General Accounting Office to study methods of adjusting the AAPCC formula to account for differences between the utilization of HMO/CMP enrollees and fee-for-service enrollees. The study will also consider means of limiting a

Medicare contractor's risk for catastrophic costs. HCFA is soliciting demonstration sites for a diagnostic cost group (DCG) payment methodology by which the rate paid to a contracting HMO or CMP would be adjusted to reflect an enrollee's prior year hospitalization status and diagnoses.[4] Those segments of the managed care industry intending to pursue Medicare business will need to monitor and influence these proposed methodology changes.

The Office of Prepaid Health Care, which regulates HMOs, has deemphasized the monitoring of HMO services to private payers and is focusing on monitoring the compliance of HMOs and CMPs that are risk or cost contractors using applicable Medicare regulations. Congressional concern with HMOs is also increasingly focused on HMOs' Medicare functions as HMOs act in the government's stead in administering the health benefits of hundreds of thousands of Medicare enrollees. Thus, risk- and cost-contracting plans might anticipate additional regulation of their enrollment practices, quality assurance programs, and insolvency protections. HMOs should consider the possibility that their business plans and projections could be significantly altered by additional governmental requirements in these areas, and they should consider building into their provider contracts the flexibility to react to the reform of benefit package requirements and the payment system.

STATE REGULATORY DEVELOPMENTS

New Focus on HMO Insolvency

The managed care industry will also need to be sensitive to state regulatory developments. The HMO product will be particularly affected by regulatory concern with HMO insolvencies. Additionally, the HMO product will be shaped in new ways as state regulators grapple with open-ended access products and triple option issues.

The much publicized bankruptcy of Miami-based International Medical Centers and Maxicare's national system as well as the less publicized failures of other HMOs have focused the attention of state regulators and legislators on plan solvency. This attention is likely to result in stronger financial controls over HMOs, the impact of which will need to assessed by those planning multistate HMOs and those making choices among managed care product alternatives.

In 1981, the National Association of Insurance Commissioners amended its model act to relate deposit requirements to the amount of uncovered expenditures by the HMO. For example, under the Model Act, an HMO is required to deposit 2 percent of its estimated annual uncovered expenditures in its second year and 3 percent in its third year. Consequently, HMO managers have, over the years, worked to increase the number of provider agreements incorporating "hold harmless" clauses so as to reduce their requisite deposits.

Several states, however, have recently increased the amounts required to be kept on deposit. For example, North Carolina requires an initial deposit of $500,000. Texas now requires that a newly operational HMO deposit an amount equal to the difference between its initial deposit and total uncovered expenditures. Multistate HMOs will find such increased requirements to be an encumbrance on their growth.

Several states supplement their deposit requirements with a reserve requirement. In some states, such as Arizona and Illinois, the reserve is determined by an income-related formula, with a maximum of $1.5 million in Illinois and $1.0 million in Arizona. In other states, such as Florida and Nevada, the reserve is calculated by the greater of an expenditure formula or a flat sum — $100,000 in Florida and $500,000 in Nevada. States such as Missouri and North Carolina have initial and/or working capital requirements. In some cases, the legislature is considering significantly increasing these amounts. For example, Florida's legislature is considering increasing its minimum net worth requirement to $400,000 and Michigan's legislature is considering a requirement that HMOs have a net worth of $1.5 million before they begin operations. The prudent managed care executive will investigate these requirements when he or she does a market analysis.

Alabama, in 1986, and Illinois, in 1987, pioneered HMO guaranty funds. HMO guaranty funds are state-administered reserves, funded by plans licensed in that state, which may pay an insolvent HMO's debts, provide continuing healthcare coverage for an insolvent plan's enrollees, and pick up additional premium charges incurred by an insolvent plan's enrollees when they seek alternative coverage. The establishment of such funds is also being considered by the legislatures of a number of additional states. Proponents argue that the funds fill the gaps left by hold harmless arrangements, insolvency insurance, and reserve requirements. Opponents argue that these funds, with contributions related to premiums, unfairly affect established HMOs. Opponents observe that it is the startup plans that have the greatest risk of failure but that under a premium-related formula, the startup plans contribute lesser amounts to the funds. Opponents also criticize the funds as protecting providers rather than enrollees. As an alternative, some opponents urge that the risk of such failures be managed by increasing initial capitalization requirements. Nonetheless, if the guaranty fund idea catches on among regulators, HMO managers will have to be prepared to absorb the cost of contributions to the funds (for example, 2 percent of premiums in Illinois).

Other areas of state regulatory focus may include (1) imposition of a premium tax on HMO products, (2) regulation of health screening, (3) regulation of open enrollment periods, (4) mandated coverages, (5) mandatory Medicaid contract participation, and (6) mandatory contracts with certain ancillary providers such as podiatrists and psychologists. When analyzing the feasibility of offering an HMO product in a particular state, managed care companies should review that state's current and proposed requirements in each of these areas. For example, mandated coverages, premium tax, and enrollment requirements can increase the costs of offering an HMO product relative to the costs of offering a PPA product where the insurance code does not contain equivalent provisions.

Regulation of Open-Ended HMOs

While they are increasing the regulation of the traditional HMO product, state legislators and administrators will be seeking to catch up to the managed care industry's move to "open-ended" HMOs. Also known as "HMOs with choice," "self-referral options," "swing-out HMOs," and plans with "indemnity wrap-arounds," open-ended HMOs are designed to reduce the negative impact a closed panel concept can have on a prospect's willingness to enroll. An open-ended plan avoids at least the perception of a lock-in by permitting a member to choose, at the time of service, to go to a provider outside the HMO's panel. The out-of-plan provider is either in a preferred provider panel or has no relationship with the HMO. The member, however, pays coinsurance (as much as 50 percent but more commonly 30 percent) and/or a deductible for the privilege of going out-of-panel.

State HMO acts commonly have required HMOs to provide at least certain basic health services directly or through "arrangements" with healthcare providers.[5] Traditionally, only out-of-area and emergency services have been indemnified by HMOs rather than prepaid. Thus, state HMO acts will require amendment or new interpretation before they will permit open-ended HMOs which, by definition, indemnify basic services provided in the service area on a nonemergency basis.

The federal HMO Act amendments will permit federally qualified plans to indemnify up to 10 percent of basic health services. The federal act's approach may be replicated by a number of states. However, other approaches are possible. Some states may place a cap on an enrollee's out-of-pocket expenditures. Others may seek to protect enrollees by requiring that coinsurance be reduced as the enrollee's out-of-pocket expenditures rise. Regulatory attention may also be given to the issue of when an enrollee can opt back into the HMO panel during a course of treatment in order to avoid further exposure to coinsurance. The HMO segment of the managed care industry will need to be vigilant in monitoring state regulatory responses to open-ended plans if it wishes to safeguard that option.

Regulation of the PPA Product

Preferred provider arrangements (PPAs) are programs in which payers (for example, insurance companies, self-insured employers, union trust funds, and nonprofit service benefit plans such as Blue Cross – Blue Shield) offer their insureds financial incentives to obtain covered services from a panel of providers (physicians, hospitals, or both) with which the payer has directly or indirectly contracted, generally at discounted rates. While this entire preferred provider arrangement involving payers, insureds, and providers is often labeled a "preferred provider organization," or PPO, the term "PPA" is used here to avoid confusing the entire insurance arrangement with one of its components, that is, the PPO, which is the organization or panel of providers.

There is no federal qualification process for PPAs. Over one-half of the states have passed PPA statutes since 1980. However, these statutes have generally been enabling acts. They are designed to eliminate statutory obstacles to PPA development, such as insurance code freedom of choice guarantees and prohibitions in insurance codes on unfair discrimination against beneficiaries in health insurance policy premiums, conditions to coverage, and benefits.

The direct regulation of PPAs has generally been through those statutes governing the PPA payer, for example, insurance codes, service benefit laws, and HMO laws. A number of other state and federal statutes, while not directly regulating PPAs, affect their operations. These statutes include rate-setting laws, antitrust laws, as well as prohibitions on fee-splitting, the corporate practice of medicine, and fees for referrals.

When the PPA payer is an insurance company, the regulation of the PPA's forms, rates, reserves, and benefits is most likely to emanate from the state insurance code and the state department of insurance. Likewise, where the PPA payer is a service benefit plan or an HMO, its forms, rates, reserves, and benefits will be dictated by the service plan statute or the HMO statute, respectively. Finally, if the PPA payer is a self-insured group or union trust fund, the primary source of regulation may be the Employee Retirement Income Security Act of 1974 (ERISA).

Accordingly, companies contemplating initiating a PPA product must assess the regulation of the PPA payer in that state. Of particular importance will be the prevailing interpretations of so-called "freedom of choice" requirements, the prohibitions on "unfair" discrimination in benefit payments, and the interpretation of the PPA's ability to exclude even those providers who are willing to participate on the PPA's terms.

For instance, PPA plans provide a higher level of payment in cases where the insured receives services from a preferred provider. This benefit differential might be regarded as inhibiting the subscriber's free choice of providers, which is safeguarded by most insurance codes and by many service plan (Blue Cross – type) statutes. Likewise, benefit differentials could be banned by the prohibition on unfair discrimination in premiums charged, policy conditions imposed, and benefits provided. Nonetheless, these insurance and service benefit plan statutory provisions can also be interpreted as not precluding PPA benefit differentials. Although there are disincentives for PPA subscribers to choose nonparticipating providers (additional coinsurances or deductibles), they still have the freedom to make such choices and the disincentives are not "unfair" as that concept has been construed under state insurance law.

Enabling acts and regulations have, to date, generally cleared the way for the organization of PPAs. However, the PPA acts in a few states, such as Pennsylvania and Michigan, also dictate the structure and/or activities of a PPA. Because of ERISA's preemption of state law, these restrictions will not apply to fully self-insured plans. However, such restrictions may apply to partially self-insured plans— those that share the risk with insurers and purchase "stop-loss" insurance.

The most potentially destructive of the new restrictions is the requirement that a PPA contract with "any willing provider." In 1986, the Rand Corporation found such clauses in seven PPA enabling acts and found that three other acts sought to promote patient "freedom of choice" by prohibiting the use of gatekeepers to regulate referrals to specialists.[6] Enforcement of this requirement has rarely been tested, but such a requirement may cripple a PPA's ability to have a restricted panel of "preferred" providers.

Related to these provisions are those mandating that the PPA contract with one or more particular types of healthcare providers. In 1988, 350 bills were introduced in state legislatures that would require recognition of a specific service or recognition of all the services performed by a licensed provider.[7] Companies interested in implementing a PPA product will therefore need to be aware of the political pressure on state legislatures from various provider organizations supporting such requirements. That pressure may increasingly threaten the PPA and other forms of managed care.

A second type of restriction appearing in PPA enabling acts limits the payment or benefit differential available for services obtained from a preferred rather than a nonpreferred provider. The theory is that large differentials unduly penalize PPA beneficiaries seeking to use nonpanel providers and result in a lock-in. Organizations that lock in enrollees may require licensure as an HMO or an exclusive provider organization (EPO).[8] In 1986, state benefit differential limits ranged from 10 to 30 percent.[9] Where the permissible differential is excessively limited, PPAs may not be able to provide sufficient financial incentive to direct their beneficiaries to preferred providers. In such cases, the PPA's forecasted savings to the payer and forecasted increased volume to the preferred providers would be compromised.

Finally, several states have adopted direct enrollee protections in the PPA context. For example, PPAs, such as those in Illinois, may be required to reimburse emergency care in or out of the service area at the preferred provider level. PPAs, such as those in Pennsylvania, may also be required to demonstrate that their service areas are adequately covered by the preferred provider panel and that they have a quality assurance plan and enrollee grievance procedures.

Many PPAs have graduated from a solely discount orientation.[10] Some are even seeking to go beyond reliance on utilization management programs to control utilization. In doing so these PPAs utilize withhold incentive systems to place some financial risk on providers. Those that share risk with providers will encounter a higher degree of regulation.

For example, if the provider panel takes a part of the insurance risk in a PPA, it may face demands from state regulators that it be licensed as an HMO or as an insurer and that it adhere to appropriate reserve, benefit, and contract requirements. In some jurisdictions, such as Pennsylvania, a panel (PPO) that assumes financial risk is subject to special licensure and reserve requirements under the PPA enabling act. Pennsylvania examines a risk-assuming PPO's corporate governance, the organization's officers and directors, the actuarial basis for its rates, as well as its utilization review, quality assurance, and grievance systems. Such a licensure process is comparable to HMO licensure. It also foreshadows the future merger, in several states, of the regulation of the HMO and PPA products. Such unified regulation would intuitively be sensible given the evolution of the PPA into a product which incorporates financial risk features and other utilization controls and in light of the merger of the two products in the open-ended HMO. Moreover, unified regulation may be the most effective way for the states to monitor the double- and triple-option products.

The Triple Option

The so-called triple-option insurance product has become an important focus of managed care activity. In this format, beneficiaries annually decide whether to receive all their healthcare from an HMO, under a PPA, or under a traditional fee-for-service indemnity plan. Under the HMO option, the beneficiary receives the richest benefit package (the highest level of coverage for the most services) and enjoys prepayment. However, all but emergency and out-of-area care must be received from a participating provider. Under a PPA option, the beneficiary is liable for a modest coinsurance amount (for example, 10 percent) when obtaining services from a member of the panel of "preferred" providers and in return for a higher coinsurance amount (for example, 30 percent) can obtain services from out-of-panel providers. Finally, under the indemnity option, beneficiaries have unfettered freedom of choice of providers but are liable for significant coinsurance amounts (for example, 20 percent or more), substantial deductibles (for example, $1000), and may have fewer services covered (for example, infertility services and well-baby care may be excluded).

Triple-option programs are designed to offer groups the administrative convenience of one-stop shopping for a variety of health insurance options. At the same time, they address a perceived need by insurers to mitigate the effects of allegedly adverse selection against indemnity products, that is, the selection of the indemnity option by a disproportionate number of poor risks. By keeping all the plan's enrollees in the same risk pool, the experience of the entire group is accounted for in rating each option. Thus, the indemnity product's competitive position is improved.

The structuring of triple-option plans can give rise to multiple regulatory issues. One issue is the ability of an HMO to contract with groups to provide indemnity services, and conversely, the ability of an indemnity company to take the legal responsibility for arranging for the provision of a product that locks in enrollees to panel providers. Moreover, issues arise as to which — reserve, board of director's composition, and enrollment — requirements should apply. Assuming cooperation between, or joint ownership by, an HMO and an insurance company, issues will also arise about consolidation of contracts, premium collections, joint marketing, and rating on an integrated basis.

The use of multiple contracts (for example, separate HMO and indemnity group contracts) can avoid regulatory problems related to having the proper supporting license for each product. However, separate contracts may lack marketing appeal and will require attention to detail in coordinating enrollment periods, premium payment arrangements, and other contractual obligations. Consolidated premium collection may promote administrative simplicity for the group, but attention must be given to specifying liability in case the administrator receives payment which is insufficient for all products. Joint marketing of HMO and indemnity products has been objected to by at least one state's regulators, and those marketing efforts would need to conform with the broker's license requirements, if any, for each product. Integrated rating poses problems where some variant of community rating is required of HMOs or where the regulators would require each product's rates to be independently actuarially justifiable.

"Point-of-service" plans raise a number of regulatory issues as well. In such plans, the employee is allowed to select a provider any time a healthcare service is necessary. Again, multiple licenses (HMO and indemnity) may be required, and the rating, marketing, benefits, and quality assurance responsibilities of each licensed organization must be satisfied.

Single-Service Plans

Single-service healthcare plans are a growing market. Generally operated along the lines of an HMO or PPA, such plans offer care or service in a single healthcare area, such as mental health, dentistry, eye care, chiropractic, or podiatry. Single-service plans are becoming increasingly visible and popular for several reasons, including:

1. Employer demand for specialty products, such as substance abuse benefits
2. Competition among insurers, including HMOs, for new products
3. The self-insurance trend, whereby employers work directly with benefits consultants to put together specially tailored healthcare plans

Single-service plans have engendered a number of complex regulatory issues at the state level. If the plan accepts insurance-type risk, a license is likely to be required. The difficult question is which statutory pigeon hole, if any, best fits for a particular plan. An HMO license is generally not available because an HMO must provide a full range of healthcare services. PPO statutes, where they exist, frequently do not allow risk-taking. Indemnity insurance statutes are, in most cases, too cumbersome and expensive with regard to capital and reserve requirements. Moreover, only a few states have broad statutory schemes encompassing single-service plans, such as California's Knox-Keene law.[11]

In most states single-service plans are left with a melange of specific single-service statutes (that is, for dental plans or vision plans) or Blue Cross–type statutes authorizing health service plans, mostly on a nonprofit basis. The specific provisions of such laws vary greatly as to capital requirements, board composition, and contract requirements. For example, some states require a majority of providers to be on the board of directors of the single-service company, while other states require a majority of consumers on the board. Other laws require all directors to be state residents. Such differences can create severe difficulties for multistate operations and often present obstacles for developing cost-effective products.

This is particularly true of some mandated benefit provisions such as required coverages in the mental health area, provider nondiscrimination provisions, and subscriber free-choice-of-provider requirements. Where nonprofit companies are required for licensure purposes, single-service plans may have to set up nonprofit, controlled affiliates which are managed through a management contract. In other words, a for-profit company is set up to serve as the sole member of the nonprofit company and to manage the nonprofit. While this is a cumbersome way to do business, it is unavoidable in some states.

In many states, single-service plans can avoid licensure entirely, or at least ease the burden, by contracting with HMOs or indemnity carriers, which then in turn contract directly with employers. However, these "license fronting" arrangements can still trigger complex regulatory issues and, perhaps more important, are often significantly less advantageous from a business standpoint for the single-service plan because a portion of the premium must be divided with the HMO or insurance company.

Impact of Hospital Rate-Setting Regulations

Another form of state regulation that affects managed care product development is hospital rate-setting legislation. Hospital rate-setting schemes emerged in response to a fear of hospital insolvency due to the strain of uncompensated care and in response to state legislative concern with growing Medicaid expenditures. The groups most frequently supportive of rate regulation have been hospital trustees interested in reducing hospital exposure to bad debt, governors interested in reducing Medicaid costs, businesses hoping to control increases in premiums or the claims experience of their self-insured plans, and commercial insurers interested in "leveling the playing field" vis-à-vis Blues plans.[12]

Commercial insurers traditionally did not have contracts with providers as did Blue Cross and Blue Shield. The insurers believed that hospitals granted discounts only to those payers they contracted with (for example, Blue Cross, Medicare, and Medicaid). As a result, the indemnity carriers felt they were disadvantaged and supported rate-setting or "all payer" legislation, which, by setting prices equally among payers, equitably distributed the bad debt burden. Under rate-setting or all payer programs, Blues plans might still qualify for discounted rates through prompt payment discounts or where they are deemed to provide affordable coverage and open enrollment periods. Nevertheless, the indemnity companies saw the all payer system as an improvement because rates have to be economically justified.

Hospital rate-setting programs persist in about a dozen states. Indemnity carriers may now feel constrained by the hospital rate-setting programs they previously supported, particularly in states where the Blues' penetration is not disproportionately high. While the rate-setting programs were largely beneficial when an insurer's business was exclusively indemnity, the programs can be a mixed blessing when the insurer is launching a managed care program. An insurer's new contractual relationships with providers might allow it to negotiate significant hospital discounts in the absence of the rate-setting law.

In some rate-setting programs, such as Maryland's and New Jersey's, PPAs and HMOs may qualify for limited discounts. Nonetheless, these programs often prevent new entrants into the managed care market from establishing managed care products where the product's success is premised on hospital discounts. Of course, the rate-setting program may also serve to protect new entrants into the managed care market in states where the program currently constrains a dominant payer from obtaining large discounts that diminish the feasibility of effective competition. In either case, managed care companies will need to keep abreast of new legislative initiatives for hospital rate regulation and proposed changes in existing rate regulation programs.

Regulation of Utilization Management Companies

Several states have recently begun to look more closely at the utilization management activities of payers and fourth-party utilization review contractors.[13] In the same way that third party administrators have become subject to licensure or other oversight in many states, utilization management companies are coming under scrutiny because their activities affect the nature and scope of healthcare services provided to subscribers. Moreover, many providers support closer regulation of utilization management companies because such companies have an important impact on payment decisions and because providers are concerned about the widespread demand for and use of medical records by such companies.

Maryland, for example, has recently enacted a law requiring both health insurers and utilization management companies (called by the statute "private review agents") to obtain a certificate of authority to engage in utilization review activity. Application for a certificate of authority will include providing evidence satisfactory to the Secretary of Health that the insurer or private review agent has appropriate standards, analyses, and procedures and employs sufficiently qualified medical personnel to conduct the utilization reviews.

LEGAL CONSTRAINTS

Liability

Managed care organizations, by definition, play some role in the provision of, or in limiting or directing access to, healthcare services. In this way, they are fundamentally different from pure payer organizations (for example, indemnity companies) and may have concomitant increased exposure to tort liability. In the future, managed care organizations may see attempts to invoke a number of liability theories against them as plaintiffs seek to reach the payer's "deep pocket." The cost of defending such actions could be significant. Thus structuring a managed care organization's procedures to minimize such liability is deserving of executive-level action.

The operational area in which the exposure to tort liability is greatest is an HMO's or PPA's utilization management program. Preadmission certifications, referral authorizations, and concurrent review are examples of processes that must be designed with an eye toward risk management. Risk is reduced by the creation of, and adherence to, sound procedures and the involvement of appropriate medical personnel. The managed care organization must devise procedures for making coverage determinations that do not interfere with the physician's right to order additional treatments on a noncovered basis. Likewise, utilization management decisions must be reached in a timely fashion, allow for "appeal" (acquisition of additional information), and inform enrollees of their right to obtain the care desired on a noncovered basis.

An allegedly defective concurrent review process was among the issues in *Wickline v. State of California*, 228 Cal. Rptr. 661 (1986). While the case turned on the physician's failure to act in accordance with his medical judgment, it was suggested that defects in the design or implementation of cost-containment mechanisms could give rise to payer liability. In *Boyd v. Albert Einstein Medical Center*, 547 A.2d 1229 (Pa. Super. Ct. 1988), a Pennsylvania appeals court reversed a trial court's determination that an IPA-model HMO participating physician could not, as a matter of law, be deemed to be an agent of the HMO. The court held that there was a genuine issue of material fact as to whether the participating physician was the ostensible agent of the HMO. The court noted that (1) the plaintiff decedent had paid her physician fee to the HMO, not the physician, (2) the HMO limited the decedent's choice of primary care and specialist physicians, (3) the HMO screened and regulated its participating physicians, and (4) the HMO's primary care physician gave the decedent no choice when he referred her to a participating specialist. While it might be contended that tort claims are preempted by the federal ERISA statute, managed care organizations should design and implement their utilization management programs with liability risk management in mind.

Another area of liability risk for managed care organizations is provider contracting. Traditional indemnity plans do not contract with providers and thus make no representations as to a provider's skill. However, PPAs give enrollees economic incentives to use preferred providers, and traditional HMOs require that all nonemergency in-service-area care be obtained from provider panel members. Thus, these organizations may be said to have a duty to their enrollees to exercise reasonable care in selecting and retaining panel hospitals and physicians.

HMOs and PPAs must therefore give careful consideration to development of a credentialing process which will verify the qualifications and competence of participating hospitals and physicians. Diligent investigation of the provider's licensure and standing, accreditation or certification, insurance coverage, and general professional history and standing is advisable.

If well documented, such a credentialing program can demonstrate that reasonable care was used in provider selection. The process should also be periodically repeated as a part of a recredentialing program. This will enable the plan to defend any claim that it was negligent in retaining a certain participating provider in light of the provider's recent professional record.

Antitrust Constraints

Antitrust concerns are an important constraint on the structure and functioning of managed care systems. Two operational areas in which antitrust concerns are particularly strong are (1) negotiations between payers and providers, especially those concerning the price to be paid for provider services, and (2) membership decisions made by provider-controlled organizations. The antitrust laws award triple actual damages to successful private plaintiffs, and even the successful defense of an antitrust case is likely to be extremely time-consuming and expensive. Thus, the attention given to antitrust issues in the design and operation of a managed care system can pay large dividends.

PROVIDER NEGOTIATIONS—INCLUDING REIMBURSEMENT DECISIONS If a managed care system is structured so that provider participation decisions, including their reimbursement aspects, are the product of negotiations between a nonprovider-controlled organization (for example, an insurer or self-insured employer) and the providers, they will, in most cases, not create antitrust concerns. This is because where provider participation reimbursement decisions do not involve negotiation between competitors, they are deemed "vertical" decisions (the result of an agreement between a buyer and a seller that do not compete), which generally fall outside the scope of the prohibition on concerted action in restraint of trade contained in Section 1 of the Sherman Act. In these cases, a provider's refusal to participate or to accept the proposed price terms is not deemed to be a "horizontal" agreement (an agreement among competitors at the same level of distribution) to boycott or the product of a horizontal price-fixing agreement. Therefore, purchaser- or payer-controlled PPAs have generally been approved by the antitrust enforcement agencies. Likewise, where the preferred provider panel is assembled by a nonprovider-controlled intermediary, the antitrust risk associated with the participation decision and the establishment of prices is modest.

However, for the many HMOs and PPAs which can be characterized as provider-controlled, the antitrust risk can be significant when it is associated with the establishment of provider reimbursement levels and with bargaining with payers. These organizations need to consider adopting measures that eliminate the potential for a Sherman Act violation in their negotiation and pricing systems.

One way to avoid liability under Section 1 of the Sherman Act is to constitute the provider-controlled organization as a joint venture within the meaning of the antitrust laws. The Supreme Court has expressly approved agreements among competitors as to price and output where such agreements are a necessary consequence of a joint venture's creation of a new product. See *Broadcast Music, Inc. v. Columbia Broadcasting Systems, Inc.*, 441 U.S. 1 (1979). Thus, for example, where physicians have formed a legitimate joint venture to offer a new healthcare financing product to a community, their collective decisions about the price paid to participating providers are less likely to violate Section 1 of the Sherman Act.

The Supreme Court, however, has not yet provided the managed care industry (or the economy at large) with a set of rules by which it can be determined when agreements among competitors will be regarded as lawful because they are ancillary to a legitimate joint venture. This ambiguity allowed the recent *Choice Care* verdict where a jury determined that the establishment of physician reimbursement by a physician-controlled HMO amounted to illegal price-fixing and awarded damages of $96 million. *See Thompson v. Midwest Foundation Independent Physician Ass'n.*, No. C-1-86-0744 (S.D. Ohio Mar. 14, 1988).[14] *Choice Care* was subsequently settled by the parties, leaving the jury's verdict and its associated antitrust determinations untested. While the settlement diminishes the case's precredential value, the managed care industry continues to wrestle with its implications.

In the infamous *Maricopa* case, the Supreme Court distinguished between the price-fixing done by the Maricopa Foundation for Medical Care and the establishment of provider compensation levels by organizations where "competitors pool their capital and share the risks of loss as well as the opportunities for profit." *See Arizona v. Maricopa County Medical Society*, 457 U.S. 332 (1982). *Maricopa*-related cases and enforcement agency guidance have suggested a number of economic characteristics which may determine whether the providers's agreements will be viewed as legitimate business decisions related to the operation of an integrated entity rather than as horizontal conspiracies to restrain trade. These characteristics include the motivation of the providers and the size of the provider panel, and whether the providers have shared the risk of business failure through capital investment, capitation, and withhold arrangements.

This type of analysis was recently employed in *Hassan v. Independent Practice Associates, P.C.,* 698 F. Suppl. 679 (D. Mich. 1988), where a federal district court found that the defendant IPA had not fixed prices in violation of the Sherman Act, in part because the IPA was a legitimate joint venture that shared the risk of loss and opportunity for profit with the HMO through capitation payments. HMOs that delegate physician reimbursement decisions to IPAs should, however, carefully assess whether the IPAs are sufficiently integrated to qualify as integrated joint ventures.

Preferred provider panels that are provider-controlled are even more susceptible to price-fixing and boycott charges because they typically involve little financial integration. The Department of Justice has, at various times, indicated that a preferred provider panel with fewer than 20 or 35 percent of an area's physicians might be viewed as a joint venture, absent evidence of anticompetitive purpose or effect, even where significant economic integration is absent. Nonetheless, the question is far from settled, as the Supreme Court's proscription in *Maricopa* was far more conservative than the Department of Justice's stance, and the Federal Trade Commission has also been skeptical of provider involvement in price setting where such involvement is arguably not absolutely necessary to the managed care organization's functioning. Those establishing managed care plans should seek the guidance of counsel in structuring the plan's activities so as to eliminate horizontal agreements on antitrust-sensitive issues. Provider panels can, for example, arrange their dealings with PPA payers so that each provider negotiates significant economic terms directly with the payer. The provider panel (the PPO or local provider unit) simply acts as a messenger between the individual providers and the prospective payer. Therefore, the panel's operations do not produce agreements between competing providers but only vertical agreements between the payer and providers.

A number of variations on the messenger approach are in use to meet the provider's and payer's administrative needs. For example, each provider may authorize the panel to contract on the provider's behalf with all payers who are willing to pay at or above a certain price. Similarly, providers can authorize a panel to make available to payers the "standing offer" as to price, with the payers selecting or assembling a subgroup of the panel that meets their pricing needs. Although the technique has theoretical flaws, it is also often suggested that PPAs attempt to avoid competitors agreeing on prices by delegating decisions on reimbursement levels to "independent" third parties, such as accounting firms or consultants.

CREDENTIALING DECISIONS Provider membership decisions made by provider-controlled managed care organizations can also lead to claims of concerted action in restraint of trade in violation of Section 1 of the Sherman Act. Again, where a nonprovider-controlled payer, such as an insurer or self-funder plan, makes the selection decisions, the decisions will generally constitute unilateral conduct beyond the reach of Section 1's proscription. Moreover, where a managed care organization is financially integrated so as to be regarded as a joint venture, its provider-contracting decisions should be beyond Section 1's scope so long as the organization has not effectively delegated the decision to a provider-controlled credentialing committee or IPA.

Credentialing decisions should be well documented. Moreover, the documentation should evidence the application of standards that have a rational relationship to the managed care organization's business and quality of care concerns. If the organization can demonstrate that a decision to exclude a provider reflected a reasonable business purpose and was not motivated by the current participating providers' fear of new competition, its decision should be upheld.

Of course, the exclusion decision is made more defensible by structuring the process to avoid a potential veto by the applicant's direct competitors (for example, physicians in the applicant's specialty and practicing in the applicant's geographic area). Additionally, managed care organizations can generally defend exclusions on the ground that they lack sufficient effect on competition, particularly if the effect on competition is measured from the consumer's view.

Due process is not a requirement under the antitrust laws. *See Northwest Wholesale Stationers, Inc. v. Pacific Stationery & Printing Co.*, 472 U.S. 284, 93 (1985). However, the common law in some states, notably California, establishes certain minimum fair process requirements. Consequently, it is generally prudent for managed care companies to adopt some standards for fair procedure by which to consider provider applications, recredentialing, and disciplinary decisions.

It should also be noted that, to the extent that a physician's or dentist's exclusion is based on quality of care concerns, immunity from antitrust and certain other claims may be obtained if the organization conforms its credentialing or disciplinary procedures to the dictates of the Health Care Quality Improvement Act of 1986 (HCQIA). Pub. L. No. 99-660, §411. The HCQIA applies to professional review actions taken "in the reasonable belief that the action was in furtherance of quality health care," if the physician or dentist involved was provided "adequate" notice and a hearing. (Id. § 412) However, the procedures that the Act deems to satisfy the notice and hearing requirements are complex, and care should be taken in structuring quality-related review processes to conform to them. It should also be noted that organizations can develop two-tiered credentialing and disciplinary procedures using an abbreviated procedure where HCQIA immunity is unlikely to be available and the more time-consuming procedures which comply with the HCQIA where immunity is available.

NOTES

1. *See generally* L. Gruber, M. Shadle, and C. Polich, "From Movement to Industry: The Growth of HMOs." *Health Affairs* **7**(3):197–208 (Summer, 1988).

2. See the section "Regulation of the PPA Product" *infra* for a discussion of the terms "PPA" and "PPO."

3. Towers, Perrin, Forster & Crosby, Inc., "Study of the Federal Employees Health Benefits Program." Contract No. OPM-87-9027 (April 22, 1988).

4. DCG payments should not be confused with diagnosis-related groups (DRGs), which are the units HCFA uses for setting the rates at which Medicare compensates hospitals for inpatient treatment of Medicare beneficiaries.

5. For example, Pennsylvania requires HMOs to provide "either directly or through arrangements with others" all emergency care, inpatient hospital and physician care, ambulatory physician care, and outpatient and preventive medical services. See 40 P.S. 1554(b).

6. Rand Report to the Department of Health and Human Services and Federal Trade Commission, p. 10. (August 1986) (hereinafter "Rand Report").

7. Woodrow Eno, "PPO Legislative Hurdles May Lie Ahead," *Health Benefits Journal.* **2**(9):5 (September 1988).

8. In California, insurers are authorized to establish EPOs—organizations where the enrollee's choice is restricted to participating providers but where the payer is an insurance company. EPOs are also often instituted by self-insured employers.

9. Rand Report, p. 11.

10. Peter Boland, "Trends in Second-Generation PPOs." *Health Affairs* **6**(4):75. (Winter, 1987). Discount-oriented plans are labeled "first-generation PPOs," whereas "second generation PPOs" are characterized by strong internal administrative controls.

11. A few other states currently have single-service–type statutes that cover more than one service. Texas is an example. Moreover, the National Association of Insurance Commissioners recently has passed a model single-service health plan statute that is likely to serve as the basis for similar statutes in other states.

12. Carl J. Schramm, "State Hospital Cost Containment: An Analysis of Legislative Initiatives." *Indiana Law Review* **19**:919–954 (1986).

13. "Fourth-party contractors" is a term used to describe companies which generally are engaged solely in the utilization management business

and which are hired by payers (insurance companies, HMOs, or employers) to review cases for medical necessity, quality, and related matters. They typically do not provide insurance or claims processing functions and, hence, are distinguishable from the third party payers or third party administrators.

14. However, the facts alleged in *Choice Care* did not simply relate to antitrust violations. Two officers of the plan were alleged to have set the plan's reimbursement payments at a low level to improve the plan's financial position in connection with the plan's conversion to for-profit status, a conversion which was alleged to benefit the corporation's officers.

POINT OF VIEW

The Future of Managed Healthcare Regulation

KENNETH J. LINDE, President

Principal Health Care, Inc., Rockville, Maryland

In the future, managed healthcare will be strongly influenced by state regulation, which is assuming the principal regulatory role as federal HMO oversight diminishes. Almost all states have enacted HMO legislation and are actively regulating HMO operations and financial arrangements. As PPOs and other managed care organizations move from simple discount arrangements to more complex utilization management and risk arrangements, it will be inevitable that these organizations will be subject to the same kinds of governmental oversight as HMOs. At the same time, there will be the pressures to increase responsibility for the quality of healthcare. In some states, legislatures have already enacted PPO legislation and in many others, bills have been introduced. Self-referral options (SROs),* exclusive provider organizations

*Self-referral options are becoming increasingly popular as HMOs require more flexibility and PPOs require control, risk, and incentive systems. An SRO is a plan in which an eligible enrollee is covered under both a HMO option and an indemnity benefit program and selects between them at point of service.

SROs have been introduced in 48 of the nations' 643 HMOs. For competitive reasons it is critical that products, such as SROs, be offered to appease consumer demand for more freedom of choice. Out-of-plan benefits usually include higher out-of-pocket costs for enrollees and often lower benefits. An indemnity insurance company usually underwrites the out-of-plan product.

(EPOs), and the other varieties and combinations of managed healthcare will be scooped into the regulatory net as they assume more and more HMO characteristics.

In today's highly competitive healthcare environment, the weaker players are being forced out. Only the strong will remain in the long run. The "shakeout" is already underway. The number of players in the competitive arena will be fewer, but those remaining will be strong and well-tempered. The challenge for managed care regulation, under these circumstances, will be to construct a regulatory environment that will facilitate the operation of sound managed care organizations concentrating on quality healthcare.

State regulators can learn many important lessons from the experience gained in the evolution of federal regulation. Paramount is the need for sufficient capital to cope with the cyclical nature of healthcare costs. The need for insolvency protection to withstand the down cycle cannot be underestimated. Limiting this protection to funded reserves not only fails to recognize the strong financial backing of parent corporation guarantees, but also depletes the available capital needed to survive the down cycle. More realistic insolvency requirements must be established for managed care organizations to be able to compete in the healthcare arena. Direction on another aspect of insolvency can be gained from the federal requirement for "hold harmless" clauses in all provider contracts between HMOs and providers. This requirement protects members from the impact of HMO insolvency by prohibiting individual providers from billing members for amounts owed to the HMO. The incorporation of this requirement into the National Association of Insurance Commissioners' (NAIC) model HMO law would strengthen the ability of state regulators to buffer members from the ill effects in the event of HMO insolvency.

Another important lesson learned in the 15 years of federal regulation is that incentive systems for providers result in high quality healthcare at reduced cost if quality assurance monitoring is adequate and effective management and data systems are implemented. State regulators tend to view these systems as shifting risk from the managed care organization to the provider. In fact, the best of these systems are designed to provide bonuses for high performance, that is, provide incentive to improve the health services to members. Developing regulations to achieve the positive effects of incentives is a challenge and requires an in-depth understanding of the intricacies of managed healthcare. This area offers a great deal of potential for improving the quality of healthcare, an issue that is surfacing as a major thrust of employers and other healthcare purchasers.

As managed healthcare becomes a mature industry with fewer, stronger organizations, each of these organizations can be expected to be operating in a number of states. For these organizations and for the states responsible for regulating them, coordinated regulation would be immensely popular. NAIC has made strides in coordinated HMO regulation and could be a vehicle for working toward real regulatory congruence for managed care organizations. NAIC might also focus on ways to coordinate reserve requirements and, thereby, avoid unnecessary capital constraints which stifle innovation and competition.

The future regulation of managed care offers many opportunities for influencing the direction of this industry. It can be an influence for good if it recognizes and supports the diversity and strengths inherent in managed healthcare.

CHAPTER THREE

Public Opinion

ATTITUDES TOWARD MANAGED HEALTHCARE

HUMPHREY TAYLOR, President
Louis Harris and Associates, Inc., New York, New York

J. IAN MORRISON, Ph.D., Director, Healthcare Program
Institute for the Future, Menlo Park, California

Public opinion and the attitudes of particular interest groups combine to help shape the evolution of healthcare. Most actors in the healthcare system recognize this, but there has been little systematic investigation of how attitudinal forces actually create change.[1] This chapter explores how public opinion and other attitudinal factors affect change in healthcare in general and in managed care in particular.

PUBLIC OPINION AND SOCIAL CHANGE

What is the real significance of public opinion? What does the study of public opinion tell us about the future? Does it matter? Does government usually follow public opinion or disregard it? Is a change in public opinion usually followed by a change in policy? There are no easy answers to these questions, except that in a democracy—which is also a marketplace for competitive products, services, *and* ideas—public opinion obviously matters.

Public opinion can operate in many different ways—particularly if a broad definition of public opinion is used that includes not just attitudes toward public policy issues, but also consumers' attitudes toward alternative choices.

In the field of healthcare, virtually all the major pieces of legislation were passed with massive public support—from the introduction of Medicare and Medicaid to the introductions of diagnostic-related groups (DRGs), COBRA, and the recent catastrophic health insurance bill. Yet the public has often supported new legislative proposals that have not passed, including the long-term care bill. Many key trends that have been changing the structure of healthcare are the direct or indirect results of consumer demand and preference or the public's willingness to accept the lesser of various evils. The recent financial fortunes of most providers, insurers, and managed care plans have been determined largely by consumer choice and consumer demand.

Public attitudes determine to a large degree the success of new financing and delivery mechanisms. In 1980, Harris predicted the rapid growth of HMO membership based on three survey findings: a high level of satisfaction, a high renewal rate among HMO members, and the appeal of the HMO concept to many nonmembers. In the mid- to late-1980s, employers would not have been able to increase deductibles and copayments as rapidly as they did if they had faced massive employee hostility. Harris surveys over the past 5 years have shown that most employees took this cost-shifting in their stride. Indeed, they showed that with good communications to employees (and that was crucial), employers could make big increases in deductibles and copayments without triggering any significant employee backlash.

Yet for all its importance, public opinion does not always prevail. Public opinion is most likely to shape public policy when as many as possible of the following conditions are met:

1. There is a large majority in favor of the policy for a considerable period of time.
2. It is an important issue that most people are concerned about. People care about it. (The polls often report majorities of the public for or against things they care little about.)
3. It is a relatively simple issue. The more complex it is, or becomes, the less likely public opinion is to be decisive.
4. It does not cost the taxpayer much money (particularly the individual taxpayer as opposed to the corporate). The more it costs, the tougher it is to pass. National health insurance is a good example of a policy that has not happened for this reason.
5. It is not opposed by a very powerful lobby. For example, any bill that confronts the American Association of Retired Persons (AARP) head on will be tough to pass. A better way to state this condition might be to say that the balance of lobbying power is not overwhelmingly opposed to public opinion. For most policies, there are interests and lobbies on both sides.

6. The policy does not conflict with other equally popular policies. For example, tax cuts meet all five of the other criteria. The public almost always favors tax cuts. So does a lot of lobbying power. It is a simple issue to grasp and communicate. It certainly does not cost the taxpayer anything. And it's a highly salient issue. But tax cuts usually mean spending cuts, and spending is only voted because the public or some other very powerful interests favors it.

Sometimes public opinion prevails when some of these conditions are not met. But the more of them that are met, the more likely public opinion is to prevail. Although these six conditions apply generally to the role of public opinion in shaping public policy, they also apply to the development of healthcare policy more specifically.

ATTITUDES AS DRIVERS OF HEALTHCARE

Public Attitudes and Pluralism

Public attitudes are a critically important driver of the healthcare system because of the extraordinary range of healthcare options available to the American public. Unlike most other advanced nations that have settled on a dominant public payer as the optimum solution of finance, coverage, and control of healthcare, the United States continues to pursue a pluralist model. With pluralism comes choice —in supporting policy and in selecting providers and health plans —and, ultimately, for some segments of the public, the choice comes down to whether to buy healthcare or some other necessity with the next available dollar. As choice remains great, so the influence of the public—as patient, family member, voter, or employee—is critical. This chapter places public opinion in the context of other influential groups: physicians, employers, government legislators, and labor unions. This chapter draws on published surveys conducted by Louis Harris and Associates and other national polling organizations and reflects current understanding of the field gained from a wide variety of survey research.

Healthcare as Public Priority

Healthcare costs in the United States are growing faster in the 1980s than they did in the 1970s—when adjusted for aging, population growth, and general levels of inflation.[2] This explosion in costs has taken place amid the rhetoric of cost containment, competition, and cutbacks. One explanation for this continued growth may lie in the simple notion that most of the users and providers of healthcare consider growth to be desirable and that these groups have political clout.

A wide variety of polls shows the public favors more rather than less spending on healthcare, but the degree to which such opinions translate into results depends on the power these opinions have in

shaping decisions. For example, a 1988 Harris survey of federal legislators and regulators shows that the elderly had the greatest political
clout concerning healthcare by an enormous margin (seven out of
ten legislators ranked the elderly as the key group). Doctors and
hospitals came in a respectable second and third place, respectively,
ahead of employers, insurers, drug manufacturers, and minorities
and the poor. If the major users and providers of healthcare are the
most dominant influence on policy, it is not surprising that the system continues to head upward.

But if there is strong support for spending money on healthcare
among certain groups, the public is not universal in its support of
healthcare as an issue deserving of increased public attention. A
recent survey by ABC/*Washington Post* placed healthcare at the bottom of a list of 12 problems that the public feels are the most important. Healthcare as a whole was not rated highly, but issues such as
drugs and AIDS were seen as extremely important (see Table 1).

Overall, healthcare has been and continues to be an important
priority with the public, but its growth is begrudged to some degree
by both the public and payers. More money is being spent, but more
health is not being delivered. To put this statement in an international perspective, Table 2 shows four key measures for the major
Organization for Economic Cooperation and Development (OECD)
countries: healthcare spending as a share of gross national product (GNP), percent of population over 65, average life expectancy, and
infant mortality. Despite the fact that the United States has one of the
youngest populations, it spends more of its resources on health,
although this increased expenditure is not reflected in an edge in life
expectancy or reduced infant mortality.

TABLE 1   Healthcare as a Policy Problem
What is the most important problem facing this country today?

RESPONSES	PERCENT
Drugs	10
Nuclear war	9
Federal budget deficit	8
AIDS	7
Communism/Soviet Union	7
Middle East	7
Unemployment	6
Other economic issues	6
Iran-Contra scandal	5
Moral decline/drugs	4
Crime	3
Healthcare/healthcare system	1

Source: ABC/*Washington Post* Poll, October 1987.

TABLE 2   American Healthcare in an International Context
Health Spending and Health Status Measure for Major OECD Countries, 1986

COUNTRY	HEALTHCARE AS A PERCENT OF GDP	POPULATION OVER 65, %*	LIFE EXPECTANCY, years	INFANT MORTALITY, rate per 1000
United States	11.1	12.0	75	10
Sweden	9.1	16.9	77	6
Canada	8.5	10.4	77	8
France	8.5	12.4	75	8
Germany	8.1	14.5	76	9
Italy	6.7	13.0	76	10
Japan	6.7	10.0	78	6
United Kingdom	6.2	15.1	75	9

*1985 data.
Source: OECD and U.N. Demographic Yearbook

New data on public attitudes toward healthcare in the United Kingdom, Canada, and the United States indicate that these differences in aggregate performance of the system are also reflected in public satisfaction.[3] Table 3 shows that lower levels of satisfaction exist in the United States, both in terms of public attitudes toward the system as a whole and toward health services used by the respondent. When asked which system they would prefer, their own or one of the other countries, the study found:

TABLE 3   International Satisfaction with Healthcare Systems and Services, 1988

	SYSTEM MEASURE	PERSONAL MEASURE
	On the whole, the system works pretty well (% agreeing)	Overall, how do you feel about healthcare services used by you or your family? (% saying "very satisfied)
United States	10	35
Canada	56	67
United Kingdom	27	39

Source: Reference 3, pp. 1–10.

- Sixty-one percent of Americans would favor the Canadian system over their own.
- Ninety-five percent of Canadians favored their system over the U.S. system.
- Eighty percent of the British favored their system over the U.S. system.

It has been assumed by many that Americans may be dissatisfied with the system but are satisfied with the care they receive. These data challenge that assumption and suggest that the managed care movement faces an enormous task in turning around an ailing U.S. healthcare system.

Cost, Quality, and Access

Healthcare arouses strong feelings in the American public. They are satisfied with the quality of care they receive (although, as seen above, not as satisfied as their northern neighbors), and yet they are less than enthusiastic in their support of the system as a whole (see Tables 4 and 5). It should be noted that the American public is particularly patriotic—when the word "American" is left out of survey questions, dissatisfaction with the system rises markedly. It is the lack of access and high costs of the system as a whole that lead to the dissatisfaction observed in public opinion polls (see Table 5). The schizophrenic "my care is good but the system has a lot wrong with it" has been observed consistently over the past decade.[4]

Surveys are consistent in showing high levels of satisfaction with physicians, hospital care, health plans, HMOs, and prescription drugs. Part of the reason for such unvariegated rapture is that the

TABLE 4   Overall Satisfaction with Health Services
Overall, how do you feel about the healthcare services that you and your family have used in the past few years?

	Year		
	1980	**1984**	**1987**
Base (number)	1543	1004	1250
		Percent	
Very satisfied	52	36	44
Somewhat satisfied	33	46	40
Somewhat dissatisfied	9	11	8
Very dissatisfied	4	5	5
Not sure	2	3	3

Source: Louis Harris and Associates, Inc., 1989.

TABLE 5   Overall View of American Healthcare System
Which of the following statements comes closest to expressing your overall view of the American healthcare system?

	Year			
	1982	1983	1984	1987
Base (number)	4796	1501	1004	1250
	Percent			
On the whole, the healthcare system works pretty well, and only minor changes are necessary to make it work better	19	21	26	29
There are some good things in our healthcare system, but fundamental changes are needed to make it work better	47	50	49	47
The American healthcare system has so much wrong with it that we need to completely rebuild it	28	25	21	19
Not sure/refused/no answer	6	4	4	6

Source: Louis Harris and Associates, Inc., 1989.

public is not fully equipped to judge the utility (or value) of healthcare services. Whereas most consumers can judge whether a shiny new BMW is "worth" $50,000 to them, most consumers are unable to determine the value of coronary bypass surgery. In that sense, healthcare is a unique commodity.

However, most consumers do not accept passively or uncritically the healthcare they receive. Differences in consumer behavior, satisfaction, and preferences can be detected in surveys when less general questions are asked. For example, consumers tend to value highly such factors as being able to see their own doctors, having a choice of physician, and being able to see the same doctor each time (see Table 6). These values are held more strongly by women than men and slightly less strongly by those who are members of HMOs.

Despite the difficulties in understanding the product, consumers do exhibit some tendency to "shop around" for healthcare, but their shopping is based more on quality than on price. A Harris survey taken in 1987 found that only 12 percent of the public had ever selected a particular doctor because of lower fees (compared to 16 percent responding this way in 1983). Conversely, when asked if they had ever stopped using the services of a particular doctor because they were dissatisfied with the quality of services provided, a full 49 percent of respondents claimed to have done so. For college graduates and people with three or more children, the proportion was even higher: 59 and 63 percent, respectively, for the two groups.

TABLE 6   Importance of Healthcare Factors, 1987

People take different factors into account when they select healthcare services. On a scale of 1 to 10, with 10 being very important, how important are each of the following items when selecting healthcare services?

	TOTAL	Sex		Managed Care		
		MEN	WOMEN	HMO	PPO	NONE
Base (number)	1250	559	651	120	88	1043
	Average Rating					
Being able to see your own doctor	9.2	9.0	9.4	8.9	9.3	9.2
Having a choice of doctors	9.1	8.9	9.3	8.9	9.4	9.1
Seeing the same doctor each time	8.8	8.5	9.1	8.5	8.9	8.8
Having some say in your treatment	8.8	8.5	9.0	8.9	9.2	8.7
Having a choice of hospitals	8.6	8.4	8.8	8.2	8.7	8.7
Cost	8.4	8.1	8.6	8.3	8.2	8.4
Having extended office hours	7.8	7.7	7.9	7.7	8.0	7.8
Having all services under one roof	7.5	7.3	7.7	7.5	7.0	7.6

Source: Louis Harris and Associates, Inc., 1989.

ATTITUDES TOWARD MANAGED CARE

A Focus on Consumers, Employers, and Providers

Growth and directions for managed care are influenced heavily by attitudes of consumers, employers, and providers. This section reviews some of the changes in attitudes that underlie this growth. Managed care plans can be described as points on a continuum from unfettered fee-for-service medicine toward completely controlled care where providers are reimbursed on a fixed-budget basis. Figure 1 provides a diagrammatic characterization of this continuum—the solid arrows indicate the degree to which public and private payers have moved by the late 1980s and the shaded arrows indicate where they may be headed for the 1990s.

If managed care is best thought of as a continuum from managed fee-for-service indemnity plans through to bricks-and-mortar HMOs, then it is important to establish the willingness of various actors to enter into various types of arrangements.

As a first step toward managed care, utilization review and increased deductibles and copayments have become increasingly popular. Increases in cost sharing have been accepted by employees, particularly where the company has done a good job of explaining these changes (see Table 7). Yet, in general, these changes have not had a great deal of effect in shaping the behavior of the employee in terms of the use of health services (see Table 8).

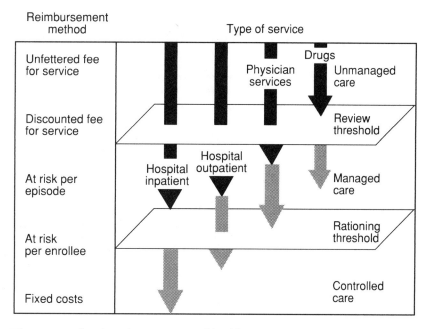

Figure 1   *The changing structure of healthcare.*

TABLE 7   Acceptability of Increase in Cost Sharing: Job Done by Employer in Explaining Changes
Base: Employees Whose Cost-Sharing Has Increased a Great Deal or Somewhat

EMPLOYEES	ALL EXCELLENT	GOOD	POOR	FAIR
Base (number)	624	99	142	171
		Percent		
Very acceptable	10	21	11	5
Somewhat acceptable	43	47	53	36
Not very acceptable	30	19	25	37
Not at all acceptable	16	13	11	22
Not sure	1	—	—	1

Source: Louis Harris and Associates, Inc., *The Equitable Survey IV,* 1985.

TABLE 8   How Much Increased Cost Sharing Has Changed Employee Behavior in the Use of Healthcare Services
Base: All Whose Plans Have Increased Employee Cost Sharing a Great Deal or Somewhat

Base number of employees	624
	Percent
A great deal	14
Somewhat	27
Not much	25
Not at all	32
Too early to say	*
Not sure	1

*Less than 0.5%.
Source: Louis Harris and Associates, Inc., *The Equitable Survey IV*, 1985.

Partly, this lack of success is due to the fact that the cost-sharing trend has a more significant countertrend—namely, greater catastrophic coverage. A recent report from the Health Insurance Association of America indicates that, in 1987, only 6.1 percent of employees in health plans faced an unlimited out-of-pocket liability, down from 41.5 percent in 1977. The true costs of the health system occur after the patient has made a commitment to enter it. Thus, user fees are really no more than a small tax on the sick and the hypochondriac, and they are unlikely to affect the overall cost of healthcare. To achieve this depends on creating controls and incentives on those who decide how much is delivered once the patient enters the system, namely, physicians!

A second example of change in corporate health plans supported by consumer attitudes is the shift toward flexible benefits. Increasingly in the 1980s, flexible benefits plans have been the framework in which managed care plans have been placed. Employees like having a choice of benefits (see Table 9), and despite the concerns of some employers, flexible benefits create few major problems in terms of the cost of administering the plan or the overall cost of the program. Rather, flexible benefits create more difficulty in communicating the details of the plan to employees (see Table 10). Flexible benefits are popular with employees, but, again, there is a significant countertrend toward inflexible benefits, where, because of cost considerations, employers limit their employees' choice of health plans.

The growth of HMOs represents a third example of how the attitudes of various groups help shape the development of the managed

TABLE 9   How Much Employees Like Having a Choice of Benefits
Base: Those Whose Employers Offer Some Choice of Benefits

Base number of employees	999
	Percent
Like it a lot	66
Like it a little	21
Don't like it	2
Don't care	10
Not sure	1

Source: Louis Harris and Associates, Inc., *The Equitable Survey IV*, 1985.

care industry. The attitudes of the public have been critical in shaping the growth of HMOs in the 1980s. Although, in the late 1980s, it is becoming apparent that the "bloom is off the rose" as far as HMOs are concerned, it would be wrong to underestimate the factors underlying their growth. In particular, five consumer-oriented factors continue to dominate as drivers of HMO growth.

• *Familiarity*   Public familiarity with the HMO concept continues to grow. Harris surveys show that 21 percent of Americans were very familiar with the concept in 1987, up from 14 percent in 1984.
• *Interest*   Interest in joining HMOs remains relatively high among nonmembers—36 percent say they would be somewhat or very interested in joining an HMO. (For PPOs in 1987, 33 percent ex-

TABLE 10   Magnitude of Problems Caused by Flexible Benefits Plans: Among Those Who Offer a Flexible Benefits or Cafeteria Plan
Base: Corporate Benefits Officers Who Describe Plan as a Flexible Benefits or Cafeteria Plan

	Percent			
	MAJOR PROBLEM	**MINOR PROBLEM**	**NOT A PROBLEM**	**NOT SURE**
The difficulty or cost of administration of the plan	14	47	36	3
The difficulty or cost of communicating the details of the plan to employees	21	50	28	1
An increase in the overall cost of the plan as a result of introducing choice	9	45	45	2

Source: Louis Harris and Associates, Inc., *The Equitable Survey IV*, 1987.

pressed such an interest, with only 6 percent being very interested.) A further point to note is that the proportion of nonmembers who are "not at all interested" has risen significantly in the 1980s (see Table 11). This is to be expected, of course, as the "interested" group actually joins HMOs.

- *Satisfaction*   HMO members are more satisfied with their health plans than those consumers in traditional indemnity insurance. For example, HIAA data show that HMO members are more satisfied with their physician care and hospital care than those in private insurance plans (see Table 12). Medicare and Medicaid recipients have the highest level of satisfaction, which may be consistent with the assertion that satisfaction is inversely related to expectations.

- *Loyalty*   HMO members are likely to remain in HMOs, since the vast majority of members continue to say they will renew their membership with the HMO (see Table 13). Even if a small minority are dissatisfied with the particular HMO they belong to, this dissatisfaction does not necessarily translate into their abandoning HMOs completely.

- *Cost*   HMO members are particularly satisfied with the low out-of-pocket costs for certain aspects of their plans. In particular, the cost of prescription drugs, costs of doctor office visits, and costs of health insurance coverage are seen by HMO members as much more reasonable compared to either PPO members or traditional indemnity plan members (see Table 14).

TABLE 11   Interest in Joining an HMO

Base: Not Now an HMO Member
From what you know now about health maintenance organizations, would you be very interested, somewhat interested, hardly interested, or not at all interested in joining an HMO?

	Year		
	1980	**1984**	**1987**
Base (number)	1462	917	1140
		Percent	
Very interested	8	8	6
Somewhat interested	31	32	30
Hardly interested	16	17	17
Not at all interested	36	40	44
Not sure	9	1	3

Source: Louis Harris and Associates, Inc., 1989.

TABLE 12   Americans' Satisfaction with Quality of Care, 1988
Percent of Respondents Who Are "Very Satisfied"

INSURANCE TYPE	HOSPITAL CARE	PHYSICIAN CARE
HMO	40	52
Private insurance	39	49
Medicare/Medicaid	49	55

Source: HIAA-MAP, Survey of 1,500 Households, 1988.

TABLE 13   Trends in HMO Renewal Probabilities

	Year			
	1980	**1984**	**1987**	**1988**
Base (number)	1089	1004	120	1000
	Percent			
Will	92	93	90	91
Certainly	75	61	63	64
Probably	17	32	27	27
Will not	3	5	7	7
Probably	2	3	6	3
Certainly	1	2	1	4

Source: Louis Harris and Associates, Inc., 1989.

TABLE 14   Impact of Managed Care Situation on Perceptions of Reasonableness of Cost of Healthcare Services, 1987
Percent of Respondents Answering "Very Reasonable" Only
Do you think the costs to you and your household of the following items are very reasonable, somewhat reasonable, somewhat unreasonable, or very unreasonable for what you get?

	TOTAL	HMO	PPO	INDEMNITY
Base (number)	1250	120	88	1043
	Percent			
Doctors' visits	22	43	17	20
Prescription drugs	21	46	24	18
Nonprescription drugs	13	10	17	13
Hospitalization	11	17	10	10
Health insurance	19	34	24	17

Source: Louis Harris and Associates, Inc., 1989.

The experience of employers also plays a major role in the development and growth of HMOs. Four key points must be noted.

- Surveys consistently showed in the mid-1980s that most employers were unconvinced that HMOs had decreased their corporate health costs. For example, a 1987 Harris survey showed that 25 percent of employers felt HMOs increased costs and 24 percent felt they had decreased costs; the balance of the sample said HMOs had no effect.
- Despite the lack of clear cost savings, employers have been satisfied generally with their experience with HMOs. In a 1987 Harris survey, 78 percent of employers were satisfied overall with their experience with HMOs (77 percent of employers with PPOs also gave this response).
- Despite research evidence claiming little or no difference in health status between HMO members and other employees, a significant minority of employers, 25 percent, have experienced adverse selection, according to a 1987 Harris survey.
- Employers have made numerous changes in their health plans: HMOs, PPOs, flexible benefits, higher deductibles, wellness programs, but no clear-cut cost saving has materialized for these early adopters. The reason why no long-term cost savings have been seen is largely because the savings from any form of managed care are one-time "step changes." Once the discount or reduction in unnecessary use has been achieved, the underlying rate of escalation in cost continues. With corporate health insurance premiums rising — in many cases by 20 to 30 percent a year in the late 1980s — few employers can be totally satisfied with their health cost experience. This predicament may aggravate employers' dissatisfaction with managed care as a solution to cost escalation.

A key set of attitudes shaping the growth and acceptance of managed care in general and HMOs in particular is the attitudes of providers, particularly physicians. Research suggests that:

- Physicians are far more satisfied with the healthcare system as a whole than is the general public. In particular, in 1983 Harris found that 48 percent of physicians thought the system worked pretty well and only minor changes were needed, whereas only 21 percent of the public shared that view.[5]
- An overwhelming majority of physicians endorse changes in the healthcare system that would reduce hospitalization, and most physicians believe that doctors order too many tests. But, at the same time, they believe the healthcare system is price-competitive and are consequently less than enthusiastic about the introduction of competitive strategies or managed care initiatives such as man-

datory second opinions for surgery or utilization review as a source of cost containment.

- HMOs, and increasingly PPOs, have been reasonably successful in recruiting physicians as contractees. For example, American Medical Association (AMA) data suggest that by 1987 approximately half of all physicians (active, nonfederal, nonresident patient care doctors) contracted with at least one HMO and almost the same proportion had contracted with at least one PPO. Anecdotal evidence suggests that there is considerable overlap between these two groups. However, this seemingly large rate of penetration belies the relatively small share of income physicians receive from HMOs and PPOs. Using the AMA data as a base, it can be estimated that, overall, approximately 10 percent of physician income was derived from HMO and PPO contracts in 1987.

- PPOs are less threatening to physicians than HMOs, which is shown by their increasing acceptance among older doctors. By 1986, physicians 56 years old or over were just as likely to have signed a contract with a PPO as physicians who were 35 years old or under (see Table 15).

Overall, the attitudes of the public, employers, and medical providers point to continued experimentation with managed care in general and with HMOs in particular, although none of these groups should go into the future with any illusions that managed care is a panacea for all their problems.

Ten Key Paradoxes

These attitudes and other trends lead to the conclusion that the prospects for managed healthcare are dependent on ten key paradoxes.

TABLE 15 Physicians Contracting with PPOs, by Age of Physician, 1983–1986

	Percent			
AGE	1983	1984	1985	1986
35 years or under	14.9	22.0	31.6	36.6
36 to 45 years	12.0	18.5	29.8	40.5
46 to 55 years	9.6	17.2	29.0	38.7
56 years or over	8.7	12.0	22.5	35.6

Source: D. W. Emmons, "Changing Dimensions of Medical Practice Arrangements." *Medical Care Review* **45**(1):101–128 (Spring 1988).

Paradox 1   Consumers are very satisfied with the healthcare services they receive but are largely dissatisfied with the performance of the system as a whole. This is the fundamental tension between how the consumers and their families perceive the care they receive (generally positive) versus the way they perceive the system as a whole (generally negative). The dissatisfaction with the system as a whole comes from concerns about cost and access.

Paradox 2   HMO members have lower expectations but are more satisfied with their healthcare plans than those in indemnity systems. The lower expectations stem largely from the demographic profile and medical needs of the HMO enrollees—younger families with children who see good healthcare as good access to primary care (especially well baby visits) with little or no deductible.

Paradox 3   Healthcare consumers seem to accept higher deductibles and copayments (when these plan changes are properly communicated), but they value low out-of-pocket costs in HMOs and PPOs as a big plus.

Paradox 4   Employers say they want to contain costs but have been unwilling to aggressively promote alternative options, such as severely limiting the choice of providers. Recent escalation in premiums may be changing the attitudes of many employers.

Paradox 5   Traditional HMO models are the most financially viable and yet their growth has been slowest. The staff- or group-model HMOs, which are capable of rationalizing healthcare delivery in a metropolitan area and providing incentives to physicians to limit use, have been steady, if not spectacular, financial performers. In terms of enrollment, they have not grown as fast because of their capital intensity and the unwillingness of employers and employees alike to enter arrangements with a strictly limited choice of providers.

Paradox 6   American doctors (especially older ones) publicly resist managed care and yet they are signing up at a rapid rate, and older doctors are just as likely to be enrolled in a PPO as young physicians. This may be the reflection of the ultimate "divide and conquer" strategy. So long as they sign up with a multiplicity of plans, only a small share of income will come from one source.

Paradox 7   Managed care was supposed to be a threat to physicians' incomes and yet the mid-1980s is proving to be the golden age of doctors' incomes. AMA data continue to show that physicians' real incomes continued to rise through the 1980s, particularly for procedure-oriented specialists. This may be a reflection of the fact that most managed care systems are still largely fee-for-service endeavors. Paying physicians on a fee-for-service system, of any form, seems to be inherently inflationary.

Paradox 8   HMO and indemnity plan enrollees under age 65 are fairly similar demographically and yet a significant number of employers claim to have experienced adverse selection.

Paradox 9 The plans with the fastest growth in the mid-1980s are not the bellwether of managed care in the long run. For-profit IPAs with fee-for-service reimbursement methods proliferated from 1984 to 1986. In the late 1980s, these plans are in the greatest financial trouble and are likely to be consumed in the coming wave of consolidation.

Paradox 10 Americans want cost containment but will not pay the price for it in terms of rationing and rationalization of services. The overwhelming irony of U.S. healthcare is that, on the one hand, healthcare costs receive enormous attention in the media, and there is almost universal acceptance that this escalation is largely unwarranted. On the other hand, the American public, employers, and government seem unwilling to introduce really tough measures—such as rationing of care, elimination of duplication of facilities and technologies, and limitations on the choice of providers—that are necessary to contain these costs.

CONCLUSION

What Does All This Mean for the Future?

What can be expected as a result of what is known about public opinion and the pressures exerted by different publics on the system, whether through consumer demand, taxpayer resistance to increased taxes, or the desire to provide a reasonable safety net for the elderly and the poor? How will these often conflicting forces shape the healthcare system and the future of managed care in the 1990s? Here are some reasonable estimates.

- Consumer demand for more and better healthcare will continue to increase because of growing consumer expectations, powerful new technologies, and changing demographics.
- At the same time, as the percentage of GNP going to healthcare continues to climb, efforts to contain this growth will become more determined and possibly more effective.
- Given their appeal to both consumers and employers, HMOs and PPOs will continue to enjoy growth for years to come. Yet, for most nonelderly Americans, managed fee-for-service plans will be the important first step away from unfettered fee-for-service.
- Given its appeal to consumers and employers, there will be more flexibility in more corporate health plans. At the same time, however, employers will increasingly introduce constraints on freedom of choice; financial incentives or penalties will be used to encourage the use of cost-effective healthcare providers.

- The pressures on both federal and state legislators to close major gaps in health insurance coverage will, within the next 5 to 10 years, lead to policies such as:

  > Long-term care insurance for either or both nursing home and home care (new government policies will not be comprehensive but will be designed to stimulate more private sector coverage). Long-term care demand is fueled by the growth in the over-75 population and the political clout of the elderly.

  > State (and ultimately federally) mandated employer-provided insurance is a likely response to the growing problem of the uninsured.

  > Expansion of Medicaid or other publicly financed coverage of prenatal and infant care will be in response to the escalating crisis in maternal health and the prevalence of low-birthweight infants in lower socioeconomic groups.

  > Further reductions in Medicare benefits, such as increased cost sharing, will shift additional costs onto many retiree health plans as the federal government continues to fight the budget deficit.

  > The need to maintain corporate retiree benefits will lead to some form of tax-deductible corporate prefunding of retiree health plans. This problem will become increasingly evident as companies are forced to account for the costs of future retiree health benefits on their balance sheets.

- Wellness programs, which are still in their infancy, will grow and, hopefully, become more effective in attracting and influencing those most in need (those who are overweight, smoke, drink too much, do not exercise, and so forth).
- Ultimately, fee-for-service care will survive in only two forms. For a privileged elite who are willing to pay for it, more or less unfettered fee for service will still be available. For everyone else, the only fee-for-service care available will be managed aggressively and will be available only with financial penalties that are designed to discourage and shrink it. In the final analysis, unmanaged fee-for-service will be available to no more than 1 in 20 Americans.

REFERENCES

1. Recent notable exceptions to this generalization are two review papers: R. J. Blendon, ''The Public's View of the Future of Health Care.'' *Journal of the American Medical Association* **259**:3587–3593 (1988) and J. Gabel, H. Cohen, and S. Fink, ''Americans' Sometimes Contradictory Views on Health Care.'' *Health Affairs* (forthcoming).

2. S. H. Long and P. W. Welch, "Are We Containing Costs or Pushing on a Balloon?" *Health Affairs* 113–117 (Fall 1988).

3. R. J. Blendon, "Three Systems A Comparative Survey: Americans are significantly less happy with their health care system than either the British or Canadians are with theirs." *Health Management Quarterly* 2–10 (First Quarter, 1989).

4. See Blendon, op cit., and R. J. Blendon and D. E. Altman, "Public Attitudes about Health Care Costs: A Lesson in National Schizophrenia." *New England Journal of Medicine* **311**:613–616 (1984).

5. Louis Harris and Associates, Inc., "The Equitable Health Care Survey: Physicians' Attitudes toward Cost Containment." March 1984.

POINT OF VIEW

How Consumers Grapple with Quality in Buying Medical Care

JOYCE JENSEN, Senior Vice President

National Research Corporation, Lincoln, Nebraska

Hospitals are joining virtually every other industry by making quality an integral component of their consumer marketing strategies. In doing so, they address potential patients who believe quality varies among hospitals and who make decisions based upon their own definitions of quality. Thus, from a marketing standpoint, quality is indeed "in the eye of the beholder." Understanding consumers' expectations and perceptions of providers which meet their criteria is paramount as hospitals develop and strive to retain the top quality position in consumers' minds.

In looking at the combination of factors which contribute most to both preferences and perceptions of quality, NRC analysis of 100,000 healthcare decision makers in individual markets of the country indicates that the top quality hospital in each market exhibits several characteristics. (1) It is perceived to have the best physicians from the standpoint of technical quality, the widest range of services available, and the most modern and sophisticated medical equipment and facilities, components which the industry has coined "high tech." (2) It is associated two-thirds of the time with being the "high touch" provider, offering a softer, more personalized approach, for example, having the most courteous and helpful nursing staff and the most personalized care. (3) It is the preferred provider for heart care. (4) It is a teaching hospital if one exists in the area. (5) It is the largest or one of the largest facilities in the market.

When using quality perceptions to actually select a hospital, consumers say the quality of the medical staff, nursing care, and emergency services are most important. Modern equipment and sophisticated technology are becoming very important characteristics. A physician's recommendation is important but ranks below the technical aspects such as equipment and emergency care. And, a previous stay at a hospital is becoming less important each year as consumers reevaluate the quality of hospitals on a periodic basis. Consumers say that out-of-pocket costs do matter, but not to the extent that they will give up technical quality. It may come into play, however, before other elective elements such as private rooms, pleasant surroundings, or proximity to their home. Quality is not being sacrificed intentionally by cost considerations.

These are the indicators of quality to consumers now, but new "scoreclocks" or ways to measure quality are on the horizon. As the healthcare industry focuses on more technical aspects of quality through release of clinical outcome data, more and more consumers could become armed with a *Consumer Reports*-type index of healthcare providers. This could eliminate the need for hospitals to understand the consumer perspective of quality since outcome data would become the leading resource for selecting high quality hospitals. Consumers are likely to become even more focused on quality as this information is disseminated to the public. Thus, input from patients will continue to hold a solid and increasing role in helping to define, monitor, and measure quality.

For example, once outcome statistics are released in a format that consumers may utilize, hospitals will fall into several segments as far as their mortality rates for various DRGs. Though there may be a great deal of difference between hospitals which fall in the top 10 percent versus those in the bottom 10 percent, there will likely be little discrimination among providers within each segment. Thus, as several facilities show equal quality in this "index," the next level of selection will be addressed in the historical manner —consumers relying on their own perceptions of quality. Consumers will no longer assume clinical quality for all providers. That assumption will be replaced by the clinical outcome data which are available to them.

The important point is that once quality factors from the consumer perspective are determined, hospitals must use this information to design, develop, and implement programs which meet customer requirements. Once consumers become patients, hospitals should measure their satisfaction with services received to determine if consumers' quality expectations are being met.

NRC research shows that in most markets, those households whose members have been hospital patients are much more likely to differentiate hospitals by quality. Their personal experience with the hospital, whether positive or negative, will determine their perceptions of quality.

Households without a recent medical care experience are also able to determine quality, but to a lesser extent. These consumers rely on information gained through marketing activities or word-of-mouth to create their quality perceptions rather than first-hand experience.

Hospitals are using "quality" as a positioning strategy in their consumer markets. They are integrating their consumers' definition of quality into these strategies. Additionally, they are assessing how their performance meets the consumers' definition of quality. Hospitals should regularly monitor their customers and implement this market feedback as a guide to changing organizational performance. Concrete market feedback helps hospitals become more competitive by indicating which services consistently meet consumer expectations and preferences.

CHAPTER FOUR

Provider Perspective

LIFESPAN — VIEWS FROM WITHIN

Three perspectives are included to illustrate the complexity and diversity of the managed care industry. Managers from each of three different healthcare companies were asked to provide, from within their own corporations, a view of the managed care industry as a whole and show how their company's strategic goals fit into that view. LifeSpan Inc. reflects a provider orientation, Lincoln National Life Insurance Company presents a payer outlook, and Honeywell Inc. expresses a purchaser point of view. Each of these perspectives —provider, payer, and purchaser—must be successfully integrated in terms of business objectives for a managed care arrangement to create a win-win scenario.

The three companies established leadership positions in healthcare and were among the first organizations in the country to develop innovative approaches to managed care.

LIFESPAN LifeSpan Inc. is a healthcare system which includes eight hospitals, a preferred provider organization, a home health company, a clinic management company, and a charitable foundation. LifeSpan corporate offices and five of its eight hospitals are located in Minneapolis–St. Paul, which is the most competitive managed care marketplace in the country.

Member hospitals range in size from 54 beds to 962 beds. The number of licensed beds for all hospitals totals 1694. Over 2500 physicians are on the medical staffs at LifeSpan facilities and their affiliates, which are located throughout Minnesota and Wisconsin. They include acute care community hospitals in rural settings as well as metropolitan-based tertiary adult and pediatric medical centers.

The LifeSpan system is unique in that it does not control its members' assets, but rather provides leadership and strategic direction to the members. It was founded in 1982 and is a founding member of Voluntary Hospitals of America.

GORDON M. SPRENGER, President and Chief Executive Officer

LifeSpan must continually update its vision of the future in order to keep members focused on the right strategic issues. The greatest contribution a CEO can make is to anticipate and always be thinking, "What if?" What if "such and such" happened, and will the organization be positioned to deal with it? This is part of a listening-reading-probing orientation.

The most significant management issue is maintaining a balance between providing quality healthcare at an affordable cost and taking care of the sick regardless of their ability to pay.

Cooperation is essential among managed care partners. Unfortunately, it usually occurs only when a crisis develops, particularly among strong independent physicians and hospitals. Despite all the managed care initiatives in Minneapolis–St. Paul, relatively few provider joint ventures have materialized, mostly because of greed on the part of all parties. Everyone wants a bigger share of the pie than the joint venture will allow. Unless there is a compelling reason to give up autonomy, cooperation does not come easily.

The conflicts which chip away at trust within an organization like LifeSpan must be dealt with. Conflicts over specific programs can sometimes be put on the back burner for a while, but not when they involve overall strategy or when they affect trust between the principal shareholders. Managed care means being held accountable for cost-effective value-driven care. It also means the ability to allow risk for a given population on some form of prospective payment system. Inherent in this idea is an adequate on-line tracking system to ensure that resources are being properly used within predetermined limits.

Tracking providers' performance and comparing it with a peer group is a prerequisite for managing risk. It changes behavior and affects practice patterns. The key is data that are accurate and handled with discretion. Insurance companies, HMOs, and PPOs have tried to be good case managers, and hospitals have tried to be actuaries and risk-taking experts. In each instance, all parties have failed. A closer relationship and partnership between the providers and the managed care companies needs to occur so that the expertise of each can be used to greater advantage.

As price among providers becomes more consistent, managed care arrangements are being forced to address quality and value considerations as a means of product differentiation. This should cause the development of genuine partnerships between providers and payers which will enable organizations like LifeSpan to deliver and allow risk for *total care* in the future.

The role of the CEO has changed dramatically as a result of managed care demands. The CEO's time is now focused on areas such as:

- Responding to broad community issues such as lobbying for increased government spending for healthcare.
- Thinking strategically, and anticipating and planning for the future. Mistakes can no longer be covered up through the historic cost reimbursement system.
- Being held more accountable by a board of directors. More and more, the complexity of healthcare delivery has pushed boards toward setting policy and demanding accountability on the part of the management staff.
- Acting as the lightening rod for new ideas, CEOs must be able to lead and push staff to try things differently.
- Providing organizational stability in time of change, and maintaining the mission of the organization. In moving from a social to an economic model, there is plenty of opportunity to wander off course and forget the basic mission of the organization.
- Taking risks, which necessitates faster decisions and streamlining the process of making decisions.
- Attracting talent with a broader base of skills.
- Being able to deal with multi-institutional issues, including multiple boards involved in diversified activities.

JOHN G. TURNER, Board of Directors, and President and CEO, Northwestern National Life Insurance Co.

A board member has two major responsibilities: (1) to provide enlightened leadership for the organization by supporting management in its effort to define a mission for the enterprise and (2) to encourage innovation and risk-taking in the organization. The board should focus on strategy, rather than operations, and reach decisions about critical business issues in spite of an uncertain and turbulent environment. The board's role is to support management in the process of sorting out and analyzing, in a strategic sense, available alternatives.

One of LifeSpan's initial managed care strategies was to develop its own PPO (Select Care). The experience of sponsoring a PPO has shown that hospital medical staff dynamics preclude developing appropriate incentives to change physician behavior. This is a prerequisite for delivering cost-effective quality healthcare. The fundamental conflict is with physician providers. While hospitals compete over physicians, a successful PPO must assure that cost-effective practice patterns prevail. The latter inevitably leads to problems in hospital–medical staff relations.

In LifeSpan's case, PPO involvement also accentuates the inherent conflict between the interests of primary care and specialty practitioners. A PPO depends upon subscriber–primary care relations for enrollment growth. This means hospitals must sense the needs of primary care physicians. In LifeSpan hospitals (that is, Abbott Northwestern, Methodist, Minneapolis Children's) the resource requirements of specialists versus primary care practitioners are frequently in conflict.

It is important to recognize that payers dealing with PPOs and HMOs look for primary care–oriented hospitals. However, an important and conflicting signal which board members receive from the market is an expectation that LifeSpan should focus on tertiary care. It is difficult to adjust strategies to fully recognize such diverse and confusing messages.

Another troubling issue is how services should be priced. HMOs have gained enough marketplace clout to purchase hospital services at prices below those paid by insurers. Such a skewed pricing patterns will eventually lead to disruption in both the hospital and insurance industries.

RICHARD J. KRAMER, Executive Vice President

Price competition and negotiated discounts are a way of life in Minneapolis–St. Paul. Approximately 70 percent of patients admitted to LifeSpan hospitals do not pay full price (including those from Medicare, Medicaid, HMO, and PPO plans). Much of the success of LifeSpan's three Twin Cities hospitals (Abbott Northwestern Hospital, Methodist Hospital, and Minneapolis Children's Medical Center) depends upon tertiary care excellence and maintaining a leading edge in medical technology and subspecialist medical staff. Technology drives up costs and presents a special challenge for these hospitals to compete on the basis of price in the marketplace. This requires hospitals to make an extra effort to contain costs and segregate out the highly specialized services when negotiating contracts.

The most important operational goals of LifeSpan's flagship hospitals are to continue to grow centers of excellence, to provide medical staff support in order to maintain a large and competitive physician distribution channel, and to further develop information systems and cost-containment strategies. These goals must be met if LifeSpan is to remain a major player in the managed care market.

In the mid-1980s, as HMO growth affected hospital revenue, LifeSpan faced three alternative managed care strategies. The most highly recommended strategy was to go into an equity partnership joint venture with a major healthcare plan or insurance carrier in the community. However, five large HMOs in the Twin Cities accounted for 30 percent of LifeSpan hospitals' revenue at that time, and hospitals were fearful about alienating any of these plans by aligning with another. For example, MedCenters Health Plan was important to Methodist Hospital since it was the major HMO plan associated with Park Nicollet Medical Center, which accounted for over half of Methodist's admissions. Minneapolis Children's Medical Center, as a tertiary pediatric facility, needed to accept all major healthcare plans. Abbott Northwestern had a majority of its physicians in Physicians Health Plan and Blue Cross.

Select Care was formed initially by the medical staffs of LifeSpan hospitals as an alternative to the Medical Society–sponsored HMO plan, Physicians Health Plan (PHP). PHP was inflicting heavy discounts and administrative controls which were unacceptable to physicians. Originally, LifeSpan physicians felt they could market a PPO without accepting discounts. Over time, Select Care was forced to introduce managed care controls to meet the demands of employers. It could no longer maintain a strictly defensive position to satisfy its member hospitals and physicians.

A second strategy was the continued development of Select Care as LifeSpan's PPO. This was less threatening to HMO plans, but it would take years to generate enough volume to be of major importance to LifeSpan.

A third strategy was to continue contracting with all plans. Essentially this is the strategy which was followed while increasing the amount of management and financial support to Select Care. However, the PPO was left to fight it out in the marketplace and was not given "favored nation" treatment on pricing. LifeSpan hospital and physicians discounts were based on volume levels which Select Care had not yet achieved. Also, the lack of exclusive commitment to Select Care from LifeSpan hospitals and doctors, who wanted to be in every plan, made it more difficult for Select Care to compete. In spite of these early obstacles, the PPO has grown to 135,000 eligible enrollees. The primary operational challenge facing Select Care is to respond to marketplace needs for low-cost healthcare while at the same time providing a fee schedule acceptable to its hospitals and doctors. It faces a natural conflict between its PPO business mission to reduce costs and hospital days by exerting pressure on physicians and the business mission of its provider hospitals to increase revenues and keep participating physicians satisfied.

Select Care has grown more independent but is still dependent upon the financial support of LifeSpan hospitals. Select Care's greatest challenge is to provide ongoing value to its hospital sponsors. This means increasing the volume of billings to reach breakeven and, at same time, reducing the amount of working capital it needs from sponsoring hospitals.

TERRY S. FINZEN, President, Methodist Hospital

Providers in Minneapolis–St. Paul face a host of competitive factors which affect managed care: the shrinking inpatient hospital market, surplus bed capacity, and competition for clinical programs and ancillary business from nontraditional hospital providers, physicians' offices, and clinics. This is coupled with increasing competition from other hospitals that are developing centers of excellence. These trends have caused Methodist Hospital to develop a higher level of technology in order to remain competitive and protect the hospital's major clinical programs.

Methodist affiliated with LifeSpan in response to competitive forces in the Twin Cities. Market demand for inpatient services was decreasing, and other competitor hospitals were forming alliances as a defensive strategy. At the same time, third party payers were beginning to dominate the healthcare market in Minneapolis–St. Paul. The hospital's interest was to strengthen its position by affiliating with other strong providers who were financially sound and high quality institutions. The structure of the LifeSpan affiliation provides minimal control at the corporate level and retains assets and operating decisions at the individual hospital level.

The most important operational issue Methodist faces is how to maintain a balance among operational autonomy and control of hospital assets and clinical programs while being part of a larger system that contains two strong competitors (that is, Abbott Northwestern and Methodist) in the same area. The challenge is to decrease the focus on competition with each other and to compete more effectively together against the other hospital systems.

One of the major reasons for coming together was to gain more leverage in negotiating with third party payers. This will have its challenges because of differences in medical staff makeup and payer mix at LifeSpan hospitals. The majority of admissions at Methodist Hospital come from a large multispecialty group practice, Park Nicollet Medical Center, while the majority of admissions at Abbott Northwestern come from numerous small group practices and individual physicians. Methodist's major third party contract is MedCenters Health Plan, the HMO entree for Park Nicollet Medical Center. Abbott Northwestern's major third party contract is Physicians Health Plan, an IPA-model HMO.

Another major issue is the different cost and charge structures found in the various LifeSpan hospitals. For example, within the Twin Cities, Methodist charges are the lowest of major metropolitan providers, while Abbott Northwestern's charges tend to be higher than other hospitals in the region. LifeSpan's challenge is to interpret these differences to third party payers when it is seeking master contracts.

A critical managed care issue for Methodist Hospital, along with Abbott Northwestern and Minneapolis Children's, is how to approach employers as quality providers with a cost-effective plan. Given the geographic sprawl of the Minneapolis–St. Paul area, a major barrier to marketing managed care is the need for geographic service points—hospitals and physicians close to the employers' plants and offices and convenient to employees' homes. An effective managed care strategy will have to address the fact that the hospital systems have not been established in response to the geographic service demands of employers and employees. This has necessitated that it "affiliate" with other providers and hospital systems to sell managed care on a wide geographic basis.

It has been proposed that in order for Select Care to be successful, LifeSpan must capitalize it and provide "favored nation" pricing to help the PPO compete in this market. This continues a "buy market share" approach which has been disastrous for providers in the Twin Cities. Instead, LifeSpan should shift the emphasis from price to quality services by capitalizing on the reputation of the provider network.

Methodist receives over half its patients from Park Nicollet Medical Center, the fifth largest multispecialty clinic in the country, with over 300 physicians and 1000 employees. This organization-to-organization relationship must be carefully managed. Park Nicollet Medical Center believes the discount required by Select Care is too great, and they refuse to participate. As a result, Methodist Hospital and Life-Span are unable to capture the market share that would be available if Methodist Hospital's entire medical staff were Select Care providers.

DAVID W. NELSON, M.D., Board of Directors

Managed care is simply a euphemism for managing cost. In its simplest and purest form, it means that some third party supervises the doctor-patient relationship.

One of the greatest sources of conflict in managed care occurs when physicians are asked to serve as "gatekeepers" for health plan members. Their income is directly related to the amount of care that is allowed.

As physicians are forced to keep an eye on their balance sheets because of declining profit margins, the quality of care diminishes—along with delays in initial diagnosis, referral, and treatment. With such delays, overall medical costs will increase as cases become more acute and complicated.

Both physicians and hospitals are now feeling such financial strain that they will be forced to join each other in an attempt to define adequate medical care and appropriate compensation. If these two groups do not unite, they will continue to be manipulated individually by the payer and pitted against each other.

As physicians and hospitals form unified delivery systems, they will need to be exclusive by definition in order to be truly "preferred." Physicians will then need to make a choice about which system to join.

WILLIAM E. PETERSEN, M.D., Vice President, Medical Affairs

In order to be successful in managed care, a major medical center must establish a comfortable relationship with its physicians. Unfortunately, physicians that overuse resources can no longer be afforded by health plans—nor should they be. One of the prerequisites of managed care is effective utilization management, which means getting physicians to buy into the idea that "less is better."

It is increasingly difficult for a hospital-based system to successfully sponsor an HMO or PPO. The major problem is not utilization review or maintaining an adequate census. The biggest problems are establishment of criteria and standards, which doctors see as "cookbook" medicine, and the inability to properly discipline physicians.

Health plans cannot tell the physicians how to practice medicine, but the plans can give the physicians adequate data and create a mind-set that leads to more appropriate utilization. But certain groups of physicians respond poorly to changes brought about by managed care. These groups include doctors 50 to 55 years of age, doctors who compulsively uncover the last diagnostic possibility with excessive testing, and political conservatives who are just too stubborn and resist change—they like the way medicine was practiced in the past. Very few physicians embrace managed care wholeheartedly, but younger doctors who are more progressive, socially conscious, and confident accept it as a necessary evil.

The single biggest factor in getting physicians to change their practice patterns is to give them all the pertinent data that are available: data broken down by DRG, by department, and by clinical specialty, and hospital costs and charges. The doctors can then compare their activity with the mean. Providing data is an extremely powerful tool. Doctors generally want to conform and do their part, but there are certain rules of the game that are cast in concrete. If these rules are not accepted, it leads to unrest, anxiety, depression, and anger. Generally, physicians want to be appreciated, and their problems need to be understood.

In presenting a "report card" of data on physician utilization, it is important not to criticize practice patterns or excessive utilization and to avoid making judgments. Data should be presented to physicians one-on-one. When physicians show up poorly, one way to soften the message is to give them a reason as to why it might have happened. Usually, they understand you are just allowing them to save face, but most importantly, they realize that in order to conform, they will have to make some changes in their thinking and practice patterns.

RICHARD STURGEON, M.D., Chief of Staff, Abbott Northwestern Hospital

Current management tools are inadequate to assess quality. A number of nonmedical variables (that is, patient personality, family dynamics and anxiety, social expectations, liability issues, physician fatigue, time of day or week) enter into treatment decisions that cannot be incorporated in standardized review protocols. Aggressive utilization management procedures assume a "best case" scenario when decisions are made. No matter how carefully programmed, these procedures are unable to address extenuating circumstances arising out of each unique physician-patient interaction. If review criteria can be accepted by all physicians, they are probably too general to be of value. If criteria are rigorous enough to be effective, any practicing physician can foresee extenuating circumstances either for themselves or for other physicians.

From a practicing physician's viewpoint, medically appropriate criteria are a matter of opinion. Aggressive utilization management is potentially antiquality. Physicians faced with the need to change practice patterns believe "efficiency" equates with profit motive. They see restricted access and reduced service level for their patients. They are convinced this represents poor quality.

Utilization review currently assesses only short slices of longitudinal health histories. Any doctor who followed all preventive care guidelines issued by such groups as the American Heart Association or the Cancer Society would be out of compliance with utilization guidelines.

Physicians actively involved in utilization management believe appropriateness equates with quality and that efficiency is a worthwhile and attainable goal. However, since medical practice is often a "best guess" situation, some clinical decisions will be wrong. Except in the abstract, a doctor prefers not to admit or publicize errors in clinical judgment or patient management. This stems not so much from a fear of litigation as from a sense of self-conscious anxiety. In the aggregate, most physicians embrace appropriateness as a goal for aggressive utilization management. One-on-one they become patient advocates.

Although providers may be willing to risk loss of income (even if they are uneasy about it) as a result of their utilization behavior, it is unfair to put providers at risk for their patient's health. Most health problems are ultimately beyond the provider's control. Financial risk from environmental, genetic, or degenerative health problems are to some extent now assigned to the provider. Patient behavior (for example, smoking or obesity) has a much greater impact on health and costs than physician utilization behavior.

Managed healthcare has forced physicians to add an unwanted additional question in a patient interview: "What insurance do you carry?" That information has always been important, but now it affects clinical decisions. Each plan has its own drug formulary, selected hospitals, approved consultants, preadmission screening criteria, second opinion contracts, case managers, and copayments. This precludes uniform treatment for everyone regardless of type of payment. Complying with utilization control guidelines can strain physician-patient relationships. By collecting copays or insisting on inconvenient morning admissions or early discharge, physicians are perceived as mercenary. Unwillingness to approve a patient-initiated referral or an unwarranted prescription causes acrimony. It is much more difficult to explain to a patient or family why a procedure is *not* necessary than to explain why it is. When a patient feels sick, the physician is expected to "do something." When the patient complains to a managed care representative about access issues, the classic response is "of course, the doctor has the final say on this," without mentioning the penalty for overruling managed care criteria.

While providers in the Minneapolis–St. Paul area have witnessed falling incomes, total health expenditures continue to rise. The alleged savings from managed care discounts have been diverted to administrative overhead. An entire industry has been developed to provide so-called managed care. Consumers have saved no money, providers are paid less, and a few entrepreneurs or stock companies have done very nicely.

JACK G. DAVIS, President and CEO, Select Care

The survival of a PPO such as Select Care does not depend on whether it is affiliated with a provider organization, an insurance company, or an entrepreneurial firm. Survival will be based on two functions: the capacity to achieve a high level of compliance from physicians and hospitals in managing utilization and the ability to establish a sophisticated information resource to communicate its performance to potential buyers.

In short, Select Care's success will be based on whether it meets marketplace needs. Select Care has to demonstrate to payers and employers that it can indeed control cost, that its providers are truly preferred (that is, efficient and high quality), and that the organization is making an impact on overall healthcare spending.

The PPO market in Minneapolis – St. Paul is still heavily focused on controlling costs through discounts. The American economy is focused on discounts, coupons, and buying products below retail. The same theme prevails in managed care. For years, the Twin Cities marketplace has been sold on the notion of broad access and freedom of choice. As a result, most employers are reluctant to limit access because of negative employee relations. However, this runs counter to controlling costs. By restricting access to a smaller group of providers (that is, smaller than wide-open PPOs but larger than HMOs), employers could further reduce costs. Select Care will succeed when it is able to balance the need for access with that of provider selectivity and utilization management.

Some employers go through the motion of shopping around from one network to another each year in an attempt to get the lowest price. This does not make much sense in managed care because employers need continuity of care and continuity of operations. They are likewise interested in ease of administration, minimal employee confusion through good communications, proper claims management, and appropriate utilization and case management, none of which can be achieved by shopping for low-cost bidders.

As the marketplace becomes more sophisticated, more attention will be given to information and provider accountability. Select Care is focusing on being able to measure results, communicating them effectively, and documenting the value for payers and employers. In the future, it will be necessary for a PPO to increase the administrative simplicity of its various payer relationships and develop a more standardized product offering. PPOs will need to use information to profile providers and manage the network. This will include varying reimbursement based on performance and outcome and establishing penalties and sanctions which could lead to termination. Payers and employers are eager to identify plans which effectively manage provider panels.

RICHARD J. FREY, M.D., Medical Director, Select Care

Managed care means financial squeeze and loss of independence to most physicians. They believe it threatens their independence by dictating how medical care can be provided and threatens their economic health by limiting fees and the scope of services covered. Hospital admissions are precertified, hospital days have been labeled nonacute, payments are denied to hospitals and physicians, the setting for certain procedures has been determined by an outside party, laboratory studies and x-rays may be judged to be unnecessary and payment denied, fees for service have been substantially discounted, and physicians may be dropped from plans because of non-compliance.

In fact, "managed care" is becoming the label for all alternative delivery systems, managed and unmanaged. Medical care in a PPO, for example, remains essentially unmanaged. The payment system is managed, but the patterns of care are largely untouched. To many physicians in the Twin Cities, managed care means that someone else (an outsider) is managing their patients' care. The majority of doctors here would like to see HMOs and PPOs self-destruct.

Physicians are increasingly aware of the need to rein in healthcare costs and to modify their practice patterns when it is shown to be outside conventional standards of care. However, such normative standards must be based on credible data. Concern is often expressed over the validity of data, not infrequently as a roadblock to change. The often-cited defense of "quality of care" can become synonymous with "private property—keep out." This is not to say that bad data are not just that, and they can inflict damage to individuals and the medical system. But, the majority of physicians will accept good data, fairly interpreted, as a guideline for change.

Even though selection is key to an effective PPO, the lack of criteria for selection was translated into an open enrollment for the staff physicians of Abbott Northwestern Hospital without their full appreciation of the dictates of a managed care system. It was presumed that the purchaser would direct employees to these physicians because of their reputation and that of the hospital. This has proven to be an unrealistic expectation. Most buyers in Minneapolis–St. Paul consider quality a given and want accountability for the dollar spent.

A loose, all-encompassing physician network cannot be managed effectively. So, a critical question arises: "How can physicians currently in the network be reselected in order to create a manageable operation?" It could be political suicide for the hospital to eliminate many of its loyal physicians because of their elaborate, high-cost practice patterns. But, it is just as deadly for the network to keep them. These physicians do not support aggressive utilization procedures because they perceive it is a threat to what independence they believe remains.

The initiative for provider selection and provider elimination must rest with the physician-oriented PPO management, thus leaving the hospital in a more neutral posture. The same division of responsibility must prevail as the PPO extends its geographic coverage to meet larger market demands. Select Care will clearly have to develop strategies and take further actions that may not be in the best interest of Abbott Northwestern or LifeSpan, at least in the short run. It must limit its physician providers; it must accommodate the broad geographic distribution of area employees; it must vastly improve its database; and it must develop a closer working relationship with large employers. This can only be accomplished with strong Life-Span support—but not at the expense of catering primarily to the interests of LifeSpan. This is indeed a compromising role for the hospital. It would be naive to think all these goals can be accomplished without conflict.

A hospital can play a key role in partnership with a restructured PPO. Risk contracts, package pricing, and performance guarantees are all possible through a close partnership between a physician organization and hospitals. The major threat to the success of such a partnership does not lie in physician unwillingness to organize or an unwillingness of physician organizations to work closely with hospitals. It lies in the narrowing window of opportunity in which providers can still take action before healthcare costs become so unmanageable that large buyers throw in the towel and demand government relief.

STEVEN G. HILLESTAD, Vice President, Marketing

There is a world of difference between what healthcare purchasers want and what providers think they want, for three reasons. First, providers hope purchasers will buy care based on a cost-benefit analysis, which implies a willingness to recognize "quality" and pay more for it. Second, providers think corporations and trust funds are going to be buying directly from hospitals, thereby eliminating intermediaries like HMOs and PPOs. The goal is to split the 10 to 20 percent fee that the insurance companies take, with part going to doctors and hospitals for patient care and part being passed back to the purchasers in the form of savings. Third, managed care issues supersede other corporate concerns such as the importance of good employee relations and morale in a declining personnel pool.

Employers still find the concept of managed care very difficult—difficult to understand, difficult to force changes in benefit plans, difficult to figure out who are the good doctors (especially if the boss's doctor does not make the list), and difficult to see what the specific benefits are. In short, managed care can be characterized as offering high hopes for providing efficient, reasonable quality care with little proof that it can, in fact, deliver what it promises.

Over the last 2 years, the Minneapolis managed care market has been pounded with negative reports on HMOs and cost-containment mechanisms designed to limit care. Major television stations have broadcast week-long prime time series on the problems with HMOs, the press has featured doctors revolting over attempts to limit their choice of medical treatment under managed care plans, numerous reports have been presented about the financial difficulties and possible insolvency of health plans, and court battles have raged over contract disputes between physicians and health plans.

Employers, particularly those in the direct firing line of buying managed care services, are very much aware of these issues. They are aware that costs continue to escalate well beyond the consumer price index, and they question whether they are getting good value for the benefit dollars being spent. However, they are also aware that channeling employees away from one health plan to another can become a volatile employee issue. As a result, making changes are difficult. Why?

Changing health plans is hard because employees seem to be satisfied with their physician. Employees generally think their doctor's care is outstanding, and they have no intention of shifting from one health plan to another. Furthermore, if they were forced to shift from their HMO, it is clear that the majority of people in the Twin Cities would switch into another HMO. The prospect of leaving their doctor in order to move into a "different managed care plan" is not something most employees take lightly. As a result, employers are having a more difficult time than anticipated implementing new and innovative managed care strategies.

In fact, one of the key variables to a successful managed care strategy in Minneapolis–St. Paul is location, location, and location. The availability of doctors near where people work and live is of utmost importance. People are not willing to drive great distances to the doctor. In areas where current managed care plans have few physicians, this factor translates directly into limited or low market share penetration.

So far, providers have not been able to sell quality successfully. Convenience and quality are both required in order to have a successful managed care strategy and to attract enrollees away from other health plans.

Lessons Learned from Managed Care Contracting

JOSEPH A. MILLER, Senior Vice President

Private Healthcare System Ltd., Lexington, Massachusetts

Private Healthcare Systems (PHCS) is a partnership of 17 midsize insurance companies that was organized in 1985 with the goal of developing a national managed care program. PHCS presently covers more than 1.4 million employees (3.0 million individuals) with its utilization review service. The national PPO has PPO networks in 40 cities and covers 500,000 employees (1.1 million individuals).

In 4 years PHCS has taken itself from a start-up to a major player in the industry by applying basic rules for developing a successful managed care corporation. PHCS believes that PPOs that survive and flourish will (1) choose the *right* providers — ones that are cost-effective and have reputations for quality, (2) negotiate competitive reimbursement rates with these providers, (3) install effective control mechanisms and utilization review programs, (4) effectively communicate the operational and administrative requirements of the PPO to all affected parties — employers, employees, and providers, and (5) successfully generate patient volume for their participating preferred providers.

These lessons should not surprise anyone familiar with the managed care industry. However, the way PHCS built a national PPO network of 400 hospitals and 30,000 physicians in under 3 years is a unique story based on common sense. The ingredients of that successful PPO building process are as follows:

- A simple, reasonable deal for providers and some degree of flexibility in the negotiation process.
- Clear communications about the programs through advertisements, publicity, and collateral material.
- A relatively small group of well-trained professionals that have the appropriate backgrounds in healthcare and experience in negotiations.
- A local approach to provider contracting — recognizing that every area of the country has its own concerns and circumstances.
- The necessary data to evaluate providers based on cost and quality.
- The willingness to ask customers, that is, providers, employers, and employees, what they want and then to listen to them.
- The necessary organizational support, well-defined milestones, and well-designed administrative systems.
- The intangibles of good management, which include creating a sense of urgency to meet deadlines, an organizational ethic of persistence and single-mindedness, a common vision of the organization's goals, and the ability to adapt and change when plans do not achieve the desired results.
- Sufficient capitalization to allow development of the managed care system with qualified people and adequate information systems. (Capitalization need not be enormous, even on a national scale; PHCS was capitalized with an initial contribution of $1 million per carrier.)

Like classic management principles, many of these tenets are recognized but ignored by developing managed care organizations. But adherence to the basic rules will, to a large degree, define which managed care corporations will be active in the marketplace in the 1990s.

Family Health Plan: Strengths of the Staff Model HMO

CONRAD SOBCZAK, M.B.A., Chief Executive Officer

Family Health Plan, Milwaukee, Wisconsin

Family Health Plan is a 73,000-member staff-model HMO which was organized 10 years ago as a nonprofit consumer cooperative. In an era dominated by the increase of IPA-model and other mixed-model HMOs, Family Health Plan owes its success to two things: (1) the straightforward implementation of the classical staff model HMO and (2) the pursuit of its intrinsic advantages. Among them are the following.

SIMPLICITY OF CULTURE

Family Health Plan and its primary care medical staff are entirely devoted to the delivery of healthcare on a prepaid basis. Thus, its physicians are compensated on a salary basis to provide care for a population of patients and not on the basis of units of service. This is consistent with the fixed-income economy of the HMO and is in contrast with many HMOs which must struggle with financial contradictions of fee-for-service and prepaid practice.

EMPHASIS ON PRIMARY CARE

At the core of Family Health Plan's delivery system is the primary care staff of 60 family practitioners, nurse practitioners, and physician assistants. It is the nation's largest example of an HMO built on family practice medicine. Family practice is increasingly being recognized as the "ideal" primary care gatekeeper because of versatility in caring for people of all ages, devotion to continuing care, and a predilection to emphasize ambulatory care.

USE OF ECONOMIC LEVERAGE

Whereas competitors use virtually every physician and hospital, Family Health Plan consolidates and delivers its referral business and hospital relationships to a relatively small number of providers. For example, Family Health Plan contracts with approximately 100 specialty physician consultants, in contrast to competitors who use over 1000 specialists. In the case of hospitals, Family Health Plan routinely utilizes less than a quarter of the area's institutions and directs significant new volume to them. As a result, Family Health negotiates capitation and per diem arrangements which generally realize cost reductions in the 25 to 30 percent range.

USE OF ECONOMIES OF SCALE

One of the intrinsic advantages of a staff-model HMO lies in its ability to exercise the "make-buy" decisions brought about by a growing membership. Simply put, a staff-model HMO can choose to provide services directly through its own clinics (make) rather than contract with outside providers (buy) as its membership grows (economy of scale). Over its 10 years, Family Health Plan has pursued this strategy and now carries out 95 percent of all ambulatory laboratory services, ambulatory imaging services (except MRI), and pharmacy services through its own facilities. As an example, the plan delivers prescription drug benefits at 66 percent of the average costs of its HMO competitors, demonstrating the power of the make-buy strategy.

Family Health Plan competes in a market which features eight other HMOs, all organized on an IPA basis, with an 85 percent overlap of participating physicians. The staff-model HMO provides Family Health Plan with a unique market niche. While its competitors have mixed the models, Family Health Plan has persisted in the straightforward staff model in the belief that sometimes mixing models results in obtaining the advantages of neither and the disadvantages of both.

Benefit Panel Services: A PPO-Sponsored EPO Product

W. MARK JASPER, President

Benefit Panel Services, Los Angeles, California

In 1985 PPOs were considered to be the ideal solution to rapidly rising health plan costs. The PPO product was flexible and offered free choice of providers without the restrictions or penalties found in HMOs. The PPO was also expected to apply medical cost controls. By 1989 the Health Insurance Association of America (HIAA) reported that PPOs are "bigger not better" and that cost control expectations are not being met by PPOs generally.

The real problem facing employers and PPOs is evaluating the impact of managed care programs on indemnity products. Evaluation is difficult because of the "swing" nature inherent in PPO option plans, that is, claimants may "always," "sometimes," or "never" use the PPO option. The risk selection and reasons for the choice at point of service are largely unknown. "Savings" are difficult to quantify because the plan incentives that encourage use of the PPO may cost more than the discounts. PPO utilization rates cannot be measured like those of an HMO because PPOs do not require annual enrollment.

Benefit Panel Services (BPS) saw that the PPO industry had created a credibility gap when it presented claims of great "savings" to employers whose premiums increased sharply despite new PPO programs. BPS expected the industry shakeout to be based on "results," that is, on the objective evaluation of impact on per capita costs and of the costs versus benefits of its managed care approach. In order to differentiate itself by product and establish a statistical basis for evaluation, BPS developed its Exclusive Provider Option (EPO) product.

At annual open enrollment, the EPO is offered in addition to the HMO and indemnity plans. If the EPO is chosen, the subscriber agrees to always use the contracted providers and facilities in the EPO network areas for elective care. Otherwise, no benefit is paid. Unlike HMOs, the subscriber may choose any contracting provider at the point of service, on every occasion! This hybrid product allows the experience (cost and utilization) of the EPO-enrolled group to be compared with the other groups.

Access to care would be greater than it is with most traditional HMOs because of the point-of-service flexibility in selecting primary care physicians. The quality of care is likely to be greater than that of an HMO because the network of physicians and hospitals in the EPO is more extensive. BPS assists patients in choosing among specialists based on the patient's preferences and geographic location as well as BPS's databases on cost and quality of network providers. From a marketing standpoint, BPS was able to offer several distinct advantages over HMOs. BPS has EPO networks in all urban areas of the state. This allows a uniform benefit for multisite employers. Within a family most HMOs require enrollment with the same primary provider, whereas the BPS EPO allows each family member to choose from the entire primary care network at point of service. The EPO is an indemnity product that allows for experience rating and for greater plan design flexibility than HMOs. For self-funder groups, the EPO allows integration of experience from a single source, which is attractive to groups for administrative and financial reasons. Usually HMOs do not have an indemnity companion coverage, so at least two plans (indemnity and HMO) must be administered by the employer. The HMO enrollees are usually a healthier group than those who enroll in the indemnity or self-funded plan. It must be assumed that there is also profit or operating surplus in the HMO premium that is recaptured by the plan sponsor in the single-indemnity EPO plan. Claims experience data are available from the EPO-indemnity plan, whereas HMOs that pay physicians on a capitation basis do not or cannot report such information to the plan sponsor.

The following are marketing advantages of the EPO product: network size and scope, point-of-service choice, better risk selection, single-plan administration, financial integration, and full experience reporting.

The EPO is designed to replace the HMO (except staff model) for a group or to enable groups who want cost controls to avoid less appealing HMO features such as restricted choice and emerging HMO issues such as barriers to care that result in poor quality. The EPO product was initially conceived as a "triple-choice" option with the indemnity and PPO-indemnity options from a single insurance carrier. Later it became clear that a choice of (1) indemnity without PPO or (2) EPO at annual enrollment would allow for greater premium and contribution incentives to choose the EPO. This is because there is greater distinction in benefits and because network penetration is 100 percent (that is, enrollment) on the richer EPO plan.

PROGRAM MECHANICS

Plan designs had to include provisions for coverage for noncontract providers' out-of-area services and in-area emergency services with noncontracted providers and for other "exceptional cases." Many of these administrative features could not be handled by insurance carriers and are part of the claims pre-processing performed by BPS.

Product pricing was initially based on the incremental cost added to the PPO (that is, a per employee per month administrative cap fee). For example, a 24-hour servicing capability was added for patient assistance. For very large groups, BPS has based its fees solely on meeting predefined "savings" objectives. Objectives are evaluated periodically, and there is a year-end accounting. The carrier's actuarial and underwriting approach was to extrapolate BPS's savings experience (30 to 40 percent penetration rate) and convert it to 100 percent penetration rate per enrollee. This often resulted in a substantial premium reduction.

CHAPTER FIVE

Payer Perspective

LINCOLN NATIONAL LIFE INSURANCE COMPANY— VIEWS FROM WITHIN

Three perspectives are included to illustrate the complexity and diversity of the managed care industry. Managers from each of three different healthcare companies were asked to provide, from within their own companies, a view of the managed care industry as a whole and of how their company's strategic goals fit into that view. LifeSpan Inc., reflects a provider orientation, Lincoln National Life Insurance Company presents a payer outlook, and Honeywell Inc. expresses a purchaser point of view. Each of these perspectives— provider, payer, and purchaser—must be successfully integrated in terms of business objectives for a managed care arrangement to create a win-win scenario.

The three companies established leadership positions in healthcare and were among the first organizations to develop innovative approaches to managed care.

LINCOLN NATIONAL Lincoln National is headquartered in Fort Wayne, Indiana. Lincoln National Corporation through its affiliates ranks among the nation's 10 largest health insurers and managed healthcare firms. The company operates in 40 major markets with annual revenues of over $2.5 billion and has more than 5 million lives under management.

Lincoln National entered the managed care market in 1985 through joint ventures and by acquiring local managed healthcare plans. Beginning in 1988, the company reassessed its strategy and acquired a number of joint venture operations in markets where a competitive advantage was possible. PPOs have been renamed Lincoln National

Preferred Plan, and HMOs have been renamed Lincoln National Health Plan. The company also divested other operations that no longer fit its strategy.

As a managed care company, Lincoln National's goal is to establish long-term relationships with providers while representing the financial bottom line and quality issues on behalf of policy holders.

EXECUTIVE PERSPECTIVE

There are five key issues facing Lincoln National which influence managed care:

1. Americans have received care when and where they want it without feeling responsible for the cost, that is, "entitlement."
2. Employers do not realize they are best positioned to apply pressure on the medical community by designing and providing plans that reward providers for making efficient healthcare choices.
3. Insurers must deal with physicians and hospitals in a positive way and dissuade them from providing care when and where they want, without regard to cost.
4. There is continuing public debate about the need for fundamental change in the healthcare delivery system. Access to care for 37 million Americans, the implications of competing in a world economy, and the unrealistic demands Americans make on the medical care delivery system have all combined to create a growing crisis. As a result, all major stakeholders in the political and healthcare system are considering ways to increase access to healthcare. Unfortunately this causes some constituents to propose universal health insurance, a national healthcare program, or other options that may not be appropriate. Everyone seems to have a political solution, most of which include compromise on the part of all parties.
5. Costs are the driving force. The cost of healthcare is going up at a rate of over 20 percent a year. That increase is attributable to medical inflation, cost shifting by the government, increased use of health services, new technology and more intensive services, catastrophic cases, and malpractice premiums.

Managed healthcare is very complex. It demands new and better data that have heretofore been unavailable. Most companies have claims systems based on 1970s technology and have not been able to create new systems to support the increased information needs of managed healthcare. It also means learning how to deal with providers in each different community. This is new, and we had to recruit business people with the knowledge and skills to operate in this new environment. Many people from the old insurance business simply were not equipped to make the transition to managed care in any company.

Organizationally, Lincoln National is well positioned to go forward in managed care. One of the critical things the company did was the integration of the different service functions and the various product options that result in managed care. Lincoln National is not an indemnity company or an HMO company; it is an integrated managed healthcare company.

The company has identified a system strategy that will be one of the tools of this integration: build a sophisticated, relational database which can deal with a high volume of claims as well as handle all the information necessary for working with HMOs, PPOs, utilization review, and all other provider contracts. Every Lincoln National employee will use the same system.

Lincoln National is the right size. It is big enough to have the necessary resources but not so big that it is difficult to get things changed relatively quickly. The skills necessary to be successful in managed care have been added over the past 2 years. Lincoln now has many more physicians and nurses as employees as well as a number of operations people who come from managed care backgrounds to assist in claims service and other managed care functions.

Perhaps of most importance, Lincoln National understands what it wants to build: a series of free-standing, local, competitive healthcare systems. On-site professionals will manage the provider relationships in each area and be backed by meaningful resources including a relational database and a management system with tight financial controls.

There is much to be done. The company is building more networks and improving those already in place. That means identifying the providers who are knowledgeable and in a position to provide efficient care in a new environment. The backbone of managing this process will be the company's data system (System for Managing and Integrating Care or SMC).

Lincoln National is changing its corporate culture. A company cannot be in the managed healthcare business with an insurance mentality. Extensive communication and education will be required to help employees understand the company's vision and what they have to do to participate in it.

As these changes are accomplished, Lincoln National will emerge among those carriers operating as managed care businesses. Although the company is a large national firm, it has decided to target key local markets and run them on a focused basis. Not many companies smaller than Lincoln National will make it in this business. Although Lincoln National is not as large as companies such as Prudential, Metropolitan Life, and Aetna, it will operate with a different model, on a more localized basis, and gain a significant market share.

Lincoln National's philosophy is that free-standing HMOs are essentially an endangered species. Customers will want their healthcare integrated from one source, and not all consumers will want to be in an HMO. HMOs that do not have other options will be in trouble.

Lincoln National is strengthening its strategic market share. It needs more clout to deal effectively with providers. That is why Lincoln National is focusing on markets where it can build market share and provide significant potential patient flow to providers. This does not mean *buying* market share. Others have tried this and lost money. Lincoln National expects to increase market share by bringing a quality product to the marketplace.

It is market differentiation. Why buy from Lincoln National? Employers will buy this product because the network functions efficiently, and the data will prove it. Also, the company is responsive to customers and provides good service. These are the ways to build market share without bowing to nonworkable pricing.

Lincoln National has learned some hard lessons in managed care. It is important to own and control businesses, as opposed to going into partnerships. In the past, Lincoln National purchased significant but noncontrolling shares in a number of HMOs and UR firms, then looked for some sort of blending of skills. It did not happen. The company then decided to obtain control of all of its strategic properties, to regain control over its destiny.

Lincoln National's message to employers is: "You can no longer provide a guarantee that employees can have unlimited access to healthcare. The fact is, this is not an affordable option. What you can do for employees is provide them a good network with physicians, hospitals, and other providers available on a convenient, local basis. If those sources are used as opposed to others, employees can expect to receive a meaningful benefit and get appropriate care. But if they choose not to use the managed care network, other reimbursement policies will need to be considered."

To the employee, the message has to be: "Traditional group insurance is too expensive, and employees must consider other means of accessing healthcare." Employees also need to be encouraged to start taking better care of themselves. This means suggesting ways to help employees stop smoking, lose weight, get more exercise, control stress, and become better managers of their own health. It will take involvement and expenditure on the part of employers and insurers to make this happen, but the potential benefits (in terms of costs and productivity) are so substantial that it makes sense to do it.

Right now the basis of managed healthcare is contracts between providers and the healthcare manager. They basically deal with price and, to some extent, an agreement to abide by utilization review protocols. Over time, there will be an increased emphasis on quality in those contracts.

As payers are able to deliver more predictable patient flow to physicians, there will be a change in the payer-provider relationship. There will be risk-sharing and profit-sharing where all parties will work together in the same environment for the same end—efficient, high quality healthcare. The issue will not be discounts, it will be quality. The discount phenomenon is transitional to the competitive healthcare networks of the future. In fact, Lincoln National is willing to pay *more* per unit to assure top-flight professional, efficient healthcare.

The relationship will be more cooperative, and there will be financial benefits to both parties for doing the job right. There will be a sharing of liabilities and responsibilities on both sides.

GENERAL MANAGEMENT PERSPECTIVE

Managed healthcare consists of bringing together the mechanisms of financing and provision of healthcare in a way that benefits the member, the provider, and the payer. This means not only paying the bills, but assisting members in gaining access to medically appropriate, cost-effective healthcare services.

Consumers are growing in their sophistication and are becoming more vocal about what they want from healthcare systems. They will become more critical in the success of new delivery systems that offer more and more choice.

Lincoln National's strength has been the development of networks that provide access to a full range of medical resources. The networks will limit provider participation to those physicians whose practice styles are conducive to managed care. Lincoln National is also restructuring incentives for both the member and the provider so as to create an environment that limits use of medical resources to those that are medically appropriate. Benefit plans are structured to focus members toward quality, cost-effective providers. Enhanced claims review procedures verify appropriateness of care within certain diagnoses.

Information is the key to success. In order to compete, the strong players in the health insurance world will need comprehensive, cost-effective delivery systems and flexible product options. They must also be able to provide a means for collecting and managing information in a timely fashion for major employers and clients who are seeking to control expenditures for healthcare. Enhanced information will aid insurance companies and employers in making better decisions about their employee health benefits plan.

Lincoln National has not been able to move as quickly as it has wished. Yet the pace of change is dizzying, and the introduction of new systems is a significant event. Some of these changes have resulted in the organization of the ways in which the work is done as well as the relocation of some of that work. It is a clear business objective to redefine the organization so that all operations are aligned to serve specific customers rather than traditional Lincoln National functions. This will require reassignment of staff and relocating some business functions to service centers which are geographically closer to the customer. These changes reflect the importance of customer service accountability. The transition to managed care is a complicated process.

Managed care is built on a variety of relationships and financial arrangements. Lincoln National is building a new corporate culture that blends the successes of the traditional indemnity insurance industry with HMO systems to create one integrated managed care company. That company can then market a full line of total replacement products under one banner—Lincoln National. This is a key aspect of Lincoln National's strategy and differentiates it from the competition. It is also integrating its offices to provide flexible managed care products and developing a common management and sales structure across the country. Lincoln National is placing heavy emphasis on what is happening at the local scene because it believes healthcare is very much a local game.

HUMAN RESOURCES PERSPECTIVE

Lincoln National has learned four major lessons about managed care. (1) Joint ventures are difficult. (2) Personnel with experience in managed care must be on board. (3) Managed healthcare involves a different definition of the business than indemnity insurance does. They might both be fruit, but one is an apple and the other is an orange. (4) Communication is critical. In a big company, it becomes very difficult. New people come in constantly and do not know the rules. There is a need for a clearinghouse organization with a genuine understanding of who does what and how it all interrelates: the necessary information has to get to the appropriate people. Awareness of required preauthorizations and approvals, and any approved exceptions is critical and requires an understanding of new functions, new roles, and clarification of the roles of each person involved in decision making.

Lincoln National needs to mesh its traditional insurance people with its entrepreneurial HMO people. There are vast differences in culture between insurers and managed care organizations. Both sides still tend to believe their way of thinking is best, and, therefore, each tries to convert the other side. In reality, both are right and both are wrong. The company needs to take a little from each.

The company has had several immediate goals. The first was to achieve financial recovery by reestablishing profitable operations. This was done through enhanced management controls, improved organizational efficiency, revised budget procedures, strengthened expense management, tightened underwriting and claims procedures, streamlined market presence, and expanded medical management. This goal has been met.

Other early-established goals continue to be important. One is the transformation to managed care. Strategies for achieving this include communicating the vision, integrating data management and operations, being a market-driven organization, increasing training, and motivating employees.

Another goal is to improve customer service. Lincoln National is implementing programs to emphasize quality performance. It is redefining service standards, providing training programs to meet those standards, and implementing a reward and recognition program to encourage superior service.

Lincoln National's vision, plan, and technology must be translated into training programs, work procedures, organizational charts, job descriptions, policies, and "to do" items. Everybody in the organization must know exactly what they are supposed to do and why.

MEDICAL MANAGEMENT PERSPECTIVE

The biggest lesson Lincoln National has learned so far is: "Don't forget the basics." Regardless of how clear a company's vision is, it must pay attention to details. Details are critical in a service organization. How they are handled can differentiate one company from the rest of the pack.

The use of technology must be improved. In addition to providing timely, accurate information, systems need to be developed to tie current providers and clients more closely to Lincoln National. One option is to implement a "smart card" with a magnetic strip on the back. Providers at the doctor's office, the pharmacy, and the hospital admissions office could run the card through a little black box and have instantaneous information about benefits. The claims could be paid electronically, eliminating claims processors and overhead. Doctors would like it because their staff would not have to handle claims forms, and they would get paid much more quickly. It could streamline the process and help tie providers into the system indefinitely. To change plans, doctors would have to reconfigure the entire electronic system in their offices.

The organization's sales people are a key part of a managed

healthcare system. They have to get the message out. This includes being well informed about what managed care is, being able to educate employers, and having data they can manipulate right there in the office to illustrate different scenarios. Good cost and utilization data about past experience must be shown to employers. Basically, the sales force needs to be trained to be managed care consultants, not just salespeople. They should be able to say to employers: "We can tell you what options you have, what the likely effect will be, and what it will cost."

PRICING AND COMPLIANCE PERSPECTIVE

How best to deliver and finance medical care is different in different locations. Each local marketplace must be evaluated separately because the provider community is different, the degree of leverage is different, and the competition is different. There is no universal solution. A different set of solutions must be designed for every location.

Lincoln National is going down the path that says there is more than one solution because there is more than one demand in the marketplace. There is a demand for cost-effective medical care, a demand for free access to providers, and a demand for options in between. Different kinds of clients require different kinds of products. The key is having the flexibility to change as the marketplace changes.

The future of healthcare really depends on three things: (1) how medical delivery systems continue to view managed care, (2) how much employers are willing to pay or what they are willing to make employees do in order to access medical care, and (3) what employees are willing to give up in terms of current wages versus using some type of closed-panel arrangement.

The day-to-day functions of the Pricing and Compliance Department have broadened with the advent of managed care. Within the pricing function, the increased level of new product development activity requires additional feasibility studies and pricing reviews. Changes within existing products, such as altering the product design or changing provider contracts, also require pricing reviews. If the marketing people for an HMO decide to increase the copay or alter deductibles, for example, prices must be set and, in many cases, rate changes filed with the state insurance department.

The key consideration in pricing is current cost trends in medical care. What is the underlying rate of medical inflation? What changes are occurring in utilization patterns and how is that going to affect costs? It is not enough to look backward and see what it has been; Lincoln National has to anticipate what is going to occur in the future, given various scenarios. A second key aspect is how to measure, quantify, and predict ahead of time what will be the impact of specific managed care actions. This entails predicting trends 18 to 24 months into the future.

Underwriting is just as important in a managed healthcare company as it was in a traditional insurance company. The role of underwriting is very similar to what it always has been: to help select appropriate risks which can be managed effectively and profitably and to set prices based on the particular circumstances of each case.

Managed care requires a different way to approach pricing questions, however. The underwriter has to understand the impact of managed care, for example:

- How the provider arrangements in a given community affect the projected costs of a given client.
- How the managed care plan the client had last year is different from the plan being proposed this year and what the impacts of the changes are likely to be.
- How this particular client and its risk characteristics will affect not just the earnings of the company but also the performance of the managed care system and the provider network in the given community.

Underwriters now have to understand a lot more about the medical side of the business and how a given risk affects Lincoln National's ability to contain those costs. Changes in products and markets are monitored to determine if and when the corresponding underwriting guidelines must be changed. The underwriting unit also generates changes by constantly evaluating the effectiveness of different underwriting guidelines and formulas for various regions and products.

Within the compliance function, developing new products and changing existing products often require filing contracts with state regulatory departments and gaining approval to use those contracts in such states. The compliance unit also must deal with the day-by-day week-by-week changes in regulatory requirements that crop up in one state or another and require changes to products offered within those states.

REGIONAL OPERATIONS AND SALES PERSPECTIVE

Lincoln National has learned that a company cannot just dabble in managed care. It must be *in* the business to be successful. Lincoln National must be a managed healthcare company rather than an insurance company that has relationships with various managed care providers. Management also must understand that there are so many changes occurring year by year that the direction in which the company started out may not be where it ends up.

The number one resource needed to succeed is people with expertise. There are big differences in terms of the expertise and management skills needed in the traditional insurance field and in the managed healthcare field. Importing new talent and reorganizing the company into large regional market groups has, perhaps, been the most difficult part of Lincoln National's transformation into a managed care company.

Lincoln National's market group organizations are working on several service and control issues. In the area of service, it means ensuring that customers receive prompt and accurate claims payment, information to properly use managed care systems, data on the status of their accounts, and all the materials that go along with managed care such as booklets, ID cards, and provider directories. To improve service, the company is restructuring jobs to fit new service requirements and making a major investment in training employees so that they can do those jobs better.

In the area of controls, the organization is trying to ensure that the best possible deals are made with providers and that all opportunities to reduce claim costs and control medical expenses are taken as they arise. To do this, a number of people with HMO experience have been brought in-house. Managers with local geographic responsibilities also have been added to work with providers in each managed care market by locating proper vendors and making direct contract arrangements. A number of doctors and nurses also have been added to review claims much more closely than in the past, using tougher definitions of medical necessity.

SYSTEMS PERSPECTIVE

Information systems are critical, especially in a service industry like managed care. Old systems for paying insurance claims were not designed for integrated managed care. The company had been using a number of independent systems which would not provide the functions needed for operating in managed care.

Lincoln National realized this and has responded with a tremendous commitment to technology. The corporation is making a major investment in an integrated database called System for Managing and Integrating Care (SMC). Parts of it are in place now, but it will not be an instant solution to all system problems.

In the meantime, there were several problems. First was the lack of data. Lincoln National needed a better way to gain and manage eligibility. Much time was spent on in-house reviews and development of new enrollment procedures. At the same time, employers had to be encouraged to cooperate with Lincoln National's greater demands for data. To do this, Lincoln National had to educate them about the value of supplying more data.

Traditional systems were built around separate functions instead of being designed and integrated for managed care. Lincoln National has a number of software systems running on different hardware configurations. It is difficult to service multioption products using a multitude of small, stand-alone systems.

Another problem was the pace of change. The division was in transition with new organizations, new products, new staff, and new expectations. People wanted to do many things and do them very quickly. The system's resources to keep up with this pace of change are very limited.

It was hard to meet all the needs of the organization and balance available resources. The systems department continues to massage the old systems on a short-term basis to serve immediate needs while also working to complete SMC to give long-term benefits.

Lincoln National is trying to respond creatively to bridge the gap between the existing environment and the future environment.

A systems committee composed of users from throughout the division was organized to assign and prioritize systems projects. The committee prioritizes those strategic projects and assigns resources according to the needs of the organization.

CLAIMS PERSPECTIVE

Within the claims department, Lincoln National's shift from claims payment into the world of managed care has required a tremendous amount of reeducation and retraining. All employees must now learn the mentality of managed healthcare, understand medical management techniques, and modify existing systems to accommodate this new environment.

Many claims employees who were comfortable in the indemnity world have been unable to adapt to the changes. The stress level has been higher than desirable and, for a time, resulted in a high turnover rate. Lincoln National is now looking for customer service staff who are better equipped to handle complex situations, the stress of operating in a demanding environment, and the more sophisticated nature of the job itself. The Human Resources department uses various methods to screen potential employees for these capabilities. Training also helps lower stress.

Another challenge is maintaining the level of customer service. As employers and employees experience the change to their new managed care plans, they must undergo a learning period. During this time, there is usually some confusion. For example, more information can be needed to process a claim, and the claims operation has to handle this increased volume of calls. Initially this can mean a longer turn around time.

MARKETING PERSPECTIVE

Communicating within a managed healthcare system is a complex job. Very little can be done on a national basis. The marketing department's audiences are diverse: Lincoln National's own employees, the sales force, clients, client employees, and providers. Each of these groups has vastly different communication needs. To be done successfully, most communication with these groups must be done on a local level.

Lincoln National's own employees require substantial training. The company is going through a major change, and sufficient training must be provided so that employees understand what is going on and why. Service people, for example, must be trained to provide quality service so that customers can get what they require. The broker network needs to understand the changes in order to sell managed care products. And the products are always changing.

Lincoln National needs to communicate effectively with employers to explain as carefully as possible—both before and after the sale— what is happening and why. Lincoln National also communicates with clients' employees to make sure they know what their benefits are, to motivate them to accept benefit changes, and to provide them with information about how to use benefits appropriately. A partnership is needed to achieve the ultimate goal—modifying the behavior of employees so they receive quality care within a financially stable program.

To some degree, elements of managed care represent "take-aways." On the other hand, they represent realistic ways to determine and access appropriate healthcare. Right now the responsibility for controlling healthcare costs falls on the insurer. Lincoln National needs employers and employees to join them in helping to keep costs in line. Within this framework, it is also vitally important to establish and maintain working relationships with the providers of healthcare. Financial incentives can be used, but education and communication are equally necessary.

CUSTOMER SERVICE PERSPECTIVE

Traditionally, insurance companies have predominately focused on two customer groups—employers and brokers-consultants. Indemnity sales are made to employers who purchase benefits for their employees. Brokers and consultants are seen as critical ties to this employer distribution channel.

HMO companies have built strong relationships with medical providers and focus on the member as the primary customer. The HMO product is based on a high quality and appealing network of physicians and hospitals. Most HMO sales activities focus on the employees through annual meetings where each HMO pitches the advantages of their particular plan.

As an integrated managed care company, Lincoln National must deliver products and services that *balance* the needs of all four customer groups.

- *Employers* who need to provide the highest level of benefits for the most reasonable cost
- *Brokers-consultants* who review and advise employers
- *Employees and dependents* who need access to quality healthcare at an affordable cost
- *Medical providers* (physicians and hospitals) who provide services under a network arrangement to gain market share and stabilize their income

Frequently, the expectations of these customer groups appear to be in conflict, although the overall objective is access to cost-efficient, quality healthcare services. For example, medical providers are looking to maximize business volume, while employers are trying to control the cost of their benefit plans. Most covered employees still believe they are entitled to unlimited medical services, while employers are purchasing managed care plans that control the delivery of care. A more tightly controlled managed care environment is one answer to controlling healthcare costs, not, however, without compromise on the part of everyone involved.

From a service perspective, managed care is distinctly different than most other financial or insurance services. Lincoln National must work with and educate each customer in order to realize the need for changing each customer's service expectations. Several examples will clarify this challenge.

- If a proposed medical service is inappropriate, Lincoln National must change the perspective of both the requesting physician and the patient to have a successful service interaction. If the insurer simply says "it is not covered," both parties will feel that Lincoln National delivered poor service.
- Employees and dependents frequently perceive managed care to be intrusive. To successfully arrange for quality and appropriate healthcare at the most reasonable cost, Lincoln National must turn utilization management into a perceived service advantage — that is, as a resource to help employees and dependents get the right care at the lowest out-of-pocket cost.

Lincoln National is striving to be customer focused by delivering the right balance of products and services. To be an integrated managed care company with service excellence, Lincoln National must constantly change customer expectations to those that can be reasonably met.

POINT OF VIEW

Insurers and Managed Care: No Easy Solutions

GARY S. WHITTED, Ph.D., Director, Health Costs Management

Employee Benefits Department, Travelers Insurance Companies, Hartford, Connecticut

Insurance companies, like all other major participants in healthcare delivery, have not succeeded in discovering any "magic bullets" to aim at escalating medical expenses. Perhaps insurers, armed with large monetary resources and an overzealous belief in their own marketing campaigns, make easy targets for "failing" to deliver on the promises of managed care. Since comprehensive managed care strategies on the part of insurers are relatively recent, it may be premature to pass judgment on their ultimate success. Expectations that insurers—or any other single group, including the federal government—could eradicate

the powerful structural forces that cause rising medical expenses have been both unfair and naive.

This preface is not to deny that insurance companies have committed a number of errors in addressing managed care. There are at least eight reasons (in no particular order of importance) why insurers have not harnessed the full potential of their managed care capabilities:

1. *Insistence on developing a "national" presence.* Both corporate bravado and the demands of large, high-profile customers induced insurers to invest too many resources too broadly, without first learning which strategies were proving cost-effective.

2. *Absence of appropriate accurate and sophisticated systems.* Until the early 1980s, insurers had virtually no data collection and analysis methodologies for indemnity medical expenses. Even when these capabilities were refined, they proved incapable of meeting the challenges of assessing such programs as utilization review, let alone new strategies such as PPOs and their

more complex brethren (for example, open-ended HMOs, triple choice).

3. *Underestimate of investment requirements.* Even with their vast financial resources, insurers inaccurately forecast the amount of capital investment necessary to establish and support managed care activities, as well as the length of time before this investment would yield a positive return on equity. Coupled with these planning mistakes were joint ventures and acquisitions of dubious conceptual or financial merit.

4. *Scarcity of seasoned healthcare professionals.* At least initially, insurers placed responsibility for the strategic direction of managed care activities under *insurance*, not *healthcare* professionals. As a result, it often took years to relearn the hard lessons learned in the HMO arena in other aspects of managed care, and innovation became shackled by too many years of preexisting bureaucracy.

5. *Lack of appreciation that healthcare is dynamic, not static.* Too many managed care programs resembled stationary arrows fired at speeding trains. Because of the absence of healthcare expertise, insurers failed to anticipate providers' reactions to managed care initiatives and the transitory nature of medical care practices. As a result, program design failed to incorporate a commitment to ongoing refinement and change. Even those programs that were moderately successful in their early stages (for example, utilization review) witnessed swift declines in efficacy, a natural evolution that could have been predicted by experienced healthcare professionals.

6. *Belated commitment to aggressive, proactive strategies.* Historically, insurers have been more reactive than proactive in healthcare. As a result, insurers were uncomfortable for a long while as they struggled to redefine their role in the medical care delivery system. Only a rapidly deteriorating bottom line and the admonitions of a small but vocal group of private sector payers convinced insurers to evolve from claims processors to active participants in the delivery and management of medical care.

7. *Overemphasis on the value of "networks" per se.* Too many resources and too much time were devoted to building delivery networks, without also establishing, performing, and enforcing disciplines of medical management (for example, standards of care, ancillary service protocols, and outpatient utilization review).

8. *Inaccurate perception of employers' commitment to, and understanding of, managed care principles.* Unlike the early TV fitness devotees, who espoused a "no pain, no gain" philosophy, most employers simply have been unwilling to realign their fundamental human resources values to be consonant with the basic tenets of managed care. Even fewer corporations have demonstrated the tenacity to enforce the imperatives underlying managed care interventions (for example, limited provider choice, cost-sharing differentials, and noncompliance penalties), in many cases for quite legitimate reasons. This tendency was exacerbated when some insurers encouraged the "you can have your cake and eat it too" for customers that balked at accepting the trade-offs inherent in managed care programs (for example, higher benefit plan reimbursement, but less freedom of choice and greater external review of services).

Fortunately, insurers today are considerably wiser (albeit poorer) for their 1980s experiments in managed care. Insurance company participation on a national scale has undergone significant erosion in the last half of the decade, and further consolidation is inevitable. Bloody lessons have been learned several times over, and a new cadre of managed care professionals has emerged. The remaining insurers are better-positioned to inaugurate further assaults against the enigma of escalating medical expenses. The first few years of the 1990s will become the proving ground to determine whether insurers' managed care ideas can overcome the inexorable demographic, economic, and social forces that continue to propel healthcare consumption and its ever higher price tag.

CHAPTER SIX

Purchaser Perspective

HONEYWELL — VIEWS FROM WITHIN

Three perspectives are included to illustrate the complexity and diversity of the managed care industry. Managers from each of three different healthcare companies were asked to provide, from within their own corporation, a view of the managed care industry as a whole and show how their company's strategic goals fit into that view. LifeSpan Inc. reflects a provider orientation, Lincoln National Life Insurance Company presents a payer outlook, and Honeywell Inc. expresses a purchaser point of view. Each of these perspectives —provider, payer, and purchaser—must be successfully integrated in terms of business objectives for a managed care arrangement to create a win-win scenario.

The three companies established leadership positions in healthcare and were among the first organizations in the country to develop innovative approaches to managed care.

HONEYWELL Honeywell Inc. is an international control company that provides products, systems, and services for the home and commercial building, industrial, aviation, and defense markets. The company is headquartered in Minneapolis and reported sales of $7.1 billion in 1988.

Because Honeywell has 78,000 employees worldwide, the provision of affordable, high quality healthcare is a critical business need. In 1983, the company began to take steps to move from being a "payer" of healthcare services, that is, covering bills as they were submitted, to being a prudent purchaser. In 1987, the company took a more active role in designing and delivering health benefits, selecting carriers and providers, and supplying health resources.

Honeywell began treating healthcare as a purchasing function. In Minneapolis, the company requested that insurers, HMOs, and other contractors bid on specifications written by Honeywell. In the Minneapolis–St. Paul area, two PPOs replaced five HMOs and one indemnity insurance plan for 12,500 Honeywell salaried employees. The HMO and indemnity options were retained for 6000 Twin Cities employees under union contracts.

Employee responsibility for selecting and financing healthcare was increased. Comprehensive coverage remained, but deductibles, a 20 percent copayment charge with a stop-loss provision, and a 20 percent contribution toward premiums for dependents were instituted.

Honeywell defines its overall approach as moving toward a "quality health management" system. The premise is that preventive services are cost-effective, and well-informed employees who share healthcare costs use the system more appropriately. A further premise is that physicians and other caregivers whose practice patterns reflect quality standards are more efficient and less costly, thus avoiding both under- and overprovision of care.

In the future, contracts with provider groups will require physicians and hospitals to specify their own standards for "appropriate and necessary care."

JOHN BURNS, M.D., Vice President, Health Management

As healthcare management moves into the 1990s, it will move away from traditional healthcare cost strategies and move toward a quality-based management system.

To evaluate quality of care, several changes will have to take place. Employers will adapt the quality lessons they already know. Most companies have quality programs for manufacturing, and some have developed comprehensive programs for their service areas. The next step in quality improvement will be in employee benefits. Such a quality improvement process will require standards for healthcare, utilization data, and a high level of participation by all parties.

Today, quality assessment means drafting detailed specifications for contracts with carriers and insurance companies so that the quality of the services purchased can be compared to the specifications laid out in the contract.

Healthcare purchasers who can describe both service specifications and the standards those services must meet are smart buyers. Purchasers who cannot describe the standards or specifications of a service are foolish buyers. When it comes to healthcare, employers must learn to buy smartly. Setting specifications for care is the first tool employers need when changing to a quality-based system. The "quality by standards" approach is proactive and starts by defining quality. It then establishes standards to judge healthcare quality.

"Smart purchasing" mimics the procurement practices of business. The employer makes purchasing decisions through a competitive bidding process that is initiated by submitting specifications of a well-defined product or service. Quality is then measured against such specifications. If the purchaser does not adequately specify the product or service, then it is difficult to assess the quality of the product.

The health benefit plan, in order to be a quality plan, should include detailed specifications which support assessing the health status (through risk assessment) of newly hired and existing employees on a periodic basis. It should also provide a "health benefit" for cost-effective health education and behavior modification for patients with existing health conditions or identifiable health risks. One incentive for healthy employee behavior would be a reduction in premium for various "healthy behaviors" such as nonsmoking and maintaining healthy weight or cholesterol levels. Therefore, a major component within the specifications should be health education and preventive services. In that way, the risk of illness is minimized or eliminated.

Prevention is a cheaper way of assuring quality than inspection and review. However, not all episodes of illness can be prevented, but 50 percent of illness can be deterred through prevention. The health benefit plan must still provide for symptom- and illness-related benefits. Business has the greatest opportunity to be a smart buyer within the area of illness care. Through specifications, Honeywell can both purchase and audit high quality medical services for employees.

In the past, quality assessment of medical care has been based on the assumption that each procedure or intervention was necessary. This assumed that quality could be determined through evaluating structure, process, and outcome. The necessity for the intervention was never questioned. Recently, a wide variation in practice style by geographic area has been reported in the medical literature. If all health services performed were necessary, there would be less utilization variation. The medical literature provides physicians with information on the effectiveness and appropriateness of various treatments. However, the recommendations in the medical literature are not always reflected in the behavior of physicians and their practice style. Large variations exist in the frequency of procedures such as caesarean section, hysterectomy, and tonsillectomy, where reimbursement incentives may take precedence over state-of-the-art medical guidelines.

CONTRACT PRIORITIES

Honeywell has found that three major areas need to be included in provider contracts: definition of quality, utilization review, and case management. Defining quality is the highest priority. If purchasers cannot define what they want, it is impossible for the provider to fill the request for quality. The provider network responds to the initiatives of customers. For example, when employers initiated utilization review systems to encourage a decrease in use of inpatient services, providers responded quickly with a variety of outpatient services. In this context employers must be careful about what they ask for; they may get it. Decisions on the definition of quality and the standards should be shared with providers, insurers, carriers, and business coalitions to explore the implications of those specifications.

Benefit design should be based on the basic premise that any medical service which is necessary and appropriate is a covered benefit. There should be no exclusions for medically necessary and appropriate interventions, either diagnostic or therapeutic. Medical necessity is addressed by evaluating all healthcare interventions from the perspective of outcome. By defining quality of care in the contract as both necessary and appropriate, the employer will limit care to just what is needed: not more, not less.

The physician's judgment determines the appropriate treatment once it is decided that treatment is necessary. Although the physician's decision is based on the details of the individual's care, treatment may still be specified to some degree to encourage the most cost-effective care.

The quality model focuses on providing the right service the first time. Closed-panel multispecialty clinics strive to develop an internal quality control and quality improvement system based on medical scientific literature. Interventions are generally limited to procedures documented to have an effective outcome. Services are provided according to the standards of published medical literature and the significant experience of the provider.

Some cost-containment strategies will continue to be viable in quality-based systems. Utilization review, employee copay, and case management translate well into the quality model of health management.

Currently, utilization review (UR) decisions are based on "norms" of allowable reimbursement, that is, length of stay, regardless of necessity. In the future, continued stay and reimbursement decisions will be based on the needs of the patient and not on the statistical norms previously derived and used for cost control. Norms will no longer drive the UR system. The contracts with providers of UR services will have quality care guidelines in place.

For example, utilization management should include specifications for discharge planning, rehabilitation, and return to work. Specifications for coordinating return to work and rehabilitation would require communication with the employer so that workplace modifications in job requirements will allow for early return to work. Concurrent utilization review should also be based on the demonstrated need for continued care in the most appropriate environment. Even the preadmission certification process will require that any proposed intervention be demonstrated to be both necessary and appropriate. This burden of responsibility is on the providers. It is not the obligation of utilization management systems to prove that intervention is not necessary.

Another important addition to employers' contracts is case management. This area, along with UR specifications for quality, forms the primary determinants of any medical coverage contract. Where UR is a preventative mechanism that ensures quality (conformance to the specifications), case management is a quality-based program that helps patients get the effective and efficient care they deserve.

The quality standards of the health benefit contract would also include specific requirements for large-case management. Highly complex cases such as spinal cord injury, severe burns, and organ transplants would be included, as well as chronic illnesses and AIDS. Also included in this group are technology-dependent patients whose need for care is unquestioned, but whose treatment setting could be changed.

Certain triggers for an "appropriateness evaluation" of the care setting are written into the contract, so that once the condition of the patient is stable, decisions on alternative care or continued acute institutional care can be made. Decisions on home healthcare, hospice care, and transitional care settings need to focus on the emotional needs of the patient as well as the medical needs.

Two further areas of contracting should be included in a quality-based contract: data requirements and selective contracting. Assessment of the quality of care given to employees is a comparison between the specifications outlined in the contract and the care given. Data from providers must be analyzed for this utilization. The service contract should include data requirements that are patient-, provider-, and diagnosis-specific.

Within a medical system based on quality standards, employer assessment of quality is reduced to an audit of health services and a determination of whether the standards have been met. A monitoring system is critical if quality assessment is to be medically sound.

SELECTIVE CONTRACTING

Special contracts with high quality hospitals should be considered when providing care to those patients with high-cost or high-severity illnesses. For example, Honeywell offers organ transplant coverage through "centers of excellence" so that employees and dependents with terminal heart and liver disease can receive transplants with increased likelihood of success. These are generally high-intensity low-frequency events. Contracting could also include high-frequency events such as pregnancy, where selective contracting with a preferred provider could guarantee higher quality services because of internal quality control systems, comprehensive protocols, provider expertise, and successful outcomes.

Selective contracting recognizes the issue of emerging technology and accommodates it within a quality healthcare system. Contracts signed by the employer, either through carriers or direct contracting with providers, should specifically allow for coverage of new technology that can clearly be demonstrated to be necessary.

Concentrating new technology in a few centers is needed to preserve quality. This type of care should be limited to "centers of excellence," since those centers have the best results and the highest level of experience. Minimum standards for both frequency of procedure and outcome should be established by the contract. The service would then be limited to those centers which meet such contract specifications. Duplication of specialized services not only dilutes experience but also causes tremendous increases in cost because of the capital investment required to test new technology. Benefit plan design and contracts should be written to provide employees with medically necessary care but limited to quality institutions specified through UR or selective contracting.

Benefit design should support shared financial participation at the point of purchase. Most companies have done this through copays such as 80-20 percent split. In a quality-based system not all procedures or tests should be subject to a copay. In some cases, copays deter preventive care. Medically necessary screenings and investigative procedures, such as mammography or PAP smear, should be paid for without patient contribution. Treatment for chronic disease, as in the case of appropriate screenings, should not be subject to copay. Treatment plans for patients with insulin-dependent diabetes, hypertension, chronic heart problems, and gastrointestinal disease are threatened by the use of copays. Treatment of ongoing chronic diseases should be exceptions to all copays, provided a protocol based on necessity is defined.

CHANGING PROFESSIONAL ROLES

One of the missing ingredients in health management has been the lack of health professionals as managers. As the benefit design becomes based more and more on the principles of medical necessity and appropriateness, health professionals will be needed to determine covered benefits. Managers with medical expertise are needed to participate in decisions regarding the contract and standards for utilization review, quality control, data reporting, audits, selective contracting, and case management.

The traditional occupational physician and occupational nurse activities are in service and program areas. They generally do not participate in benefit design, contracting, service audits, or data evaluation. The occupational nurse may be trained as an employee advisor and advocate with the responsibilities of initiating case management and facilitating referral of candidates for high-technology procedures. This new role is critical in a quality-based system. The input from the full-time occupational health nurse (functioning as a health service manager) is imperative to the assessment of the level of quality in employee care. Training nurses to be health managers enables the company to institute quality assessment at the level of employee interaction.

The contribution of the company physician is also required in a quality-based system. Corporate America can no longer afford to use physicians strictly in service functions. The best use of company physicians would be to remove them from primary care functions and put them in charge of healthcare quality assessment. The physician should work closely with the professionals in benefits, risk management, and personnel. The physician should also serve as the liaison with the provider community to get feedback on possible contract specifications.

TOM SEUNTJENS, Director Corporate Insurance and Risk Management
HARRY ROSAASEN, Manager Group Insurance

In 1987, Honeywell changed their fee-for-service medical benefit design from a first dollar coverage to an 80-20 coinsurance plan on a companywide basis. Honeywell also reduced the number of medical plan options in Minneapolis from six to two. Five HMOs and one fee-for-service plan were eliminated and replaced by two PPO plans (Blue Cross–Blue Shield and Physicians Health Plan).

In 1988, Honeywell published their Long-Range Health Management Plan. This comprehensive plan covers all areas of health — employees, internal Honeywell management system, and the external health system. For the employees, the plan specifies good health habits, how to be an informed consumer, and the need to understand their benefits. The internal health management system requires continuation of Honeywell's health promotion and employee assistance programs. The new aspect is training the company nurses as Health Service Advisors (HSAs). This training requires that the HSAs not only know the benefit plans and support the management of claims and large-case management but that they also act as employee and dependent advocates.

The external health system changes are being implemented in two phases. The first phase, in 1989, addressed detailed specifications for all fee-for-service contracts. These specifications require "standards of care" to be implemented by the fee-for-service carriers to support the utilization review activity. Triggers for large-case management were also specified as well as detailed descriptions of data required from the providers in these cases. These specifications, when fully implemented, will require the maximum possible "quality of care" from all carriers. The second phase, which began in 1990, requires the implementation of new quality-based arrangements replacing some of the existing HMO offerings. These quality-based arrangements that would normally be considered preferred provider organizations (PPOs) will be named exclusive provider organizations (EPOs) by Honeywell. The number of fee-for-service carriers will also be reduced.

When purchasing healthcare in the future, the company plans to have a PPO-EPO based on a closed-panel staff-model HMO or multispecialty physician group. This PPO-EPO would compete with the indemnity plan and the eventual goal would be to have most employees in this plan. Both would be fee-for-service plans, so adverse selection would not be an issue, and their prices would be based on their cost to the company. Besides lower premiums, there would be added benefit incentives to the PPO-EPO for preventive and chronic care.

With this quality PPO-EPO model, Honeywell would receive the quality control benefits of these staff-model organizations. Employees would benefit because of the reduced number of external quality controls that will increasingly be necessary in fee-for-service plans (that is, ambulatory utilization review, service exclusions, and other restrictive benefit designs).

The EPO-PPO physicians would not be subjected to many of the external quality controls found in the fee-for-service plans. This provider group would have the freedom to practice medicine based on their own clinical standards for management of chronic illness, high-intensity services, and ancillary services. The standards would be developed by the physicians within the organization but based upon and supported by the scientific medical literature. The group's activities would be monitored through data analysis and internal actions taken to improve the quality of services provided to Honeywell employees. For example, physicians would stop ordering tests that do not prove to alter the course of treatment or improve the outcome, such as routine chest x-rays prior to surgery.

Honeywell will benefit from this type of arrangement because employees and dependents will receive high quality care without many of the excesses inherent in the fee-for-service system or the questionable level of care in some capitated HMO networks. Improved quality of care translates into cost control and improved services. This plan should cost significantly less than the fee-for-service indemnity plan. This model has been implemented in Minneapolis and potential arrangements are currently being considered in Albuquerque, Phoenix, and Clearwater, Florida. These locations have large employee concentrations which make it easier to work with existing institutions to form EPOs for Honeywell. In other areas, Honeywell will work with business alliances or other networks to implement new networks.

Honeywell has gone beyond the basic managed care offerings to concentrate on quality-based arrangements. By ensuring quality healthcare with the delivery of only necessary and appropriate care, the employee and Honeywell will benefit and at reduced costs.

BRAD McDONALD, Corporate Director of Health Systems

Honeywell is currently participating in most types of managed care systems but would like to return to simpler times. For Honeywell, this means returning to the base transactions in healthcare: an informed employee deciding on his or her own healthcare in consultation with a knowledgeable and skilled physician. Ideally, this transaction would take place without the interventions of "managed care." While this is an optimistic view of evolution and change in the healthcare system, Honeywell has this vision as a long-term goal for its employees.

The immediate plan at Honeywell is to get a handle on the many health benefit plans, health plan administrators, and other managed care services it purchases. Honeywell will continue to have comprehensive indemnity plans, PPOs, and HMOs among its managed care options, but it can no longer function in a "business as usual" mode. Healthcare is now the third highest cost category ($150 million or $1.80 a share) in the corporation after salaries and raw materials. Development of closer working relationships with fewer vendors is the goal, the primary purpose of which is to maximize customer services that are obtainable through a continuous quality improvement process. Honeywell will accomplish this through the development of specifications and by auditing the quality improvement process of the vendor.

QUALITY CONTROLS The long-term strategy that is being piloted in Minneapolis is a PPO built around a group practice of physicians. This group practice could be a part of a staff-model HMO. Recognizing that discount PPOs and most IPA HMOs are primarily reimbursement schemes, Honeywell is attempting to control costs through quality control. Honeywell also recognizes that while the costs of care are primarily inpatient costs, the physician is the one who determines the true cost of most inpatient and outpatient care.

Honeywell intends to maximize the formal and informal quality controls that already exist in a group practice of physicians. It would like to see more effort placed on a continuous quality improvement process rather than on the traditional quality assurance process that already exists. Being self-insured, Honeywell would prefer to pay for this care on a fee-for-service basis, which is not always easy for a group practice HMO to accommodate. Other funding mechanisms will be explored, but the company has always tried to avoid the incentives for underservice that occur in capitated plans. Generally, Honeywell would prefer to be charged for services on a fee schedule with negotiated adjustments.

These quality-based PPOs would have certain benefit incentives such as 100 percent payment for scheduled preventative screenings and for chronic care. These incentives are designed to encourage participation in the plans and to reduce copayment disincentives to appropriate preventive screens for follow-up of chronic conditions.

Marketing such quality-based plans is made more difficult by messages that bombard employees from managed care firms selling "choice" of physicians. Honeywell feels it is battling Madison Avenue because employees have received the message that having the choice of any provider is the ideal. HMOs in the Twin Cities have been very effective in communicating the freedom of choice message. Group practices would limit the choice. They may also be perceived as unwilling to do all the tests an employee requests or to actively treat self-limiting acute illness.

The bottom line is that there is just too much care being provided. In 1980, Minneapolis–St. Paul families made 2.3 visits to physician offices. This figure jumped to 4.7 visits per year during 1987. Getting a full workup has become the norm, and illness prevention has been taken to the extreme.

MONITORING Honeywell's main role in the quality purchasing model is to do a quality job of setting up the monitoring system, that is, process-control monitoring. If this is done correctly, divisional managers will be able to tell the company on a quarterly basis what action has been taken. This will include a review of the internal quality control systems and actions taken to correct quality problems. Monitoring will be a cooperative process with Honeywell looking for ways to help the providers do their job by, for example, assisting the provider with information to capture coordination of benefits (COB) or subrogation.

INDIRECT COSTS The company is beginning to realize that the indirect costs of healthcare are probably 3 to 4 times greater than the cost of current employee health benefits. Indirect costs include the expense of replacing an absent worker, lost productivity, sick pay, and further medical costs from unexpected medical complications that result from surgical procedures and that could have been avoided had the case been better managed medically.

For example, 30 to 40 percent of carotid endarterectomy surgeries have been shown to be unnecessary and ineffective. In fact, 11 percent result in a stroke or death as a consequence of the procedure—exactly what patients try to prevent by seeking care. Unnecessary procedures are costly in terms of both the actual and disability costs. Changes in the way Honeywell specifies purchasing care through its quality-focused PPOs will begin to address these indirect costs.

An even bigger problem is that 3.8 percent of Honeywell's employees account for 50 percent of medical expenses at an average cost of $20,000 per case. Honeywell is continuously exploring ways to recognize high-intensity high-cost cases and manage them efficiently.

COPAYMENT   While Honeywell generally has 80-20 copay plans, it recognizes the limits of copayments in affecting costs. Fifty percent of employees have no claims and are unaffected by copayments. Very few "max out." As healthcare costs go up each year, the relative value of the copay declines. For Honeywell, copayments serve the following functions:

1. Involve the employees in the buying decisions
2. Tie employee contribution levels to the cost of healthcare services used (for example, $160 of a $800 nuclear magnetic resonance imaging)
3. Protect employees in terms of copayment maximums

Many employees do not know who to go to for care and take objection to being "herded." As a result, benefit differentials should not be made too great and the employer should be aware of the legal ramifications of doing too much directing.

FUTURE STRATEGY   Honeywell's goal to improve service over the next few years will be accomplished by reducing the current offering of 120 HMOs and redefining the 5 major indemnity plan sponsors. Because most of these HMOs service fewer than 50 employees each, Honeywell spends too much of its healthcare budget on overhead. The future agenda is to specify the company's needs and then develop a tracking system to monitor them.

Unfortunately, Honeywell cannot "go it alone" with this model or go too far out on a limb. It still needs a competitive benefits package for recruitment purposes. Honeywell is working with other corporations to encourage them to develop a quality focus and specify their needs to providers.

Honeywell is getting smarter as a company. It can no longer afford to test out different cost-containment techniques with different vendors and then choose the best ones in a "mix and match" sort of fashion. There is not enough time and energy available for this approach. The company needs to form long-term provider relationships and work with them in a business relationship.

POINT OF VIEW

Why Employers Are Not Using Quality to Select Providers and Plans

LAIRD MILLER and JOANNE MILLER
Health Systems Management, Inc., Minneapolis, Minnesota

Healthcare cost and quality often have an inverse relationship. While many employers find this difficult to understand, others quickly recognize how healthcare costs can decrease when physicians diagnose patients correctly (the first time) and provide appropriate services effectively and efficiently. Often, companies that have reduced their own costs of doing business by improving quality can more easily see how this might work in healthcare. Others, of course, have difficulty accepting that physicians and hospitals, just like everyone else, can make mistakes or practice inefficiently.

Although many companies understand how improving quality has decreased the price of their own goods or services, few have applied this knowledge to purchasing healthcare services. These are some reasons employers resist using quality as a criterion for selecting plans and providers:

- *Employers believe it is easier to use price as a criterion for selecting plans and providers.* Price, after all, is a concept most businesses understand. And purchasing services from plans or providers that appear to offer the most services for the least cost seems intuitively simple. Unfortunately, few employers know that purchasing healthcare based on price may negatively affect the quality and availability of these services.

- *The experience of many employers with the health-*

care delivery system is limited. These employers may view providers and plans as authority figures who should not be questioned. Some do not believe it is appropriate for business to ask questions about healthcare quality nor do they feel capable of using available tools and information to assess quality.

- *Often employers do not understand (and others do not believe) that quality healthcare services can be defined and quality providers can be identified.* Even companies that subscribe to the industrial quality model and define quality as *conformance to customer requirements* often do not see how this model can apply to purchasing healthcare.

- *Employers who have not worked in healthcare environments often do not know that providers in their communities can be more effective and efficient.* Some assume that all physicians in "their town" provide quality care and that "therapeutic misadventures" occur elsewhere.

- *The community's culture may make it difficult for employers to evaluate quality of healthcare services.* In many communities, people do not believe it is "proper" to question whether providers deliver quality care. Employers who challenge providers to prove they deliver quality care may quickly find themselves—*and their businesses*—shunned by the community.

- *Many managers, including healthcare benefits managers, believe their company rewards employees for avoiding controversy.* They perceive taking innovative approaches to controlling healthcare costs (like providing incentives to improve quality) could hurt their careers.

- *The philosophies, cultures, or value systems of some*

corporations clash with the notion that employers are responsible for evaluating healthcare products and steering employees to quality providers. These employers believe company payments for healthcare services are an "employee benefit." They contend a company should not choose providers for employees any more than it directs them where to live—or how to spend their paychecks.

- *Many companies do not have a staff that feels qualified to determine which providers deliver quality healthcare.* Even when reports and analyses describing efficiency and quality are available, most benefits managers do not have time to learn how to use this information effectively.

- *Employers do not know that one or two energetic dedicated individuals, with strong support from their company's CEOs, can positively affect a community's healthcare delivery system.* Some mistakenly believe that it takes many people (or companies) to effect change.[1]

Purchasing healthcare services using quality as a criterion is not an easy task. If it were, employers would have done it long ago. By some accounts, half of the rejections [due to quality problems] are the fault of the purchaser. Hopefully, as more and more employers recognize their responsibility and power as healthcare purchasers, they will form partnerships with providers to better manage and improve health.[2]

1. *Value Managed Health Care Purchasing: An Employer's Guide Series.* Midwest Business Group on Health, Chicago, Illinois, 1989.

2. Philip B. Crosby, *Quality Is Free.* McGraw-Hill, New York, 1979.

CASE STUDY

Xerox: Healthcare Purchasing Strategy

PATRICIA M. NAZEMETZ, Director,
Corporate Benefits

Xerox Corporation, Stamford, Connecticut

How can a large corporation that purchases healthcare benefits for tens of thousands of employees and their dependents in hundreds of locations in virtually every state and territory in the United States purchase smarter? A good place to start is to look at techniques used for other major expenditures. Leverage, focus, supplier oversight, and management are a few techniques that seem to spell success in purchasing. Xerox has embarked on a healthcare purchasing strategy that will use all of these "smart" purchasing tools.

In addition to its self-insured fee-for-service plan, Xerox currently purchases healthcare benefits from about 140 suppliers. With so many suppliers, purchasing power is diluted, management of suppliers cannot be achieved, and purchaser (or customer) requirements are often unmet and usually not well defined.

One objective of Xerox' healthcare purchasing strategy is to move from being a mere payer of the bills to being an intelligent purchaser of healthcare needs of employees and their dependents. To meet this objective, Xerox is defining its purchaser requirements and will limit the suppliers from which it purchases healthcare programs and services. Fewer suppliers translate to increased market share for those selected and increased purchaser leverage in ensuring that requirements are addressed and met. Fewer suppliers also means better opportunity for Xerox to manage supplier performance.

While establishing fewer, larger, more focused purchaser-supplier arrangements is critical to the success of an intelligent purchasing strategy, there are many facets of the healthcare delivery system that may not respond well to a national or centralized approach. Xerox recognizes the importance of preserving many of the characteristics of the local healthcare delivery system. It recognizes, too, that managing such a system requires a great degree of skill and experience in the process and structure of healthcare delivery. This is an area of expertise that Xerox has not developed internally. With all of the changing dynamics and complexities of the system, this is best left to the experts.

Xerox' goal is to find the experts—managing partners—who can be engaged to establish and manage a system of health plans that will deliver healthcare to the company's employees and dependents. To do this, Xerox must establish its requirements for the selection, purchase, and management of health plans and programs throughout the country. These requirements must address the levels of benefits and service; the quality of care; and the cost, administration, and community impacts of purchasing programs and services from healthcare systems. These requirements must represent the needs of users, that is, patients as well as the corporation.

The basis of any good partnership is a mutual and clear understanding of the objectives of the venture. Program requirements must be realistic and achievable. To assure that the program can be accomplished and sustained over the long term, Xerox has engaged a limited number of potential partners in discussions meant to help focus and refine customer requirements.

In an effort to correctly identify the requirements of employees and dependents participating in company health benefit programs, Xerox surveyed all employees late last year to establish the basis of their needs and expectations for health benefits. The survey results indicated that some involvement in the choice of healthcare provider is very important to employees and their dependents. Survey respondents also indicated that limited and predictable out-of-pocket costs is important and that uncertainty or concern about quality of care would be the main reason for leaving a plan.

The results of the employee survey, compiled and analyzed by an independent market research firm, are being provided to all prospective partners along with the company's official request for proposal (RFP). Through the company's RFP and the network managers' response, customer requirements will be translated into supplier specifications. Managers (that is, potential partners and suppliers) will tell Xerox, in their terms and within their scope of abilities, how the requirements can best be met. Provider performance will be assessed according to these specifications.

Xerox will select several managers who will be asked to establish and/or maintain a network of managed health plans — possibly like HMOs — to deliver health services to Xerox participants at a local level. The plans will provide for a full range of services to meet participants' healthcare needs. They will be reimbursed at a prospectively established, community responsive, capitated fee. At major sites, Xerox will encourage some network managers to compete with others through local plans in their respective systems. In other words, Xerox employees should, when feasible, have more than one health plan to choose from. Employees will be required to chose a plan annually.

With this healthcare purchasing system in place, Xerox can hope to regain control over the quality and cost of the healthcare benefits they buy. The management of health benefits has moved beyond the control of the corporate purchaser. Establishing control over the health programs and the expenditures associated with them must be a priority. Xerox needs a model that enhances the opportunity for control, allowing it to manage the process. Reducing the number of players to a few carefully selected network managers presents several opportunities. First, it allows Xerox to focus on managing a small number of "suppliers." It also spreads market share among fewer systems, thus making Xerox a major customer on a national basis, even if relatively small on a local basis. Finally, it allows management and administration to be centrally focused while still preserving the local character of the delivery system. Within these systems, the network managers will be responsible for assuring that the local health plans are performing according to specification. Since managers will be selected for their expertise in the area of managed healthcare, they should be up to this task.

A critical role for Xerox is in the inspection process. The company must determine if customer requirements are being met. Measures of conformance to program specifications will be developed and agreed to by all parties as part of the partnership agreements. Measures will be established for all specifications, including patient satisfaction, level of service, quality of care, cost and spending levels, and finally, health outcomes. Measures must be objective and quantitative. Where performance falls short of specification, corrective action plans will be developed and applied. The long-term goal is 100 percent conformance to specification — the true measure of quality.

Xerox is investing its resources in the development of these partnerships with the intention of building quality in at the front end. It hopes to increase the *value* of healthcare spending — not necessarily to spend less. If inefficiencies can be reduced and quality of care and health status can be improved, then future spending should be more manageable.

General Electric: Regional Healthcare Management

CHARLES R. BUCK, Jr., Sc.D., Staff Executive

Health Care Management Programs, General Electric Company, Fairfield, Connecticut

The organizational structure and strategy of GE's Health Care Management Program is based on three basic factors:

1. The healthcare system is organized regionally.
2. GE, to a large extent, is decentralized.
3. While healthcare purchasing must be tailored to each regional marketplace, there is a set of strategies, support activities, and expertise which is common across healthcare marketplaces.

GE AS A DECENTRALIZED ORGANIZATION

Like many large organizations, GE operates largely on a decentralized basis. This structure facilitates a region-specific approach to medical care purchasing. It also is a key to ensuring the active involvement of each GE business in local healthcare purchasing activities and in bringing critical employee relations and local healthcare marketplace issues to bear in structuring specific purchasing strategies.

Three of the most important elements of the healthcare management purchasing organization strategy are:

1. All actual medical care benefit costs for employees are directly charged to one of the 14 major GE businesses, such as GE Appliances, GE Lighting, and GE Aircraft Engines.
2. Each GE business has a lead healthcare manager.
3. The performance of each GE business in managing its healthcare costs is measured relative to other GE businesses and is reported to each business and to the CEO.

GE-WIDE STRATEGIES AND SUPPORT

The Corporate Health Care Management Program provides overall leadership for GE's medical care purchasing activities. Some of its main functions include:

1. A broad purchasing strategy which identifies a range of preferred approaches has been developed. This provides a framework within which local healthcare managers can shape specific strategies to take advantage of local healthcare marketplace opportunities and to meet immediate business requirements.
2. A companywide medical claims information system is maintained which incorporates all medical benefits claims. It is available, on-line, to all GE businesses for their direct use in analyzing local marketplace conditions such as overall hospital admission rates and hospital-specific prices.
3. Corporate healthcare managers work with local healthcare managers in partnership to develop and implement region-specific purchasing programs such as PPOs, managed mental health programs, and employee education programs.
4. One GE-wide medical benefits plan has been established. Negotiated changes to this plan are driven in part by the overall medical care purchasing strategy.
5. The medical claims information system is used to evaluate the results of regional purchasing strategies and the performance of specific vendors; the results of the evaluation are used in planning subsequent actions.
6. GE's medical benefits plan is administered by several carriers. They have been assigned to specific geographic areas to complement the regional purchasing strategy. Carriers are evaluated based on their support of regional purchasing activities in addition to the usual utilization and price controls and administrative activities.
7. Outlines for employee communication programs on healthcare issues are provided to the businesses.
8. GE undertakes a continual process of reviewing new programs being offered by vendors, new

strategies adopted by other companies, and "best practices" within GE regions. Successful programs are then communicated throughout GE's healthcare network.

9. Regional performance targets, usually in terms of projected savings, are negotiated with each healthcare manager, along with an action plan for implementation. They are used as a guide for ensuring and measuring overall progress.

REGION-BASED APPROACH TO PURCHASING

Within the overall corporate structure, there must be broad flexibility at the regional level to optimize healthcare purchasing. The relative strength of carriers, HMOs, PPOs, and other provider organizations and vendors varies greatly from region to region. The competitive situation and related employee relations issues vary greatly among GE businesses and by location. Similarly, GE's relative leverage in the marketplace varies in relation to GE's own size and the size of the marketplace in general. Thus, a great deal of flexibility is provided in selecting specific programs for implementation. However, the local programs have several uniform characteristics:

1. Each major GE business has a healthcare manager who generally reports to the manager of human resources.

2. These healthcare managers have the additional responsibility for regionwide GE purchasing in major GE locations where they represent the predominant GE business.

3. The healthcare managers manage the on-going relationships with local vendors, including HMOs and PPOs, and draw on support from the respective GE carrier for their particular region.

4. The local healthcare manager, in concert with local employee communicators, is looked to for leadership and coordination in shaping and implementing employee medical communications.

Programs implemented within this framework, such as managed mental health programs, managed care systems based on enrollment, and carrier changes based on local marketplace leverage, appear to be setting the stage for important cost savings. Those programs which succeed will be replicated in other settings where there are similar opportunities.

Tenneco: Select Provider Program

KAREN E. MILLER, Dr.P.H., Health Care Administrator

Tenneco Inc., Houston, Texas

Corporations generally manage healthcare by purchasing "prepackaged" programs, such as HMOs, PPOs, and utilization review, from an outside agent. Tenneco Inc., a conglomerate headquartered in Houston, took a different approach. It developed an in-house management program called the Select Provider Program (SPP), which provides access to specific medical services for cancer, heart disease, neurosurgical complaints, and psychological disorders in children and adolescents.

Developing and managing an in-house program is a formidable task. Although Tenneco's SPP is essentially a one-person operation, its development required the cooperation of the medical, benefits, finance, and legal departments. Support and acceptance from upper level management, providers, and employees were essential to its success. The program was designed to benefit all participating parties.

Over 250 subscribers have used the SPP in the last 4 years and perceive it as a bonus to the existing medical plan. They are directed to high quality medical care, and because the usual deductible and coinsurance are waived, all covered services are provided at no expense. There are no claims forms for subscribers to complete, as payments are handled directly between the providers and the insurance carrier. Employees are free to use other providers, but the copayments apply.

In exchange for price considerations, the providers are assured referrals and rapid payment of fees. Although no set volume of referrals is guaranteed, the SPP maintains or increases the providers' patient load.

Providers are chosen on the basis of quality and cost rather than on cost alone. If a corporation can demonstrate that it has diligently selected providers based on quality criteria, it can parry possible legal complications and minimize adverse employee relations. For instance, there is a strong positive correlation between the volume of certain surgical procedures performed by a hospital, such as coronary artery bypass, and better clinical outcomes. Contracting with such high-volume hospitals may lead to better results in terms of reduced mortality and morbidity rates, lengths of stay, and costs.

Since most managed care programs have an additional function of containing costs, below market fees can be negotiated. Tenneco has found, however, that high quality providers are often the less expensive providers because of their ability to manage healthcare services more efficiently. Analysis of the first 2 years of experience with the SPP revealed that significant savings from discounted fees and the cost-effectiveness of the providers were realized, especially in cardiovascular care. Tenneco determined that the average cost of coronary bypass surgery in the SPP was $16,500 in comparison to $30,000 for the same procedure performed outside of the program.

It is important to contract with physicians as well as hospitals in order to manage the total spectrum of care. Physicians should have the capacity to offer comprehensive, coordinated care and to make appropriate referrals when necessary. Some purchasers negotiate only with hospitals, leaving to chance the selection of physicians. This is not advisable since preferred hospitals can have both good and bad physicians on staff. Likewise, the quality of treatment of a preferred physician is highly dependent on the technology and staff of the admitting hospital. In some cases, an influential physician can assist in negotiations with the hospital, thereby facilitating the participation of all parties involved.

It may be necessary to develop more than one kind of reimbursement structure. Package pricing, an all-inclusive fee for a particular treatment such as coronary bypass, is basically limited to uncomplicated, elective surgeries. Since it is inevitable that an employee will require a procedure for which no set price exists or extensive services which fall outside the scope of the package price, it is essential to negotiate fee schedules to accommodate all possible situations. A discounted fee-for-service or per diem rate, for example, may work better for the treatment of complicated illnesses, such as cancer, which do not always follow a predetermined protocol. It is important not to deny employees access to the select providers because they do not "fit the mold."

Selective contracting must be incorporated into a managed care program. It is destined for failure if it is left to itself. An important determinant of success is the relationship between the providers and the corporation. A partnership must be formed which fosters open communication and trust. If all sides involved establish a symbiotic, rather than an adversarial, relationship they can better provide high quality medical care to the corporation's covered individuals.

CHAPTER SEVEN

Negotiation Strategies

THE NEGOTIATING PROCESS FOR MANAGED CARE PLANS AND PROVIDERS

ERIC R. WAGNER, Senior Manager
Price Waterhouse, Washington, D.C.

Managed care plans combine aspects of the financing and delivery of healthcare services into a single organization. In most cases, the mechanism for combining financing and delivery of services is through contractual agreements between the managed care plan* and providers† of healthcare services. These agreements must be negotiated and renegotiated, often on an annual basis.

The negotiating process is a very important factor in determining the success of managed care plans because the results of negotiations — the terms of its agreements with providers — largely determine whether the plan can compete successfully in the marketplace. A managed care plan that fails to obtain participation agreements from a sufficient number of providers or that fails to negotiate favorable reimbursement arrangements with its providers will find it very difficult to attain its financial and market objectives.

This chapter provides an overview of the negotiating process, including competing theories and components of negotiating, and describes the negotiating process from the different perspectives of the managed care plan and the provider.

---

*The term "managed care plan" encompasses HMOs, PPOs, insurance companies, and employers who contract directly with providers.

†The term "provider" encompasses physicians, hospitals, nursing homes, and other institutional and professional providers of healthcare services.

OVERVIEW OF THE NEGOTIATING PROCESS

The negotiating process has been described as having the following characteristics:

- A give and take between two or more parties
- A friction or level of discomfort between the parties resulting from the constraints and motivations of the parties
- An important issue that the parties wish to resolve
- Conflict between the positions of the parties to the negotiations[1]

In the context of negotiating managed care provider agreements, parties approaching the bargaining table have only one factor in common—the desire to provide healthcare services to a particular population. This common need is the factor that spurs negotiations. Overall, the parties are in conflict over most of the details concerning the provision of those services. The managed care plan seeks to spend as little as possible for this obligation, while the providers seek to maximize their reimbursements. The myriad terms and conditions that constitute a provider agreement place many obstacles in the path of the parties who are attempting to forge an agreement.

Levels of reimbursement, timing of payments, exclusivity provisions, and patient volumes are aspects of potential agreements that heighten frictions between the parties and are capable of scuttling once-promising negotiations. Given these predictable sources of conflict, managed care agreements can be reached by accommodation of the parties. Each party must approach negotiations with the expectation of giving and taking for the mutual benefit of the parties. Truly successful negotiations result in the parties believing that they fared as well as they could expect considering their relative constraints.

The effectiveness of negotiations results from a combination of the styles of the negotiators and the way in which they prepare for negotiations.

Negotiating Styles

Those who have been involved in any form of negotiations, from purchasing a car or home to negotiating complex agreements, know that there are a variety of styles and tactics used by negotiators. Some negotiators appear to combine different styles and tactics during a single negotiation as they evaluate and adapt themselves to the needs of the moment. Although preparations for negotiation are usually the key factor in determining success, the style or tactics employed during negotiations can also have a major influence on the outcome.

Negotiators tend to use one of two broad types of style: confrontational or collegial. Many negotiators believe that an aggressive and confrontational approach is appropriate. These negotiators tend to focus on the real or perceived differences between the parties at the bargaining table. Negotiators may be particularly aggressive when the party they represent is perceived by both sides to be dominant.

Confrontational negotiators often overlook the fact that the parties are attempting to reach an agreement that will govern their ongoing relationship. A confrontational and overly aggressive approach can poison the relationship between the plan and its providers from the outset and lead to long-term distrust between the parties.

One example of problems that can arise from applying a confrontational approach is provided by Maxicare Health Plans, which used this style in its negotiations with providers. Those same providers were unwilling to give Maxicare any consideration when it encountered financial difficulties. Perhaps the situation would have been different if Maxicare had chosen to pursue a less-combative negotiating style.

The second negotiating style seeks a collegial relationship where the negotiators attempt to build a consensus between the parties through the give and take of negotiations. This style is well suited to the concept that the outcome of the negotiations (that is, the agreement) represents the beginning of the relationship between the managed care plan and its providers.

A collegial style does not imply that negotiators are weak or that they give up important positions without a valid quid pro quo. It does mean that the dominant party refrains from unilaterally imposing its position on its opponent. It also means that the negotiating sessions themselves are conducted in a cordial fashion and that the negotiators try not to allow personality conflicts to influence the outcome of negotiations.

Negotiating style also encompasses such issues as the number of people who should participate in the negotiations and whether the negotiators have the power to bind the party they represent.

Some negotiators believe that they should bring a team to the negotiating table. There are definite advantages to a team approach, including a division of labor and the ability to add special expertise to the negotiating process. A team of two people is ideal for many negotiations. One person can direct the negotiations and serve as the spokesperson for the team while the other person can take good notes of the discussion and agreements reached during meetings. Care must be taken in forming the team to make it clear that only the chief negotiator can articulate the team's positions to the other party.

The team approach generally should not be used if the other party is represented by one individual. The danger of using a team approach against a single negotiator is that the other party may feel as though the team is attempting to gain dominance through numbers. These feelings can create an adversarial atmosphere. On the other hand, the team approach works very successfully if both parties agree at the outset to use this approach.

Some successful negotiators have advocated what they view as a completely different style of negotiations. Instead of bargaining over the *positions* of the parties, these commentators believe that negotiations should be *principled* and should take place on the merits of the issues.[2] To accomplish this goal, the following is advocated:

- Separate the people from the problem.
- Focus on the interests of the parties, not on their positions.
- Generate a variety of possibilities for solutions before agreeing on a particular solution.
- Agree to apply an objective standard for selecting the appropriate solution.[3]

One benefit of the principled method of negotiation is that it eliminates the problem of confrontational versus collegial styles of negotiating. Both parties are attempting to reach a common goal of attaining the best possible solution. The principled method can also foster the sense that agreement between the parties represents the beginning of a relationship and not the end of a disagreement.

One example of using an "objective standard" is an agreement between a hospital and an HMO that the hospital is entitled to a "fair" level of return, or contribution margin, from its HMO patients and that the HMO is entitled to reimbursement rates that are no less favorable than offered to other, similarly situated payers. The fair level of return could be defined as the hospital's average contribution margin per patient day for all classes of patients. Once these objective standards were agreed upon, the HMO and the hospital could determine whether various combinations of reimbursement rates and exclusivity provisions would satisfy the standards. The focus on these standards can help both parties to understand one another's concerns.

Preparing to Negotiate

Lack of adequate preparation is cited frequently as a reason for failed negotiations. Fortunately, this key success factor is within the control of negotiators. Preparation for negotiations should include developing an understanding of the organization's goals and objectives, understanding the other party's goals and objectives, drafting a proposal, preparing the negotiating team, and conducting the negotiations.

UNDERSTANDING THE ORGANIZATION'S GOALS AND OBJECTIVES It sounds self-evident that a negotiator should understand the goals and objectives of the organization he or she represents. In many cases, the negotiator is a high-level executive with the organization and thus should be intimately familiar with its goals and objectives. Perhaps because of this sense of familiarity, however, some negotiators fail to formally clarify their organization's objectives before entering into direct negotiations. The organization's goals and objectives should be reviewed prior to beginning negotiations so that all internal participants have a common understanding.

The following issues should be considered to develop an understanding:

- What does the organization hope to accomplish through the negotiations? A complete list of the items the organization hopes to gain from the negotiations should be prepared and the value of each item should be assessed. This "wish list" will serve as a guide during the give and take of negotiations. Some examples of motivations for managed care negotiations include:

  A physician who has recently moved into a community may want to attract patients covered by HMOs or PPOs in the area to help build the practice.

  A hospital may want to obtain a participation agreement with a managed care plan to preclude its competitor from negotiating an exclusive agreement.

  A PPO may want to obtain the participation of a specific hospital because certain employer groups have told the PPO that they will not offer it as a benefit option if the hospital is not included on the provider panel.

- What are the organization's strengths and weaknesses, and how will they affect negotiations? Organizations almost always view themselves favorably and convey this positive impression to their outside negotiators. This can leave their negotiators unprepared to confront the organization's weaknesses as they are presented by the other party. The negotiator must understand both the strengths and the weaknesses of the organization because the other party will have uncovered many of the weaknesses during its preparations. An understanding of the weaknesses can also help place the emphasis on offsetting strengths during discussions with the other party.
- What is the "corporate culture" of the organization and how will this affect its relationship with the other party? Is the organization perceived as trustworthy by its employees and outsiders or as overly aggressive and always seeking to achieve its own advantage regardless of the impact on other parties? Does the organization give meaningful authority to its line managers or is all power centralized with a few top executives? These factors will influence how negotiations are conducted, how the other party reacts to

proposals, and whether the negotiator is perceived as credible by the other party.

- What is the organization's "bottom line" for negotiations and how much is it willing to give up to obtain an agreement? This issue must be discussed before commencing negotiations so that management is not forced to address the issue during the heat of the negotiations. The negotiator must be given a clear picture of how much the organization is willing to give up and what it wants in return.

An alternative to determining the bottom line is to understand the organization's "best alternative to a negotiated agreement" (or BATNA).[4] Instead of focusing on an artificially defined bottom line, the BATNA addresses the issue of what the organization's options are if agreement is not reached. For example, a managed care plan might see the alternative to failing to negotiate an exclusive agreement with one hospital in a community at favorable rates is to obtain agreements with several other hospitals at slightly higher rates. The inclusion of these other hospitals may allow the plan to be marketed more successfully, generate higher enrollment, and provide higher margins. These issues should be considered by the plan in defining its BATNA.

UNDERSTANDING THE OTHER PARTY'S GOALS AND OBJECTIVES Good negotiators attempt to understand as much about the other party's goals and objectives as they do about their own organization's. While gaining this understanding is more difficult, it can be accomplished through review of publicly available information about the other party. A good negotiator will attempt to view the issues from the other party's vantage point.

The issues described for understanding the negotiator's organization should also be evaluated for the other party. One important issue to consider is the other party's strengths and weaknesses and how they may affect the relationship. A more effective proposal can be prepared if it specifically includes solutions to offset the other party's weaknesses.

For example, a PPO may be attempting to offer its services to employers throughout a metropolitan area. Employers may be reluctant to offer the PPO because its panel of providers does not include a well-regarded hospital within a geographic area where many of their employees reside. A well-regarded hospital within that area would have an opportunity to offset a major shortcoming of the PPO by offering its participation. In return, the hospital could demand higher payment rates than other hospitals within the metropolitan area.

In summary, a good negotiator should understand as much as

possible about the other party before beginning discussions. This understanding is important for preparing an attractive proposal and for conducting the negotiations. At the same time, however, the negotiator should listen carefully during discussions to ensure that new information offered by the other party is incorporated into the proposals.

THE NEGOTIATING TEAM In preparing for negotiations, the identification and preparation of the negotiating team is an important success factor. The first step in this process is to identify who will be members of the negotiating team.

From the provider's perspective, contracting with a managed care plan is largely a financial issue, so the negotiations tend to focus on financial issues. As a result, most providers should plan to include their chief financial officer on their negotiating team.

Some providers have so many managed care agreements that they have appointed a vice president for managed care. This person should clearly be included on the negotiating team. Other providers have little experience with negotiating third party agreements and infrequently conduct negotiations. For these providers, it is both valuable and cost-effective to include consultants and lawyers who specialize in managed care. Such outside advisers can bring broad experience to bear on negotiating the few managed care agreements required by the provider.

Larger institutional providers may find it useful to include internal legal counsel to help other members of the team understand the legal issues surrounding potential agreements. In addition, counsel often can provide an objective view of proposals put forward by the other side.

Managed care plans typically include their provider relations personnel on the negotiating team because they are expected to understand the local marketplace and the concerns of the provider community. Many plans also include at least one financial staff member because of the impact that reimbursement rates have on premium rates and financial results. Some managed care plans include their chief executive officer on the negotiating team, at least at some meetings, to demonstrate the importance of the agreement to the plan.

The negotiating team's preparation should include thorough review of the parameters of the proposal, acceptable trade-offs, and an understanding of the alternatives available to the other party. If discussions are being held to renegotiate a current agreement, the team should review all aspects of the existing agreement to determine problems caused by the current agreement, changes that should be made, and changes that are likely to be requested by the other party.

During preparations, the negotiating team must clearly define the agenda for the negotiations for both the team as a whole and for individual members. The role of each member of the team should be specified. Weak negotiating positions can result if team members decide to "play it by ear" during the negotiating sessions.

Limits of authority should be established for each member of the team to define the extent to which they are allowed to set forth the organization's positions, make counteroffers, or critique the other party's proposals. The team must try to avoid that sinking feeling that comes when a member of the team becomes a "loose cannon" who makes overly generous offers or unsupported statements. The process of defining the role and authority of each team member during negotiations helps make them aware of the organization's expectations for performance. Members of the team will perform better when they understand their performance expectations.

While preparing, members of the team should familiarize themselves with the characteristics of the other party's negotiators. The team members can research the positions and roles of the other party's negotiators, their professional backgrounds and training, the universities or graduate schools they attended, and their philosophical approaches. Some of this information may be available through professional directories,[5] while other information can be obtained by talking with colleagues who have dealt with the other party's team members. Books, articles, and presentations by members of the other party's negotiating team may also provide insights into their styles or philosophies.

Understanding of the other team's characteristics can help during the negotiations in several ways. First, it allows anticipation of the style of negotiations that will be used by the other party. Adjustments in approach can be made in response to this information. Second, better predictions can be made about the other team's focus for negotiations. For example, if the other team includes legal counsel, it would be safe to assume that a major part of the negotiations will revolve around terms and conditions of the resulting agreement. With this knowledge, it would be appropriate to add a lawyer to the team (if counsel has not already been included). Finally, identification of common interests or backgrounds (for example, the same graduate school) can allow negotiators to establish a better working relationship and foster more congenial communications.

CONDUCTING THE NEGOTIATIONS One of the first decisions about conducting negotiations concerns the location. Some people believe that in negotiations, as in real estate, the three most important factors are "location, location, and location." While the site for negotiations can be important, it usually will not be the decisive factor in success or failure.

Nevertheless, the selection of an appropriate site can provide one side or the other with a slight advantage. In most cases, it is preferable to have a "home-field advantage." Team members typically are more comfortable in familiar surroundings, and this increased comfort level can provide a small edge in conducting the negotiations. It would be a mistake, however, to fight a protracted battle to have negotiations conducted at a favored location. A fight over location will distract both parties from the primary reason for their discussions and could poison the atmosphere for the substantive negotiations.

It is very important to probe for the limits of the other team's authority early during negotiations. Some parties to negotiations believe that they should not allow their representatives to bind them to agreements. Instead, they maintain that their negotiators should convey to the other party that they have to clear all agreements with a "higher authority" before the agreements are binding. This technique is intended to provide a safety valve for rejecting agreements after they are examined more closely. Some negotiators only reveal that they must appeal to a higher authority after they have obtained significant concessions from the other party, thereby giving themselves a "second bite at the apple."[6]

Unfortunately, most negotiators expect that the other party will be able to conduct a give-and-take exchange without checking each point with an outside authority. Otherwise, negotiations could be conducted more easily by an exchange of letters. Both parties will probably make final agreement subject to corporate approval, but approval should be based on the entire package, not on every individual point covered during the negotiations.

Both negotiating teams should maintain accurate records of the discussions. If the team includes more than one person, one member should be designated to take notes. The notes should reflect the following information:

- Date and location of the negotiating session.
- Names and titles of all participants and observers.
- Salient terms of all proposals that are made by either party, including who made the proposal.
- Key points made during discussions of proposals, including who made the points.
- Agreements made by the parties, including conditions and contingencies related to the agreements.
- Areas of disagreement between the parties.

The records of the negotiating sessions are valuable for at least two reasons. First, they will allow the parties to draft documents that accurately implement the agreements reached during negotiations.

Second, they may be useful if the parties become involved in litigation concerning the agreements or negotiations. In this context, the record of negotiations may be subject to the discovery process and could be available to the other party. They may also be released in open court and available to the general public. For these reasons, notes taken during negotiating sessions should be as factual as possible and should not express opinions that could be damaging or embarrassing if they were released in public.

It is often helpful to prepare a written proposal for distribution at the initial negotiating session. A written outline establishes a framework and baseline for future negotiations; future offers and counteroffers are made in the context of the initial proposal. The outline can set the tone for the balance of negotiations. The proposal should outline the organization's position on all issues subject to the negotiations.

NEGOTIATING FROM THE MANAGED CARE PLAN'S PERSPECTIVE

An important success factor in negotiations is understanding the positions and motivations of the other party. The following information is presented to help providers understand negotiations from the managed care plan's perspective. In addition, the information may be helpful for managed care plans that have limited experience in negotiating agreements with providers.

Objectives of Negotiations

The typical managed care plan has four major objectives for its negotiations with providers:

- Acceptable provider panel
- Reasonable reimbursement
- Framework for future relationship
- Favorable contractual terms

ACCEPTABLE PROVIDER PANEL What constitutes an "acceptable" provider panel varies with the type of managed care plan involved and the type of product offered. For example, an acceptable provider panel will be very different for a network model HMO versus a nongatekeeper model PPO. The PPO will probably seek to include many more physicians and hospitals in its network than the HMO because choice of providers will be more important to its product. The most important factors include:

- *Availability* Are all services covered by the plan available through its panel of participating providers? This factor may limit the ability of some providers to demand exclusivity if they are unable to provide all covered services under their exclusive arrangement.

- *Accessibility* Are the services offered by participating providers accessible to the plan's covered beneficiaries? The plan's view of what constitutes accessible varies depending on the type of plan. In general, however, routine services would not be considered accessible if patients were required to travel more than 30 minutes to a provider. This factor may also limit the ability of providers to demand exclusive arrangements with managed care plans.
- *Specialty coverage* Most managed care plans attempt to negotiate participation agreements with physicians representing all major specialties and subspecialties.
- *Perceived quality* Despite the difficulties inherent in measuring quality, managed care plans attempt to align themselves with providers who enjoy good reputations. Conversely, significant price concessions may not be sufficient to entice a managed care plan to align itself with a provider that is perceived to deliver a lower quality of care. The bottom line is that the perceived level of provider quality may influence the reimbursement levels offered by a plan.

REASONABLE REIMBURSEMENT The definition of reasonable reimbursement largely depends on whether it is being viewed from the perspective of the managed care plan or the provider. From the managed care plan's vantage point, reasonable reimbursement generally has two qualities:

- Reimbursement rates should be set as low as possible.
- Reimbursement amounts should be predictable.

There are definite trade-offs between predictability and rates. For example, a plan might project that its members will use 350 days per year of inpatient hospital care per 1000 members. If a hospital offers to provide care for a $750 per diem reimbursement, the plan would expect inpatient hospital costs of $21.88 per member per month. Under this system, the plan would be at risk if the actual number of days of care exceeded the expected number of days.

Because of this risk, the plan might decide to accept a capitated proposal from the same hospital of $22.50 per member per month. Although the expected value of the capitated arrangement would exceed the expected value of the per diem arrangement, the capitated arrangement results in more predictable costs for the plan. In this case, the plan would do better under capitation if actual patient days exceeded the expected number of days by 10 days per 1000 members (a variance of less than 3 percent). Naturally, any proposal will be evaluated by the plan in the context of its premium rates.

FRAMEWORK FOR FUTURE RELATIONSHIP   Most plan managers would prefer to establish longer-term relationships with their providers. Renegotiating all the salient points of provider agreements requires personnel and produces friction. Annual changes of reimbursement rates and service terms may mean climbing and unpredictable costs for the plan. Plan members and their employers resent interruptions in the doctor-patient relationship that result from changes in the provider panel. As a result, most plans hope to establish long-term relationships with providers when they negotiate participation agreements.

FAVORABLE CONTRACTUAL TERMS   Another objective of negotiations for managed care plans is to obtain favorable contractual terms with participating providers. Plans usually propose terms where the providers must agree to the following:

* Abide by and cooperate with the plan's utilization management and quality assurance protocols.
* Look solely to the managed care plan for the payment of claims, even in the event of insolvency (the provider "hold-harmless" clause). This provision is often required by state regulations.
* Submit claims in a format that is acceptable to the plan.
* Continue serving the plan's members after termination until the anniversary date of the member's group agreement.
* Refrain from encouraging the plan's beneficiaries to change coverage to another plan.
* Refrain from derogatory speech and publicity concerning the plan and its sponsors.
* Use binding arbitration to resolve disputes between the provider and patients or the plan.

This list is representative but not exhaustive of the possible terms.

Negotiating Styles

Managed care plans tend to adopt one of two opposite styles in conducting their negotiations. The first style can be characterized as "provider bashing" and confrontational. The second style can be characterized as either "provider friendly" or neutral.

CONFRONTATIONAL   Some managed care plans have adopted a very aggressive and confrontational approach to negotiations with providers. These plans behave as if the providers will be devastated if they fail to obtain an agreement with the plan. In many cases, these plans try to influence the provider's negotiating position by emphasizing the number of individuals for whom they provide coverage and may threaten the provider with a loss of these patients. These plans tend to overstate the extent of their market clout.

As an example, when a large indemnity insurance carrier was in the process of establishing its PPO, it emphasized the number of employees and dependents it covered in particular service areas during negotiations with potential providers. In fact, the insurer did cover an impressive number of beneficiaries. What the insurer did not focus on, however, was that only a small proportion of these covered beneficiaries would be shifted into its PPO product. The PPO product design did not contain strong incentives for beneficiaries to use participating instead of nonparticipating providers. Consequently, the insurer greatly overstated the market impact of its PPO during negotiations with providers. The providers were disappointed by the patient volume delivered by the PPO and were unwilling to extend large discounts in subsequent years.

The negotiator's rationale for using a confrontational approach is that there is sufficient provider competition within the market area. Thus, if one provider is antagonized during negotiations, other providers are available. When provider "good will" is lacking, the result can be devastating to the plan, as Maxicare discovered during its negotiations with medical groups and hospitals. The unwillingness of Maxicare's providers to extend further credit or good faith to Maxicare was a factor in the plan's bankruptcy.

NEUTRAL The neutral or provider-friendly approach, which is compatible with the collegial approach described earlier, has been adopted by many plans for their negotiations with providers. The neutral approach is consistent with the plan's objective of establishing longer-term relationships with its providers. The basis for such relationships is mutual trust and respect, not intimidation and antagonism.

Negotiating Tactics

Regardless of the negotiating style, there are a variety of tactics used by managed care plans to negotiate favorable agreements. These include the following:

- *Threat of competing proposals* The managed care plan may indicate either explicitly or implicitly that competing proposals on the table offer more advantages to the plan. Sometimes such proposals exist, but often this threat is a bluff intended to obtain more favorable pricing terms.
- *Threat of lost market share and reduced income* Plans may threaten to move their covered patients to other providers if the

parties fail to reach agreement. It is important for providers to understand the implications of this threat prior to entering negotiations by assessing the number of patients covered by the plan, what those patients contributed to the provider, and whether the plan can actually move the patients to other providers. Unrealistic threats can then be deflected at the bargaining table.

- *Whip-sawing providers*   Some managed care plans play hospitals and physicians against one another in an attempt to get one or the other to participate despite their reluctance. Plans have recruited key physicians from a hospital's medical staff and then forced the hospital's participation at reduced reimbursement rates. This tactic can be avoided when hospitals and physicians work closely together on their managed care relationships.

- *"Last chance" offers*   Managed care plans sometimes indicate to providers during negotiations that this will be their last chance to participate with the plan. Even though the plan currently may not have many covered individuals, the plan implies that if the provider fails to participate immediately at favorable rates, then the provider cannot participate when the plan becomes successful.

- *Use of information*   Some managed care plans prepare detailed analyses of provider cost and/or charge information for their market areas before they commence negotiations. For example, one large insurance company prepared for each market area briefing books that contained charge information by Diagnosis-Related Group (DRG) and payer for each hospital in the area. Their analysis projected the number of their patients who would fall into each DRG category and what their total costs of care would be based on the use of different hospitals in the market area. This sophisticated information allowed them to evaluate and counter proposals by hospitals that had been accepted by other, similarly sized payers.

NEGOTIATING FROM THE PROVIDER'S PERSPECTIVE

Just as it was important for both managed care plans and providers to review negotiations from the perspective of managed care plans, it is important to examine the objectives, styles, and tactics for negotiations from the perspective of providers.

Objectives of Negotiations

Providers usually have one or more of the following objectives for their negotiations with managed care plans:

- Market share
- Competition among managed care plans
- Satisfaction of other provider needs

- Favorable reimbursement
- Framework for future relationship
- Favorable contractual terms

MARKET SHARE Many providers view participation with managed care plans as a mechanism to protect or expand market share and the income associated with managed care patients. These providers fear that if they fail to participate with certain plans, they will lose some of their patient base. Other providers view managed care plans as a way of attracting new patients and expanding their market share. Generally, these providers insist on some measure of exclusivity as a way of guaranteeing that they will receive incremental patient volume (that is, patients who otherwise would not have used their services).

COMPETITION AMONG MANAGED CARE PLANS Some providers believe that they should participate with as many managed care plans as possible to prevent any single plan from becoming as dominant a player in their market area as Blue Cross has been in many markets.

SATISFACTION OF OTHER PROVIDER NEEDS Hospitals sometimes participate with managed care plans because their physicians have joined and need to admit their patients to participating hospitals. This objective is related to preventing loss of market share; the hospitals that participate to satisfy their physicians' needs do so to protect their own loss of market share if their physicians were to move their practices to other facilities.

FAVORABLE REIMBURSEMENT From the provider's perspective, favorable reimbursement means maximizing rates and enhancing predictability. In contrast to the managed care plan's perspective, predictability to the provider implies a fee-for-service–based reimbursement approach with prompt payment.

FRAMEWORK FOR FUTURE RELATIONSHIP Providers would prefer to consider their relationships with managed care plans on a longer-term basis. Assuming that other aspects of a provider's relationship with a plan are satisfactory, it is desirable not to have to continually renegotiate agreements and fight over terms and conditions. As a result, an important objective is to provide a satisfactory framework for the future relationship between the provider and the plan.

FAVORABLE CONTRACTUAL TERMS Another objective of providers is to obtain participation agreements with favorable contractual terms. Among the desirable terms are the following agreements by the managed care plan:

- Work within the provider's established policies and procedures for implementing utilization management and quality assurance activities.
- Pay undisputed claims within 30 days or less.
- Obtain consent of the provider before using the provider's name in marketing material.
- Minimize the involvement of hospital personnel in implementing the managed care plan's procedures.
- Eliminate the managed care plan's ability to retroactively deny legitimate claims.
- Provide adequate protection for the provider in the event of insolvency.

Negotiating Styles

The negotiating styles used by providers for their relationships with managed care plans fall into three broad categories:

- Nonexistent
- Emotional
- Objective

NONEXISTENT   The provider with a nonexistent negotiating style simply signs all, or virtually all, managed care participation agreements that are offered. In many cases, these providers believe they do not have sufficient market clout to force legitimate negotiation on issues of importance to them. Many of these providers believe that any business is good business.

Unfortunately, providers who fail to negotiate before signing agreements may be giving up important concessions that they could retain. Most managed care plans are willing to bargain about some aspects of their participation agreements (for example, utilization management procedures), even with providers holding little power. The provider's failure to negotiate may send the message that plans can take advantage of the provider. In the long run, this message will place the provider in an even weaker position.

EMOTIONAL   Some providers react to proposals by managed care plans in an emotional fashion. They view requests for discounts and imposition of utilization management and quality assurance programs as affronts to their expertise and honesty. In some cases, these providers insist on their positions out of a sense of righteousness.

Emotional negotiators generally do not achieve good results for their organizations. Most successful negotiations require both parties to view the other's proposals somewhat objectively. An emotional style does not facilitate the give and take required during negotiations.

OBJECTIVE The objective negotiating style corresponds to the collegial approach advocated by many successful negotiators. It requires the negotiators to separate themselves from the issues at hand and to evaluate proposals based on their merits. Objectivity follows preparation of relevant business data.

Providers who adopt an objective style of negotiations typically evaluate participation proposals from many managed care plans. Each proposal is assessed based on its relative benefits and is accepted if it offers business advantages to the provider.

Negotiating Tactics Providers adopt many different tactics in their attempts to gain negotiating advantages. The following negotiating tactics are among those used by providers:

- *Joint physician-hospital negotiations* Some hospitals have formed joint ventures with their medical staffs for the purpose of participating with managed care plans. These provider groups, which may be known as MeSHs (medical staff–hospital organizations), PHOs (physician-hospital organizations), CPUs (combined provider units), or LPUs (local provider units), are intended to blunt the ability of managed care plans to whip-saw providers by negotiating separately with hospitals and physicians. The combined provider unit evaluates and negotiates participation arrangements for both the hospital and the affiliated physicians concurrently.
- *Use of information* Some providers prepare their own analyses of the alternatives available to the managed care plan in an attempt to predict the offers that will be made by competing providers. For example, a hospital negotiating with a PPO sponsored by a large insurance company prepared an extensive analysis of charges and utilization by DRG for itself and for competing hospitals. This hospital was able to prepare a proposal that met the needs of the PPO and could demonstrate, using actual utilization data and the proposed rates, that its proposal was superior to other offers.
- *Threats not to participate* Some providers have sufficient market clout that their lack of participation can place a managed care plan at a competitive disadvantage in the market. These providers use the threat of not participating as a means of obtaining concessions from the plan.
- *Analysis of the managed care plan* Some providers use analysis of the managed care plan to their advantage during negotiations.

One example of this technique is the analysis of financial statements and premium rate requests filed by HMOs with state regulators. Among the items that can be estimated from these reports is the average amount paid by the HMO to hospital providers for inpatient care. Hospitals have used this information to their advantage during negotiations when representatives of the HMO claimed that their average hospital payments were below the hospital's proposal. The hospitals were able to respond by showing that the HMO's own reports indicated that the amounts were much higher. The use of this information allowed some hospitals to obtain higher reimbursement rates, which more than offset the cost of obtaining and analyzing the regulatory reports.

Providers are most successful in their negotiations with managed care plans when they adopt an objective and collegial negotiating style in combination with tactics that rely on the analysis of information about their competition and about the managed care plan.

CONCLUSION At the base of negotiating participation agreements between managed care plans and providers is conflict. For many, the process of negotiating an agreement is a learning experience. Managed care plans and providers alike discover their own requirements and attitudes while they explore their bargaining positions. As negotiations occur, parties may strike, alter, and abandon several positions. Changes in bargaining positions may result from manipulative forethought, but may just as well be rational reaction to both self-discovery and dialog among the parties.

The way to resolve the basic conflict and to forge agreements between managed care plans and providers is to seek an agreement that allows all concerned parties to believe that they are faring as well as they have a right to expect. This collegial approach means the parties must set aside their customary desire to score big against their "opponents." Each party must attempt to understand and accommodate the fundamental needs of the other. Where all parties are at least content with the terms, an agreement can result. Satisfied parties are easier to deal with during the life of an agreement. They treat the end-users of their services better than they might otherwise. And contented parties are apt to renew their agreements from year to year.

The likelihood of finding satisfactory terms is increased enormously with proper preparation for negotiations. Preparation starts with identifying the organization's own needs, constraints, and corporate climate. It then proceeds to selecting negotiators who can function effectively when confronted by aggressive parties. Following that, preparation means understanding external parameters such as market conditions and the needs and constraints of the opposing party. It also means knowing in advance what tactics are legitimate and what defenses are feasible. Finally, proper preparation means knowing when the proposed terms of an agreement are too onerous to live by. Negotiators must not commit to an agreement because they believe that any business arrangement is better than no business.

REFERENCES

1. Donald B. Sparks, *The Dynamics of Effective Negotiation.* Gulf Publishing, Houston, 1982), pp. 3–5.

2. Roger Fisher and William Ury, *Getting to Yes.* Penguin Books, New York 1986, p. 11.

3. Ibid.

4. Ibid., p. 104.

5. One example is the *Biographical Directory of the Membership*, published by the American College of Healthcare Executives.

6. Fisher and Ury, op cit., p. 138.

New England Medical Center: Negotiating Contracts with HMOs

LYNNE J. EICKHOLT, Director of Managed Care

PETER VAN ETTEN, Executive Vice President, Chief Financial Officer

New England Medical Center Hospitals, Boston, Massachusetts

New England Medical Center (NEMC) is a 460-bed tertiary care facility with a full array of pediatric and adult residency and research programs. The hospital is closely affiliated with the Tufts University School of Medicine. Located in downtown Boston, NEMC competes with five other major teaching hospitals affiliated with Harvard Medical School and one hospital affiliated with the Boston University School of Medicine. All are high-cost teaching and research centers; however, NEMC is more expensive than some because it maintains a comprehensive teaching program on a relatively small bed base.

Competition among these hospitals is fueled by a state rate control system that severely limits hospital price increases but richly rewards volume increases. Competition for patients has intensified over the past few years as the population enrolled in managed care in Massachusetts approaches 25 percent and these organizations increasingly negotiate exclusive deals with hospitals in return for discounts. Managed care business will probably continue to rise sharply as indemnity plan premiums in this market increased 40 to 60 percent in 1989.

PAST EXPERIENCE WITH MANAGED CARE CONTRACTS

Several years ago, NEMC began to aggressively pursue managed care referrals with the belief that this would be the key to future growth in a competitive market. The hospital presently has 17 managed care contracts, and 16 percent of its admissions are gener-ated by these contracts, up from 9 percent 3 years ago. Most of the hospital's growth in admissions during 1989 resulted from increased managed care admissions.

One of NEMC's principal strategies has been to play a key role in establishing Tufts Associated Health Plan (TAHP), a network individual practice association (IPA) affiliated with 16 community hospitals located throughout eastern Massachusetts. NEMC is the sole tertiary facility in the network and has the largest and fastest growing IPA in the network. Admissions from this HMO constitute over 6 percent of the hospital's activity. NEMC has recognized, however, that the hospital must aggressively market to competitors of TAHP since it is unlikely that TAHP will be able to provide the significant number of tertiary referrals needed to fill NEMC's beds. Moreover, the hospital has realized that to capture and retain market share, relationships should be established that go further than simply offering discounts that could be met by other hospitals.

Another key strategy has been to develop a management information system that has enabled NEMC to examine all aspects of the hospital's activities including costs of services and patterns of care. By understanding marginal costs, the hospital can effectively price services and adjust practice patterns to become more cost competitive. The information system also enables the hospital to include practice pattern changes as part of the annual budget process and to closely monitor activity on a concurrent or monthly basis.

Still another strategy has been to concentrate on contracts with IPAs rather than with closed-panel or staff-model HMOs. IPAs of particular interest have been those affiliated with group practice plans. If a doctor with a large number of fee-for-service patients could be induced to refer their IPA patients to NEMC, it seemed likely that the doctor might also be interested in sending fee-for-service patients to NEMC. NEMC can then afford to give significant discounts to attract IPA patients if other patients with more favorable insurance might come to NEMC as well.

NEMC was the first hospital in the state to offer a number of innovative contracts, including discounts for volume, fixed-price packages for various surgical procedures including physician fees, and capitation agreements to handle all the tertiary business from one HMO. The results of these efforts were generally successful as NEMC's volume has grown compared to other teaching hospitals and the institution has a balanced referral base in that it is not dependent on one HMO. Knowledge of the hospital's costs has given NEMC negotiators more credibility than representatives of other hospitals. In a number of cases HMOs chose to sign contracts with NEMC rather than a competitor who offered to match NEMC's price because the HMO had confidence that since NEMC understood the hospital's costs, NEMC would not undercut a competitor to gain a contract and then significantly raise prices once the HMO had marketed its relationship with the hospital.

CHANGES IN CONTRACTING STRATEGIES

Recently NEMC has reevaluated the hospital's managed care contract strategy. The innovative programs described previously only involved a small portion of total HMO referrals. Managed care contractors complained about the hospital's standard contracting system, a combination of per diem rates and of percentage of charges for blood, operating room, and pharmacy, which HMOs found unpredictable. Moreover, as the hospital improved its cost effectiveness and reduced length of stay, the per diem system often resulted in less revenue for NEMC, even when the per diem payments increased.

During contract negotiations, the hospital discovered its fixed prices for cardiac surgery admissions were higher than some other hospitals by about $3000 per case. An additional concern to HMOs was that the hospital exempted patients from the fixed price based on subjective postsurgical clinical criteria such as neurological catastrophes or renal insufficiency, which some HMOs found difficult to interpret or to monitor. Several other Boston hospitals had established fixed prices, whereas NEMC billed a combination of per diems and ancillary charges. The hospital had stopped taking on the risk of fixed prices for various procedures, such as major joint replacements, because the volume did not seem to warrant it. To address these problems and continue to attract profitable managed care business, NEMC has crafted a new strategy for managed care contracting.

NEMC'S FIXED PRICE STRATEGY

1. Be proactive—by, for example, taking on risk for high-cost high-volume procedures or diagnoses and for episodes of illness rather than just one inpatient admission.

Hospitals have traditionally avoided risk—viewing a contract based on percentage of charges as the most desirable relationship with HMOs. Medicare Diagnostic Related Groups (DRGs) are viewed as an unfortunate reality and a fact of life, acceptable only because of the power and volume delivered by the federal government. However, the risk of fixed prices offers the opportunity for profit that a charge system does not. Risk commands a higher rate of reimbursement. The savings from cost-effective innovations in treatment are retained by the healthcare organization that developed them, not captured by the payer. Another benefit of accepting risk is in the reduction of utilization review over length of stay and ancillary resource use.

Finally, contracts based on risk-sharing forged a closer relationship between provider and HMO that could not be easily upset by another hospital offering discounts, often below cost to gain market share.

For these reasons NEMC began to examine how to develop more innovative fixed-price packages, targeting several high-cost illnesses over the entire course of treatment. Initially, these include transplants, adult and pediatric leukemia, and neonatal care. One of the most aggressive efforts by NEMC was to package 2 years of treatment for pediatric patients with acute lymphocytic leukemia (ALL). This package would include anywhere from one to ten inpatient episodes, routine outpatient maintenance, all professional fees, and even home health, if necessary. ALL treatment costs over 2 years can be quite high—in the range of $120,000 to $250,000, or even more if the child requires a bone marrow transplant.

2. Package treatment in those areas where treatment can be controlled. Being proactive does not mean accepting risk irresponsibly.

This means working in clinical areas where:

• The clinical team has significant experience with treatment protocols.

• The clinicians are interested in examining the

costs of treatment approaches and believe there is room for improvement.

- The hospital exerts control over most aspects of care.
- There are good cost data.

When NEMC began developing the pediatric ALL package, the chief of the pediatric hematology-oncology service and the clinical team had over 1 year's experience with the treatment protocol. The team, including nurses and a social worker, were stable and had developed written educational materials and special programs for families of leukemia patients. In contrast, brand new experimental protocols for bone marrow transplants were being developed for adult leukemia patients, making creation of a package very risky.

The pediatric hematology-oncology service chief had a special interest in analyzing the cost of treatment and believed that, given the right incentives, it was possible to make more improvements in the cost effectiveness of care. Continued reductions in length of stay only squeezed profits from the per diem contracting system. While home health may be desirable for some patients, the revenue for this service simply reduced outpatient clinic revenue for which the hematology-oncology chief was responsible. With a fixed-price package, any surplus remained with the service so the chief would have the incentives to prescribe the most cost-effective treatment possible. Finally, the entire service was eager to reduce what they viewed as extremely onerous utilization review requirements for these patients.

With pediatric leukemia it was possible for the hospital to place itself at risk for all aspects of care for 2 years. Unlike the treatment of some illnesses, the tertiary hospital manages all aspects of care for pediatric leukemia patients. A family's primary care pediatrician may be involved in some of the routine monitoring, but this is closely coordinated with the tertiary hospital team. On the other hand, this same degree of control does not exist, for example, with neonatal care, so it is much harder to develop a comprehensive package for that service.

Control over the risk of a fixed-price package was increased by the state-of-the-art clinical cost information system that was developed in-house at NEMC; this system permitted analysis of patient- and diagnosis-specific "true" costs of treatment. This system captures extensive inpatient diagnostic and proce-

dural information on each patient admitted. Analysts discussed with physicians the incidence of expected complications for pediatric leukemia patients and then used the system to cost these complications. The linking of diagnostic and cost information permitted NEMC to make adjustments to expected costs based on expert knowledge of the likely occurrence of certain complications. With a low-incidence disease, such adjustments are critical in managing risk, because the experience of a large volume of patients is not available.

Routine feedback on costs of treatment compared to norms could easily be provided to the team on a concurrent basis. These norms are budgeted average length of stay and cost that may be entered in the system and reported along with actual experience and diagnostic information that helps to explain variances. At this point, the information system provides protocols regarding actual cost, length of stay, and profitability information on a per admission basis. Enhancements will be necessary to accumulate data on treatment over a period of time.

3. Design fixed-price packages to give clinicians positive incentives to substitute low-cost care wherever it is equal in effectiveness to a higher-cost alternative. Give them flexibility in treatment planning.

The treatment of pediatric leukemia is a good example of one area where fixing a price for a single admission could have perverse effects. The treatment begins with an inpatient admission for induction-intensive chemotherapy and radiotherapy. Complications often occur which can lengthen admission. This admission is followed by outpatient maintenance of chemotherapy.

Home administration of this therapy is also possible. Complications of the compromised immune system may require admission at any point along the course of treatment. Physicians in charge of treatment use a great deal of judgment about when and for how long to admit the patient, and how capable the family might be of supporting the home administration of chemotherapy. Incentives to limit a patient stay may simply result in complications and greater expense later on.

4. Design fixed prices that reflect clinical reality and reduce the risk of treating more severe cases of an illness.

One often criticized problem with the DRG system is its failure to adequately adjust for differences in severity of illness, except through outlier policy. In creating their own fixed prices, hospitals have the opportunity to reduce their risk by setting prices according to severity of illness. For pediatric leukemia treatment, three prices were set, based on the patient's age and white blood cell count. These criteria both determined the protocol used by the clinical team and had a major impact on the length of the first hospital stay, number of complications, and readmissions. The criteria that determine the cost of treatment for many illnesses may not be as obvious or as simple as they are for pediatric leukemia. However, the criteria should be objectively measurable and set prospectively. In the past, many hospitals, including NEMC, set prices based on postprocedure outcome. A fixed-price package would also include a list of patient conditions for which the fixed prices did not apply. This reduces risk for the hospital, but in a way that can have a negative impact on patient outcome, in that the hospital is reimbursed for negative outcomes.

CONCLUSION

NEMC has developed a managed care pricing strategy designed to increase its market share by balancing increased profitability with acceptance of reasonable risk. The availability of data regarding costs, practice patterns, and the ability to monitor whether expectations have been met are essential aspects of the NEMC contracting strategy.

PART TWO

PRODUCT CHARACTERISTICS

CHAPTER EIGHT

Healthcare Plans

EVOLVING MANAGED CARE ORGANIZATIONS AND PRODUCT INNOVATION

PETER BOLAND, Ph.D., President
Boland Healthcare Consultants, Berkeley, California

The five most prominent types of managed care vendors are health maintenance organizations (HMOs), preferred provider organizations (PPOs), utilization review organizations (UROs), insurance companies, and third party administrators (TPAs). Hospitals, physicians, other caregivers, and healthcare suppliers play pivotal roles in providing managed care, but they are not primary distribution channels for the full set of services which make up a managed care system.

Each type of managed care vendor is discussed below in terms of its operational characteristics, evolving product lines, and marketplace innovation. The final section presents an overview of "third generation" delivery system characteristics, which will likely generate truly *managed* healthcare in the future.

HEALTH MAINTENANCE ORGANIZATIONS

HMOs are in a crucial transition phase. The industry shakeout underway is a result of increasing competition among HMOs and among a variety of other delivery systems. In some regions of the country, there is a surplus of HMOs on the market, many of which are losing money with little prospect of gaining enough new enrollees to survive. However, the industry will be strengthened by market consolidation and the improved financial performance of "winners" that emerge from the shakeout.

The winners' defining characteristics are apt to fall into two categories: cost-effective performance and one-stop shopping service.

Cost-Effective Performance

Cost-effective performance is seen in health plans with a strong local or regional base and characterized by experienced management, adequate capital, effective cost controls, and a genuine service orientation.

Until recently, IPA-model HMOs were expected to emerge as the industry winners because of their access to convenient physician offices and relatively low capital requirements for market entry and expansion activities. But lack of internal controls, halfhearted physician loyalty, inadequate management information systems, and sometimes small size have led to relatively poor financial results to date for many (but not all) IPAs in numerous markets.

Group- and staff-model HMOs, on the other hand, have the advantage (that is, economic leverage) of channeling business to a limited number of physicians and providing (and managing) most services in-house as a result of economies of scale.

How an HMO is designed and managed is a far more important barometer of its success than its legal structure (that is, group, staff, or IPA model). Among the best indicators of success is that the hospitals and physicians have the common goal (and ability) to deliver cost-effective healthcare and act cohesively to achieve it.

One-Stop Shopping Service

Many employers want to streamline their health benefit options, which means using fewer vendors. This varies by size of employer. Larger corporations want to offer employees choice, but not as wide a selection of health plans as before. Midsize and smaller firms generally do not want to handle more than one health plan option. As a result, many employers will be cutting back on the number of vendors by 50 to 95 percent over the next few years. This reflects a general corporate trend toward greater quality control and product accountability. It will also increase an employer's leverage over the remaining providers.

Thus, purchasers may be far more selective in choosing a few health plans (or only one) in each region. This will give a competitive edge to HMOs and PPOs that have multiple product lines which can provide all necessary services under one corporate roof. It is important for plan sponsors to include at least one other health plan alternative (that is, dual option) or out-of-plan option.

Some HMOs are attempting to require "exclusivity" in return for offering dual choice or triple options to employers. EPOs and PPOs may meet this need, as do point-of-service options. The latter is particularly attractive for HMOs to sponsor, and some employers like it because it usually requires only moderate reconfiguration or additional resources.

Health plan exclusivity can be difficult to sell to many employers because of patient loyalty to other plans, lack of proven efficiencies to justify the change, and reluctance to give one vendor a monopoly on their business. In such situations, purchasers are nervous about how to guarantee future health plan performance when the threat of competition has been largely removed.

One-stop shopping also means offering a complete line of healthcare services and utilization review features, which should include comprehensive psychiatric and substance abuse management services. To date, few HMOs have placed enough emphasis on managing mental healthcare benefits despite a growing recognition of its soaring costs and relationship to other medical conditions.

The most typical response of capitated plans has been to restrict benefits for psychiatric and substance abuse to a limited number of hospital days and outpatient visits rather than truly managing the case. This means the plan prescribes varied treatment regimens, alternative care settings, and a limited range of resources which are appropriate for the treatment of psychiatric and substance abuse–related medical problems.

Many HMOs, particularly IPA models, lag far behind specialized behavioral healthcare systems in meeting customer needs and employer demand in this area. Some employers want HMOs to completely "carve out" all psychiatric and chemical dependency services. However, federally qualified plans are required to maintain a certain level of basic mental health services. As a result, some HMOs are shifting to mental health carve out arrangements where the management of mental health services is subcontracted to specialized vendors.

Marketplace Challenge

Utilization review presents a dilemma for the HMO industry. Since most HMOs are based on capitation and thus assume full risk for care, they rely on a number of cost control mechanisms (for example, underwriting guidelines and gatekeeper requirements), only one of which is utilization review. As a result, many HMOs have not developed state-of-the-art utilization management capability other than what is needed for internal peer review purposes.

In terms of UR, some HMOs continue to rely on physicians to voluntarily monitor their own practice patterns without the aid of sophisticated utilization management procedures and feedback. This approach has achieved mixed results, at best, so far. Until recently there has been little incentive for group and staff models to develop sophisticated data collection and reporting abilities on utilization for corporate customers.

As a result, many HMOs are not adept at capturing the inpatient, outpatient, and ambulatory care data necessary for comprehensive UR as well as for client reporting. To deal with this weakness, capitated health plans should view UR as both an internal administration function and an external customer service function.

This lack of consistent performance data, reports, and product accountability represents the Achilles' heel of many HMOs. Without purchaser-oriented data, many HMOs are not able to overcome criticism about shadow pricing and alleged marginal quality. Perception defines reality in managed care arrangements, and HMOs have not dealt adequately with growing corporate unrest about service, quality, and cost issues.

Organizational Structure

HMOs have adopted more complex organizational structures to support the range of healthcare products they now must offer in order to be competitive. This has spawned multiple operating divisions within many medium to large HMOs.

Operating departments can be based on key functions such as claims, finance, marketing, member services, provider relations, referral services, medical and utilization management, management information systems, provider contracting, and Medicare departments. Or they can be clustered around broad functional areas such as acute care, diversified services (for example, durable medical equipment, home healthcare, transportation, and collections), medical affairs, and managed care. In turn, managed care can include provider contracting and network development, vendor services arrangements, and information production and management.

Benefit Design

While the range of benefit-plan structures varies according to how the HMO is organized (that is, group, staff, or IPA) as well as local market characteristics, these plans often employ insurance company–type of benefit incentives and disincentives. HMOs are currently trying to reduce premiums (and discourage unnecessary utilization) through higher copayments for hospital stays, emergency room episodes, physician office visits, and prescription drugs, that is, shifting cost partially back to members.

Some plans shift even more costs to users by charging $5 for urgent care and sometimes for maternity care visits. Emergency room copayments range from $15 to $50, depending on whether the case was judged to be a true emergency. Prescription drug copays range from nothing to $10 per refill.

Additional services such as vision care, eye wear, and durable medical equipment may also require a copay from users. A few HMOs offer physician house calls at $5 to $10 a visit. Periodic physical exams may also be offered at those same rates. Therapies such as physical, occupational, and speech often cost about $10 a session.

Most acute care services are included in the benefits package, plus a $3, $5, or even $10 charge per physician office visit and for certain ancillary procedures such as laboratory tests and x-rays. Higher benefit packages customarily waive such fees.

Inpatient copay rates and deductible percentages in some plan options are moving away from first dollar coverage to $100, $200, $300, or $500 per stay with an annual ceiling for each family (for example, $1500). Outpatient surgery can have a copay of up to $30 for each procedure. These types of packages, however, have not been widely accepted to date.

The most restricted HMO benefit remains psychiatric and substance abuse treatment. Typical inpatient care fees are either no charge or $15 for a limited number of days (for example, 5, 30, or 45 days). Some offer 60 or 90 days of partial hospitalization in lieu of 30 or 45 days of inpatient hospitalization without charge, respectively. However, some HMOs are adopting 50 percent copay formulas for 30 days of care a year, depending in part on the level of mandated benefits required by different states.

Outpatient coverage for chemical dependency and mental health has a very wide range of benefit designs. Twenty visits a year without charge is common, as is $10 to $20 per session (or half that for group therapy) for the same number of hours. After the 20-visit level is reached, a copay of $20 per visit or 50 percent of charges (whichever is less) is widely accepted, if there is any coverage at all. The focus is predominately on crisis intervention.

Services   Typical comprehensive health coverage includes the following:

- Complete range of physician services, including inpatient and outpatient coverage
- Inpatient hospital stays
- Full range of ancillary services such as laboratory tests and x-rays
- Emergency services and out-of-area coverage
- Mental health and chemical dependency treatment
- Skilled nursing facility or convalescent care
- Outpatient prescription drugs

Most traditional HMOs do not unbundle their core services because federally qualified HMOs have been required to provide most of these services. Some plans offer certain options like senior care, dental, vision, behavioral health, and Medicare supplemental coverage as separate riders.

A few IPA plans now include laboratory tests and x-rays on site in neighborhood offices that remain open every day and evenings. Some offer pharmacy services. The growing number of relationships with TPAs are enabling some HMOs to design complete employee benefit programs for fully insured and self-insured employers.

Most HMOs use standard quality assurance mechanisms such as appropriateness evaluation protocols for inpatient stays, prior authorization, generic screening systems, medical records and chart reviews, discharge planning and coordinating, and ambulatory UR and QA review.

Reimbursement and Cost Controls

Risk-sharing techniques serve as one of the mainstays of cost containment for many HMOs. The most common approach to risk sharing among IPAs, for instance, is to withhold 15 to 30 percent of provider claims from the approved payment. This amount is placed in a risk pool as a buffer against unanticipated price increases or excessive utilization in the future. An increasing number of IPAs directly capitate their physician groups; some capitate them individually.

When hospital expenses come in over budget, that excess can be split between the health plan and its IPA physicians, drawing from the withheld funds. Some plans have methods to share profits with physicians over and above withhold amounts. Thus, both deficits and surpluses can be shared according to predetermined formulas. In order to "spread the risk" back to the health plan, HMOs sometimes offer reinsurance to participating primary care groups to guard against adverse selection and the occurrence of catastrophic cases.

Capitated fees usually cover referral care, ambulatory services, and some ancillary services under typical "gatekeeper" approaches. These services, in turn, can be IPA-based as well as staff-, group-, or facility-based. In such arrangements, some physicians can be paid directly by the HMO on a modified fee-for-service basis, or they can be capitated directly. Modified fee-for-service is also the typical payment mode for services outside the capitation agreement.

Hospitals are typically paid according to a set per diem rate, per case rates, or negotiated discounts off charges. As a general practice, HMOs try to negotiate away from "all payer DRGs" when their membership base is large enough to warrant lower reimbursement rates. This ensures that the HMOs will continue to benefit from any decrease in hospital lengths of stay. Percentage discounts remain the norm for hospital-based outpatient services.

Successful HMOs usually attribute cost control to at least 10 principal factors:

1. Capitation modes of provider payment
2. Realistic premium development

3. Strict underwriting guidelines
4. Provider risk-sharing through withholds and sharing in hospital pools
5. Effective utilization management controls, including prior authority and concurrent review
6. Tight physician and physician group membership criteria
7. Stringent "gatekeeper" requirements
8. Rigorous financial controls
9. Low administrative expenses as a percent of aggregate revenue
10. Efficient data systems

To be effective, the HMO must integrate these factors into a complete management systems package. This requires additional features such as: competitive fee structures (for example, discounted RVS schedule), tiered per diem hospital charges, outpatient provider fee schedules and discounts, patient monitoring and referral procedures (which include designated tertiary care providers), and a comprehensive management information system to tie all the components together.

In some IPA plans, physicians may be targeted for further review and increased withholds when their practice pattern statistics rise 15 to 25 percent above their respective specialty averages within the plan. Above-average profile data can also indicate a more difficult case mix. However, in the absence of such documentation, outlier physicians can be warned, monitored for a period, and required to repay the plan for the difference between peer practice statistics and their performance. In rare cases, these physicians may be asked to resign.

A few HMOs have gone so far as to temporarily impose a 30 percent fee withhold and to levy stiff financial penalties against physicians who fail to provide appropriate medical care. This situation is likely to occur when an HMO is forced to make unusually tough decisions to protect its financial viability.

New Services   The lexicon of HMO acronyms now includes "point-of-service" plans (also known as open-access HMOs) which enable enrollees to opt out for services with nonpanel providers. Far higher copays and deductibles are applied in such instances, although not as stiff as the financial disincentives of a traditional "hard lock-in" HMO plan. The intent is to provide a feasible alternative which is not unduly punitive to enrollees nor economically harmful to the plan overall.

Related to that option is an integrated HMO and PPO product offered to employers as an exclusive program with a particular company. It can be experience rated and requires a significant degree of administrative coordination for proper plan support.

A few HMOs (often insurance company–owned) also offer EPOs designed for the small-group market. EPOs require such plans to retool their physician networks in terms of geographic access, depth of coverage, and documentation of the cost-effectiveness of participating physicians. This model can be a fully insured dual-option approach.

A variant of both the HMO-PPO and HMO-EPO approach is triple-option capability, typically offered by an insurer. It would include a managed indemnity plan (that is, strong UR and high copays) as a third option.

A number of plans are also developing at least one or more of the following options: HMO benefits for individuals who pay directly (rather than the employer), CHAMPUS supplemental programs, low-option senior products, and Medicare supplement coverage.

Stand-alone services offered by specialty providers are becoming more commonplace, particularly for psychiatric and substance abuse services. The latter is important because it largely relieves primary care physicians (and HMO UR departments) from managing a service which they do not understand well and consequently cannot control as much as other medical areas. It such cases, the HMO becomes a purchaser of these services on behalf of its enrollees.

In order to offer behavioral health services through fully capitated and preferred provider arrangements (and be financially successful), HMOs must either subcontract these services out or upgrade both utilization management and quality assurance capabilities.

Many HMOs are currently offering more analytical and interpretive services to self-insured employers, trust funds, and insurers. Some have added sophisticated forecasting and computer-modeling capability to aid in benefit redesign activities.

Marketplace Opportunity

Both the market and health plans should carefully consider what types of performance incentives and criteria are most appropriate for different delivery system models. Some cost management approaches and quality assurance measures, for example, will be more appropriate (and effective) for PPOs and IPA-model HMOs than for EPOs and group- or staff-model HMOs.

At present, HMOs are largely competing with other HMOs (and PPOs with other PPOs) for managed care business. But in the next few years, HMOs and PPOs will compete directly against each other. As the lines blur between HMOs and PPOs, purchasers and payers will increasingly evaluate different managed care organizations at the same time, rather than one particular delivery system mode or organizational structure (that is, HMO or PPO).

HMOs are in a better position than PPOs—in terms of resources
—to develop new delivery system options because many plans already have sophisticated cost controls in place. What is sometimes
missing is the business commitment and political will of many group-
and staff-model HMOs to embrace organizational diversity in order to
meet new customer demands.

HMOs should generate more data across a broad range of clinical
and administrative functions to improve their competitive position
and satisfy employer needs. HMOs should streamline their information operations in order to produce *focused* data sets for customers.
If the data do not enhance decision-making, then they have little
value. If they do not enable employee benefits managers and trust
fund administrators to make choices about resource allocation and
benefits design that could not have been made without them, then
the effectiveness of data collection is reduced. Current HMO data
practices, however, may have substantial value for internal management purposes.

HMOs can capitalize on the market's need for increasingly sophisticated utilization management procedures. A number of group- and
staff-model HMOs, as well as some IPAs, know how to hold down
costs because of internal management controls such as tight admission criteria, efficient patient triaging, and aggressive discharge planning. Crucial to these procedures is an effective utilization review
system. It is important for HMOs with good UR systems to advertise
them; others should improve their utilization management system so
that it becomes a marketable asset.

However, HMOs have not demonstrated to customers *how* their UR
and case management process works and, therefore, have not gained
adequate market recognition for it. It must be presented explicitly as
a state-of-the-art resource rather than as one of many program components that cannot be distinguished from each other. Otherwise, an
HMO's ability to control utilization will be attributed to financial
disincentives for physicians and enrollees. This information can be
presented in a series of "impact reports" which document the effect
of each measure on cost and utilization.

Unless HMOs can separate the impact of stringent financial controls (for example, capitation, low reimbursement for out-of-plan
services) from medical management controls such as UR, customers
will continue to take for granted one of its most significant resources
—the ability to direct care and use of resources by patients and
physicians.

HMOs have a strategic opportunity to position themselves as market leaders in terms of utilization management resources. This expertise must be explicitly demonstrated and reported in a purchaser-
oriented format in order to be credible.

PREFERRED PROVIDER ORGANIZATIONS

PPOs are beginning to take on the characteristics of a mature industry, particularly in major metropolitan markets where first-generation models are being replaced by more sophisticated products.

A shakeout among preferred provider organizations is emerging, only a couple of years behind the HMO market constriction. Narrowly based provider-sponsored plans which were originally established to fill hospital beds and channel patients to physician offices are no longer competitive. Organizations which were thinly disguised marketing shells were forced to either develop control systems to manage utilization and costs or get out of the market. More and more PPOs are emphasizing their capacity to control overall costs and resource consumption rather than focusing on discounts per se.

The result has been market consolidation, similar to the HMO industry, to the point where there are relatively few free-standing provider systems or independently sponsored PPOs without significant insurance company affiliation. Insurer-backed plans are now the dominant PPO force in many markets in terms of supplying patient volume.

Type of sponsorship and form of organization, which were important market factors a few years ago, are no longer key criteria for selecting a PPO for most purchasers and payers. At the same time, the stability and commitment of the sponsor is vitally important. At a minimum, however, an individual PPO should cover an entire area. Some are now statewide or regional, and a few will have national service capability within 2 years.

National coverage was a goal of a handful of insurers and hospital management companies until finite resource and lack of market demand focused their sights on more local and regional markets. There is still relatively little demand for true national capability, particularly when most potential sponsors have been unable so far to demonstrate adequate cost savings at the local level. Very few employers are large enough and have sufficiently decentralized employee populations to warrant doing business with a national delivery system company.

A growing number of PPOs are forming regional affiliations and referral relationships with other delivery systems in adjacent or nearby states. This is occurring most often among organizations with similar affiliation (for example, religious) or nonprofit hospital status. It will provide a further marketing edge to dominant PPOs.

Services

At this stage in PPO development, purchasers require preferred provider organizations to include a full range of inpatient, outpatient, and ambulatory services. What is distinguishing some PPOs is product line diversification, which is occurring in four areas:

1. Availability of comprehensive utilization management resources for ambulatory review, high-tech procedures, specialty monitoring, and provider profiling, particularly for physicians
2. Ability to capture, analyze, and report focused claims and utilization information which is useful for employer decision making
3. Willingness to develop new service components like workers compensation and disability management, home healthcare, and psychiatric and chemical dependency treatment
4. Presence of innovative product designs such as EPOs as well as the capacity to share risk, which means alternative funding arrangements and different pricing mechanisms

Plan Design   Plan design features and financial incentives drive PPO participation. The degree of plan penetration within employee groups is directly related to the differential between the indemnity or swing-plan option and the PPO rate of copayment and deductible (as well as availability of providers). Since most PPO plans build in only a 10 to 20 percent out-of-pocket differential (for example, 80-20 versus 90-10), PPO penetration has been only moderately successful in plain-vanilla type models. Low penetration is also due to lack of employee education.

In fact, uncertain savings have resulted from low penetration (for example, frequently less than 30 percent), benefit incentives which often outweighed savings from discounts, and inadequate utilization management procedures for high-cost areas like ancillary services and psychiatric and chemical dependency cases.

In PPOs where there is a 20 percent or more benefit differential from the indemnity option, use of preferred providers has been far higher. However, plan design is more a function of employer or insurer decisions rather than of a particular PPO's preference. So far, most employers, insurers, and TPAs have been reluctant to implement more than modest cost differentials. Aggressive channeling of more employees into preferred provider networks requires larger benefit differentials than many employers, insurers, or brokers are ready to accept at this time.

This timidity in benefits design will likely change because of growing corporate pressure for increased cost-savings performance. Inadequate cost savings have also been hampered by lack of aggressive financial incentives to appropriately use PPO services rather than standard indemnity services. Unfortunately, there is very little information that documents the extent of out-of-network use or what savings could have been achieved through greater network utilization.

Disincentives are widely used to discourage unnecessary inpatient hospitalization and to encourage second opinions, but few controls have routinely been placed on misuse of ambulatory services such as physician office visits and ancillary services like laboratory tests, x-rays, and outpatient diagnostic tests. As a result, ambulatory care costs have escalated rapidly because of increased frequency and intensity of services.

Review resources are currently focusing on ambulatory services because costs are growing faster than other medical expenses. Ambulatory care cost escalation is being fueled by a combination of factors:

- Benefit plan design and financial incentives for outpatient care
- Increased reimbursement for outpatient care
- Growing acceptance of treatment in ambulatory care settings
- Ability of providers and vendors to increase ambulatory care utilization patterns
- Aggressive inpatient utilization management review procedures
- Application of new technologies

Just as the pendulum veered too far in favoring inpatient care—in terms of employee benefit coverage and provider reimbursement—it is also likely to swing too far toward ambulatory care, regardless of cost-benefit and treatment-efficacy considerations. What is needed is greater flexibility on the part of payers and providers in deciding which treatment settings are most appropriate for specific medical conditions and for family or social support situations which can aid patient recovery.

Exclusive Provider Organizations

One of the newest managed care features is the development of exclusive provider organizations or EPOs. While it is referred to as a PPO and HMO hybrid, it more resembles a preferred provider organization in terms of administrative controls and structure. There is relatively little financing risk (compared with HMOs). It limits consumer choice to a restricted group of providers (but usually not as much as HMOs do) and offers an integrated set of cost-management controls in order to assure greater cost predictability and, therefore, potentially lower premiums than traditional PPOs. Medical care received out of the network is generally not covered.

EPOs are designed to be an HMO "alternative" or "replacement" product in tandem with the existing PPO. EPOs enable an employer to offer plan options with substantial freedom of choice (PPO) and more restricted choice (EPO) alongside a wide-open plan (standard or managed indemnity). In so doing, the EPO would potentially undercut or reduce the appeal of a standard HMO option.

One of the most positive characteristics of an EPO is the enhanced capacity of the sponsor to collect data on all healthcare utilization if employees are restricted to EPO and PPO or indemnity choices. This approach to benefit control enables the organization to collect data on employees and family members who always use EPO and PPO services, sometimes use them through "swing-plan" provisions, or never use them.

EPOs have moderately strong financial incentives (that is, a moderate lock-in) to discourage out-of-network use, but they may not be as strong as those of HMOs. EPOs tend to be developed by mature regional or statewide PPOs which face significant HMO pressure. To be successful, they require substantial infrastructure resources in terms of utilization management, financial forecasting, and information systems. Some state laws, however, currently prohibit EPOs unless they become regulated as an HMO.

EPO administrative fees (including network access with full utilization review and administrative support services) can be up to twice as high as regular PPO fees or can be paid for on a percentage of savings basis.

Reimbursement

Payment for PPO administrative fees are generally on a per employee per month basis, much like standard indemnity coverage. However, fees are often unbundled in relation to network access (that is, $1.00 to $2.50 per employee per month) and utilization review ($0.75 to $2.50 per employee per month). Specialized services like claims prepricing and case management are usually priced separately, often on a per transaction basis (for claims) or on an hourly rate basis (for case management). A growing number sell services according to percent of savings off billed charges or percent of claims billed.

A few plans have taken the step of guaranteeing that network access fees will not be larger than network savings and that each claim will be a least 10 percent below current market rates for hospital charges in that area. Physician reimbursement is generally a percentage discount off a fee schedule or, in aggressive situations, a fixed cap on specific fees. RVS (relative value scale) schedules are also used in physician contracting. PPOs generally realize up-front price discounts of 5 to 20 percent on physician charges, depending on the locale and medical specialty. These "savings" must be evaluated in terms of appropriateness standards and medical necessity criteria in order to judge whether the discount actually resulted in true savings.

Hospital payment is primarily based on a percentage discount from billed charges, which ranges from 10 to 35 percent for inpatient services. More sophisticated approaches use per diems or multiple per diem schedules and DRGs. Hospitals have largely resisted more stringent capitation formulas from PPOs. Some hospitals are beginning to talk about risk-sharing mechanisms with PPOs, particularly

EPO models which show more of a capacity to channel predictable volume to fewer facilities.

Outpatient services are often discounted up to 10 to 15 percent, particularly for high-volume customers, and package prices are becoming more frequent for certain high-cost procedures in both inpatient and outpatient settings.

Allied Healthcare

As with HMOs, allied health services such as mental health, chiropractic, podiatry, and rehabilitation are being offered on a PPO "carve-out" basis by specialty vendors which offer one or more services. This has been the case for vision and dental care plans for years, and more recently for prescription drugs as well. Managed mental health or "behavioral healthcare" is a particularly high-growth service at the present time. While these medical services are sometimes offered on a capitated basis, they are more often provided on a fee-for-service basis and structured as a PPO.

Many of these companies began as specialty-oriented utilization review organizations and built a service base to include other functions such as medical case management, workers compensation, data analysis, and hands-on patient care management.

However, the trend toward specialty carve-outs is likely to reverse itself for three reasons. First, on the employer side, many corporations are trying to reduce the number of vendors in order to simplify administration. Offering numerous health plans and medical service options has not paid off in terms of cost savings and has added a great deal of administrative burden. That strategy has not worked. The recent move to streamline operations will increase the pressure on delivery systems (HMO, PPOs, and indemnity options) to offer "one-stop shopping," which includes a full array of "managed" specialty services like behavioral health, rehabilitation, home healthcare, chiropractic, and podiatry.

Second, major insurers are moving into these fields quickly, either by developing their own resources internally or through acquisition. Insurance company PPOs have been losing managed care business to specialty vendors because they were slow to develop and integrate the requisite "piece parts" of a comprehensive delivery system. This is changing and will substantially undercut the appeal of many single-service vendors.

Third, stand-alone service vendors which are successful eventually run into the problem of how to build a national organization with limited capital and retain a competitive edge in terms of price and technology. These firms are finding it difficult to support a national sales force, to maintain an adequate administrative support structure, and to adequately fund research and development on a shoestring all at the same time. Small entrepreneurially driven companies are ordinarily not equipped to manage rapid growth successfully on their own.

Each of these factors points to further consolidation in the field as the industry shakeout continues. Nonetheless, some sophisticated "niche" vendors, particularly technology-driven companies, will survive and prosper.

Workers Compensation

Occupational medicine and (more broadly defined) workers compensation PPOs are breaking ground in numerous states which have favorable regulatory environments for workers compensation and disability management services. This field is one of the last bastions of truly *unmanaged* care and lends itself to multiple managed care interventions.

Workers compensation PPOs are experiencing rapid growth because employers are desperately seeking solutions to check escalating compensation claims, which are now outpacing medical plan expenses in rate of increase. These PPOs generally follow the same development course as the first wave of medical PPOs with one exception—the focus is on ambulatory care, where the bulk of treatment occurs, rather than on hospital services.

As with other early PPOs, they are characterized by an emphasis on discounts, relatively weak utilization review and reporting capability, and little quality assurance activity. Payment is most often based on a straight percent of savings (for example, 25 to 30 percent) or on a per case basis.

There are at least five principal reasons why workers compensation PPOs are not as sophisticated as other medical PPOs currently on the market. First, plan sponsors generally lack management depth or experience in what works and what does not in terms of managed care approaches. That has not usually been their chosen field or training ground.

Second, the workers compensation industry is relatively narrow and focuses primarily on turning claims around efficiently (that is, productivity equals success). So the administrative systems involved have not been designed to collect crucial information about basic medical facts: type of service and setting, severity of illness and injury, provider practice profiles, or appropriateness of care. Since these data are not collected on a routine basis and linked to a patient record, they cannot be integrated or accessed by medical software which supports utilization management and quality assurance procedures.

Third, employers are generally ill-informed about what they can do administratively to decrease the occurrence of unnecessary claims or to facilitate appropriate medical care when it is needed.

Few employers are looking beyond immediate "quick fix" approaches like discounts to remedy systemic healthcare problems.

Fourth, many states have legislation which protects the right of employees to choose their own provider rather than employers having the "right to direct" injured workers to preferred providers. Some states allow such direction for designated periods only (for example, initial 30 days).

Fifth, there is more opportunity for providers and employees to "game" the workers compensation system because relatively few effective controls have been instituted so far.

Workers compensation and disability management functions are handled in the risk management side of a corporation rather than in the employee benefits department. This means that risk managers, who are usually in charge of workers compensation services, are not familiar with managed care approaches or technology on the market which can address many facets of the problem.

Too often, an employer's internal workers compensation policies act at cross purposes with other employer policies and are contrary to effective claims prevention (that is, medical and legal) and case resolution.

The awareness level of risk managers has not reached that of many employee benefit managers who have been struggling for years with how to ask the right questions in order to get practical answers. When risk managers begin to demand documentation and results from workers compensation vendors, they will begin to see the development of second- and third-generation products on the market.

In many respects, the workers compensation and disability management field is 5 years behind managed care cost-containment technology and application. The surest way to narrow that gap is by embracing state-of-the-art technology which offers a systems approach for analyzing the quantity, cost, and necessity of medical service and the medical justification of lost work time. This must be joined with cost-effective intervention techniques, like PPOs and fee schedules, to control workers compensation and medical disability claims and to increase worker productivity.

Network Criteria

The single biggest obstacle to long-term cost management is the inability to select and motivate the right doctors for panel membership. However, state-of-the-art techniques for assessing provider performance through sophisticated medical software are expensive. They require substantial data collection and provider cooperation in order to maintain and forward appropriate data on physician practice activities.

The "name of the game" is physician profiling, and at this stage, it is rudimentary at best. But without adequate profiling mechanisms, which can be used as a basis for selecting doctors, PPOs will be forced to patch together networks with few meaningful standards about who is and who is not a good provider.

The key to profiling is accurate data, and managed care organizations with comprehensive claims systems already contain much of the required information. In order to be useful, however, the data must have been entered in a meaningful format, such as CPT codes and ICD-9 codes.

The usual process for network formation is to enlist a percentage of providers (for example, 25 percent) or by location, by hospital staff privileges, or by specialty—and then apply screening criteria. The most frequently used criteria include current state and specialty licensure, Medicare violations, malpractice coverage, and the circumstances surrounding pending or past malpractice litigation.

While some data are generally available concerning Medicare violations and malpractice history, it is difficult to gather useful or accurate information about physician performance prior to forming a network.

A number of PPOs now call for medical board certification, namely, that most (for example, 90 percent) or all doctors be board certified in their particular field (as listed in the PPO directory). In such cases, PPOs may allege higher quality physician care than delivery systems which do not require this.

While board certification is a useful network selection standard (as a proxy for quality rather than efficiency), many other traditional criteria are inadequate for assuring better-than-average care. At best, they may screen out some of the worst practitioners, such as the bottom 10 to 15 percent. This is a significant accomplishment, but it does not begin to focus attention on above-average doctors, let alone outstanding ones. This is one of the chief purposes of *preferred* provider organizations.

Until this is done, PPOs will have to continue relying on after-the-fact utilization review measures to reduce unnecessary admissions and catch outliers. Payers and purchasers will continue to "take their chances" with minimally screened physicians.

Some employers realize this is an untenable approach to cost management, because it essentially ignores quality assurance. Aggressive purchasers are formulating their own agenda to "buy on quality" based on performance specifications which dictate what they want to happen as a result of provider intervention, but the mode of delivery and treatment protocols are left up to participating providers.

Employers want assurance from PPOs that adequate quality controls are built into the delivery system to minimize exposure to risk (for example, rigorous physician credentialing standards) and the unintended consequences of poor medical judgment (for example, QA system protocols). Only a handful of preferred provider organizations have seriously addressed this issue so far.

Hospital selection criteria are much more straightforward, if not formalized. With some notable exceptions, and despite a great deal of rhetoric about selecting hospitals based on quality, they are picked largely on location, name recognition or community reputation, availability of acute care and specialty services, and price. This last factor remains by far the most important network selection criteria.

Attention is also given to where particular employees and families go for care. Employers seek to minimize resistance to using a restricted hospital network and often put pressure on PPOs to include certain hospitals patronized by their work force and dependents. More nebulous issues like "general reputation" are often used as a proxy for specific quality standards. The adage about "everybody knows who the best hospitals are" often prevails in evaluating providers.

Utilization Management

PPOs are under criticism for failing to manage utilization, particularly outpatient and ambulatory services, and for relying too much on discount pricing as the chief means to restrain costs.

Utilization management is a critical factor for PPOs to provide value for customers. Purchasers expect PPOs to provide a full array of utilization review services. PPOs lacking comprehensive utilization management capacity will not be competitive. The most aggressive PPOs have moved into specialty review activity such as mental health, chiropractic, and podiatry as well as medical case management.

State-of-the-art delivery systems now offer ambulatory review, outpatient review, high-technology procedures assessment, and allied health services review, including home health, mental health, rehabilitation, and DRG (utilization) management.

Unlike utilization review organizations (UROs), however, most PPOs have not kept pace with state-of-the-art advances in utilization review in terms of protocol development, medical software, or technology. In other words, many utilization review companies are developing PPO capability faster than PPOs are developing state-of-the-art review capacity.

If this trend continues, traditional PPOs will suffer market share loss over time to emerging URO-PPO companies which have invested heavily in infrastructure resources. A further market advantage of URO-PPOs is that they have regional or multistate network development capability. Thus, they cover wider geographic areas than locally based PPOs.

One of the dividing lines between second- and third-generation

PPOs is the extent of ambulatory review and management expertise. It will clearly differentiate market leaders from the pack. Before long, PPOs in a metropolitan area will not be competitive without it. In order to be successful in the 1990s, PPOs must invest now in ambulatory review capability.

Unfortunately, utilization review—as it is being performed today—is a short-range or stop-gap measure to constrain unnecessary costs. It reflects a "gotcha" approach to snaring bad doctors and weeding out the rotten apples from the barrel. An increasing number of good physicians are growing weary of cumbersome and sometimes irrelevant compliance procedures (in relation to quality care). For some, the aggravation and time required is simply not worth the incremental value of another patient, whose fee has already been discounted.

As a cost-containment device, utilization review has been successful in reducing length of stays and attacking fraud and abuse in the system. But in the future, there will be less "fat" in the system, fewer "convenience" inpatient days, and less opportunity for sustained savings due to usual UR procedures. PPOs will be forced to retool their UR procedures in order to emphasize quality management techniques generated through quality control devices.

In essence, utilization review is moving into utilization management. This is the most feasible short-term answer for PPOs to control misutilization until efficient means are developed to select the right doctors in the first place.

Client Reporting

PPOs often produce so much data that purchasers cannot make sense out of it for decision-making purposes. Many PPOs generate cumbersome reports for two reasons. First, useful reports, which are geared to customer decision-making needs, require sophisticated data collection and retrieval systems—as well as payer cooperation. They are expensive and necessitate a corporate commitment to product accountability. It means a client *service* orientation in addition to a traditional provider orientation.

A major data collection issue is lack of combined in-network and out-of-network reporting with separate analysis for each category. This is due to a lack of claims detail (for example, "unassigned" claims) and pricing based more on claims ratios and trends rather than on specific network costs.

Another data-tracking problem is that insurers frequently pay different percentages on different reimbursement schedules. For example, they can pay 80 percent on a contracted schedule and 60 to 70 percent of "usual and customary" (U&C). In many instances, the lower percentage of the U&C is much greater than the higher percentage of the contract rate.

Second, PPO reporting is limited to the delivery system's ability to provide cost-effective services. What purchasers and payers want is specific information on utilization, costs, cost savings, and quality. If a PPO does not have quality indexes and has only superficial cost-savings measures (for example, difference between requested and authorized hospital days), it will be limited to baseline data.

It is very difficult to evaluate whether most PPOs generate substantial "real dollar" savings. Typical savings information like network discounts and hospital days denied often evaporate when the statistics are more critically evaluated in relation to frequency of services, appropriateness of care setting, medical necessity for procedures and admission, and outright billing and coding errors. Also, cost avoidance (that is, lower level of care) is hard to quantify as "savings."

However, unless a system collects this type of information, it cannot report it. The key indicator for employers is savings per covered life. Larger employers and insurers are now taking a more serious look at how to measure and more accurately document genuine cost savings. This is difficult, but far less so than coming to terms with how to demonstrate and document quality assurance.

Monitoring providers for quality, not just utilization, will inevitably lead to a new standard of quality-based reports. These will be used both as a clinical support tool for judging the delivery of care as well as a report card on individual caregivers. The most important application of quality data is as an educational tool for medical directors to use in discussions with specific physicians.

UTILIZATION REVIEW ORGANIZATIONS

The utilization management field has grown from a handful of private review firms and a large number of professional standards review organizations, established to monitor provider activities on behalf of Medicare beneficiaries, to over 200 monitoring services.

Utilization review organizations now offer a broad array of not only review functions but also management support services and healthcare programs themselves. The more aggressive UROs have crossed the line from providing an arm's-length monitoring service to providing hands-on care and delivery system management.

Many UROs have aggressively moved into PPO functions like network development and contract administration. Some are now competing directly with PPOs by offering a one-stop service bureau to self-insured employers and insurers. The shakeout occurring in the healthcare industry as a whole is also affecting UR vendors. The market for review services cannot support the burgeoning number of vendors indefinitely. Nor do many vendors have the necessary profit margins or access to capital for ongoing research and development to upgrade current review procedures.

The industry is reaching the point where average UR products will no longer be competitive except with unsophisticated buyers, even if they are underpriced. Purchasers and payers are looking for results-oriented (that is, savings) vendors which tend to be at the forefront in criteria development, systems integration, and administrative support features. Such vendors are competitive in terms of price but are rarely low-price leaders except in large volume situations.

Numerous specialty UR companies arose in the last 4 years in response to market demand for greater cost management expertise in mental health, workers compensation, and specialty areas such as dental, chiropractic, podiatry, and prescription drugs. While these service niches initially provided wide-open opportunities for specialized firms, the market is shrinking as a result of at least four trends:

- Utilization review as an industry is entering the "mature phase" in the product life cycle. Continued growth dictates that companies must develop new products (such as PPOs, workers compensation, and data analysis) which both expand and complement core business lines.
- Insurers are expanding UR protocols to include more specialty services, particularly psychiatric and chemical dependency, to stem employer and trust fund losses in those areas.
- Employers are cutting back on the number of healthcare vendors —of all types—as a way to reduce overhead, increase quality, and keep better track of vendor performance.
- General utilization review firms have quickly developed expertise in specialty areas and are aggressively marketing these services, even on a stand-alone basis.

As a result, most specialty UR firms will likely expand to become multiservice vendors, be acquired by existing UROs and insurers, or form joint venture (and marketing) relationships with others who provide larger distribution channels than those of stand-alone companies.

Organizational Structure In terms of ownership, vendors of utilization review services reflect the diversity of the managed care industry as a whole. Recent mergers and acquisitions have led to a variety of ownership structures, such as those shown in Figure 1.

Services Until a few years ago, utilization review services could be divided into fewer than a dozen core services, which could not be unbundled, and optional procedures, which could be purchased à la carte. Now, the number of basic services is extensive, and many UROs offer most services on an unbundled basis.

Insurance carrier or brokerage company

Investor group–venture capital firm

Hospital management company

Health maintenance organization

Preferred provider organization

Foundation for medical care (physician)

Third party administrator

Healthcare consulting company

Other UR organization

Independent

Figure 1 *Typical utilization review organization ownership.*

Major UR companies offer combinations of the following services for inpatient and ambulatory care (including supplemental services):

Inpatient: Review

Preadmission review (also known as precertification)

Emergency and urgent admissions review

Medical or surgical second opinion (also referred to as selected, discretionary, focused, or managed)

Concurrent hospital review (sometimes referred to as continued-stay monitoring or length-of-stay determination)

Case management (including terms such as medical, large, catastrophic, individual, and chronic disease management)

Discharge planning

Retrospective hospital review, including severity of illness and intensity of treatment analysis

Hospital bill review (or screening, audit, and validation)

Physician bill review

DRG validation (or review)

Psychiatric and chemical dependency (substance abuse) review for adults and adolescents

Inpatient: Supplementary Programs

Severity of illness and intensity of treatment analysis

Quality assurance services

Alternative care funding (that is, per case authorization limits)

Prepayment claims screens review (that is, for fee and appropriateness of care)

Fee negotiation

Fraud and abuse investigations

Medical information help line (or hot line)

Ambulatory (Including Outpatient): Review

Medical and surgical service predetermination (or certification)

Diagnostic tests (for example, CT scans, MRIs, angiograms, myelograms, allergy testing)

Highly discretionary prospective procedures (for example, arthroscopy, endoscopy)

Procedures with a high degree of geographic variation, large differences in billed charges, divergent use of assistant surgeons and other ancillary services, and routine occurrence of nonconfirming second opinions

Psychiatric and chemical dependency (or substance abuse) and psychiatric case management

Case management

Dental review (prospective and retrospective)

Chiropractic review

Podiatry review

Optometric review and other vision services

Extended care facility and skilled nursing facility review

Home healthcare review

Hospice review

Private-duty nursing review

Medical necessity and appropriateness screening

Ambulatory Care (Including Outpatient): Supplementary Programs

Pregnancy screening programs and high-risk pregnancy management

Fee management in conjunction with prospective procedure review

Procedures in which nonconfirming second opinions routinely occur

Case management, like ambulatory care UR, has become an integral part of the utilization review process. When utilization review flags cases in the high-risk category (for example, terminal illness, stroke, heart attack, premature birth, and organ transplantation) or high-cost conditions (for example, major head trauma, spinal cord injury, cancer, and AIDS), it focuses attention on finding appropriate alternative care settings.

Case management significantly reduces indemnity and medical costs while improving quality and daily functioning skills of patients. This requires preservice and ongoing follow-up and assessment which involves patients, families, friends, and various caregivers.

The most innovative new services involve both utilization review and delivery system functions, including:

- Workers compensation and disability management
- Specialty provider services
- Claims administration
- Delivery system support
- Employee benefits consulting
- Quality assurance

Workers Compensation and Disability Management

Medical review

Claims verification (that is, for proper diagnostic and procedure codes)

Independent medical examination review

Case management

Fee schedule analysis

Safety consulting

Rehabilitation case management

Rehabilitation specialty management programs (including medical and vocational services)

Short-term and long-term disability review

Disability management

Specialty Provider Services

Prescription drug review

Drug utilization and cost analysis

Therapies review (for example, physical, occupational, speech, and vision)

Durable medical equipment precertification, review, and discounts

Private-duty nursing review

Home healthcare review and network access

Skilled nursing facility review

Long-term care review

Hospice review

Specialty provider PPOs (for example, dental)

Ancillary services networks (for example, laboratory or pharmacy)

Organ transplant facility networks

Centers of excellence

Employee assistance programs (EAPs) and services

Health promotion services

Claims Administration

Claims pricing service, including informing claim administrator of negotiated fees on each claim

Complete claim administration, including eligibility verification (of claimant, provider, and service), review of fee levels and appropriateness of services, proper application of plan provisions, coding, payment (or denial), and communications with claimants and providers

Integrated review and claims management systems (internally or in conjunction with claims processing company) that include treatment protocol screening to identify abnormal practice patterns before claims payment

Electronic claims transmission and receipt

Delivery System Support

HMO and PPO administrative services (for example, utilization review, case management, quality assurance, claims, provider relations, and reporting)

PPO contract administration (for example, contracting, provider discounts, and joint marketing arrangements)

Fee negotiation with noncontract providers

Provider contracting (that is, primary care and specialty services)

Employee Benefits Consulting

Employee benefits consulting, including plan design, financing, administration, vendor selection, and communication

Interactive medical benefits software (for example, ad hoc claims research and report generation)

Client education programs

Data and claims analysis

Normative databases (for example, length of stay and provider charges analysis by diagnosis and location)

Medical criteria development

Quality Assurance

Provider credentialing and recredentialing

Quality of care studies

Assessment of provider conformance with appropriateness of care standards

Outcome measurement

Member satisfaction surveys

Member and provider grievance procedures

Pricing   There are few rules of thumb about how to price utilization review and management services or what is included in a specific service or package.

In the last 2 years, different vendors have adopted remarkably similar pricing schemes despite the fact that their internal costs, such as research and development, technology, and payroll, varied widely. About the only dictum that seems to prevail is to price UR according to "what the market will bear."

Services can be purchased in at least five ways:

1. Per case
2. Hourly fee
3. Capitated rate (that is, fixed rate per employee per month)
4. Either of the above at a discount

   a. If multiple services or packages are purchased

   b. If a large volume is involved

5. Percentage of savings

Basic inpatient review services generally run between $1.10 to $2.75 per employee per month. Case management services can vary from $55 an hour to $175 an hour when board-certified medical specialists are involved. Case management is often broken down into a per case rate for screening and an hourly fee for ongoing assessment and follow-up.

Product Diversification   Many successful utilization review organizations are taking on more and more characteristics of a new hybrid service company, which includes many of the following features:

- On-site patient medical management
- Preferred provider contracting and network administration
- Group medical benefits review and property casualty benefits review (for example, workers compensation and disability management)
- Utilization review and claims payment (for example, as an integrated system in-house or through joint venture arrangements with claims administration companies)
- Proprietary medical, surgical, and ambulatory care criteria as well as in-house specialty physician reviewers
- Data analysis and coding verification software
- Joint marketing agreements with managed care organizations, claims payment and administration systems, and allied health services companies (for example, home health agencies and durable medical equipment suppliers)

Utilization management organizations are well-positioned to capture clinical data on provider quality with two limitations: insufficient norms are available for judging quality and the type of data collected is limited to their URO-specific cases, which does not necessarily reflect general population characteristics. The capacity to develop quality indicators and reporting procedures will greatly enhance URO competitiveness.

The "integratability" of services, administrative support systems, and payment mechanisms will likely be the key to reaching wider markets for utilization review organizations in the 1990s.

However, one issue which UR companies (as well as other managed care vendors) have not dealt with is an agreed-upon methodology for establishing cost savings. Utilization review organizations have not historically collected real dollar information on savings but rely instead on "projected" savings. As a result, many purchasers and payers are beginning to question the favorable cost-benefit ratios and cost-savings assertions made by UROs about their services.

This may be difficult to accomplish in the short run because few review organizations directly capture claim data which provide useful information on costs for savings analysis.

INSURANCE COMPANIES

The managed care goals of insurance companies have changed markedly in the last few years. Bold assertions about "national coverage," "triple-option capability," and "state-of-the-art data processing" have given way to more modest assertions among all but the largest carriers.

The lessons learned along the way have been sobering and very expensive. In many cases, loss ratios have forced a number of insurers from the field. Their commitment to group health as a line of business and the resources required to compete in managed care were inadequate. The industry shakeout demanded both "deep pockets" and the corporate resolve to stay the course despite the cyclical nature of the field and its degree of uncertainty and chaos.

Basically, insurers have faced three strategic choices in managed care:

1. Invest heavily in infrastructure resources and delivery systems (for example, data technology, HMOs, and PPOs).
2. Develop relatively low-cost network rental arrangements with existing PPOs.
3. Adopt a "wait and see" strategy with an added emphasis on managed indemnity options (that is, cost-containment features and benefit restructuring).

Choice 1 was high risk and will likely yield the best result in terms of market positioning, product uniformity, geographic placement to match market demand, and effective cost controls. In this scenario, the actual delivery of medical care is strongly influenced, if not governed, by payer objectives and administrative controls.

For those carriers which spread their money quickly and tried to buy business through hasty acquisitions early on, the price of the "learning curve" will be steep. In fact, initial early errors in judgment and lack of readiness to enter the market are contributing to more focused (and modest) managed care strategies as a consequence.

Choice 2 was cautious and, if the right linkages were established, could prove to be a relatively low-cost vehicle for garnering managed care market share. However, if the PPOs selected do not have the vision or resources to become truly managed care organizations (for example, third generation PPOs) they will not develop into effective network management companies such as exclusive provider organizations (EPOs).

It will be a challenge for first and second generation PPOs (owned or backed by insurers) to develop EPO capability and thus offer an HMO alternative or replacement product. This may be required in some markets to compete head-to-head with HMO companies (also owned or backed by insurers) which develop "open-ended" and "point-of-service" options.

Choice 3 underestimated the rate of change taking place throughout the industry and how difficult (and expensive) it will be to catch up. In retrospect, the biggest risk of all was to do nothing. The "price of entry" is now much higher for medium- and small-size carriers because most managed care relationships have been formed. Relatively few high quality delivery systems are still unattached and available to choose from on a contractual basis.

Insurance companies attempting to affiliate with credible HMOs and PPOs for the first time now have to demonstrate "pulling power" and be willing (and able) to divert a substantial book of business into their networks. Carriers must also demonstrate aggressive benefits-design and product-pricing techniques. The administrative expense of bringing on and working with a new carrier must be more than offset by what the insurer's business contributes to the PPO's bottom line.

As the market further constricts in terms of reimbursement and the number of delivery systems offered by employers, insurers in this category will probably be precluded from the market except as modified indemnity plans.

The overall mood of insurers at this stage—even aggressive ones —is to solidify their managed care assets and to tighten up existing programs. For example, there is now more of an emphasis on reversing poor loss ratios in current HMOs rather than buying new ones. PPOs are being directed to expand their network coverage and, in some areas, to lay the groundwork for EPO-type dual options.

In essence, the insurance industry thrust heading into the 1990s can be summarized by management phrases like:

Consolidate resources

Prioritize markets

Integrate organizational units

Fine-tune new products and services

Focus management information resources

Develop system linkages

The new marching orders are realistic and make sense in terms of meeting customer objectives. They focus more on providing appropriate medical care within existing networks than expanding rapidly into new geographic markets. The early emphasis on external growth has shifted to building far greater internal capacity to control costs through utilization management techniques and plan design.

Highly sophisticated insurers are grappling with the dilemma of how best to support individuals who make treatment decisions about medical care. These carriers realize that physicians, for instance, are the lifeblood of managed care and largely determine—through countless day-to-day decisions—cost and quality.

The conclusion that many insurers have come to is that these medical decision-makers need better information and access to alternative treatment options in order to practice cost-effective medicine. There is a growing consensus that enhanced information is the glue that cements a managed care strategy.

Geographic Coverage Insurers split between wanting to be in as many "primary" markets (or "secondary" markets as a strategy for some medium-sized carriers) as possible. With the exception of Blue Cross–Blue Shield, which can offer national coverage through its affiliated state plans, even the largest carriers have abandoned 50-state marketing strategies in favor of more focused activities. This ranges between a high of 70 markets in over 20 states to as low as a handful of cities in a few states.

Triple-option capability is more limited and EPOs are restricted to one, two, or three service areas or demonstration sites at the present time. Assuming changes in state regulations, the number of EPO sponsors and sites may mushroom in the next few years as some indemnity plans move away from triple choice back to dual choice, that is, indemnity versus EPO.

There are no easy-to-define categories for size of employee groups eligible for HMO and PPO coverage. Insurers market both options to as few as 1+ covered lives and as many as 100,000+ in jumbo accounts. Coverage options are limited below 50 lives and very limited below 25 lives (or below 10 in some markets).

Ownership Insurance company affiliation with managed care organizations run the gamut from full ownership to ad hoc case-by-case marketing relationships (see Figure 2). As a rule of thumb, the largest insurers prefer to own delivery systems rather than rent them. They have both the capital and internal program resources to build networks from scratch, buy significant equity positions in existing HMOs and PPOs, or form joint ventures. Medium-size carriers have hedged their bets through minority ownership and leasing arrangements. Smaller insurance companies have predictably chosen low-cost affiliations or, in one case, banded together to leverage their purchasing power through a national managed care contracting company.

---

100 percent ownership

Majority

Minority (for example, joint venture)

Shared gain (nonequity)

Network rental (that is, access fee) or subcontract

Marketing only (that is, license agreement) or comarketing

Case-by-case

Figure 2 *Insurer managed care organization affiliation.*

Delivery System Options

A number of carriers now offer multiple option plans with a lock-in or a point-of-service arrangement. This is largely dependent on network availability (and related control functions). Such HMO opt out products are intended to preserve the cost-containment features of HMOs and freedom of choice options through PPOs and reduced indemnity coverage for out-of-network services. It also results in most of the medical care going through the network rather than only 20 to 40 percent of it. The mechanism may also reduce the biased risk selection by putting the "pool" back together.

But multioption means different things to many different audiences. It can include comprehensive, wrap-around, or supplemental major medical coverage. It can likewise refer to different degrees of provider choice and benefit design (see Table 1 for common delivery system combinations).

Plan Design

The demarcation lines between alternative delivery systems (and managed indemnity plans to a lesser degree) are blurring to such an extent that it is difficult to distinguish an HMO from an EPO, an EPO from a PPO, and a PPO from an HMO in some cases. Criteria for defining HMOs and PPOs according to funding arrangement, plan design features, and scope of services are no longer adequate indices to tell them apart.

Fully capitated HMOs, where a set premium is paid in advance, can pay physicians in different ways: salary, an amount per patient minus a withhold, or on a fee-for-service basis often combined with a percentage of fees set aside. Thus, while front-end premiums are capitated, physician reimbursement is not always on a capitated basis in IPAs and group-model HMOs.

Product differentiation becomes even more confusing in the case of EPOs which can reimburse physicians on a reduced fee-for-service basis and then further compensate them later with a bonus payment if utilization and cost-containment goals are met. The effect of this mechanism is virtually identical to HMO physician withholds. Both pay less than full rates up front and reward good physician performance after the fact. EPOs use this means to get around placing physicians "at risk."

Benefits coverage has shifted from the standard 80-20 plan with full inpatient coverage to a variety of "incentive" and "disincentive" arrangements. Incentive-based PPO mechanisms range from 100 percent coverage for in-network services and 80 percent reimbursement for nonnetwork care to 90 percent and 70 percent, 85 percent and 70 percent, 80 percent and 70 percent, 80 percent and 60 percent, and even 80 percent and 50 percent.

Disincentive-based approaches can go as low as 50 and 40 percent reimbursement for eligible services given by nonnetwork providers.

TABLE 1   Common Delivery System Combinations

PLAN OPTION	BASE SYSTEM	ALTERNATIVE SYSTEMS*
Dual	Indemnity Indemnity	HMO PPO
	HMO HMO	PPO EPO
	PPO Workers compensation PPO	EPO PPO (medical)
Triple	Indemnity	HMO or PPO
	PPO	EPO or indemnity
Multiple	Indemnity	PPO (standard and 50% copay for out-of-network care) HMO look-alike
	Indemnity	HMO (standard and point-of-service) PPO
	Indemnity	PPO PPO (ancillary-specific services, for example, dental and vision)
	PPO	Workers compensation PPO Indemnity
	PPO	EPO Workers compensation PPO

*It should be noted that not all EPOs are designed to be HMO alternative products as was originally the case. EPOs may emerge as a strategic hybrid product in highly competitive markets.

This approaches "hard lock-ins" typically used by HMOs, except for dual-coverage families who can still obtain 100 percent reimbursement through standard coordination of benefits.

There is a growing trend (among a number of insurers, TPAs, and employers) away from incentive approaches in favor of straight disincentives to maximize network penetration.

As with HMOs, it is becoming more common for PPOs to charge a $5 to $10 office visit fee. Likewise, the occurrence of "no copayment" for in-network care (that is, first dollar coverage if preferred providers are used) is giving way to PPO deductibles (and coinsurance) of $100 to $2000 for individuals and $4000 per family, for example. In such cases, the deductible for nonpreferred provider use (or a mixture of PPO and non-PPO services) could be $3000 to $5000 per family for the year. In each situation, 100 percent of care is covered after the individual family's limits are reached during the benefit period.

Some insurers use different "corridors" for deductible and copayment options, such as 80 percent of the first $2000 to $5000 of services or $100 to $500 deductible per hospital confinement.

Stiff penalties are also being phased in for not complying with preauthorization guidelines. Examples include:

- 50 percent reimbursement for eligible expense or $500 penalty (whichever is less)
- $200 penalty for not calling the UR precertification number for hospitalization or surgery

Plan limits on mental healthcare still reflect standard indemnity approaches. Inpatient psychiatric and chemical dependency care is generally covered at 80 percent, while outpatient service coverage ranges from 50 to 70 percent. Insurance company HMO and PPO plans have developed relatively few creative plan designs for psychiatric benefits which reward early detection and intervention approaches (outpatient) or least-intensive treatment settings (alternative community-based sites). As a result, costs continue to escalate more rapidly in this area than for other medical benefits.

Payment Mechanisms

The insurance industry vacillates between wanting to put providers at risk and recognizing that placing physicians and hospitals at total risk threatens their participation. Thus, some approaches include a corridor of "free care" wherein physicians and hospitals are at risk; but when it reaches 125 percent of premiums, the insurer picks up the remainder in full. The flip side of not wanting to put providers at total risk is that insurers do not want to share all the savings either.

On the employer side, rate guarantees for 12 months are commonplace, and there is a growing demand for multiyear caps. For small-group indemnity plans, 6-month rate guarantees are becoming common; whether this will extend to managed care plans remains to be seen.

The most prevalent forms of payment in PPOs are still discounts from hospital-billed charges and physician fee schedules or "usual, customary and reasonable" (UCR) charges, particularly for medical, surgical, anesthesiology, and pathology. Hospital discounts generally run the gamut from 15 to 35 percent for well-regarded institutions and higher still for borderline facilities. The range for physician discounts is not as broad, but usually begins around 7 to 12 percent and tops out at 20 percent or more.

Hospital per diems are gaining wider acceptance for general acute care, acute psychiatric care, rehabilitation, outpatient, and other specialty services like cardiovascular care.

Services   A range of utilization review services (standard and specialty) are available internally as well as through independent vendors.

In addition to the usual major medical services, many HMOs and PPOs have broadened their product base to include personalized health assessment, health promotion, and disease prevention. This amounts to an effort to institutionalize health education as a legitimate benefit.

A number of specialty services are also available. The most traditional ones are dental and vision care. The latter, when part of a specialty PPO, is often available to subscribers who have not signed up with the vision care PPO itself. Thus, PPO vision centers pass on savings to a wider audience of insureds.

Three of the newer insurer-sponsored services in managed care include:

- Psychiatric and substance abuse (integrated and as a stand-alone)
- Workers compensation and disability management, including short-term (STD) and long-term (LTD)
- Long-term care

Senior care and youth care are also stand-alone features in some PPOs.

The growing number of service configurations and health plan options have led some managed care organizations to offer consumer advisory services and benefit consulting. A number of insurance company health plans include health information help lines which are staffed by registered nurse reviewers. They give routine information about hospital preadmission tests, outpatient surgery, home healthcare, second opinions, skilled nursing facilities, and hospice care.

Some medical help lines go so far as to coach employees and dependents on what questions to ask providers. This generates patient compliance, which should, in turn, translate into greater cost savings.

Utilization Review   Managed care organizations, particularly PPOs, do not readily unbundle most utilization review services. HMOs cannot. However, market pressure from insurers and large employers who want to retain their own UR programs is forcing PPOs to accommodate requests for independent UR. This often leads to duplication and "unused capacity" within the PPO. However, a national or multiregion insurer cannot readily integrate different PPO utilization management programs, particularly when the insurer has its own internal program.

In cases where the carrier uses an outside utilization review organization and where the PPO's UR program is strong, the insurer will be more likely to adopt the PPO's UR program locally.

The decision to "bundle or unbundle" utilization review is often a deal breaker in terms of insurer-PPO relationships. It is an important issue and goes to the heart of program integrity and data capture capability. If a PPO cannot control utilization internally or retain basic information on day-to-day transactions, it will be at a distinct competitive disadvantage. In cases where UR is unbundled, PPOs must be able to retrieve that information in order to build an adequate database for ongoing business functions.

The most typical core UR services offered by insurers (directly or through their affiliated managed care organizations) include the following:

- Precertification
- Second opinion
- Concurrent review
- Retrospective review
- Discharge planning
- Large claims case management
- Healthcare information

Other review services which are listed less frequently are:

- Preadmission testing
- Preservice procedure review
- Outpatient and ambulatory facility surgical review
- Home health
- Birthing center
- Hospice
- Nursing home
- Hospital bill audit

Some of the newer review procedures include such specialty areas as:

- Mental health, including substance abuse
- Dental
- Chiropractic

- Podiatry
- Private-duty nursing
- "Managed" case management (which focuses on specific illness and injury episodes)
- "Managed" second medical opinions (which correctly identifies cases that benefit from such review and waives the second opinion requirement for others)
- Prospective fee negotiation (which occurs during the UR process)

A number of insurers are becoming more flexible in interpreting and administering utilization management guidelines. At the same time, many new specialty review functions are being added. One of the most important utilization review changes is that insurers are beginning to enforce "medical necessity" criteria regardless of place, price, or plan.

Three services which are receiving new-found emphasis are case management, ambulatory UR, and psychiatric and chemical dependency review.

Case management is intended to control the high costs of treating catastrophically ill or injured individuals. It usually begins with triggers for certain diagnoses and procedures which occur during the hospital precertification process (that is, through system linkages). The next step is to evaluate alternative care options.

Ambulatory UR incorporates professionally based benchmarks for how frequently services should be provided in nonhospital settings. These services include physician office visits, laboratory tests, diagnostic procedures, and x-rays.

Psychiatric review has become a major focus, since 10 to 20 percent of total medical benefits are spent in this category. Likewise, it is a major contributor to short- and long-term disability as well as workers compensation claims.

Insurers are currently undecided about whether it is best to provide psychiatric and substance abuse UR internally or contract it out to independent specialized vendors. When the latter is done, insurers can also take advantage of the vendor's mental health networks on a discounted basis.

The employer trend is toward "one-stop shopping" in terms of utilization review. For instance, this often means integrating psychiatric UR as a complement to existing company employee assistance programs (EAP). To the extent that insurers are able to incorporate specialty UR vendors as a "transparent" resource which does not involve extra client effort, they will continue to be able to carve out such functions.

Psychiatric UR vendors which also offer network services emphasize outpatient treatment alternatives such as residential treatment centers, partial and day hospital programs, and halfway houses.

Local referral and evaluation teams are often available with 24-hour phone access and face-to-face service.

New Products

One of the ways in which managed care organizations differentiate themselves in the market is by offering new products and services on a regular basis. What seemed innovative only 2 years ago (for example, focused second opinion, mental health precertification, and ambulatory review) is becoming more commonplace today and will be the accepted norm in the early 1990s.

Examples of new product lines include:

- High-risk pregnancy and maternity care management, usually first identified by nurse reviewers during ambulatory or hospital review
- "Centers of excellence" required for high-cost difficult procedures such as coronary artery bypass operations and organ transplants
- Specific disease management providers who specialize in treating chronic or intermittent illnesses such as cancer, AIDS, and Alzheimer's disease
- Exclusive provider organizations (EPOs) designed to achieve utilization levels comparable with effective HMOs — often marketed in multioption settings which are more familiar with restrictive networks and can include on-site peer group review
- "Managed care" dental services which rely on limited networks and preauthorization requirements on all treatment subject to fee schedules (which are capped)
- Electronic claims submission that go directly to paid claims, thus avoiding rekeying and postage costs; will likely lead to electronic funds transfer
- Comprehensive ambulatory care control through stepped-up utilization review services such as frequency determination, precertification of numerous outpatient medical procedures and surgeries, per case reimbursement (rather than discounts on billed charges), and benefits design changes

The development and implementation of new service products will intensify the demand for enhanced data capability. As the role of payers — particularly insurers and Medicare — changes from distributing risk to reducing risk, the need for new information technology will multiply.

Managed care is increasingly becoming an information-driven industry, especially for insurers. The task ahead is to translate voluminous data into useful focused information. This requires capturing different data and generating better information from managed care administrators.

Once useful data are identified, they must be interpreted correctly. For example, HMO renewal activities will require greater experience reporting and analysis. PPOs and other hybrid plans will need to integrate utilization, cost, and quality data in order to project credible savings estimates. Rigorously analyzing utilization patterns is a prerequisite for financial forecasting.

Thus, the information system challenges facing insurers are formidable and will likely spell the difference between managed care success and failure.

THIRD PARTY ADMINISTRATORS

Third party administrators are far less organized, cohesive, or predictable than their chief competitor — insurance companies. While most TPAs are small and many can still be classified as "mom and pop" businesses, the largest claims administrators process from $400 million to over $1 billion in medical benefits a year.

Their client base, like insurers, is diverse and can encompass over 3500 employers at the top end and fewer than 20 for smaller TPAs.

Plan administrators are not new to medical benefits, but they are new to managing medical benefits in addition to claims adjudication functions. There are few rules of thumb about TPAs involved in the managed care industry.

Third party administrators tend to broker or arrange delivery system services (other than claims adjudication) rather than own them. Some of the largest TPAs are becoming managed care companies, while others are forming joint ventures with a variety of vendors where there is a compelling client need or business opportunity. The limiting factor has much more to do with resources and potential liability or regulatory constraints than ideology or habit. A few TPAs have formed subsidiary companies for their managed care product line as well as a not-for-profit PPO spin-off for labor-management health plans.

Plan Design

TPAs rely principally on benefit designs adopted by employers and trust funds to control medical costs. Since benefit design is a function of what the client wants and is willing to implement, it varies greatly from TPA to TPA depending on their client base. However, many purchasers rely on TPAs for benefits-design advice, just as a large employer might rely on employee benefits consulting companies.

For employers who want to maximize overall plan savings, third party administrators can provide relatively "lean" benefit structures, which place more of the cost burden on the employee. This often amounts to greater plan deductibles for physician services and for hospital care than are present in most health insurance plans. Levels of coinsurance can likewise be higher and include variable "corridors" of reimbursement for nonnetwork services.

In other words, tighter plan design controls frequently associated with TPAs are a function of the plan sponsor. Generous benefit plan features can just as easily be included if desired by the employer.

For example, hospital or physician care outside the network may involve:

- $100 to $200 deductible per person and $300 to $900 per family per year
- 30 percent coinsurance to a maximum out-of-pocket expense of $1000 per year
- 10 percent coinsurance thereafter

In general, the "differential" between network care and out-of-network services is greater in TPA plans than those sponsored by insurers or other delivery systems.

Likewise, mental health services are more narrowly defined and subject to more financial disincentives than in typical carrier plans. For example, a $100 deductible per hospital admission for psychiatric care is common with a maximum benefit of $5000 when network care is given. A 20 percent coinsurance rate for the first $2000 is sometimes built in with an out-of-pocket family maximum of $1500. However, outpatient and office-based services are often set at a 50 percent coinsurance level with a maximum benefit of $1000 per year. Substance abuse treatment can be limited to $500 a year.

In cases where utilization review is mandatory prior to hospitalization and the patient does not comply, an additional deductible of up to $250 can be imposed. Or up to 50 percent of the cost of a particular claim can be applied.

Cost-Containment Services

Most TPAs offer limited utilization review and management services through subcontracts with local or national UR organizations or via insurance company "partners." Many TPAs now have UR medical specialists on staff. The range of review services can be roughly categorized as minimal, average, or advanced as outlined below:

Minimal

Preadmission certification

Preadmission testing review

Concurrent or continued-stay review

Discharge planning

Retrospective review

Second surgical opinion

Average (in Addition to Minimal Services)

Emergency admission review

Focused surgical review and referral

Large case and/or medical case management

Hospital bill audit

DRG validation

Health information services

Advanced (in Addition to Minimal and Average Services)

Focused outpatient services review, including admissions to skilled nursing facilities and nursing homes

Outpatient precertification on psychiatric and substance abuse treatment

Predetermination of high-cost medical services and complex dental claims

Chiropractic peer review

Podiatric peer review

Rehabilitation and physical therapy review

Even within these arbitrary categories, there are significant differences in UR capability. Three examples are mental health, discharge planning, and bill audit. Some TPAs are moving quickly into psychiatric and chemical dependency services, for instance, in terms of both monitoring, and administration functions. These services include UR, case management, discharge planning, peer consultation with clinical providers, and quality assurance.

Discharge planning can be as comprehensive as the plan administrator or clients want it to be. It can cover initial case review and evaluation of numerous alternatives to inpatient care, such as ambulatory or outpatient services, therapeutic or diagnostic care, rehabilitation and restorative services, extended care, home healthcare and nursing, and medical supplies and equipment.

Case management also encompasses alternatives to inpatient settings, which include home healthcare and homemaker services, professional nursing, speech therapy, nutritional counseling, extended care facilities, and hospice.

Hospital bill audit services are not all the same. The usual process is to compare a hospital bill with the medical record and then determine the accuracy of the charges, that is, were the services ordered and were they actually rendered? However, this does not determine the "medical necessity" of the rendered treatment or whether the charges were reasonable. Nor does it take into account whether the diagnosis coincides with the length of stay and the treatment, a factor which is becoming increasingly important in workers compensation cases. Each of these features is crucial.

Without the qualitative dimension built into the audit process, TPA clients will not be getting more than an "automatic pilot" approach to hospital and physician audits. Sophisticated plan administrators are incorporating indices of medical necessity and appropriateness of care.

Additional services offered by some plan administrators include the following:

- Employee assistance programs
- Prescription drug card programs with incentives for using generic drugs
- Early-detection and disease-screening services
- Wellness programs

Marketplace Challenge

Like utilization review organizations, insurers, and delivery systems, TPAs are being called upon to perform more data analysis for clients who do not have such in-house ability. TPAs have an opportunity to fill a tremendous market need for integrating claims data with utilization review information. They are positioned to move into a leadership role by synthesizing a broad range of information categories, such as:

- Utilization rates across the board
- Specialty care and ancillary services in terms of age and gender
- Provider practices and physician profiles
- Cost management services—impact and cost savings per service, including benefit design features
- Modeling and simulation—plan design and rate options

Very few have the technical capacity or have committed adequate resources to produce comprehensive and focused reports so far. One of the features that clients are most concerned about is how their experience compares to other similar companies (intra-industry), regional norms, and national averages. This requires access to normative databases and the ability to fine-tune aggregate data to the point that useful and accurate comparisons can be made efficiently.

What some TPAs have found is that many small employers do not take the time to read reports. This presents a client education and communication challenge. Unless employers can learn how to use and interpret data for decision-making purposes, a TPA's operational efficiency will not have as full an impact on cost management.

Large third party administrators, who want to compete for managed care business with insurers and delivery systems, will have to become managed care companies. That means being able to document cost savings and appropriate utilization management. This requires:

- Enhanced capability in claims administration using state-of-the-art technology and flexible repricing mechanisms (for example, DRGs, per diems, discounts), including variable package pricing
- Internal utilization management capability or contracting with sophisticated review organizations with comprehensive services and transparent (to the client) administrative procedures
- Provider network development (for example, through PPOs) and management (for example, direct provider-employer arrangements) for general book of business and on a client-specific basis for acute medical services, specialty care, and ancillary services
- Information services and data analysis resources which can be unbundled and offered as a stand-alone service
- Customer service functions, including problem resolution between enrollees, providers, and the health plan
- Member communications, including on-site activities tailored to individual clients

CHAPTER NINE

Market Research and Product Positioning

DEVELOPING, IMPLEMENTING, AND USING MARKET RESEARCH

PAUL H. KECKLEY, Ph.D., President
The Keckley Group, Nashville, Tennessee

An "effective" HMO or PPO provides value for three major groups in the local health delivery system:

1. Value to providers in maintaining or increasing usage and thereby providing incremental revenue and income
2. Value to participating companies in controlling health costs and employee utilization without adversely affecting the quality of the healthcare services delivered
3. Value to participating consumers (either as company employees or individual consumers) in providing a "better" healthcare benefit than previously available

The concept of value simply implies that a benefit accrues to the purchaser of the product, in this case a managed care arrangement between providers of care (doctors, hospitals, and others) and payers and users of these services (businesses and their insured employees). Value research in managed care circles has traditionally focused more on the providers and companies. This chapter focuses on the third group — consumers, the end user of the managed care system. Specifically, it addresses ways and means of identifying the value associated with a managed care plan and the usefulness of this information for getting and keeping consumer participation. It examines both the process of researching the consumer market and the usefulness of this information in the decision-making process.

CONSUMERISM IN HEALTHCARE AND IMPLICATIONS OF THE RESEARCH PROCESS IN MANAGED CARE

The starting point for this discussion is a snapshot of the current role played by consumers in the health delivery system, including managed care systems. Four major observations are:

1. Most consumers are not well-informed users of the health delivery system. Only 17 percent of U.S. adults read any healthcare literature on a regular basis, and these tend to be better educated white collar young mothers, or senior adults over 65 seeking diagnosis-specific information. Most (89 percent) do not know what DRG means, and even more (94 percent) do not know whether their personal physician is licensed or board-certified.

   Research implication Market studies which rely solely on the *opinions* of consumers will be misleading. An *uninformed* consumer provides little insight in some critical areas of managed care, such as comparisons of clinical protocols. Therefore, any consumer study must be highly focused, targeting a select segment of the population with the intent of exploring in-depth only a few issues. This allows sufficient time in the process for the researcher to *inform* while soliciting feedback. What consumers *say* is based on what they have observed and experienced. Since most consumers have no direct experience with managed care plans, it is unlikely that consumer surveys of opinion will provide definitive information about the particular plan.

2. Most consumers are becoming more aware of healthcare issues. Though current levels of understanding and awareness are low, there are clear indicators that consumers are becoming more aware of health choices. For instance, in 30 percent of all childbirths in the United States, mothers-to-be participate in classroom discussions, often with "dad." Healthcare is now the single focus of two network television programs, and more than 700 local television stations carry at least one weekly healthcare report. The impetus for this growing awareness appears to be a surge in concern relating to both healthcare costs and public policy issues such as healthcare rationing and indigent care.

   Research implication Consumers are accessible to market researchers. They are willing collaborators in the information gathering process vis-à-vis surveys, focus groups, and panels. So, getting information from consumers is an important component in the process, and they are increasingly better informed and thereby helpful.

3. Most consumers of healthcare are not price-driven. They are, however, price-sensitive. The most valid indicators of price sensitivity in consumer healthcare research are those behaviors (not stated opinions) which correlate statistically to a high level of price sensitivity. Some of these behaviors include:

- Calls made to doctor's offices to get information about the office charge rate
- Calls made to hospitals requesting prices for procedures and for amenities such as private rooms
- High levels of employee participation in company-sponsored programs to identify billing errors by hospitals or doctors

Perhaps the most vivid price sensitivity measures are those daily negotiations in unionized companies where management has repeatedly faced union negotiators intent on maintaining a fee-for-service, first dollar coverage plan, even conceding hourly wages in the process.

Price sensitivity in the healthcare arena is far from its driving force. It is a secondary factor in the selection of a doctor behind the perception of the doctor's skill (gained from word of mouth) and accessibility of the physician (office location, ability to get a commitment).

For hospitals, price sensitivity is more pronounced. Consumers are more inclined to use a particular hospital because of a lower price than a particular physician in the same scenario (see Table 1).

Research implications Consumers by and large do not know what health costs are. They know only their out-of-pocket expenses and their monthly insurance premium. As a result, a researcher seeking to ascertain the level of price sensitivity must first define the behavioral indicators: do consumers check bills, make calls, comparison shop? A researcher must also project levels of price consciousness on a scale which correlates to an eventual price-driven consumer healthcare decision. If a managed care plan chooses to present itself to consumers solely on the basis of its lower price, most consumers will be receptive but not sold. Therefore, in the research process, measuring the price sensitivity of the consumer market is more complex than asking simply, "Do you care about health costs?" or "How important is savings?" The researcher must provide *specific* dollar savings scenarios and gauge changes of use which result.

4. Most consumers purchase healthcare services on the assumption that the quality of care is essentially the same. Therefore,

TABLE 1   Consumer Price Sensitivity

INSENSITIVE	PRICE SENSITIVE	PRICE DRIVEN	PRICE
Percentage of all adults	30%	55%	15%
Consumer behaviors	Use of private rooms Never ask about charges Purchase fee-for-service insurance	Inquire about charges Purchase generic substitutes Avoid physician office visits unless absolutely necessary	Join closed option plans Purchase the low-priced plan Select minimum benefits from menu Join HMOs, PPOs
Consumer attitudes	"You get what you pay for." "I want the best." "Healthcare is not something you can price." "Price doesn't matter."	"It's too expensive, but what are my options?" "The hospitals and docs make too much money."	"I can't afford everything." "The quality is all the same." "If I need something, I can get it and worry about paying for it later."
Most prominent groups	Affluent upper and upper middle class Younger seniors 65–75 with pension benefits	Younger, middle-class households Older seniors 75+	Working poor Young single males under 30 Young families in lower or middle class

the differentiation for a provider is a function of service, price, and program package.

Consumers believe most doctors are competent, and most hospitals are good. They believe bigger hospitals have an advantage in technology, but do not associate a smaller hospital with inferior care. Therefore, the value of a managed care plan can be presented to a consumer in such a way that it relates more directly to three other points of comparison.

- *Service* How quickly can the consumer get an appointment? Are employees helpful and courteous? Are operating procedures reasonable and understandable? Are waiting times tolerable? Are locations convenient? Is the enrollment process simple?
- *Price* Price per se is not the driving force. Out-of-pocket expenses, payment terms, and the extent to which monthly premiums or fees fluctuate are points of comparison.
- *Program packaging* Which doctors are participants? Which hospitals? What is not covered in this plan? How flexible are the components of the plan?

Though consumers are not well informed, they nonetheless discriminate in choosing options or plans which address rudiments of all three points. As they become aware, they will become increasingly more sophisticated in discriminating among *all four.* And what triggers an advantage today will inevitably change tomorrow (see Table 2).

Research implication Measuring the value of any managed care option at the consumer level will ultimately lead to specific attributes which are in each of these four categories: quality, service, price, and packaging. In a study to determine the position of any managed care option, consumers must see evidence of the plan's performance in all categories before the plan is marketable. Increased economic pressures on the household budget and the likelihood that outcome-specific quality measures will be publicly accessible bodes well for a managed care option which provides a high quality low-price plan.

TABLE 2 Managed Care Option Discriminating Factors

	1989–1990	1992–1993
Quality	Perception of providers	Clinical outcome
		Performance of providers
Service delivery	Staff attitude	Efficiency of operation
	Location accessibility	Location accessibility
		Operational protocols for use
Price	Competitive pricing	Lower pricing than competition
Packaging	All inclusive	Unbundled menus

Against this backdrop, the next sections address the use of consumer research in the evaluation of the market for a *new* managed care plan followed by its application in an existing plan.

EVALUATING THE CONSUMER MARKET FOR A NEW PLAN

Most hospitals, physicians, or insurance companies assessing the market potential for a plan in a local market use the ample supply of already available information to assess the environment. If these data indicate favorable conditions, stage II of their research usually involves individual interviews with several opinion leaders and gate-keepers (see Figure 1).

At stage III in the process, the object of the research shifts to the consumer. The most important issues raised at this point are:

- Do consumers perceive a need for an alternative approach to health delivery? If yes, which segment of the consumer market does so? Why is it receptive?
- What would motivate these potential enrollees to choose one plan over another? How can a specific plan maximize its competitive advantage in terms of price, service delivery, the program components, or quality?
- How should the proposed plan promote itself to these targeted potential enrollees? What are the key message points and channels of communication?

It is not possible to develop a pro forma analysis of the potential for any plan unless it is accompanied by consumer research. To assume market acceptance of a plan without consumer research is as risky as assuming that *all* who say they are interested in the plan will actually enroll. (For consumer managed care research the conversion rate is the number of consumers who actually enroll expressed as a percentage of the total number of consumers who expressed interest.) As the process outlined in Figure 1 indicates, the consumer research is preceded by fact gathering (stage I) and opinion leader interviews (stage II).

Consumer research is expensive. The out-of-pocket expense involved in stage III is probably $20,000 to $25,000, which is usually more than has been expended up to that point. The best method for conducting a survey of consumer opinion about an HMO option in a market is the telephone survey of a random sample of households whose members have lived in the market for at least 1 year prior to the survey. This questionnaire will capture sufficient information about existing health providers in the market.

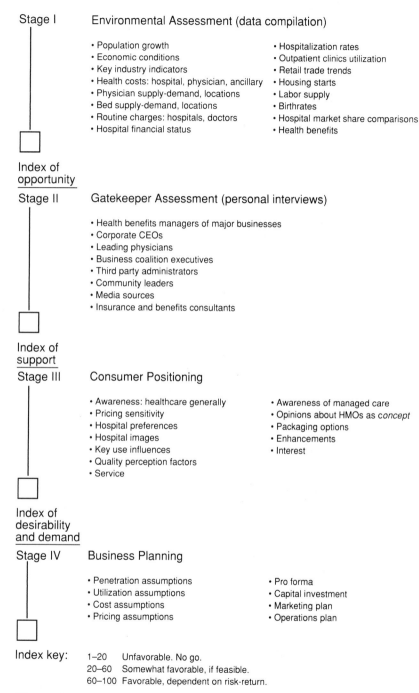

Stage I — Environmental Assessment (data compilation)

- Population growth
- Economic conditions
- Key industry indicators
- Health costs: hospital, physician, ancillary
- Physician supply-demand, locations
- Bed supply-demand, locations
- Routine charges: hospitals, doctors
- Hospital financial status
- Hospitalization rates
- Outpatient clinics utilization
- Retail trade trends
- Housing starts
- Labor supply
- Birthrates
- Hospital market share comparisons
- Health benefits

Index of opportunity

Stage II — Gatekeeper Assessment (personal interviews)

- Health benefits managers of major businesses
- Corporate CEOs
- Leading physicians
- Business coalition executives
- Third party administrators
- Community leaders
- Media sources
- Insurance and benefits consultants

Index of support

Stage III — Consumer Positioning

- Awareness: healthcare generally
- Pricing sensitivity
- Hospital preferences
- Hospital images
- Key use influences
- Quality perception factors
- Service
- Awareness of managed care
- Opinions about HMOs as *concept*
- Packaging options
- Enhancements
- Interest

Index of desirability and demand

Stage IV — Business Planning

- Penetration assumptions
- Utilization assumptions
- Cost assumptions
- Pricing assumptions
- Pro forma
- Capital investment
- Marketing plan
- Operations plan

Index key:
1–20   Unfavorable. No go.
20–60   Somewhat favorable, if feasible.
60–100 Favorable, dependent on risk-return.

Figure 1

Before questionnaire design begins, however, an important precursor is the use of at least two focus groups to determine prevailing attitudes and awareness of the notion of managed care plans. In fact, the most important investment in consumer research is the focus group because it provides the research team with an opportunity to hear firsthand the mindset of the consumer to whom the market strategy will ultimately be aimed. In the group setting of a focus group, the interaction between consumers is an important observation, since most consumers rely on word-of-mouth information in assessing delivery system issues.

Focus groups represent an art form that involves careful screening and recruitment, a professional facilitator who is capable of extracting needed information from a group of strangers in a neutral but provocative manner, and a setting where the consumer opinion process is explored in depth without outside interference.

A focus group about an HMO or PPO should probe several key questions:

- How sensitive are healthcare consumers to healthcare cost increases? Are they concerned? What are they doing to reduce their healthcare expenses?
- What do consumers know about HMOs and PPOs? How sophisticated is the market?
- What is the best source of information that is useful in changing the mind of the consumer in the market? How important is the family physician in positioning the HMO?
- What is the consumer's reaction to the concept of an HMO? Do they like one model more than another? How do they process the differences? What terms do they use?
- What are the optimal ways in which a managed care plan can deliver better service, better prices, better programs, and better outcomes? Which of these is the driving force?
- What is the role of the corporate health benefits plan in altering consumer preferences? Do employees of particular companies prefer specific features or benefits?
- Which local providers are considered essential participants in the plan? Why?

The screening interview to recruit participants should elicit information about the participant's employer, age, and length of residence in the market area, and the names and locations of the doctors and hospitals used in the past 12 months.

It is best to segment these groups into younger adults under 40 and those 40 to 59, since the healthcare needs of these generational groups are quite different. It is commonly held that the younger consumer is more concerned with the affordability of care and is attracted to price, while older ones are thought to be more hesitant and more cautious about nontraditional care choices.

If HMOs or PPOs already exist in the market, it is prudent to recruit only nonenrollees. Separate interviews with groups of enrollees in competing plans may provide insightful competitive intelligence.

Since the overriding purpose of these groups is to bring to the surface critical issues needed for the telephone survey, it also functions as a means of assisting the research team in the development of the survey instrument itself. It is usually not necessary to do more than two or three groups, provided the protocols of random recruitment are followed.

From a budgeting standpoint, the guidelines given in Table 3 fall within the expected ranges for most focus group operations around the country.

So, for two focus groups, it would not be unusual to pay $5000 to $8000 plus travel expenses.

A focus group does not provide projectable data useful in making a go–no go call on the consumer strategy best for a particular market. It will provide insight for the actual design of the telephone survey questionnaire, and it will sensitize the research team to the mindset of the market prior to undertaking the survey.

The telephone survey is the bread and butter tool used in gauging consumer receptivity to an HMO. It provides immediate reactions, much the way the consumer would respond under normal conditions such as in regular conversation with a coworker or in discussing the idea with an acquaintance in a shopping mall or social setting.

The advantages of the telephone survey method are many:

- It provides information quickly.
- It provides spontaneous information, top-of-mind reactions.

TABLE 3 Typical Focus Group Expenses

	FEE PER GROUP
Recruitment cost	$800–1200
Participant incentives (8–10 per group)	$250–400
Facilitator	
Including report	$1000–1500
Excluding report	$2000–2500
Room rental	$200–300
Taping	
Audio	Included in rental
Video	$200–250
Refreshments	$100

- It provides geographically and demographically projectable sample segments if properly executed.
- It allows the researcher to probe opinions and test trade-offs and options.

The disadvantages of the method must also be understood:

- It is expensive—about $30 to $40 per interview for a 15-minute interview with a normal sample population.
- It excludes those households which do not have telephones (it does include the 15 percent of the population which is unlisted because the telephone numbers are obtained by random digit dialing).
- It usually requires an outside firm using trained interviewers with experience in probing and coding complex questionnaires.

A common mistake made in testing the market for an HMO is in the questionnaire design itself. Some basic rules of design for managed care market research include:

1. Never assume the consumer understands the terms HMO, PPO, or any other acronym. Use the terms in their long form, that is, health maintenance organization, and explain the term to the consumer early in the questionnaire so as to elicit a valid response.
2. Always use a scale for responses that the consumer can easily remember and easily use. For instance, on the telephone, consumers are time-sensitive. They want to get off the telephone as quickly as possible. So a suggested response using a number is usually better than a response that requires a verbal reply. Use of the 1 to 10 scale is among the best techniques because the consumer has a predisposition to think in such terms. However, a 1 to 6 is not usual and might cause problems.
3. Always use open-ended questions sparingly and in strategic locations in the questionnaire. The most critical information needed from current HMO or PPO members relates their satisfaction with the HMO or PPO. This information follows a direct question about how satisfied the person is; in this case the interviewer is prompted to ask, "Why do you rate it this way? Can you tell me more?" Logistically, the most expensive part of a telephone questionnaire is the open-ended question, so the inclusion of no more than two or three key questions will save time and money.

4. Always use a questioning sequence which does not effect a self-fulfilling prophecy in the responses. Often, the questions themselves suggest answers which are not valid.

5. Always withhold the name of the sponsoring organization from the respondent. Consumers are inquisitive; they want to know why the caller wants the information. In almost every test for a new program, product, or service, consumer responses will be shaped and swayed by their perception of the sponsor. There-fore, a good rule of thumb is that interviewer should always tell the consumer that (1) the information is confidential, (2) the sponsor's instructions are that its identity is not to be revealed, and (3) the results will not be made public. If the firm employs experienced interviewers (which many do not), the consumer will agree to the interview.

When the interviews are completed, there are other quality control factors to keep in mind:

- Any analytic effort should use simple statistical tools such as the *t* test and chi-square test to determine the significance of the quantitative information. Often, too much is made of minor differences that prove to be statistically insignificant.
- The open-ended comments are as valuable as the numbers, so they should be carefully coded and reviewed intensely by the researchers.
- Cell sizes, that is the number of people included in each group in the sample population, should be scrutinized with caution before in-depth analysis proceeds. For instance, projecting HMO penetration to a zip code where only six individuals were interviewed would be inappropriate and prone to much error. One general rule of thumb is that a cell size of 30 is "safe" for assumption and interpretation.
- Keep in mind that any survey is only a picture of the current event. Timing may have an important influence on the findings, so be careful in preparing by noting current advertising and news events in the market. A telephone survey is a picture of a market at a point in time. It can and will change.

EVALUATING THE CONSUMER MARKET TO MODIFY AN EXISTING PLAN

The 600 PPOs and 650 HMOs in the market already use consumer market research in three principal applications.

1. Market penetration research
2. User satisfaction research
3. Program enhancement research

Application 1:
Market Penetration
Research

This is consumer research targeted to nonenrollees in the market-place for the purpose of determining ways and means of increasing current enrollment by attracting new enrollees to the plan.

Usually, these studies involve a combination of two primary research methods: First, two to four groups get the "feelings" and "predispositions" of the nonenrolled market. Then a telephone survey of potential enrollees follows.

Example A 320-bed acute care hospital in a three-hospital Carolina market wanted to enroll more companies in its PPO but feared resistance from the corporate leadership, who were predisposed to think that their employees wanted to make their own choices of providers without interference from the companies. The hospital identified sample populations of households employed by 11 targeted companies using company personnel office assistance. Four focus groups were conducted: two with male heads of household, one with female heads of household, and one with spouses of employees. These issue-identification sessions provided valuable insight into the price, service delivery, program features, and outcome (quality) expectations and concerns. Clearly, the market did *not* believe local provider quality differed, and most were not interested in new programs, thinking the local capabilities were complete. Therefore, the differentiation would need to focus on price and service delivery.

Four weeks later, the results of a follow-up telephone survey verified the findings. The PPO would have strong acceptance if positioned by and through the company as a lower price (out-of-pocket cost) but, more important, a better service (after-hours primary care) option. This information was used in concert with pro forma analysis of the incremental costs involved to build a stronger PPO. The result: a 13 percent enrollment increase in 7 months.

Application 2: User
Satisfaction
Research

Retaining enrollment by reducing member turnover for preventable reasons (a change of location out of the market due to a job change is not preventable) is a second major area of consumer research in managed care plans.

Traditionally, the costs of acquiring an enrollee have been 3 to 4 times the marketing costs associated with retaining the enrollee. Knowing when an enrollee or participant is likely to disenroll, the reasons associated therewith, and the creation of a defensive strategy can mean substantial returns for an HMO or PPO.

The most customary method for obtaining enrollee satisfaction information is a direct mail survey of members. Direct mail affords the advantage of targeting geographically by zip code or census tract, demographically by the sex, age, and related characteristics of members, and member class, that is, length of enrollment.

The process of user satisfaction research is widely used in managed care to improve service delivery, evaluate new programs, or develop information used by the sponsoring HMO or PPO in recruiting companies to the plan.

Example A northern California closed-panel HMO of 55,000 enrollees experienced an annual turnover rate of 35 percent. It noted that the percentage was especially high for enrollees who had been in the plan less than 1 year but did not know how to explain the situation.

In response, the HMO began sending a quarterly survey to all new enrollees in the plan for less than 1 year and an annual survey to the rest of the enrollment panel. Using a mail drop date, which meant the mailing was to be delivered on a Wednesday or Thursday (the best response days for consumer mail surveys), the HMO successfully achieved a 55 percent response rate. The changes that have resulted have reduced the turnover rate to 14 percent in 16 months, and the HMO has initiated an internal restructuring plan to facilitate increased responsiveness to the consumers it serves.

Application 3: Program Enhancement Research

Both applications above provide meaningful insight for managed care plans seeking to add or modify their services. Yet, on occasion, it is useful to probe deeply into a *specific* program alteration or enhancement.

The operative concept in program enhancement research is the focusing of consumers on a specific program enhancement. Rather than making a futile attempt to cover several possibilities, the effective study limits the possibilities to no more than three options, details them to the consumer, and probes for immediate reactions. The most prevalent research method is focus groups, since they permit the explanation of a "new" enhancement by the facilitator and lively, immediate discussion by attendees.

Example A major Chicago area IPA-model HMO was interested in offering its own prescription drug discounting program, contracting with a local discount chain with multiple locations in the area. It postulated that the availability of the 20 percent discount would more than offset the inconvenience to many who did not live close to an existing location. Three options were proposed: (1) maintenance of the current system, (2) change to the 20 percent program, or (3) change to distribution through participating physicians' offices at a 10 percent discount. To the amazement of the plan administrators, having the service available in the physicians' offices was the top choice—and not as a result of any discount. They perceived the convenience (service delivery) advantage first and foremost.

CONCLUSION   The role of the consumer acceptance in the process of managed healthcare delivery is certain to increase. As a result, the HMO or PPO which maintains an aggressive research program targeted to the needs and wants of potential enrollees and current members will have a competitive advantage.

POINT OF VIEW

Managed Care Marketing Requires a Broader Understanding

ROBERTA N. CLARKE, Associate Professor, Department Chair

Boston University, School of Management, Boston, Massachusetts

The period from 1985 to 1990 represents a period of significant transition for managed care industry marketers. With expanding primary demand for managed care of all kinds through 1985, the marketer's job was merely to help the organization participate in this growth market. The marketer's task was to sell, promote, and encourage a trial of a managed care system and to seek enrollment.

In contrast, the 1990s offer a different, if not more difficult, marketing challenge. The managed care market no longer promises rapid expansion of market demand; instead, managed care systems will have to fight for selective demand or market share to grow. They have done so increasingly in the 1980s, but the battle for share will become far more intense as the market size stabilizes. One delivery system's growth will come only at another's expense.

The implication is not that selling and promotion must become even more aggressive to seek greater enrollment or "trial purchase." The primary marketing issue will be viewed semantically as "disenrollment" or lost sales. With managed care systems experiencing annual disenrollment rates of 20 to 30 percent and sometimes higher, managed care organizations will start to recognize that no matter how fast members are pushed in the front door (enrollment), the house cannot be kept full if they are running out the back door (disenrollment).

The word "disenrollment" hides the complexity of the underlying problem. Disenrollment itself is merely the manifestation, the most visible symptom, of the organization's disease — that *the organization is failing to satisfy the customer.* Classical marketing assumes that, if the customer is satisfied, trial (enrollment) will lead to continued repeat purchase (reenrollment).

However, the decision to repeatedly purchase the same product or service will swiftly change once the consumer is no longer satisfied (disenrollment). Customer loyalty is only as strong as the customer's satisfaction with his or her most recent purchase.

The underlying rationale for an organization to exist is to create a satisfied customer. Since this is now becoming the very essence of successful marketing for managed care systems, the structure of the marketing function will have to change. Marketing now has to encompass or transact with all those activities that not only attract but retain members by creating satisfied customers. In other words, the activities of the whole managed care system become marketing activities in that they directly affect members' retention and disenrollment.

Marketing can no longer be limited to promotional activities plus forays into market research and strategic planning. Marketing must now be seen as a crucial component of the day-to-day operations of the managed care system. Line managers must be assigned marketing responsibility and be held accountable for customer satisfaction with the specific services they manage. A service mentality must be introduced throughout the organization so that each and every employee, from the bottom to the top, realizes that he or she is to create a satisfied customer. Without this broader understanding of marketing, the symptom of high levels of disenrollment could signal a terminal disease for the managed care system.

CASE STUDY

Preferred Health Network: PPO Marketing Strategies

JERRY T. PAYNE, Vice President Marketing
Preferred Health Network, Monterey Park, California

The first step in packaging PPO services is to segment the marketplace. Different approaches are required to sell to each market segment. Since PPO sales resources are limited, it is imperative to prioritize segments based on their product needs and ability to generate members.

MARKET SEGMENTATION

The simplest way to segment the market is according to *funding mechanisms* and *distribution systems*. Groups are either fully insured (paying a carrier for coverage) or self-funded (funding their own liability). The products offered to insured and self-insured groups differ and are sold through separate distribution systems. Table 1 shows the different parties involved in such a distribution system.

TABLE 1 Distribution System by Market Segment

FUNDING MECHANISM	DISTRIBUTION SYSTEM
Fully insured	Broker or employed agent of insurer
Self-insured	Consultant, third party administrator (TPA), stop-loss carrier, or stop-loss broker

Payer (or market) segments are ranked in order of importance, that is, ability to produce the greatest number of lives. A typical ranking is shown in Table 2.

INSURANCE COMPANIES

To determine the priority for qualifying prospective carriers, identify licensed carriers in the target area, their size, and PPO linkages if any. First, array them by the amount of accident and health insurance premium each has in force. The state insurance commissioner or reports such as *A.M. Best* can provide this information. Next, estimate the number of lives covered using a rough rule of thumb that one life represents $1000 in premiums, which is based on current industry estimates. The amount will vary up or down depending on the average healthcare costs in a state compared to the national average. Target the largest ones for earliest contact.

The existence and strength of one or more PPO linkages between other networks and payers should

TABLE 2 Payer Ranking by Importance

1. Insurance companies
2. Large companies (>1000 employees)
3. Unions
4. Medium and small groups (<1000 employees)
5. Workers compensation carriers
6. Federal programs
7. Brokers and consultants
8. TPAs

also be assessed. There is a variety of PPO directories which list networks and payers they contract with, for example, local hospital associations, American Medical Care and Review Association (AMCRA), or the American Association of Preferred Provider Organizations (AAPPO).

The fact that a carrier already has a PPO linkage is not an absolute barrier to overcome. Through the initial sales interview, dissatisfaction may be discovered with that PPO's service, or niches which can be filled may be identified. For example, a carrier which develops its own networks nationally may make an exception and contract with an established local network if it feels the network is superior in terms of quality or price or if it cannot be replicated without incurring significant costs. Remember that regional networks are a viable alternative to national efforts which have difficulty ensuring a quality delivery system in each local market.

A PPO can attempt to segment the insurance company marketplace by dividing it according to funding mechanisms and distribution systems. For insurance companies, there are three distinct systems: (1) national brokerage firms for groups of 1000 or more employees, (2) regional brokerage firms for groups of 100 to 999 employees, and (3) independent brokers networked by general agents (GAs).

In practice, the national firms will handle accounts with fewer than 1000 employees and regional firms will handle those with over 1000 employees, but these group sizes are a convenient boundary between the two types of firms for the sake of this discussion.

KNOW THE LOCAL MARKETS

Spend the time to make the PPO known to and accepted by the local distribution system of the carrier prior to contacting its headquarters. This step should give the PPO the advantage of having been recommended by the local sales force of a carrier.

By identifying holes in the carrier's PPO service, a network can offer services to fill that niche. Cost-savings reports are an example. The medium-size carriers tend to form joint ventures like Private Health Care System. By combining their insureds, the carriers leverage their negotiating power with providers and gain access to a common utilization management (UM) program. Joint ventures typically have not yet developed cost-savings report mechanisms other than utilization management reports. This provides an opportunity for PPOs having such reporting capabilities to enter a market that may otherwise have been closed.

IMPORTANCE OF MASTER GENERAL AGENTS

When contracting with carriers who underwrite multiple employer trusts (METs), the role of the master general agent (MGA) needs to be appreciated, because this role does not exist with larger carriers. Generally, the MGA has designed a product, found a carrier to underwrite it, acquired exclusive marketing rights for the product, and may collect the premium and even process the claims. The MGA controls the product and will move the block of business from one carrier to another to gain a competitive edge. That edge may be more underwriting control, a larger commission override, or better rates.

PPOs may find that an MGA has moved its product from the carrier with whom they have a contract to another with whom they have none. Therefore, strong relationships need to be developed with MGAs to ensure that the PPO will be included with the next carrier. The PPO's part of that relationship will involve supporting the MGA during such a move by maintaining confidentiality and being willing and able to react promptly to such a change. For its part, the MGA needs to keep the PPO appraised of its intent to move and of the identity of the new carrier, and it needs to advocate the PPO to that carrier. Because timing is critical in these situations, the MGA will want a great deal of control, which the PPO should relinquish only if sufficient trust has been earned through previous experience.

The general strategy PPOs should adopt when approaching carriers is to seek the support of their local sales manager and brokers before contacting the headquarters. Large carriers will be more interested in the network and less interested in UM or cost savings reports, whereas the interest of the medium and smaller carriers in all three products will increase inversely with the size of the carrier, as shown in Table 3.

SELF-INSUREDS

The trend toward self-insuring continues to grow, particularly with insurance premiums increasing so rapidly. Add to this the growing impatience of large employers for more effective cost containment and the stage is set for a great deal of experimentation. This translates into opportunities for flexible PPOs. For example, a group may want a PPO in the state where its costs are highest and only want precertification of hospital admissions elsewhere in the country.

The recommended strategy for this market segment is to contact the group directly, impress them with the ability of the PPO to create savings, and help design a benefit plan with financial incentives and disincentives.

UNIONS

Factors which can be encountered when marketing to unions are listed in Table 4. With these points of

TABLE 3   Insurance Company Priorities

	Products			Strategies	
MARKET SEGMENT	NETWORK	UM	MIS	SUPPORT	CONTACTS
Large	Offer	Unbundle	Unbundle	Sales and headquarters	Brokers
Medium	Offer	Offer	Offer	Sales and headquarters	Brokers
Small	Offer	Offer	Offer	Sales and headquarters	Brokers

TABLE 4   Points to Qualify when Prospecting Unions

- Benefit plan: Is it part of the collective bargaining agreement, or can it be amended at any time?
- Trustees: Who are they, who represents labor and management, what is the length of their terms of office?
- Benefits committee: Who are they, who represents labor or management, what is the length of their terms of office?
- Consultants: Who are they, who represents labor or management?
- Funding mechanism: If insured, by which carrier; if self-funded, is plan self-administered or administered by a TPA?
- Degree of flexibility: Are they willing to modify benefits?

define the average size of each contact (for example, number of covered lives per insurer, average number of employees per large- or medium-size employer group, and average number of members per union). Note that every employer must file a Form 5500 with the Internal Revenue Service which details each type of benefit plan it offers. Commercial services as well as Employee Retirement Income Security Act (ERISA) sell directories recapping this information. It is the most comprehensive source for this type of information. Unfortunately, the information can be outdated, for example, a new carrier may be in force, but it provides essential data such as number of employees, renewal date, and the name of the decision maker.

PRODUCTIVITY ASSUMPTIONS

Once a PPO has defined the total number of contacts, it must develop a series of assumptions which pre-

clarification in mind, a PPO is better prepared to anticipate the flexibility or rigidity to be encountered when it offers a new PPO approach to a particular union.

Be aware that benefit disincentives can be construed by union membership as a loss of hard-won benefits. This problem arises because seniority is the basis for increased benefits, and apprentices would receive the same preferred benefits as senior journeymen.

RECAP

Having ranked the market segments by importance and having discussed several segments, the next steps are to define the universe, create productivity assumptions, apply assumptions to the universe to determine the number of salespeople needed, and design the sales incentive and compensation plan.

UNIVERSE

Table 5 illustrates sources for defining the total number of contacts in each market segment. They include state agencies, industry publications, and commercial directories.

Besides the number of contacts, a PPO needs to

TABLE 5   Sources Used to Define Universe

SEGMENT	SOURCE
Insurers and workers compensation	State Department of Insurance, *A.M. Best* state license
Self-insureds	Form 5500, listings showing employee size (>100), state filings to self-insure workers compensation
Unions	Department of Labor, International Foundation of Employee Benefit Plans
TPAs	State regulatory agency, Society of Benefit Plan Administrators
Consultants, brokers, and general administrators	Special issues of *Business Insurance*, state insurance agency, local chapter of NAHU, PIMA, and MI2.

dict the productivity of the sales force by market segment. Those assumptions should include:

1. How many contacts must be made to produce a qualified prospect (prospecting ratio).
2. How many qualified prospects yield a sale (closing ratio).
3. How long this entire process takes (sales cycle).
4. How many sales will be produced each month (selling rate).
5. What percentage of covered lives will use the PPO during the first and second year (penetration rate).

STAFFING

Applying these assumptions to the universe in each segment will yield the number of salespeople needed to reach that market. An example appears in Table 6. Table 7 shows the results that can be expected from a single salesperson.

Who makes the best PPO salesperson? It depends on the positioning strategy of the PPO. If that strategy is a rigid HMO-like maximum cost saving model, the salesperson must be an expert with that model. If the looser, more market-driven flexibility strategy is used, the answer is money-motivated individuals with sales backgrounds in group insurance, brokers, TPAs, employers, and the healthcare industry.

TABLE 6 Staffing Derivation Assumptions

Universe	500 insurers, of which 260 represent 80% of the accident and health premium in force in a service area
Prospecting ratio	One qualified prospect per ten contacts per salesperson, assuming five contacts per week
Closing ratio	One sale per ten qualified prospects per salesperson
Sales cycles	One sale per 9 to 12 months per salesperson
Penetration	
First year	30%
Second year	50%

TABLE 7 Staffing Results for One Salesperson

Universe	260 insurers
Prospecting ratio	26 qualified prospects (10% of 260)
Closing ratio	Three sales (first sale in ninth month, second sale in tenth month, third sale in eleventh month)
Penetration	
First year	22,500 lives (25,000 lives per insurer × 30% × 3 insurers)
Second year	37,500 lives (25,000 lives per insurer × 50% × 3 insurers)

Where are these people found? HMOs. With sales leveling off for many HMOs, there are more productive salespeople looking for new opportunities. At a minimum, they should know employers and should have a fair exposure to brokers and group insurance.

INCENTIVE COMPENSATION

Too many PPOs offer just a salary and a small bonus for each contract, providing no real incentive for good producers. Ultimately, good people leave because they can earn more elsewhere through a higher commission. This leaves an unmotivated sales force of average producers who can live on the salary provided and have no incentive to produce more because of the small bonus.

An effective approach to incentive compensation includes a relatively low base salary, a bonus for each contract, and a commission based on the revenue that each contract produces. The salary should be too low to subsist on, thus providing the incentive to sell.

Next, take away any excuses for not being able to sell; for example, the excuse that the access fee is too high relative to competition offering the same services or marketing literature is inadequate. Because it takes quite a while to make a sale, the PPO should pay a bonus once the contract is produced. In addition, the commission should be a percentage of the access fee. Finally, there should be no cap on the amount of commission which can be earned by a good producer. This is not a problem because it comes from earned revenue. For example, the base salary should be roughly equivalent to that of an insurance or HMO sale representative with 2 years of experience (for example, $18,240 to $30,000 depending on the section of the country), the bonus $250 to 500 per contract, and the commission 5 to 10 percent of the access fee.

SUMMARY

Once a marketing and sales plan has been developed, the PPO should be prepared to make adjustments to the plan. Changes made need to be made in the incentive compensation plan to spur more sales production. Prospects which are sluggish may be reassigned to another salesperson to stimulate activity. A sales contest can generate sales by offering a bonus on top of the commission plan for a certain period of time. Ultimately, a continuing series of adjustments to the original plan will create a successful program which matches the unique features of a local marketplace.

CHAPTER TEN

Strategic Planning and Implementation

DELIVERY SYSTEMS, STRATEGIES, AND TECHNIQUES

HOWARD R. BERRY, Principal Associate
LOU PAVIA, Senior Vice President
McManis Associates, Washington, D.C.

It is no secret that the way healthcare is delivered and financed in the United States is undergoing a dramatic upheaval of epic proportions. Providers, payers, employers, government, and patients are all feeling the impact of this revolution as the industry grapples with the need to provide increasingly expensive, state-of-the-art healthcare services in a cost-effective manner to an expanding and more demanding population base while maintaining the solvency and integrity of the healthcare financing system.

The pressure on providers and insurers to manage healthcare—both cost and quality—will continue and intensify. By the year 2000, nearly 90 percent of all patients will be in some type of managed care plan or managed indemnity program. But what does it take to create an effective and successful managed healthcare plan?

There is no pat answer or single, simple solution for success in managed health. However, the chances of being a winner in the managed care business can be significantly enhanced by effective, market-based strategic planning and management. Too often, providers, insurers, businesses, and others enter into managed care without clearly defining their long-term goals and objectives and assessing the implications of their actions. They "forget" that the development of managed care strategies, like other strategies, is a process — a systematic but political and organizational process — that should involve the board, management, and staff in order to be successful. They ignore the importance of gaining an understanding of the unmet needs of their customers and the likely response of their competitors. They "forget" to develop management, business, and financial plans, and human resource plans in tandem with the strategic plan. Further, they fail to recognize that the implementation of new strategies often requires changes in the organizational structure and culture, current management practices, and decision-making processes. Figure 1 shows the basic elements of strategic planning.

This chapter explores how to prepare a successful managed care strategy that fits with an organization's goals and how to develop a business plan that is based on a sound and thorough examination and analysis of the market, the customer, and the competition. It also addresses some of the keys to successful implementation and the need to frequently reevaluate and update strategies and plans.

Figure 1   *Strategic planning.*

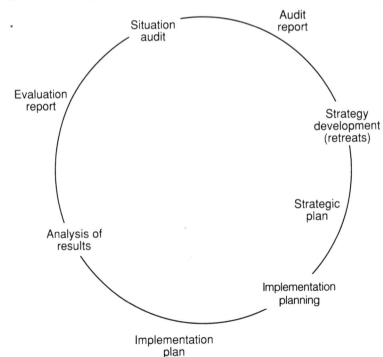

WHY PLAN? Planning is not an easy task. Given the pressures of day-to-day business survival and the need to move new ideas quickly, it is far too easy for action-oriented executives to skip or slight the strategic planning process. Too many fall back on instinct or simply follow the pack and count on the latest trend of the day. Another mistake is the practice of relegating responsibility for developing the strategic plan to staff or strategic planners. Common justifications for ignoring this important management responsibility are the lack of time, fear that the strategic plan will get into the hands of a competitor, or the lack of faith in predications about the future. "How can I plan 3 years out when I can't even plan for tomorrow?" is a common lament.

While no one can predict with absolute certainty what the future will hold, particularly in today's dynamic business and healthcare environments, having an overall strategy is still a necessity. Without an overall direction and goals an organization is far too vulnerable to any change that might come along, be it from environmental forces, new legislation, or economic trends.

In addition, one of the most important reasons for planning is the *process*. In many ways, the process of strategic planning is even more important than the end product or document. Developing a database of hard facts, brainstorming strategy with the management team, articulating vision and objectives, understanding competitors and customers, communicating the plan, and building consensus are all valuable to the success of an enterprise, regardless of the final document produced.

No strategic plan should be considered cast in concrete. It needs frequent periodic course corrections and updates. However, an organization that has gone through the planning process is much better prepared to address the unknowns and uncertainties of the future as they arise than one which has not. Studies to evaluate the effectiveness of strategic planning in corporations have concluded that companies with strategic plans are generally more successful than those without. Moreover, the fact that companies which do not strictly adhere to their plans are also more successful, proves that the real value of strategic planning is the process. Figure 2 describes some of the elements of strategy development.

There are compelling reasons why a strategic plan should be developed before entering a new managed care venture or when evaluating the future of an existing venture. The strategic planning process is the ideal vehicle for articulating mission, goals, and objectives.

Articulating Mission, Goals, and Objectives Before entering any new venture that will require significant resources or play a key strategic role in the organization's mission, it is important to carefully think through and articulate the project's objectives. The strategic planning process forces management to

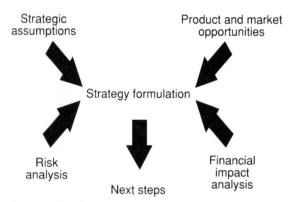

Figure 2   *Strategy development.*

carefully consider objectives of a new venture and how that new venture will fit with the overall mission and vision of the organization.

If a hospital is considering an investment in an HMO or PPO or is considering starting one from scratch, the first important points to consider are the reasons for getting into the business, the expectations of the effort, and the specific yardstick that will be used to measure the success of those expectations. Is the goal to capture additional patients, sustain existing market share, or make a return on investment? A clear understanding of these objectives by all who will be involved in implementation is critical to the success and the ability of the new venture to stay on course when the going gets tough.

Elements of a Mission Statement

- Product-market scope
- Market position
- Basis of differentiation
- Geographic scope
- Financial objectives
- Key values of the organization

Assembling Facts   Developing a "winning strategy" depends on strategic thinking which is founded on fact, not supposition. Carefully research the market, the customer, the competition, and the environment. Be honest and objective about the strengths, weaknesses, and capabilities of the organization. Today's demanding competitive environment leaves little room for error and requires fact-based analysis (see Figure 3).

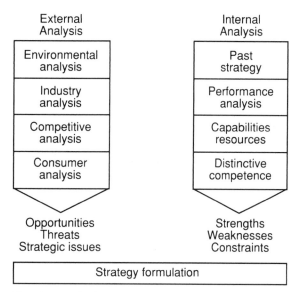

Figure 3 *Situation analysis.*

The situation assessment phase of the strategic planning process is the vehicle for uncovering the facts necessary to develop an effective strategy. However, be careful not to suffer from "analysis paralysis." Be selective in gathering facts and use them to stimulate, not get in the way of, creative thinking. Be thorough, but do not become inundated with extraneous data or let the analysis become an end in itself. It is important for the strategist to identify key variables which have impact on the decision-making process. The data collection process should appropriately address these variables.

Building Commitment

Successful implementation of a managed care strategy depends on the efforts and cooperation of many people in different parts of an organization. For instance, human resources, finance, marketing, and operations all need to be committed to the success of the strategic plan. Unfortunately, this critical factor is often overlooked and thus, the strategic plan is too often viewed by the rank and file as a lengthy and lofty document prepared by "the powers that be" and then foisted on the rest of the organization.

The *process* of developing the strategic plan is more important than the plan itself. Involve those key individuals who will be responsible for implementation from the beginning of the planning process. If the key players do not understand or buy into the strategy, how far will the strategy get? A critical function of the strategic planning process is the involvement of the key constituent groups in the decision-making process. People will perform better if they understand why they are being asked to do something and have input into the tasks they will be asked to undertake. Building consensus and gaining commitment come through participation in task forces (small groups which focus on key strategic issues such as competition, product design, and pricing strategy and report results back to the main planning body) and strategy retreats (which offer a forum for key constituents to identify, discuss, and reach consensus on the major planning assumptions and next steps) that form the core of the strategic planning process. These types of participatory activities enable people to feel they are part of the process; therefore, they buy into the outcome.

For example, an insurance carrier developing a strategy to enter the HMO field or a third party administrator (TPA) that wants to develop a PPO network will require the cooperation and commitment of many people within the organization. Some will see this strategy and potential changes as threatening to their careers, others will feel that resources are being siphoned from their operations, and others might just outright disagree with the strategy. The battle will be tough enough on the outside without having to worry about internal strife and dissension and lack of dedication from employees.

Marshalling Resources

Developing a managed care organization or even developing a new managed care product is not for the faint of heart. Implementing a managed care strategy often takes far longer, requires greater resources, and yields far less return than expected. Some have found managed care to be a proverbial "black hole." Therefore, it is critical to get a solid handle on the resource requirements in terms of capital, skills, person hours, and management time from the outset. Do not underestimate the resources that will be needed; few new ventures come in ahead of schedule and under budget. Anticipate and expect the unexpected and put some flexibility in the plan and a cushion in the budget to be prepared for contingencies.

The strategic planning process should estimate the resource requirements for implementation of the strategy and include specific action plans identifying who will do what and when. A detailed financial plan delineating start-up costs as well as ongoing revenue and cost projections is an important element of any strategic plan. The resource and financial plans must be prepared for the board of directors to assure that adequate funds are appropriated to the total project. They should also be woven into the annual budgeting process to assure that funding is available to the right operational department at the right time. Equally important is their use in human resource planning to assure that the right people are available for the project when needed.

Guiding Actions   The strategic plan should provide a vehicle to orchestrate and coordinate the efforts of the many people required to implement the strategy as well as monitor progress of the implementation. Each individual involved must know what is expected, what must be done, and when it must be done. A "winning" strategic plan will carefully break down into tasks the total effort required to implement the plan, including specific responsibilities and time frames. Typically, Gantt charts and other project management techniques will be used to manage the implementation of the strategy and to provide a mechanism for progress reports to management. This will also help to identify trouble spots, such as critical areas where additional resources may be needed, unexpected delays in the process, and other issues which may need management attention. As each task is completed it should be checked off on the master schedule, and if tasks are delayed, the reason for the delay and the revised due date should be logged in on the master schedule.

For example, a provider developing a strategy for building a preferred provider organization will give careful consideration to the overall effort involved, which should be broken down into tasks and subtasks. The major tasks might include:

1. Developing the provider network and negotiating provider contracts
2. Establishing a sales and marketing organization
3. Developing a utilization management and quality assurance capability
4. Developing a management information system
5. Establishing an organizational infrastructure

Each of these major tasks then would be broken down into individual subtasks. The major task of developing a provider network could be further broken down into subtasks that might include:

1. Analyze provider admission and cost information
2. Identify desired providers
3. Develop model provider contract
4. Negotiate provider contracts
5. Establish ongoing provider relations function

Understanding the Risks   Every strategy has inherent risks. There will be hundreds of things that can go wrong. The downside risk of possible adverse outcomes should be recognized and discussed before embarking on the strategy. In some cases the maximum exposure may be limited and quantifiable, such as losing the start-up capital. In other cases the risk may be nebulous but serious, such as damaging physician relations. In either case, recognize and be prepared for risks. Try to address and therefore neutralize risks and be sure that potential rewards outweigh the potential risks.

Strategic planning is an important tool for management to set objectives, assemble facts, gain commitment, marshal resources, guide action, and understand risks. This is not to say that a managed care organization cannot be a winner without one, but the chances of winning are greatly enhanced by using the techniques of strategic planning that have been developed and tested in the corporate world and applying them to the managed healthcare environment.

BUILDING COMPETITIVE ADVANTAGE AND STRATEGIC OPTIONS

In formulating a "winning" strategy for a managed care organization, strategists have a wide array of strategic options at their disposal to skillfully craft a strategy that differentiates it from the competition and builds a sustainable competitive advantage. The strategy formulation process is inherently a creative endeavor and certainly an iterative process, and the building blocks of strategy can be assembled in numerous combinations and permutations. It is the job of the strategist to assemble and articulate a cohesive strategy for the organization which addresses the needs of the marketplace and its customers, recognizes the strengths and weaknesses of the competition, and considers the capabilities and limitations of the organization itself.

The task of strategy formulation, however, is made easier by a thorough situation assessment that builds a database of factual information on the environment, market, customers, industry, competition, and the organization itself. Once there is a solid, realistic grasp of the facts and there is input from a wide range of sources, both internal and external, the task of building a strategic plan can begin.

The building blocks of strategy for managed care organizations can be generally focused in several major categories. Some of the primary strategic options include the following areas.

Product Offering

Today the design of managed care products is limited only by imagination and available resources. Healthcare benefit products are no longer as simple and as clear cut as indemnity plans, HMOs, and PPOs. Variations of all three forms have proliferated to the point where there is a blending of the basic products and it is difficult to differentiate them. Products will vary in the breadth of benefit coverage, the degree to which the consumer can freely choose a provider, the constraints put on the delivery of care, the assignment of risk, copayments and deductibles, and the premium. Decisions about which product to offer should be made on the basis of sound market research, careful competitive assessment, and thorough financial analysis. In other words, do not design the product in a vacuum. Be mindful of customer needs and wants, the need to differentiate or improve upon the competition's offerings, and the financial realities. To be successful in today's competitive marketplace, the product mix must be unique and at the cutting edge, and it must provide both health and financial benefits.

Another key strategic variable is the *breadth of the product offering*; the decision to offer one, two, or three products; and the number of variations of each. Employers such as Xerox and Allied Signal are currently looking to suppliers of health benefit programs to provide a portfolio of integrated products such as indemnity or managed fee-for-service, HMO, PPO, comprehensive ambulatory care, or Medicare risk products. They seek "one-stop shopping" so they can reduce the number of suppliers they must deal with and gain efficiency in their procurement and administrative processes. On the other hand, the broader the product line, the more difficult it is to focus resources, avoid costly confusion internally and externally, and fend off niche competitors. However, based on the fact that employers are trying to rationalize their employee benefit programs and consolidate business to a few suppliers that offer a wide range of integrated products, it is more prudent to go broad rather than narrow with product lines. In the future, there will likely be few single-product-line companies.

The people aspects of offering a wide range of services must also be considered. Many large indemnity carriers which have been strategically broadening their product offerings with managed care programs have been greatly frustrated by the lack of understanding and enthusiasm for managed care plans on the part of their field sales force. The sales force, in most cases, has not received adequate training regarding the needs of the market and the benefits of cross-selling to their customers. In addition, the sales force recognizes that managed care products require a double sell, once to the employer and then to the employee, thereby making it a more difficult and time-consuming sale. Consequently, managed care plans may not be well launched and the field sales force may not focus on actively promoting these products.

Target Market Segments

After products, the next major strategic decision is the selection of markets. When developing a strategy, it is important to identify the various segments of the market, target those that offer the greatest opportunity, focus on priorities, and develop individual strategies for each target segment.

For example, depending on the assessment of the market and the product's features and capabilities, specific target markets might be large, midsize, or small employers; local, regional, or national employers; governmental units, associations, industrial firms, or service organizations. Remember that each target market will have different needs, different buying behaviors, and different competitors. Small employers usually buy on price while large employers buy price, service, and quality. National firms look for national or at least regional provider networks and a strong service orientation. Industrial firms may want an integrated workers compensation product, and governmental units will probably open their doors to a smorgasbord of competitors. Pick target markets that are substantial in size, enjoy strong growth, have little competition, and play to the strengths and capabilities of the product.

Marketing and Distribution

A marketing and distribution system must be designed to support the particular type of product and the markets that are being targeted. For instance, the distribution options available include direct marketing to the employer, utilizing an insurance company to market the product in conjunction with their products, or utilizing a third party administrator to market the product to their client base. As mentioned earlier, managed care services must be sold twice; once to the employer to get on the list of available options and then to the employee who will select from many options and plans. In both cases "the sell" can be difficult and expensive, involving extensive education to both customers. Because the buying considerations of each of these potential customers are different, this can be a very labor-intensive process for the sales force. Generally, indemnity salespeople cross-sell other products such as group life and pension fund management to help spread the cost of the sales effort.

Depending on the design of the managed care product and how the business is defined, it might be sold directly to employers, union trusts, insurance carriers, benefit consultants, TPAs, or even to other managed care organizations. Managed care is characterized by its need for a multichannel distribution network which allows for a variety of distribution points.

A strong sales force is worth its weight in gold. Hire good people and support them with the proper marketing tools, extensive educational programs, and attractive incentives. Marketing and sales is not the area in which to skimp. Regardless of how wonderful a product or the provider network in place might be, if the sales force is not adequately prepared to sell that product, it will not sell.

Provider Network

Developing a network of high quality, cost-effective, and cooperative providers is another important task. Start by identifying the geographic coverage, types of specialties, and number of specialists necessary to support the strategy and plan. Then decide on first, second, and third choices of providers in each specialty.

Treat the recruitment of providers into the network as an important sales effort. Sell the *benefits* of being part of the organization; most providers contract with numerous managed care organizations and are deluged with opportunities to join many more. To gain a competitive edge in attracting providers, document the plan's ability to channel patients to their facilities and make a commitment to prompt payment of claims. Approach providers armed with facts, such as a brand design which shows how the product will channel patients to specific providers and data which identify the additional market share the provider will be able to capture, and demonstrate how participation in the plan will increase their patient volume. Be prepared to offer equity participation (profit sharing, cost savings, or equity shares in the managed care corporation) and possibly a governance role (a board seat, ability to vote on key issues, advisory board participation, or some reserve powers) to bellwether providers.

In developing the provider network, think broadly and aim for a full continuum of managed healthcare services. Include not only acute care hospitals and physicians but other providers covered under employers' health benefit programs, such as outpatient care, psychiatric and rehabilitation services, chemical dependency programs, prescription drugs, vision, dental, and workers compensation.

Another key strategic factor in developing a provider network is the type of contractual arrangement with the providers. How will they be paid — fee-for-service, discounted charges, per diem payments, per case payments, or capitation? These are important decisions that have a direct bearing on the future profit potential of the plan and the amount of risk each constituent will be asked to shoulder. Where possible, strive for "attorney-in-fact" contracts that offer the flexibility to freely negotiate price with a customer without having to seek continuous approvals from myriad provider groups.

Utilization Management and Quality Assurance

Utilization management and quality assurance go hand in hand in the managed care environment, and both are key strategic variables. Quality care is cost-effective care. In addition, there is a perception on the part of the public that when the utilization of healthcare is managed, the quality of care suffers. However, it is important to realize that more care does not equate to better care and get that message across to the customers. Do not settle for anything less than quality providers and services and put in place programs that continuously monitor and control quality. If the necessary programs or tools to monitor quality are not in place, they must be developed.

Utilization management is where the "rubber meets the road" and is a key module in providing value to the customer. Cutting edge managed care organizations will have comprehensive, expert system–based, utilization management capability, including preadmission review, second surgical opinion, concurrent review, large case management, discharge planning, retrospective review, and bill auditing. Utilization management should be broad in scope, covering not only inpatient acute care but also outpatient care, prescription drugs, vision, workers compensation, disability, and the full range of healthcare services financed by employers and third parties.

Utilization management is a function that can be developed in-house or can be contracted for externally. However, as the tools of utilization management become more comprehensive and sophisticated, the cost of developing an in-house system is rising. There are increasing numbers of independent utilization management organizations which offer computerized systems, technological capability, and tested protocols. These organizations tend to have large databases and significant expertise in utilization management; therefore, many managed care organizations find it more effective and cost efficient to contract for these services. Further, many employers like to have a choice of utilization management options and may be skeptical about having a provider-owned managed care organization policing itself and doubtful of the wisdom of having "the fox watch the hen house." In addition it is imperative that managed care organizations substantiate benefits to employers and providers by providing data to current and potential customers which document savings and demonstrate a successful track record and high quality services.

Management Information Systems

Employers have thus far been extremely frustrated by the lack of meaningful cost and utilization information provided by managed care organizations. They are accustomed to receiving this information from their indemnity carrier or their claims administrator and want the same from their supplier of managed healthcare services. Employers' health insurance premiums have been rising at an average annual rate of 20 percent in recent years. In addition, corporate America is being forced to recognize a nearly $2 trillion unfunded liability in retiree health benefits. So expect the pressures for this type of information to be stronger than ever.

Advances in computer and information technology offer an opportunity for managed care organizations to use technology as a source of product differentiation and a competitive advantage in the marketplace. Collecting the proper data and then presenting it to the client in a meaningful manner using state-of-the-art graphics showing trends and comparative data is a way to add real value. Employers want cost and utilization information by employee, provider, and key procedure. They want to follow these trends over time and compare their experience with that of other employers.

Take advantage of the opportunity to use information systems as a means of continuously informing employers about savings on their healthcare bills. The same goes for the ability to document to providers how much new business is being channeled their way. Use technology as a key source of differentiation and competitive advantage.

Member Services

Make member services a key module of the strategic plan. Managed care organizations have multiple customer groups, and constituents not only have to be sold initially but must also be serviced continuously. Convincing employers to include the products as an option in their health benefit programs is only the first step. Next, the employee must be convinced to select this option and then to stay with the plan. The fact that employees show satisfaction and loyalty to a particular managed care plan is a good reference in terms of renewal by the employer. Key service enhancements which may help to bond employees to a plan include toll-free health information hot lines, benefits coverage information hot lines, or electronic eligibility verification.

In addition, make it easy for members to enroll in the plan, to get information on the benefit coverage, and to identify themselves to a provider. Some managed care organizations include an emergency medical records service and patient scheduling as part of their member services "bag of tricks." Remember the customer is king; make customer service a key strategic initiative. Be "user friendly" and easy to do business with.

Pricing

Formulating an effective pricing strategy depends on having solid product cost information, knowledge of competitive pricing, and an understanding of the price sensitivity of the market. It is crucial to have a solid analysis of the costs associated with the managed care product. It is imperative that cost be considered when formulating a pricing strategy because it has a significant bearing on the ability of the organization to endure short-term losses for long-term gains. Moreover, it assists the planner in determining capital level requirements to sustain the managed care product while building market share. Many managed care organizations have used a strategy of "buying market share" by setting a low price in a highly price sensitive market to stimulate revenue growth. The objective of this strategy is to sacrifice near-term profits for fast growth as a means of quickly building critical mass and establishing a market position. This is a relatively high-risk strategy, and careful consideration must be given to determining capital requirements and ensuring that capital is available to sustain the organization through this high-growth low-profit stage. However, caution must be exercised to avoid a price war in which the competition simply matches the low price and thus lowers the price level of the entire industry at the expense of industry profits.

Another pricing strategy frequently used is "market skimming." Under this strategy, the highest price possible is established given the comparative benefits of the product versus those of the competition. Even at this relatively high price, certain segments of the market will still buy the product. Each time sales slow down, the price is lowered to draw in the next price-sensitive layer of customers. This strategy results in slower growth. The significant risk inherent in this type of strategy is the limited market available to the product. Clearly, the product must be substantially differentiated from that of lower-priced competitors to justify its higher price in the eyes of the consumer.

Where possible, try not to sell on price alone. Try to establish a reputation as a high quality, service-oriented organization and demand a premium price for a superior product. It is wise for the managed care provider to pay careful attention to consumer perceptions of quality care and quality service. Consumers tend to judge the level of quality of providers by the appearance of facilities, the existence of amenities, and the amount and type of high-technology equipment. However, it is important to continually and effectively monitor the attitudes and opinions of consumers regarding the managed care product and track this over time. To be successful, a managed care company must be aware of the requirements and needs within its market and must have the flexibility to change with the market.

Strategic Partners

Given the magnitude of the task and the skills, time, and resources needed to develop an effective managed care organization, consider building a network to facilitate implementation of a managed care strategy via strategic alliances. Look for partners that complement the business, have a good reputation in the marketplace, are financially viable, and share similar visions and values. These alliances may take the form of joint ventures, license agreements, comarketing arrangements, or subcontracting. Whatever form the alliance takes, make sure the partner(s) complement the organization's skills and product mix to enhance and better position the product and its ability to tap into new markets. For joint arrangements to succeed, the venture must be a "win-win" situation for all parties. Clear benefits must be derived by all participants (managed care plans, employers, and employees) to ensure success.

Strategic alliances may also offer opportunities to expand the network geographically or by specialty, to round out product offerings, to bolster operational capabilities, or to leverage sales coverage. Think through what partnership will best add value and create synergy.

PEOPLE: THE VITAL LINK IN STRATEGIC PLANNING

Organizations do not implement strategies, people do. Yet the most frequently neglected aspect of strategic planning is human resources. An organization needs more than a vision of where it is going and supporting strategies and plans to get there. It needs the organizational capacity and the appropriate human resources to address the changing dynamics of the market. The organizational climate must be conducive to appropriate levels of risk-taking by its staff to implement these strategies and, therefore, the organizational climate must be able to accommodate the successful as well as unsuccessful endeavors by its employees.

An organization needs the commitment of the key players—board members, top management, middle management—to successfully implement a strategy. But this commitment will not emerge on its own. Commitment comes from ownership, and ownership comes from participation. There will be little buy-in or perceived ownership of a plan if it is developed solely by the board and CEO. Instead, planning must be linked with strategic management and human resource planning and employees must have incentives to buy into the fulfillment of the strategic vision. Employees must understand the logic behind their role in attaining the strategic vision by defining with management clear objectives which relate to their roles in the strategic vision of the organization. These objectives should also be tied to the employee's compensation level and performance reviews.

Senior management has a responsibility to consider a strategic plan's impact on the entire organization. As part of the overall planning process, the organization's structural and management capacity to implement the plan must be carefully assessed. The business strategy must be linked to departmental and individual goals, management by objective programs, and performance appraisal systems (see Figure 4).

Recently, the President's Council on Management Improvement (PCMI) commissioned a study to identify exemplary human resource practices in the corporate world. The PCMI is now adapting the best of these practices for use in the federal government, and the results have applications for the healthcare industry as well. Many of these top corporations, such as IBM, AT&T, and Exxon, are repositioning themselves in highly competitive, restructuring industries, and have experienced problems similar to those in healthcare. These corporations are being forced to undergo a transition from a highly regulated

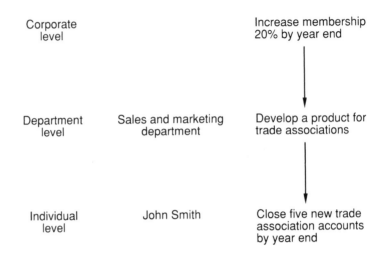

Figure 4 *Linking of strategic goals.*

environment to a consumer-oriented environment. A clear need for market-based strategies has caused these organizations to rethink their basic core strategies and their approach to determining human resource requirements.

The study discovered a common practice among these successfully repositioned organizations—the integration of strategic planning with management and human resource planning. In tandem with the strategic plan, they prepare a formal human resource plan which details how many and what kinds of people with what types of skills and backgrounds will be required to get the organization "from here to there." Moreover, the plan details how to structure the organization, reorganize and retrain existing staff, determine if, and what type of, additional staff will be needed, and integrate working units to accomplish the stipulated goals and objectives. In other words, they link together staffing, recruitment, management succession, management development, performance appraisal, and compensation and benefit decisions so that the performance and individual behavior of corporate employees optimally support the goals of the strategic plan.

Few healthcare organizations have done an effective job of integrating management and human resource planning with strategic planning; the majority have yet to begin. The new directions healthcare organizations are currently considering, such as corporate restructuring, mergers, diversification, vertical integration, product line management, and joint ventures, clearly demonstrate the need to address this vital issue in the planning process.

Healthcare organizations have identified the need to become market-driven in their planning and program development. They are segmenting and targeting their markets, developing new products and services, and modifying or repackaging existing ones. All of these strategies are designed to build sustainable competitive advantage and to position the organization for the future. However, each strategy has direct and profound implications for the organization's human resources and management structure.

All too often, senior management underestimates the effect of external trends and proposed strategic initiatives on their management and staff. Many new strategies require significant changes in attitudes and basic ways of doing business. A company which has traditionally been able to operate successfully with little feedback from its customers may have difficulty becoming attuned to and responding to the needs of its clientele. Some may shift away from the traditional, hierarchical structure and its separate functional units to a matrix management system that fosters increased cooperation and communication among and within various units and departments (see Figure 5). Any change, good or bad, in management structure is usually accompanied by a period of confusion and disorientation within the organization. This turbulent period may have a significant bearing on the ability of the organization to respond effectively to any proposed strategy.

New strategies and product lines may also require new expertise —managers with skills and abilities that may not be available from within the current organizational framework. Sometimes this expertise must be recruited from other service industries, importing into the current environment a very different type of individual with

Figure 5 *Matrix management.*

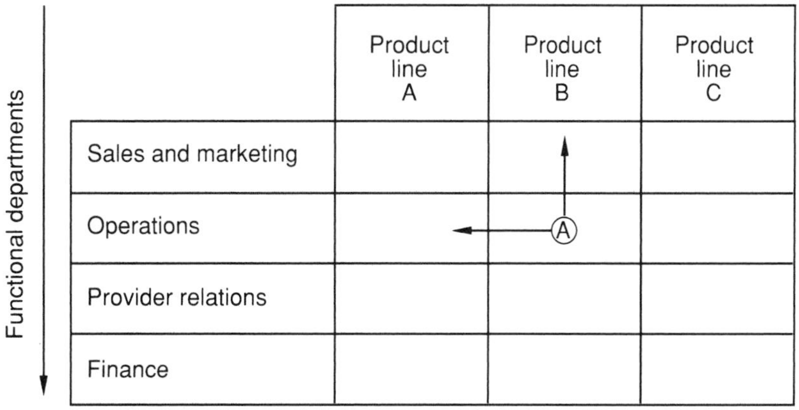

	Product line A	Product line B	Product line C
Sales and marketing		↑	
Operations		←Ⓐ	
Provider relations			
Finance			

Functional departments

Employee A has a dual responsibility to the product line manager and to the operations manager skills in marketing and a more businesslike, risk-oriented perspective.

The healthcare industry is becoming increasingly complex. The leadership of these new organizations must be prepared to commit themselves to new management structures, systems, and tactics that will support and revitalize their organizations and the people in them.

The challenge to senior management goes beyond simply ensuring that the organization has a strategy to cope with a changing environment. They must also recognize that they need to make a sizable investment in time, money, and energy to put into place the human resource skills and capabilities that are needed to successfully implement the strategies.

UPDATING STRATEGIC PLANS

With changes in competition, technology, legislation, and the healthcare environment occurring almost daily, many executives have been tempted to scuttle strategic plans. But planning is still a valuable tool for coping with future uncertainty.

To help keep strategies alive and on track, update them at least once a year. There are two critical reasons for doing so.

First, the environment *is* fast-paced and many events beyond senior management's control can have a sudden and dramatic impact on how business is conducted. A periodic reassessment and adjustment of strategies is necessary to put executives back in the driver's seat and regain control. Rather than simply being buffeted by the winds of change, use updates to manage change and capitalize on the opportunities it presents.

Second, and worth repeating, the strategy should not be a lofty document that sits on a shelf, but a plan that can evolve and help keep an organization headed in the right direction. And, as with the original strategy development, the process of updating strategies is what keeps the vision alive and keeps people interested. It is the update process that gives senior managers and others time to think strategically and creatively and to reach a consensus on revised strategic objectives and how to achieve them.

Brief annual reviews of strategic plans also help to identify problems being encountered in the implementation of the strategies and help people refocus their thinking on long-term objectives. After all, when executives get wrapped up in putting out the fires in day-to-day operations, it is far too easy for them to lose sight of the big picture.

Updating a strategy, a strategic management assessment, does not mean going back to square one and rehashing all the old data, statistics, and research that led to the development of the strategy in the first place. Nor should the assessment be a lengthy and involved process. What the assessment should do is force the organization's senior management team to examine the organization and its vision from the standpoint of its strategy. It should provide executives with an update and an objective reassessment of the organization's current position and identify course corrections needed for the future.

In addition, the assessment will help to identify implementation problems or the reasons for a "stalled" strategy, enabling the organization to get back on track with the right programs and directions for long-term success.

Key Steps Start with an analysis of the major environmental forces that are having an impact on the organization. Take a look at the information that was gathered at the original strategy development process and update it to reflect recent events and changes. Are the original strategic assumptions still valid? What has happened on the legislative front? What are the recent and expected medical and information technology advancements that could influence major lines of business? How will these changes affect the bottom line?

Second, conduct a diagnostic review of the organization. Examine the structure, management capacity, support systems, and information systems that are so often vital to implementation. Does the organization really have the right people, systems, and programs in place to implement the strategy?

Then, take another look at the company's competitive position and its customers. What is happening in the market and how might the recent moves of competitors affect the company's competitive position and its customers?

Finally, based on this updated information, evaluate the original strategy against the backdrop of developments during the past year to measure progress in implementation. At this point executives will be able to determine whether any changes and course corrections need to be made in strategies and plans.

The entire assessment process should take no more than 45 to 60 days. Do not get bogged down in old data, or even new data. Use the update process as a valuable tool for promoting creativity and innovation. Use this opportunity to assess new directions, focus discussions, bridge differences, and build consensus among key players.

THE FUTURE OF MANAGED CARE The managed healthcare organization of the future will focus on and revolve around the providers. That is where the care is delivered, the costs incurred, and the key decisions are made. The providers have the direct contact with the consumer, and traditionally any bonding that occurs is between the consumer and the provider.

Employers will be compelled to get heavily involved in healthcare as a way to tame the raging monster of runaway healthcare costs and will seek help from managed healthcare organizations that offer a comprehensive solution to the problem and a track record to back it up. Employers will seek long-term relationships that address the full continuum of their healthcare dollar. They will look for provider networks that manage not only inpatient acute care but also outpatient care and the full range of health and preventive services. Employers will also increasingly contract directly with providers, cutting out the intermediaries and building long-term partnerships with providers for the total health management of their employees.

The managed care organization of the future will offer the employer an array of ancillary services that are both fully integrated yet modular and include utilization management and quality assurance, management information services, fully electronic claims administration, financial services, member services, proven treatment protocols, and benefits consulting. The new generation of managed care organizations will be flexible and responsive to the needs of the employers and will be able to demonstrate that they can improve the quality of care while increasing its cost effectiveness.

Managed care is going through an upheaval, as is the whole healthcare industry. What worked in the past will not necessarily work in the future. The survivors will be dedicated to satisfying their customers, will keep an eye on their competitors and not underestimate their strength, and will realistically understand their own distinctive competence and the value they add.

CASE STUDY

Group Health: Integrated HMO Options

GEORGE C. HALVORSON, President and Chief Executive Officer

Group Health, Inc. Minneapolis, Minnesota

In 1961, Group Health, Inc. (GHI) was a fledgling 3-year-old staff-model "prepaid health plan" (the term used prior to the early 1970s before "HMO" was coined). Group Health's enrollment was relatively small and its market position was promising, but fragile. Every enrolled group was important to Group Health's survival.

The insurance companies who dominated the Minnesota healthcare market at that time had been generally tolerant of Group Health's relatively small penetration into their groups. Group Health was always offered as a second (that is, dual) choice, alongside an insurer or Blue Cross plan and was expected to continue using that strategy for the foreseeable future.

That expectation was badly shaken, however, when a Group Health representative showed up to renew a large group and was told that the GHI coverage was to be canceled at the insistence of the fee-for-service insurer who shared the group with GHI. The insurer had given the group an ultimatum: either cancel Group Health or lose the insurance carrier's coverage.

Group Health challenged the decision and suggested that an equally appropriate way to resolve the dilemma was for the employer to cancel the insurer and give the entire group to Group Health. The employer explained that approach was impossible because a number of employees had a strong preference for their current non-Group Health doctor.

Group Health's CEO resolved the issue by developing a choice plan that would offer full benefits to covered persons who used Group Health clinics and lesser benefits for those who elected to seek care from non-Group Health doctors. The care location decision could be made at the time that care was needed, rather than at an annual renewal date. This decision-making flexibility justified the word "instant" in the new product's name, "Instant Choice."

The employer decided to accept Group Health's proposal, thus creating a new concept in managed care. This new two-tier benefit approach encouraged members to receive care from Group Health's medical center. However, it also gave members a choice of continuing long-standing relationships with their current physician. Because the flexibility of Instant Choice allowed patients to make provider choices, the product significantly decreased employee resistance to accepting a closed-model plan as the only plan offered by the employer.

In a marketing sense, Instant Choice met the needs of both the employer and employees. The original Instant Choice group is still with Group Health on an exclusive basis and has grown from 400 to 4000 members.

For the next two decades, the Instant Choice product was made available by Group Health but was used almost exclusively in a defensive mode. Even though the approach was financially successful and very marketable, Group Health's standard product was also successful. The standard "locked-in" approach was the philosophical product of choice for the HMO. As a result, Instant Choice was not heavily promoted by the plan.

Through the 1970s and 1980s, Group Health grew to almost 200,000 members and built a strong multispecialty group practice using a strategically located network of clinics. Then in the early 1980s, other local HMO plans began to have great marketing success with IPA-types of provider configurations. The marketplace began responding very favorably to the competitor's "freedom of choice" ad campaigns and marketing themes, and Group Health lost much of its marketplace momentum. Competitors also become more price competitive with Group Health's traditionally lower rates through a combination of improved cost controls, very deep provider discounts, and "zero margin price war" rating strategies.

Group Health's strategic response was to pull the Instant Choice product out of mothballs in order to offer its own "freedom of choice" alternative to the market. The original Instant Choice product had been underwritten solely by Group Health. Over time—and due to regulator concerns that the original product may not have been entirely legal due to the "insuring" out-of-network benefits—Group Health evolved into offering the plan on a competitive basis with a Minnesota-based insurer. (Further

233

regulator concerns also caused Group Health to form a subsidiary state-licensed HMO called GroupCare to offer freedom-of-choice health benefit plans.) In the mid 1980s, Group Health also entered into a new joint venture with Prudential Insurance Company to offer an improved Instant Choice approach called CareSpan. Like the older Instant Choice plans, Care-Span is offered by Group Health's Group Care HMO subsidiary. The Prudential insures the out-of-network care.

CareSpan has become very successful in the marketplace by enrolling more than 50,000 people since 1985. CareSpan and Group Health's continuing Instant Choice plans now represent about 20 percent of Group Health's total patient base of 270,000 members.

CareSpan has been particularly successful in helping Group Health respond to the current employer trend of reducing the number of health plans offered in a given group. CareSpan resolves employer concerns about risk selection and employee-provider relationships. This has helped Group Health move into a position of being the only surviving health plan in more than 380 of its 750 groups. In almost 30 others, Group Health has used these product approaches to survive a reduction in the number of plans offered. Less than 25 groups, representing a few hundred contracts, have canceled Group Health coverage in favor of other plans over the past few years.

The CareSpan/Instant Choice approach also has another very beneficial impact on the HMO. Group Health clearly wants to "treat patients—not take captives." In the groups where Group Health is the sole surviving insurer or health plan, any employee who wants to seek care elsewhere can do so, albeit, with reduced benefits. That means patients are not forced to seek care from Group Health doctors if they prefer another care setting. As a result, Group Health's member relations stay friendly and positive.

Enrollees do elect to receive their care through Group Health's medical centers and provider network. Typically 90 percent or more of care is received in-network. The percentages of in-network care are somewhat lower for new groups, but these numbers move upward rapidly and typically meet Group Health's goals after 2 to 3 years for any given group.

Out-of-network hospital care and major cases are managed using the types of techniques typically utilized by IPA, HMOs, PPOs, and a few of the more progressive indemnity insurance company managed care plans. As a result, employers who purchase CareSpan not only receive the basic efficiency advantages of a staff-model integrated care system, but, at worst, the out-of-network care efficiency approximates the better efforts of other, less integrated managed care systems.

Group Health works at bringing all the care for CareSpan enrollees into Group Health's provider networks. The out-of-plan benefit differential starts with a $200 deductible. Group Health contacts each choice plan member annually to encourage in-plan provider use. Additionally, Group Health's integrated care delivery system is targeted at encouraging in-plan use. For example, Group Health offers a special "answering service" that is available evenings and weekends to offer care advice over the telephone and directs members into Group Health settings. Group Health's answering service is staffed with specially trained nurses and physicians and is far more convenient, efficient, and popular than independent physicians' clerical answering services for off-hours care. As a result, it serves as an efficient feeder system for in-network care and is used frequently by new members who might otherwise have sought care elsewhere.

The Instant Choice solution created in response to market competition 28 years ago has become the cornerstone of Group Health's marketing thrust today.

CASE STUDY

SELECT Health: Failed PPO Promise

THOMAS J. DAVIES, Principal

Claremont Business Group, Inc., Oakland, California

SELECT Health began as one of the most promising California PPOs launched in the tumultuous wake of selective hospital contracting by MediCal and Blue Cross's Prudent Buyer plan in 1983. It was established by six leading northern California hospitals with a commitment to involving their medical staffs in policy making and service delivery. By targeting self-insured employers, labor trusts, and small market share insurance companies, SELECT Health looked like a sure winner. Yet within 4 years it had run its full course and, as an alternative to closing its doors altogether, merged with Preferred Health Network of Los Angeles.

Many credible analysts argue quite forcefully that provider-owned PPOs are inherently doomed to failure. This case study suggests, however, that it is the aggregate mix of corporate structure and behavior, not ownership alone, that over time determines the success or failure of an enterprise.

Ironically, the decision to merge came on the heels of SELECTS's most successful 9 months' performance—income was up dramatically, overhead had been cut, and sales were on target with the company's recently completed marketing plan—resulting in a doubling of paid enrollment during SELECT's last year and a projection of break-even operations within 6 months. So, what had gone wrong? How could an organization with such a bright future fail to succeed?

Initially it appeared that SELECT Health's owners had lost interest and confidence in it as a vehicle for their individual patient acquisition strategies. SELECT had not produced "enough" patient days to justify continuing subsidy assessments. Clearly, the owners felt "tapped out" financially. Furthermore, much of the common ground in which SELECT had been rooted had been eroded by the rub of conflicting competitive strategies, new alliances and priorities, mergers, and management changes involving some of the owner hospitals.

The deterioration in owner interest and support was likely a manifestation of underlying business problems that plagued the organization from its inception. At the time, SELECT Health seemed to make good business sense. In addition, it enjoyed adequate financial backing and a head start in the marketplace. But in retrospect, more subtle, yet critical, ingredients appear to have been slighted or missing in SELECT's makeup. Among them were:

1. A solid, well-conceived business concept or mission
2. An appropriately constituted board of directors
3. Continuity of capable executive management
4. Businesslike operation and decision making
5. A more complete hospital and physician network
6. A sound business plan and marketing strategy

THE CONCEPT

SELECT Health's most fundamental flaw was its concept of trying to serve as the collective marketing arm of its owner hospitals. It was actually organized as a "consumer" cooperative in which the owner hospitals were the consumers of SELECT's marketing services. In a very real sense it was viewed as an extension of the hospital business, and its strategies were driven by shareholder and physician desires as healthcare providers rather than by market needs of the health benefits industry. In this vein, SELECT was expected to "sell" beds for higher per diem prices than owner hospitals themselves were charging competing PPOs and insurance companies.

Initially SELECT did not charge third party payers a per member per month PPO network access fees. Relying entirely upon monthly owner assessments —which were treated as income rather than capital —SELECT Health slipped into a "cost center" mentality rather than a profit orientation. While it was expected that in time assessments might decline as fee income developed, financial independence from owner assessments was never an important business goal. Yet, ultimately, it was the financial drain of these assessments that triggered SELECT's demise.

SELECT Health could have been designed to stand on its own feet financially and to compete as a separate but related business. Its natural mission would have been to facilitate preferred provider contracting arrangements between third party payers and an outstanding network of highly respected northern California providers, emphasizing economy and quality of care and requiring effective patient channeling mechanisms.

BOARD OF DIRECTORS

SELECT Health was governed by a large and often difficult to assemble board of directors. Members were selected as representatives of hospital, physician, and community interest groups. As such, they quite naturally exercised their policy-making authority in the interests of those they represented. Unfortunately, this too often resulted in the subordination of SELECT Health's own business needs to the parochial interests of individual owners, as in the exclusion of rival, but needed, hospitals from the PPO network.

In fairness, whether this particular problem reflected a flaw in the makeup of the board or a failure of management leadership, or some of each, is a matter of perspective. However, it illustrates the conventional wisdom that large "representative" boards usually work best when their function is to balance and blend policy with constituency interests and to keep management within those bounds. In contrast, the boards of successful start-up businesses are more often characterized by their relevant business expertise, manageable size, and riveted focus on the bottom line and success of the enterprise.

MANAGEMENT

In 4 years of operation SELECT Health had two interim and two permanent chief executive officers. This discontinuity of executive management was unfortunate, and undoubtedly reflected the inherently frustrating circumstances in which SELECT soon found itself. As comfortable as they may have been with hospital and healthcare issues, SELECT's CEOs were unable to marshal sufficient board resolve and commitment to tangible and realistic business goals or staff knowledge and understanding of marketing in the health benefits industry to successfully launch this new business.

BUSINESSLIKE OPERATIONS AND DECISION-MAKING

Making decisions on the basis of likes and dislikes and how they affect constituencies may be appropriate in healthcare industry associations and profes-

sional societies, but it does not work well in business. An economic decision-making model, focusing on market realities and the financial impact of decisions on the core business, is imperative for sound business operations.

Equally important is the need for commitment to the goal of operational and financial self-sufficiency. With management's reliance on assessments for operations, SELECT took on the flavor of a government agency supported by "taxes." And, when the owners lost patience, what followed seemed to some more like a taxpayers' revolt than a businesslike cost-benefit assessment.

HOSPITAL AND PHYSICIAN NETWORK

In general, the SELECT Health network was very attractive, consisting entirely of well-respected hospitals and physicians. Yet, after 4 years, gaping holes in service coverage still remained. Two problems hampered network development. The first was a classic "chicken and egg" proposition. Nonowner hospitals understandably were reluctant to pay required network participation fees until substantial enrollment had been achieved in their communities, and enrollment generally lagged most in areas not adequately covered by the provider network. Participation fees were eventually waived for hospitals in areas lacking enrollment, and this seemed to help. The second problem was SELECT's practice of allowing a single owner to veto a needed hospital's participation in the network. This problem was never solved and cost SELECT the opportunity of being offered to thousands of potential enrollees.

BUSINESS PLANNING AND MARKETING STRATEGY

SELECT's operations were never characterized by a sophisticated understanding of its markets. Although a planning process was utilized which facilitated important dialog among staff, physicians, and hospital representatives, it was not effective as a process for fine-tuning products or for understanding how target markets operated. The result was confusing. For example, third party administrators were mistakenly seen as "customers" rather than "distribution channels," and sales personnel were given incentives accordingly. Signing up TPAs became an end in itself even though not all TPAs were suitable as distribution channels and no attempt was made to qualify, categorize, or prioritize them.

Adding to the confusion was a lingering notion that hospitals, too, were customers of sorts because they were the "consumers" of SELECT's marketing services, paid for through owner assessments and network participation fees.

An earlier and more accurate picture of SELECTS's markets, channels, and products would have revealed its true customers to be those bearing the *risk of health benefits expense.* It was those customers — insurance companies and self-insured employers (not hospitals and third party administrators) — for whom SELECT's products provided added value.

SELECT's planning efforts would have benefited from two important features: greater focus on differentiating its product offerings from those of competitors and an earlier commitment to price competitiveness. It must be remembered that at the outset, PPO products competed against conventional health benefit plans. Any plan offering a good provider network and *any* discount from billed charges seemed to have a competitive advantage in certain market segments. But, by year 3, SELECT found itself competing increasingly with other PPO offerings in addition to conventional benefit plans. To its credit, SELECT quickly hammered out a policy commitment intended to achieve price competitiveness for the network as a whole by demanding of network hospitals their "best" PPO per diem prices.

Sophisticated purchasers had known all along, however, that the discounted per diem prices could actually increase health benefit outlays, depending on which hospitals were patronized. If patient channeling incentives redirected patients from hospitals with low billed charges to ones with higher (though discounted) prices, group benefit costs could actually increase.

The point is that providers generally have been slow to recognize the need for long-term strategies to compete effectively not just on the basis of price alone, but also on the basis of quality as measured by medical outcomes. SELECT's providers were no exception. Sensing such a need, the staff initiated board

discussion of available outcome monitoring systems. But it failed to first establish an understanding of and secure a commitment to the basic concept. Not surprisingly, the discussion focused on the technical aspects of individual systems, never actually addressing the strategic issue of competition among PPO networks based on medical outcomes.

The single factor which contributed most to SELECT's demise was probably its lack of relevant, realistic goals and expectations for evaluating individual and organizational performance in terms meaningful to its owners. Such goals as were employed were just not particularly useful in describing or measuring business success. No expectations were set out in terms of how many patients might have been "enough" or what level of assessment might have been tolerable. The owners had a clear sense of what success was not, but in the end they were beyond caring about what it might have been.

CONCLUSION

By early 1987, credibility among its backers had so declined that SELECT itself had become "the problem" to be solved. As a significant financial drain on its owner hospitals, it no longer was viewed as a key element in any of their strategies. Even among some owners who might have supported SELECT's continuation, there was no confidence that a sustainable turnaround had been achieved.

Happily, an affiliation that had existed for several years between SELECT Health and Preferred Health Network (PHN) for purposes of serving statewide accounts seemed to offer a possible solution. At different times in the past, this arrangement had been viewed as a possible step toward merger. However, real movement in that direction had always been inhibited by faint management interest, operational problems, conflicting styles, and a mixed view of the benefits of merger. In 1987, as the board considered its alternatives and the commitments required to revitalize SELECT, merger with PHN appeared to present a number of compelling advantages and quickly emerged as the consensual course of action.

LifeLink: Closed-Panel Behavioral Health Program

ERIC E. ANDERSON, Ph.D., Chief Operating Officer

LifeLink, Laguna Hills, California

Early product development for LifeLink concluded that a comprehensive behavioral health program must be characterized by several critical features.

- The system must have the ability to successfully manage risk through a financing mechanism that incorporates a rational design of behavioral health benefits.

- The provider system must be a closed panel (EPO or HMO) rather than an open panel (PPO) of directly contracted providers.

- The case management and utilization control systems must be both comprehensive (covering all cases) and individualized (per each patient utilizing care).

LifeLink offers a variety of benefit programs for treatment of substance abuse (chemical dependency) and psychiatric care (mental health). It underwrites accounts of 1000 or more employees, taking into consideration the demographics of the group to be covered, previous claims and benefit experience, and regional and industry variations.

Plan benefits usually have limited or no copayment or coinsurance (for example, 100 percent paid by the plan) and high lifetime maximums (for example, $50,000 lifetime maximum). They cover any services authorized by LifeLink case managers and delivered by contracted providers. Benefits are considered as inventory for use by case managers on behalf of patients. Benefit restrictions (that is, low hospital day, office visit, or dollar limits) per se are not the primary mechanism for cost containment. Rather, cost containment is achieved through the efforts of aggressive case management in conjunction with provider discounts. There is a deliberate effort likewise to provide benefits across a full continuum of care, so that every patient can receive the type of service indicated by the diagnosed medical disorder. Concurrent reviews and related authorizations for services are conducted throughout each treatment episode (for example, every 5 to 7 days for inpatient hospital care and every few weeks for outpatient care).

Providing the full continuum of care has been critical in building the foundation of LifeLink, characterized by five levels of care ranging from intensive care and detoxification for mental health and substance abuse (Level 4) to outpatient office visits and formal outpatient substance abuse program (Level 0).

PROVIDER SYSTEMS

LifeLink uses an exclusive provider organization (EPO). Benefits specify that services *preauthorized* to contracted providers are covered, but no services to noncontracted providers are authorized or covered except in *narrowly* defined emergencies. Provider networks within each region are broken down into service areas and each provider is assigned to one or more area. New patients are quickly directed by the case manager to the appropriate service area of the provider network based on corresponding Zip codes.

Provider contracts are negotiated directly with facilities for each program level. Site visits are conducted by case management staff to assess each program and determine whether it meets LifeLink criteria for that type of service and level. Facility contracts are based on all-inclusive per diems at each approved program level, and they are usually discounted by 25 to 35 percent from usual and customary daily rates. They also include ancillary charges, so the actual discount from billed charges may exceed 30 to 40 percent. Practitioner agreements are standard contracts with regional fee schedules using RVS procedure codes and different scales for each professional group (M.D.s at one rate, Ph.D.s at another). This fee structure acknowledges both clinical training and local marketplace considerations.

CASE MANAGEMENT AND UTILIZATION CONTROLS

It is important to emphasize several key aspects of LifeLink case management.

1. All new cases go through intake procedures where eligibility is determined.

2. All services are preauthorized by case managers.

3. Each case is assigned to a case manager who follows the case throughout its duration.

4. Case managers use LifeLink proprietary criteria for admissions and treatment planning as the basis for authorizations.

5. Case managers maintain direct knowledge of patient status, including on-site case management for patients receiving care in facilities.

6. Services are authorized in small allotments (four or five inpatient days or office visits) so as to require regular involvement in each case.

7. Case managers monitor cases and authorize benefits; they *do not provide treatment services*.

8. LifeLink case managers are not given quotas; rather they are charged with directing patients to the most appropriate type of service. Throughout the course of treatment, they monitor the match between the need of the patient and the services authorized.

Inpatient utilization is approximately 80 hospital days per 1000 lives for both substance abuse and mental health. These 80 days are spread across all levels of "hospital" care including partial hospital (that is, day treatment). An overall range of 30 to 100 is experienced depending upon demographics, region, and benefit structure. This compares with targeted 110 to 120 days per 1000 lives achieved by similar companies which use a PPO delivery model. Outpatient visits typically run 300 to 500 visits for substance abuse and mental health combined.

Case managers are charged with knowing the status of their patients at all times, asking, what does each patient need now? The underlying philosophy is that patients should get what they *need*; no more, no less. Using the level system and treatment planning criteria, case managers are instructed to authorize the level of care justified by the *current needs* of patients. Treatment which begins at one level often concludes at a less intensive level of care.

PREMIUM CONTROL

Annual premiums in the introductory year for a new client typically run 10 percent below the claims experience for the previous year. Rates in the first year amount to an effective savings for the client of 25 to 30 percent from projected claims for the implementation year had LifeLink not been involved.

Contract savings apart from case management cannot achieve lasting savings for behavioral health care. But by reducing the lengths of stay and using less intensive levels of care as appropriate, costs are held down. The physician gatekeeper model, typical in the HMO environment, is replaced by case management.

Vantage Direct: Managing PPO Mental Health and Chemical Dependency Services

WILLIAM D. ZIEVERINK, M.D., Chief of Psychiatry, Executive Director

Emilie Gamelin Institute, Providence Medical Center, Portland, Oregon

JACK A. FRIEDMAN, Ph.D., Executive Director

Vantage PPO, Sisters of Providence, Portland, Oregon

This case study examines the experience of a preferred provider organization, known as Vantage Direct, in delivering managed mental health and chemical dependency services in greater Portland, Oregon. Early program results suggest that there are four essential components to successfully managing such services. They include a select, multidisciplinary team of mental health and chemical dependency providers; a system of vertically integrated inpatient, partial hospital, residential, and outpatient services; a management information system tracking *all* services rendered; and a clinical intake and placement function.

The Vantage Direct program is accessed only by calling an intake coordinator (a psychiatric nurse practitioner) who clinically evaluates the case and then directs it to the most appropriate provider. The nurse practitioner spends 15 to 20 minutes discussing the nature of the problem, eliciting information about the emotional state of the patient, whether drugs or alcohol are involved, whether the problems are influencing family relationships or work performance, and other clinical information. A determination is made regarding whether these problems are having any related physical manifestations such as affecting sleeping, eating habits, or sexual functions. This line of inquiry helps the intake coordinator to form an accurate diagnostic impression.

If drug or alcohol use is not the primary issue, the intake coordinator will recommend a mental health provider based on several criteria. These criteria include matching the person to the specific subspecialty of participating providers and satisfying patient requests for specific provider characteristics (for example, gender, geographic location, clinical emphasis on a particular style of therapy, and in some instances, the provider's religious background). The intake coordinator has met personally with each of the 48 Vantage providers and maintains current information regarding their subspecialty skills and patient preferences. Several of the providers, for example, specialize in eating disorders, adolescent psychiatry, sexual dysfunctions, phobias, and specialized care following chemical dependency treatment.

Once the referral is made, the provider sees the patient for two visits, after which a detailed authorization treatment plan must be submitted. The treatment plan includes the DSM III-R criteria diagnosis, a detailed description of the presenting signs and symptoms, treatment objectives, and specific number of outpatient visits required to realize those treatment objectives. In one case, for example, the diagnosis was described as dysthymic disorder, in which the patient was experiencing deepening depression and loss of concentration. The treatment goal was to involve the patient in short-term psychotherapy and return her to a functional level to complete her school term. This short-term goal was to be accomplished within 10 outpatient visits.

The medical director and intake coordinator review each authorization request before granting the requested number of visits. If the medical director disagrees with the number of visits requested, the provider is called to discuss the nature of the problem and to reach agreement on a treatment plan. If the issue cannot be resolved at this level, the provider is asked to present the case to the Vantage Direct Utilization Review Committee. This group is composed of the medical director, three psychiatrists, a psychologist, and a family therapist and has final authority over authorization of treatment regimens.

The program is not yet capable of assigning a specific number of outpatient visits to a specific DSM-III-R code. Diagnoses-specific utilization criteria have not been developed, and it remains questionable whether such criteria can be formalized. The Vantage Utilization Review Committee will analyze first-year data, comparing providers' case mix, diagnoses, and treatment regimens to determine if regionalized and formalized utilization criteria can be applied to a specific set of diagnoses.

For the first three months of 1989, the intake coordinator made 210 outpatient mental health referrals from a population of 94,000 Vantage participants. Nearly 60 percent of these referrals required 10 outpatient visits to meet treatment goals, 20 percent required fewer than 10 visits, and another 10 percent required between 15 and 20 outpatient visits. Ten percent of the referrals were not acted upon since those members opted not to seek treatment following the initial intake call. All requests for more than 10 visits are reviewed after the tenth visit, at which time additional visits may be granted.

Early results from the Vantage Direct program suggest that controlling outpatient psychiatric costs depends largely on the provider's commitment to goal-oriented therapy. Providers have been selected based on a demonstrated ability to diagnose a problem and return the patient to a functional level. Problems have arisen when a provider seeks to work with long-standing psychological disorders that require long-term psychotherapy or when specific treatment goals were not formulated prior to beginning treatment. The issue of treatment philosophy is an ongoing problem, which is addressed through quarterly meetings with providers, the medical director, and senior management from the health plan. This issue is especially significant among the panel's child psychiatrists, who have received several adolescents requiring long-term, intensive treatment.

First quarter experience with inpatient psychiatric services showed 17 admissions to the program, with an average length of stay of 7.5 days (5.8 days for adults and 12.5 days for adolescents). That compares favorably with 1988 data from Vantage PPO, in which average length of stay for all psychiatric admissions was 12.2 days. These lower length of stays are due largely to more focused concurrent review and to more aggressive management of the hospital-based delivery system.

Vantage Direct has intentionally restricted inpatient, outpatient, and residential mental health and chemical dependency programs to its affiliated Sisters of Providence hospitals, with the exception of two other hospital programs that were included to serve specific geographic areas. The Vantage Direct medical director has line management authority over all Sisters of Providence mental health and chemical dependency programs. This has enabled the program to apply effectively stringent cost controls and managed care principles to these hospital-based programs.

Vantage Direct has been less successful in controlling chemical dependency costs, especially when these services are delivered outside the Sisters of Providence network. Initial results indicated there were 22 admissions to four participating residential chemical dependency programs. When the patient was admitted to the flagship Providence Medical Center program, the average length of stay ran 14.9 days on eight admissions. The remaining 14 admissions were spread between three other participating programs, where the average length of stay ran between 26 and 29 days. The Providence program attempts to help the patient realize the severity of their addiction within the hospital setting and then relies on specialized outpatient programs for follow-up care. Several of the Vantage providers specialize exclusively in postaddiction therapy and work in concert with hospital program staff.

Detailed management reports have been designed to evaluate the cost effectiveness of the various hospital-based mental health and chemical dependency programs. These data show comparative length of stays, use of hospital ancillaries, and readmission and recidivism rates. Participating providers are also profiled to determine their case mix, average number of visits, average cost per case, and overall compliance with the utilization review and quality assurance protocols and criteria. These reports serve as objective recredentialing tools and establish a valid frame of reference for measuring provider performance.

CHAPTER ELEVEN

Organizational Structure

IPAs AND PHYSICIAN-OWNED PPOs: LEGAL IMPLICATIONS OF ALTERNATIVE FORMS OF ORGANIZATION

J. PETER RICH, Esq., Partner
McDermott, Will & Emery, Los Angeles, California

Over the past decade, the independent practice association (IPA) has become the primary vehicle through which physicians and other healthcare professionals—aside from those in multispecialty medical group practice on a full-time basis—are able to participate in managed care contracting.[1]

An IPA is no longer just a vehicle for physicians in private practice to contract on a capitated or other at-risk basis with health maintenance organizations (HMOs). Rather, the contemporary IPA—and particularly the common form of hospital-affiliated IPA—is a part-time group practice that also enters into the same types of discounted fee-for-service contracts that once were the exclusive domain of physician-sponsored preferred provider organizations (PPOs), sometimes using two or more panels of contracting physicians to accommodate those physicians who do not wish to accept capitation or other financial risk arrangements. Indeed, "plain vanilla" physician-owned PPOs which do not contract with HMOs on an at-risk basis are fast becoming obsolete, except in certain situations where a hospital or its physicians may prefer, for operational or "political" reasons, to have a relatively small and select hospital-affiliated IPA coexisting with a large and relatively open hospital-affiliated PPO. Under these circumstances, for all intents and purposes the larger entity is referred to as a PPO rather than an IPA, primarily to distinguish it from the smaller physician organization and to indicate that the PPO's participating physicians do not enter into risk contracts.

This type of dual approach has begun to prove problematic, however, because increasingly PPOs have seen the handwriting on the wall: If they are to compete effectively in the managed care market, they must enter into some at-risk contracts, at a minimum those with more limited withhold risk pools and primary care case management obligations, if not capitation contracts. Thus, a hospital with both types of organizations may well find that its affiliated PPO is competing with its affiliated IPA for the physician services component of a particular managed care contract. Unsurprisingly, such competition within a hospital's medical staff may prove harmfully divisive. Moreover, since payers and brokers generally rely upon the hospital to designate the appropriate contracting physician organization, the hospital is likely to be faced with a Hobson's choice between its IPA and PPO (and perhaps even other affiliated physician groups), inevitably damaging hospital-physician relations.

The resulting dilemma for the hospital is an unnecessary one. The preferred approach is to have a single hospital-affiliated physician organization for managed care contracting which is flexible enough to perform all of these functions; if relatively few physicians wish to accept risk, then their contracts with the IPA can so specify. Thus, such an IPA may have two or more physician panels, with one consisting of physicians who have agreed to be bound by all risk-sharing contracts, another of physicians who desire to have the right to "opt out" of individual risk-sharing contracts as well as not-at-risk contracts, and perhaps still another of physicians who will accept only not-at-risk contracts on a case-by-case basis. With this type of flexibility, IPAs can successfully serve as vehicles for physicians to enter into provider agreements with HMOs as well as all types of payer- or broker-sponsored PPOs or exclusive provider organizations (EPOs) (hereinafter collectively referred to as "plans"), and particularly with plans that offer more than one of these options to their members.

While a particular managed care contract may still require that a difficult decision be made with respect to the appropriate physician panel, that decision is likely to be much easier under this organizational form, and, most importantly, the decision will rest with the board of directors of the IPA rather than being forced on the hospital. Unless a fundamental change occurs in the American healthcare system which reverses the current path toward managed care contracting, it would seem likely that by the mid-1990s, if not sooner, the vast majority of hospitals, and perhaps nearly all, will have a single affiliated IPA organized along these lines.

In this regard, it should be noted that while some hospitals or medical staff may be tempted to organize the entire medical staff as an IPA, it is strongly recommended, for liability and other legal reasons, that IPAs be formed as separate legal organizations independent from the medical staff. This recommendation does not mean that it is unwise to engage in other appropriate activities aside from managed care contracting; rather, it is based on the view that the legally mandated and other appropriate activities of a medical staff may conflict with those of an IPA. In particular, the legally mandated "fair hearing" requirements applicable to medical staff credentialing have not as yet been made applicable to IPAs, which therefore have much greater freedom in choosing their membership. IPAs that are separate from the medical staff will not be forced to accept everyone who may meet the minimum standards for medical staff membership; conversely, not everyone who joins the medical staff will be required to participate in managed care contracting.

Regardless of the type of IPA, many existing IPAs have been organized in a legally appropriate manner. As a result of an apparent failure to appreciate the implications of federal tax rules governing the tax-exempt status of pension plans, as well as applicable federal and state securities laws, some or all of the physicians who own shares of stock in an IPA may be exposed to disqualification of their pension plans' tax exemptions, as well as potential fraud liability under the securities laws. This risk should be a cause for concern but should not immediately strike terror in the heart of every physician who owns shares in an IPA; it does not appear that any such adverse consequences have occurred thus far. Nevertheless, the potential risk is a real one; while the current level of probability appears to be low, this situation could conceivably change for the worse in the future. Given the potentially devastating consequences, IPAs that have not been formed in such a manner as to eliminate or at least minimize this risk should consider converting to taxable nonprofit corporations, for the reasons discussed in detail in this article.

Such a conversion is particularly advisable if the physicians who purchased shares in the IPA were not fully apprised of the potential risk to their pension plans in a detailed prospectus or investor disclosure letter provided to them prior to their purchase of stock in the IPA. Those physicians who were not fully informed of the potential risk in this manner may be able to bring lawsuits against the IPA's promoters for damages under securities "antifraud" laws in the event that their pension plans are adversely affected by the manner in which the IPA was organized. Physicians who were so apprised may still experience an adverse impact on their own pension plans, but at least the IPA's original organizers and board of directors should not have to face securities fraud lawsuits from other angry physicians whose pension plans are similarly harmed.

To reiterate, because the risk that pension plan tax exemptions will be disallowed is relatively small, physicians who purchase stock in IPAs may make a reasonable informed business judgment to do so in spite of this apparent risk. However, if an IPA issued stock in the past without providing these physicians with legally appropriate written information concerning this risk, that IPA should immediately either inform the physicians in writing of this risk and offer them an opportunity to rescind their original purchase, with the IPA returning to them the full amount of the purchase price or, preferably, convert the IPA into a taxable nonprofit corporation.

This chapter is divided into four parts. Part I discusses the potential application of Section 414(m) and the Internal Revenue Code (IRC) "affiliated service group" rules and the impact of these rules on the choice of organizational form for the IPA. Part II reviews the alternative business forms available to the IPA. Part III deals with funding and management alternatives. Finally, Part IV discusses physician participation issues, including relevant antitrust principles.

The term "IPA" is used throughout this chapter because it is fast becoming the most common term for a partially integrated physician-owned organization that negotiates and/or enters into PPO, HMO, or other managed care contracting arrangements on behalf of its affiliated physicians. All of the legal issues discussed in this article are, therefore, equally applicable to essentially similar physician arrangements often referred to as "PPOs."

PART I. IPAs AND THE IRC AFFILIATED SERVICE GROUP RULES

The threshold issue that must be considered in structuring an IPA is the potential application of Section 414(m) of the IRC and the regulations issued by the Treasury Department thereunder, which are generally referred to as the "affiliated service group" rules.[2] This section discusses the current status of applicable law and the possible courses of action that may be taken by the IPA with respect to these rules.

Affiliated Service Group Rules

BACKGROUND Section 414(m), which was enacted in 1980 and amended several times thereafter, broadly defines the term "affiliated service group" for purposes of determining whether a retirement plan (for example, a pension or profit sharing plan) is "qualified" for tax purposes. Qualification of the plan is essential in that it permits the deductibility of employer contributions and the deferral of an employee's obligation to pay income tax on plan contributions, earnings, and benefits until such employee's actual receipt of the benefits.

If an IPA and one or more professional corporations, medical groups, partnerships, or individual physicians are deemed to constitute an affiliated service group, they will all be treated as a single employer for purposes of determining whether the retirement plan of any member of the affiliated service group complies with applicable antidiscrimination, eligibility, vesting, contribution, and benefit limit requirements under the IRC—even if the IPA has no employees of its own. Section 414(m) also applies to medical reimbursement, cafeteria, and certain other benefit plans (IRC §414(m)(4); Prop. Reg. §1.414(m)-3).

Although these rules were enacted by Congress in an effort to prevent certain abuses—principally those involving doctors and lawyers who formed multiple professional corporations in order to discriminate in their own favor, and against their nonprofessional employees, in regard to plan benefits—the statute and the proposed regulations elaborating on the statute have been written to encompass a broad range of transactions and also contain numerous ambiguities. While Section 414(m) may well be interpreted or amended to except IPAs and similar organizations, the Treasury Department and the IRS have thus far been unwilling to clarify this issue in a definitive manner. Thus, regardless of the IPA's business form, it is conceivable that the IRS could seek to apply these rules to the IPA as well as its investors, officers, and any persons characterized as "highly compensated employees."

APPLICABLE TO IPAs An IPA may fall within one or more of the definitions of an "affiliated service group," regardless of whether the IPA has any employees, if the IPA has one or more of the following individuals:

1. Any owner (that is, shareholder or partner) who "regularly performs" services for the IPA, if the IPA is a professional corporation
2. Any such owner who is "regularly associated" with such an IPA in performing services for third persons
3. Any owner of the IPA, whether or not it is a professional corporation, who is characterized as a "highly compensated employee" of the IPA (which, in general, includes persons who own 5 percent or more of the IPA, persons who earn more than $50,000 per year as employees of the IPA, and officers of the IPA who earn more than $45,000 per year from the IPA for their services as officers) and whose income from the IPA for services rendered to third persons in association with the IPA exceeds 5

percent of the physician's total annual income derived from the performance of patient services.

If such an owner or employee is found to be part of an "affiliated service group" with the IPA, the physician owner's professional corporation or partnership may also be included in that group if the physician owns 50 percent or more of it, either individually or collectively with other IPA owners.

If the affiliated service group rules were to be successfully applied by the IRS to an IPA and the IPA's owners or "highly compensated employees," the tax-preferred status of their retirement plans would be jeopardized. In that event, the retirement plans of those physicians (including their professional corporations or partnerships) could be disqualified by the IRS, as a result of their association with the IPA, causing them to incur substantial tax liability.

Therefore, it is extremely important that the scope of Section 414(m) and its possible implications be considered when determining the legal structure of an IPA.

Alternatives   The affiliated service group rules are unusually complex, and the IRS has provided no definitive guidance as to the circumstances, if any, under which an IPA and its owners and highly compensated employees will be treated as members of an affiliated service group. However, an analysis of the rules results in the following conclusions:

1. To be completely safe, there should be either no IPA shareholders or only shareholders who have pension plans that are comparable to the IPA's. Any shareholder who does not meet this test is at risk.

2. No IPA officer or other employee should earn more than $50,000 as an employee of the IPA. This latter situation will rarely if ever occur, except possibly in the case of an IPA medical director, who should not be at risk if either (1) he or she has no pension plan or "freezes" a preexisting plan prior to joining the IPA or (2) the IPA has no pension plan of its own and the medical director is the only employee who makes over $50,000, which is likely to be the case.

Under one possible approach to deal with this issue, an analysis could be undertaken of all the plans of all such IPA shareholders and officers (and their respective professional corporations and partnerships) in order to determine whether the coverage, discrimination, and other requirements are satisfied in the aggregate. If the plans do not meet the statutory requirements, the plans could be modified.[3]

However, this process is likely to be costly and time-consuming; therefore, this approach is disfavored.

The preferred options, and the ones that are chosen most often, are either a sole shareholder professional corporation (if the IPA has no employees, or if the sole shareholder is a physician who does not maintain a plan, who "freezes" his or her plan prior to purchasing stock in the IPA, or who has a plan that can easily be made comparable with the IPA's) or, preferably, a taxable nonprofit corporation, either with statutory members or, as authorized under state law, without such members.

If the investing physicians fully appreciate the risks, they may instead choose to structure the IPA as a multiple shareholder professional corporation [preferably with no physician owning 5 percent or more of the stock, to at least reduce the Section 414(m) risk]. While a significant percentage of IPAs have been formed as multiple shareholder professional corporations, this alternative is not recommended because of the risk under Section 414(m). In this regard, if an affiliated hospital sponsors the formation of the IPA, IPA physicians theoretically could bring legal action against the affiliated hospital if their plans are disqualified as a result of the IPA's structure. Although proper disclosure of the risk to prospective shareholders or members should make it likely that the affiliated hospital would prevail in any such litigation, the litigation cost may well be high and, more important, there could be serious damage to the affiliated hospital's relationship with its physicians.

The basis for these recommendations is discussed in Part II below.

PART II. BUSINESS FORM OF THE IPA

The basic alternative forms of legal organizations that could be used in the formation of the IPA are (1) a general business corporation, (2) a professional partnership, (3) a professional corporation with multiple shareholders, (4) a sole shareholder professional corporation, (5) a taxable nonprofit corporation with one or more statutory corporate members, or, when authorized under state law, and (6) a "memberless" taxable nonprofit (taxable) corporation.[4]

Because of concerns with respect to the corporate practice of medicine, liability, securities law compliance, and Section 414(m), it may well be legally inadvisable, depending on the laws of the state where the IPA is to be formed and operated, for the IPA to be organized either as a general business corporation, a professional partnership, a professional corporation with multiple shareholders (particularly if any shareholder has more than 5 percent of the stock), or a nonprofit corporation with statutory corporate members (if there are enough members to require registration under the securities laws).

In regard to the general business corporation form under the laws of most states, the corporate practice of medicine doctrine provides that medical services generally may only be provided by licensed persons, individually and in medical groups, and by professional corporations.[5] Since the IPA would be arranging for the provision of medical services to plan members, the IPA would appear to be engaged in the unlawful corporate practice of medicine if it is organized as a general business corporation rather than as a professional corporation or professional partnership or, possibly, a nonprofit corporation.

With regard to the professional partnership form, unlimited liability makes this an unattractive vehicle, particularly if some of the physician partners are not incorporated.

Therefore, this section of this article discusses only the advantages and disadvantages of using a professional corporation or a nonprofit corporation without members.

Professional Corporation

If the IPA were formed as a professional corporation, the risk of violating the corporate practice of medicine prohibition would be eliminated because the doctrine permits professional corporations to practice medicine. Further, as opposed to a professional partnership, shareholders in a professional corporation generally have more limited liability for the debts and obligations of the corporation, except with respect to each shareholder's own individual malpractice. In addition, the offer and sale of stock in a professional corporation generally is exempt from registration requirements under state securities laws. For these reasons, the professional corporation has historically been by far the most common form of IPA legal organization.

A disadvantage of a professional corporation (as with any corporate form), as opposed to a partnership, is that the profits of a professional corporation are subject to double taxation. However, the practical impact of this disadvantage on the IPA should be minimal, particularly in the initial years, and are outweighed by the disadvantages of operating an IPA as a partnership, which can result in unlimited liability for all of the partners.

The major legal issue, however, has arisen relatively recently under Section 414(m), as discussed above, and appears to make it legally inadvisable to use this traditional IPA form of organization, at least if these are to be multiple physician shareholders with separate plans. If the IPA were formed as a professional corporation with only one shareholder who is not covered by a retirement plan (or, if the one shareholder has a plan, the IPA has no employees, or the IPA's plan is comparable to the shareholder's), the risk under Section 414(m) should be minimized. A disadvantage of this approach is that only one physician could be an investor in the IPA, which could create political problems with the other participating physicians, despite the fact that IPA "profits" typically are distributed through risk pool arrangements or held in reserve, rather than being paid as dividends, and are thereby subject to double taxation unless the corporation qualifies for a Subchapter S election. In contrast, in a sole shareholder professional corporation, the participating physicians may be assessed a "membership fee," but there is no possibility of their receiving a return on investment in the form of stock dividends. Control issues may also be raised, though the IPA's corporate documents may be drafted so as to place control of the IPA in a broadly representative board of directors that is made up of contracting physicians and thus minimize any possibility that the sole shareholder could personally profit from his or her investment.

For these reasons, despite the greater risk that the affiliated service group rules may adversely affect the pension plans of the shareholder physicians, many IPAs have been formed as multiple shareholder professional corporations. In order to reduce this risk, in general the shareholders or officers of these IPAs each hold less than 5 percent of the IPA's stock and intend to derive less than 5 percent (and in no event more than 10 percent) of their total annual professional fee income from the IPA—although, as they should be made aware, in practice the IRS may choose to apply a greater or lesser standard. These physicians often take the position that if the IPA becomes successful enough to generate income to them in excess of the supposed 5 percent (or at least 10 percent) threshold, they can reassess the risk based on any new developments concerning Section 414(m).

In view of the apparent absence of past or current IRS enforcement against IPA physicians, some physicians have chosen to ignore the risks of Section 414(m) altogether and to derive more than 5 percent and even 10 percent of their fee income from IPAs of which they are shareholders. If physicians decide to proceed on this basis, they should do so only after they fully understand the risk based on reviewing an IPA "investor disclosure letter" with their own attorneys, and then willingly choose to go forward and accept that risk. However, a hospital affiliated with the IPA may reasonably take the position that a particular structure entails too great a risk for the affiliated hospital to be associated with it in any way, particularly since the affiliated hospital may be sued by any physicians whose plans are disqualified. Therefore, the affiliated hospital may decide to deny its financial and other assistance if the physicians proceed to implement the IPA.

Taxable Nonprofit Corporation

The IPA could be formed as a nonprofit corporation. Such a nonprofit IPA would be a taxable organization. Because IPAs are formed and operated for the benefit of their affiliated physicians, it is highly unlikely that they could qualify for tax-exempt status, at least without radical changes to their typical structure which would not be acceptable to most prospective physicians.[6]

The primary reason for using such a nonprofit corporation would be to eliminate the risk of being subject to the affiliated service group rules under Section 414(m), because the IPA would then have no owners and an affiliated service group can only be formed among an organization and its owners. A recent amendment to Section 414(m) has made it unnecessary to resort to the use of a "memberless" nonprofit corporation, as opposed to one that issues corporate memberships (which are similar to voting stock in that members have the power to elect the IPA's board of directors and receive a distribution of net assets upon the IPA's dissolution, but, unlike stock, entail no dividend rights). Before this amendment became effective on January 1, 1989, Section 414(m) could have been interpreted to combine all corporate members of an IPA into an affiliated service group. With this amendment, it is clear that only those corporate members who are "highly compensated employees" (that is, those who are paid in excess of $50,000 at a minimum) face this risk. Therefore, IPAs may now safely be formed as either nonprofit corporations with members or "memberless" nonprofit corporations. However, as discussed below, depending upon the interpretation of state securities laws and the number of IPA members, it may still be most expedient to form an IPA as a memberless nonprofit corporation.

If there are no statutory members, a nonprofit IPA may be capitalized by loans and/or dues and other contributions, with any assets remaining on dissolution going to loan repayment or a designated nonprofit purpose (for example, the affiliated hospital that provided the initial "seed money" for the IPA). In the absence of statutory members, who would normally make "contributions" to the organization in exchange for their membership interests, physician "investment" in the IPA would be limited to payment of annual dues or participation fees by the physicians participating in the IPA. Any such payment should be carefully solicited and structured to minimize any risk that it might be deemed to constitute a "security" requiring registration under the securities laws. In a few states, if statutory memberships in a nonprofit corporation are sold to more than a certain number of physicians (for example, 35 in California or Texas and most other states, 34 in Nevada, 10 in Oregon), such sales may need to be registered under the securities laws; this would involve additional time and expense. This risk and expense can be eliminated by forming the IPA as a "memberless" nonprofit corporation.

Finally, in some states, such as California, statutory memberships of a nonprofit corporation cannot be terminated without according the member certain statutory notice and hearing rights. This process may make it more cumbersome for the IPA to terminate participating physicians who are also members. The "memberless" nonprofit corporation, if available under the laws of such a state, may be preferable for this reason alone or in combination with the securities issues discussed immediately above.

It should be noted that adopting any IPA corporate format other than that of a professional corporation may involve some risk of violating the corporate practice of medicine doctrine, which is applicable, to varying degrees, under the laws of most states.[7] In this regard, it may be argued that an IPA, which "arranges for" but does not itself "provide" medical care, would not be a corporate vehicle "by or through" which professionals practice, and that an IPA which merely provides certain contract negotiation and related business management services to participating physicians would not violate the corporate practice of medicine doctrine.

In addition, the nonprofit corporate form is an unfamiliar organizational structure for physicians to use in the practice of medicine. On the other hand, the nonprofit form may be preferable, in order to emphasize to physicians joining the IPA that their financial rewards will be based upon their professional performance rather than a return on their investment.

Recommendation Unless the prospective participating physicians desire to terminate their existing pension plans and form a new joint plan, the IPA should be formed as either a sole shareholder professional corporation or a nonprofit corporation. These forms appear to face the least exposure to application of Section 414(m) affiliated service group rules, and also tend to have the major advantages and to avoid the primary disadvantages associated with other possible organizational forms. Accordingly, the balance of this article assumes that the IPA will be either a professional corporation or a nonprofit corporation, either with or without members.

PART III. FUNDING AND MANAGEMENT

Start-Up Costs

As noted above, the initial source of funding could be (1) application or participation fees paid by participating physicians, (2) the sale of membership interests to participating physicians if the organization were formed as a nonprofit corporation with members, (3) a line of credit and/or direct contribution from an affiliated hospital or HMO, or (4) a combination of these funding methods. The level of initial capital required will depend on the objectives of the IPA and the range of activities in which it will engage. An affiliated hospital often provides at least half of the required funding in amounts ranging from $50,000 to $150,000, though sometimes the physicians insist on retaining primary or even sole funding responsibility. To the extent that the activities of the IPA do not require capital expenditures for such items as space and equipment, the minimum required amount could be kept closer to the lower end of that range.

Strong arguments can be made that these expenditures are consistent with a nonprofit tax-exempt hospital's charitable purposes and thus should not jeopardize its tax-exempt status as "inurement" or a "private benefit" to the physicians who form the IPA. Nevertheless, in view of recent IRS general counsel memoranda involving payments or loans to hospital-based physicians,[8] it would be safest for tax-exempt hospitals to structure their funding as a loan with rates of interest and other terms that are commercially reasonable.

In addition to legal, consulting, and other start-up costs related to forming the IPA, the IPA might incur costs in connection with, for example, (1) engaging a medical director to be responsible for managing the IPA's network and related utilization review and quality assurance, (2) contracting with a management company (which may be a hospital or one of its affiliates) to be responsible for the business aspects of the IPA, including billing, collection, and risk pools, (3) computer rental and software necessary to monitor the ongoing performance of the IPA, (4) advertising, (5) other promotional activities, and (6) the establishment of a referral service. Some of the initial capitalization could also be used to create a reserve that would be available in the event that the IPA's income under its contracts with plans is insufficient to cover operating expenses.

Operating Expenses

The IPA's contracts with plans to provide medical services to plan members will provide the primary source of income to defray operating expenses. Another source of revenue to be used for this purpose may be initial and ongoing physician membership dues or other fees.

Management

IPAs are expensive organizations to manage and operate because of the amount of information which they must process in order to allocate the funds which they receive from the plans to their participating physicians. Many IPAs enter into management contracts with their affiliated hospitals to provide these management services. Typical management contracts for these services include the provision of (1) administrative personnel to manage the IPA and assist in negotiating contracts with the plans, (2) billing and collection services to obtain funds from the plans for services rendered to plan members and allocate the funds received to the participating physicians, (3) computer hardware and software to monitor the performance of the IPA, (4) accounting and legal assistance, and (5) marketing and promotional assistance. These contracts generally provide for compensation from the IPA based on a percentage of the collections of the IPA. These services are sometimes provided by the affiliated hospital at below cost, at least at the outset, in order partially to subsidize the large administrative expense associated with operating an IPA.

The management services and financial support provided to the IPA can come either from a hospital or its affiliate or from an independent company that specializes in this area. If the IPA chooses to contract with an independent management company, it should insist on some form of incentive arrangement based upon measures of the management company's performance. The IPA should also pay heed to the contractual provisions for ownership of computer software and control of MIS outputs so that if the management contract is terminated, the IPA will be able to carry on its MIS functions.

PART IV. IPA PHYSICIAN PARTICIPATION

Selection of Physician Participants

Medical staff membership at one or more local hospitals will be a prerequisite for providing services to the IPA. To minimize possible antitrust exposure, the IPA should be certain that its own credentialing process incorporates legitimate business and quality of care criteria. An IPA is highly unlikely to face antitrust liability for denying membership to physicians, particularly if the IPA does not wield significant market power, but the potential for such liability may arise as the IPA grows to dominance in size and market share, particularly if denial of participation is motivated by an anticompetitive purpose. Careful attention to the criteria for physician participation can minimize this risk.

A related issue concerns possible limited immunity from most legal, including antitrust, liability under the Health Care Quality Improvement Act of 1986 (the Act).[9] Should the IPA fall within the terms of the Act as a "group medical practice," it may qualify for the Act's safe harbor if its credentialing and peer review activities meet the Act's notice, fair hearing, and reporting requirements. If the IPA chooses to contract with a separate organization to perform credentialing and other peer review services, which generally is not necessary or advisable in view of the additional expense, the IPA might not fall within the terms of the Act. If the IPA performs these tasks itself, it must ensure that its peer review process is fair and reasonable. As a legal matter the IPA need not provide a "fair hearing" as required of hospitals or even "notice and an opportunity to be heard," since IPAs are essentially just medical groups and should be held to the same liberal standards in this area.

Another antitrust issue related to the selection of physicians is the potential risk of liability for monopolization or conspiracy in restraint of trade. As the IPA grows, so does the importance of attending to this risk. In particular, if the IPA requires that physicians participate on an exclusive basis, those participants no longer compete with one another. If those physicians represent a sufficiently large share of the market for health services in the relevant geographic area, the exclusive arrangement might be deemed to be an unreasonable restraint on competition. A useful rule of thumb for exclusive contracting is 20 to 30 percent of the market; exclusive participation of physicians with a larger total market share — in any subspecialty — materially increases the risk of antitrust liability. On the other hand, nonexclusive contracts with physicians representing up to 50 to 60 percent of the relevant market in their subspecialty should pose no such antitrust problems, because they are still free to compete with each other for non-IPA patients. To the extent those percentages are exceeded, antitrust risk increases. Thus, it may well be legally advisable to turn down certain physician applicants for IPA membership.

Eligibility to Provide Services to the IPA

Careful evaluation of the professional qualifications of physicians seeking to provide services to the IPA will be crucial to the success of any IPA. Particularly as the IPA increases in size, it must carefully evaluate potential participants to assure that they are high quality, cost-effective providers.

The IPA should set certain objective standards for participation and solicit information from applicants in order to evaluate their qualifications for participation. The criteria could be based on such attributes as the physician's staff category, proclivity for ordering hospital and ancillary tests, thoroughness and timeliness in completing medical records, board certification or eligibility, fee level, willingness to participate in committee work, referral patterns, attitude toward peer review, malpractice history, and general reputation. Additionally, the IPA should take into account whether the plan's enrollment levels necessitate the participation of physicians in that particular field of medical practice or geographic area before contracting with a particular physician.

It is essential that the criteria established for providing services be rationally related to the objectives of the IPA and uniformly applied to all applicants and that the procedures for determining eligibility be reasonable. This is particularly important if the IPA is to be shielded by the Act from antitrust and other liabilities. Deficiencies in these areas could result in physicians who have been excluded or expelled bringing suits against the IPA or its affiliated hospital based upon claims that the IPA's actions were the product of anticompetitive or other impermissible motives. There will generally be a lesser risk of liability if a physician is excluded at the outset, as opposed to being expelled.

The criteria for participation must also be related to the further-ance of quality healthcare if the IPA is to be protected by the Act from antitrust and other lawsuits. Even if the IPA does not fall under the terms of the Health Care Quality Improvement Act, the IPA's use of participation criteria related to quality of care can minimize the risk that anticompetitive motives will be ascribed to its peer review activi-ties. As the IPA grows, the importance of basing participation on quality measures increases, as financial and political pressures to add participants may tend to overcome the legal and operational advan-tages of restricting the number of physicians who can participate in the IPA.

Control of the IPA

It may be desirable to include certain controls in the structure of the IPA that will help to promote its objectives. For example, as the IPA increases in size, new members of the board of directors may not share the goals and values of the initial IPA members. The IPA could provide for staggered terms of directors in order to make it more difficult for a block of physicians to achieve control of the IPA, while also assuring that there will always be a majority of experienced board members.

If the IPA is organized as a professional corporation, the share-holders of the corporation will have the right to elect the board of directors. If a sole shareholder professional corporation is used, that right will belong to the sole shareholder. If the IPA is organized as a nonprofit corporation with statutory members, the members will elect the board. On the other hand, if a "memberless" nonprofit corporation is used as a matter of law, the board of directors will be "self-perpetuating," that is, the current board members will have the collective right to elect their successors. To the extent that it is important for physicians participating in the IPA to have control over the members of the board of directors, a nonprofit corporation with members has the advantage of giving participating physicians who are corporate members the right to elect the board of directors. If a "memberless" nonprofit corporation is used, however, a physician advisory committee may be formed, consisting of all contracting physicians, to "recommend" some or all new board members. Of course, the existing board would depart from these "recommenda-tions" at its peril, since IPAs require broad support from their partici-pating physicians in order to succeed.

Professional Fees

A variety of compensation methods can be used by an IPA. For example, third party payers may pay a capitation fee to the IPA calculated on a per member per month basis; the IPA would then compensate its physicians according to a fee schedule. Alternatively, physicians might be paid on a capitation basis. Physicians can share the risk that the IPA will not be able to provide services within the capitation budget by agreeing to have a certain percentage of their reimbursement withheld and placed in an accumulating fund. At the end of the contract term, any excess left in such a risk incentive fund is shared; if the IPA lost money on the contract, the entirety of the withhold might be lost. There may be separate risk incentive funds for primary physicians and specialists. The IPA and its participating physicians may also share in separate risk incentive funds for ancillary and hospital services.

There is a risk that the IPA's activities in negotiating fees to be paid participating physicians may lead to antitrust liability for horizontal price fixing. There are three general approaches to minimizing this risk. First, the IPA might function merely as a "conduit" or "messenger" of price information to the physicians, negotiating with third parties only on nonprice contract terms, such as utilization review, quality assurance, or billing practices. Each physician would then separately agree to the proposed rates or attempt to negotiate different ones. This approach, while safest from an antitrust perspective, is highly unwieldy in practice and thus has been avoided by providers and payers alike.

Second, and probably the best approach at the outset, the IPA could adopt a proposed blended professional fee schedule, or sign third party payer agreements proposing such a fee schedule so long as each individual physician has a period of time (for example, 10 days) within which to "opt out" of this limited "attorney-in-fact" arrangement. Silence is contractually presumed to mean conclusive consent. This approach is most popular among start-up IPAs that are not yet ready to accept the risk-sharing arrangements of the third alternative (that is, the joint venture approach, discussed below) but wish to negotiate professional fees collectively with third party payers, at least on a conditional basis. While not entirely free of risk, this approach should withstand a price-fixing challenge, particularly when combined with a collective agreement not to balance bill enrollees, to take assignment where required, to accept utilization review restrictions, and to follow other dictates of the IPA as well as any third party payer contracts entered into by the IPA with respect to which the individual physician does not opt out. The IPA also should otherwise be formed and operated for procompetitive and not anticompetitive purposes. It should represent no more than 50 to 60 percent of the physicians in the applicable service area, if possible (or 20 to 30 percent if the IPA is the exclusive contracting organization for those physicians), in order to minimize other potential antitrust risks.[10]

Third, the IPA physicians may agree among themselves as to fees so long as the IPA is deemed a legitimate, integrated joint venture as demonstrated by financial contributions and risk sharing. The joint venture approach shields the IPA from antitrust liability on the theory that a new product is being offered as to which price requirements are integral. To establish integration under the joint venture approach, the physicians *must* undertake some risk of loss if the IPA cannot operate within budget for services rendered.[11] At a minimum, the physicians should be subject to a 20 percent or greater withhold of their professional fees, to be paid to them after the end of the contract year only to the extent that certain financial and related utilization management targets have been met by each physician as well as by the physicians collectively.

Liability The provision of medical services by the IPA involves a certain risk that the IPA may be held liable for the malpractice of a contracting physician. IPAs may also be held liable for improper physician credentialing decisions and negligent utilization review determinations. The IPA should purchase malpractice insurance to cover these risks and require contracting physicians to maintain adequate malpractice coverage. The IPA also should maintain director's and officer's liability insurance. A combined IPA/PPO professional liability and director's and officer's liability insurance policy, including coverage for utilization review decisions, has been available recently at a rate of approximately $10,000 per year for $1 million per occurrence and $1 million annual aggregate coverage. This insurance includes coverage for liability that may result from utilization review activities but not for antitrust liability, reportedly because of the recent large insurance company pay-outs in connection with HMO conversion-related litigation, particularly in the ChoiceCare case.[12]

CONCLUSIONS IPAs should generally be structured as either a sole shareholder professional corporation, a taxable nonprofit corporation with statutory members, or, if permitted under state law, a "memberless" nonprofit corporation. The advantage of a sole shareholder professional corporation is that it eliminates the risk of an affiliated service group being formed and avoids any requirements of qualification of the sale of its stock under state securities laws. However, the disadvantage is that the physician who is the sole shareholder will have a disproportionate degree of control over the election of the board of directors of the IPA and, as a result, the management and operation of the IPA.

The advantage of a nonprofit corporation is that it appears to avoid the affiliated service group problem completely. However, in certain states it may face onerous statutory restrictions limiting termination of members or, depending on the size of the IPA's membership, securities law registration requirements. In order to avoid these problems, a "memberless" nonprofit corporation may be utilized if provided for under state law. Although the board of directors of such a corporation would be self-perpetuating as a legal matter, the contract physicians could be given the right to recommend new board members, thus allowing the physicians who participate in the IPA to control its management.

NOTES
1. Although the acronym "IPA" originally stood for "individual practice association," over time the more descriptive "independent practice association" has prevailed.

2. Internal Revenue Code §414(m)(2)(ii), as amended, effective January 1, 1989, by the Tax Reform Act of 1986, §1114(b)(11).

3. After January 1, 1989, it is doubtful that some plans would satisfy IRC Section 401(a)(26), which requires each plan to cover the lesser of 50 employees or 40 percent of the employees of the group.

4. See, for example, Cal. Corp. Code §§ 7110 et seq.; Ore. Rev. Stat. §61.091.

5. There is a wide variety of state laws governing the corporate practice of medicine. See, for example, Calif. Bus. & Prof. Code §§ 2400 et seq.; Mass. G.L. c. 156A; Minn. Stat. ch. 319A; N.C. Gen. Stat. §§555b-1 et seq; Ohio Rev. Code Ann. §1737.01 et seq; for a general compilation of state laws in this area. See E. S. Rolph, J. P. Rich, P. B. Ginsburg, S. D. Hosek, K. M. Keenan, and G. B. Gertler, State Laws and Regulations Governing Preferred Provider Organizations, 89–162 (1986).

6. See, for example, Rev.Rul. 86-98 (August 18, 1986), holding that an IPA does not qualify for tax-exempt status under either Section 501(c)(4) or Section 501(c)(6) of the Internal Revenue Code.

7. See supra, note 5.

8. See, for example, GCM 39498, GCM 39670, and GCM 39633; but also see *Rev. Rul. 8419071, Rev. Rul. 73-313*, 1973-2, CB 174.

9. 42 U.S.C. §§11101 et seq.

10. See, generally, the unpublished May 15, 1987 Federal Trade Commission advisory opinion letter to Charles E. Rosolio regarding Maryland Medical Eye Associates, P.A.; see also, the remarks of Charles F. Rule, Assistant Attorney General for the Antitrust Division, to the Connecticut Health Lawyers Association, March 11, 1988.

11. Where a group of ophthalmologists contributed $10,000 and participated in a capitation program for some services, the FTC found "significant integration among . . . physicians shareholders" where the physicians "made capital contributions and assumed a degree of risk and created a product none of them could produce alone." See the unpublished FTC advisory opinion letter, supra note 10.

12. Thompson v. Midwest Foundation Independent Physicians Ass'n. d/b/a ChoiceCare, no opinion (S.D. Ohio, March 14, 1988).

CASE STUDY

Summa Health Plan: Why HMOs Fail

PAUL M. KATZ, Senior Management
Consultant

Millimen & Robertson, Inc., San Francisco, California

HMOs rapidly expanded across the country in the early 1980s. More recently, many have failed. Although growth in the number of new HMOs has now slowed, most continue to prosper despite a number of dramatic failures. For HMOs that were operational for more than 3 years, 56 percent showed a profit in 1986, with profits ranging from 2 to 10 percent of revenues. For HMOs in a start-up phase (under 3 years of operation) only 14 percent showed a profit. The question remains: Why do some HMOs fail while others succeed?

Summa Health Plan (SHP) is typical of many HMOs that were started in the mid-1980s, but this plan presents a worst-case picture of why HMOs fail. Summa Health Plan was organized in California in 1983 and after 5 years of operation went into bankruptcy. As an initiative of the Medical Society of Fresno and Madera Counties, it had the largest provider base of any HMO in its service area. At the outset, there were no other large HMOs practicing in the area, and the market was wide open to a locally run and managed HMO. Nearly 100 local physicians invested in the health plan.

When SHP began operations in 1984, utilization review on outpatient services was not enforced, physicians were able to refer cases to themselves, and there were no checks on referrals among physicians or ancillary providers. Specialists were allowed to act as primary care doctors. With most of the physicians in town participating in the HMO, and the plan not enforcing HMO-type utilization review and prior authorization programs, the health plan appeared to operate more on faith than on sound implementation of HMO policies and procedures to assure its viability.

In 1988, the HMO filed for bankruptcy reorganization under Chapter 11 of the federal bankruptcy law. It was unable to control costs, the 35 percent withhold on its physicians had never been returned, and it faced default on numerous debt obligations (some of which were guaranteed by members of management and investor physicians). The bankruptcy court required the HMO to continue to operate as long as patients remained or until its funds were depleted.

THE SUMMA MARKETPLACE

In 1984, when Summa was granted its operating license from the State of California, only one other HMO operated in the area. With a two-county population of 500,000 lives, the total HMO enrollment at the time was only 8000 members, which clearly indicated an opportunity for HMO growth. Kaiser entered the marketplace in 1986. With an established employer base among federal and state employees, and unions, Kaiser was able to quickly grab the largest market share among the HMOs. In 1987, three additional HMOs entered, and in 1988, two more. Summa never reached its optimistic enrollment projections. As the market became increasingly competitive, they were forced to target the higher risk individual and small case groups.

For HMOs to develop and survive, they need to demonstrate four key criteria: management capability, access to capital, marketing position, and high quality and efficiency of the provider system. An HMO in a highly competitive market must constantly evaluate and upgrade its criteria.

SUMMA MANAGEMENT

A prerequisite for HMO success in competitive markets is a core group of seasoned managers who understand the business. When Summa Health Plan began operations, very few management personnel had previous HMO management experience. By conventional standards, neither the CEO, CFO, director of marketing, or other managers had any experience in the HMO industry. As a result, Summa's management reports, for example, were produced on a cash basis at the outset and were often inaccurate. The industry standard is to use accrual accounting with an estimate of incurred but not recorded (IBNR) expenses for outstanding claims based on a claims lag study. Management was not knowledgeable enough about industry standards to use the financial tools necessary for operating an HMO on a businesslike basis.

SHP also bought administrative services, including

claims processing, from outside organizations that were affiliated with the Medical Society. Such administrative services were contracted from providers inexperienced in the HMO industry, and these services were purchased at noncompetitive rates. At the end of fiscal year 1986, SHP claimed to have achieved breakeven. Yet after an audit, substantial losses were found.

Summa Health Plan established itself as a limited partnership, with the management in the role of general partner and physicians invited to participate as limited partners. In this arrangement, the limited partners were asked to personally guarantee the original debt. In the case of a limited partnership, the limiteds are taxed on the full amount of recorded profit. This occurs even if a profit distribution is not made to the limited partners because the profits are reinvested into the company.

CONFLICT BETWEEN PROVIDERS AND OWNERS

As both practitioners and investors, the physicians could view their investment as a vehicle to guarantee cash flow by providing medical services. They expected to be paid as providers, even when as owners, they knew that the money was not available. Because it paid physicians almost as much as their usual and customary rate, the health plan paid more for services than other HMOs in the same area.

When a company enters bankruptcy, two options are available: First, under a declaration of Chapter 11 bankruptcy, the company can restructure its debts and operations and continue in business. Organizations that successfully restructure have productive assets that are able to generate products and services that satisfy a market. The whole organization is worth more in future revenue than can be obtained by selling the assets on a short-term basis. The second option is filing for Chapter 7 bankruptcy and results in liquidation of the company by sale of its assets.

An HMO has a very difficult time with both of these options since its only assets are group insurance contracts. Employer groups are not interested in paying money for their employees to an organization that has filed Chapter 11, which indicates it is not able to pay bills that have been incurred. There has yet to be any indication that a bankruptcy court can force the insured groups to stay with the HMO.

When Summa Health Plan filed for Chapter 11 bankruptcy, the largest employer groups (those with the ability to easily find another HMO to underwrite their business) moved their employees to other HMOs. This reduced Summa's future earning power and depleted its ability to eventually pay back its creditors and owners. As a result, SHP has entered Chapter 7 bankruptcy.

When an HMO enters Chapter 7 and dissolves, there is also no easy solution. Since the assets are the group contracts, which cannot be guaranteed as part of a sale of assets (since the employer group has the right to seek coverage elsewhere), there is very little left of the HMO to sell.

LESSONS LEARNED

The case of Summa Health Plan presents several lessons for the HMO industry. First, HMOs must be developed and managed with the long-term goal of building a successful healthcare business, rather than short-term objectives of securing market share, income to providers, or financial write-offs. The following recommendations are intended to avoid the pitfalls of groups similar to Summa.

RECOMMENDATIONS

1. An HMO is a unique business which demands the full-time attention of experienced professionals. It must guarantee proper utilization and quality of care and, at the same time, manage financial risk of an insurance product. Summa attempted to do this with inexperienced part-time staff. Finance is the biggest weakness of most HMOs. Too often, HMOs are surprised when they think that their financial performance is good, and in fact it is quite poor. A secondary need is strong leadership at the top that can work effectively with providers.

2. If physicians and other caregivers are also owners of the organization, specific rules on the terms of fees for providing medical services need to be set in place. The creditors and owners of the HMO are required to subordinate their respective liability and equity to the overall equity needs of the organization. The same rules should apply to a provider that has a significant ownership in the organization. This

would also encourage the provider-owners to set fees at a rate that makes the most business sense for the organization. Summa fees were set to maximize short-term personal gain.

3. All transactions with affiliated companies should have obligations incurred by the HMO subordinated to equity needs. In the case of Summa, the organization had administrative contracts with three other businesses associated with the local medical society. Some of these were run by the same officers and board members as Summa. By subordinating the HMO's obligations, the affiliates are forced to see that their activity is necessarily in the best interests of the health plan.

4. The HMO should be required by law to make full disclosure in its state or federal reporting about the nature of the transactions between the HMO and affiliates, as well as to identify the financial interests of board members and the company's officers in affiliates or other organizations contracting with the HMO. In the case of Summa, they were not asked about potential conflicts of interest concerning administrative service contracts with affiliates. This proved to be a serious financial problem.

While the situation outlined in this case study describes a worst-case scenario, the future of the HMO industry appears strong. As some HMOs cease operation or are acquired, the remaining firms will have a stronger market position from which to prosper.

CHAPTER TWELVE

Benefit Design

MANAGED CARE BENEFIT DESIGN

LINDA J. HAVLIN, Flexible and Group Benefits Consultant

LARRY J. TUCKER, Flexible and Group Benefits Consultant

Hewitt Associates, Lincolnshire, Illinois

Early efforts to control medical benefit costs emphasized the importance of cost sharing as a key to controlling both the use and cost of health services. More recently, it has been recognized that the most effective way to control medical benefit costs is to manage not only the scope of benefits provided, including cost-sharing provisions, but also to manage the appropriateness of utilization, control the price paid to healthcare providers, and encourage the use of efficient providers. These objectives underlie the benefit design of managed care plans.

HISTORICAL PERSPECTIVE
Today's managed care plans are an outgrowth of plan designs that inadequately controlled the cost and use of services. In the 1960s and 1970s, benefit managers assumed that costs could be controlled through cost sharing, education, second opinions for surgery, and incentives to use lower-cost sites of care (for example, outpatient surgery). Another assumption was that physicians would modify their behavior if they were provided, on a retrospective basis, with information about questionable patterns of care.

Assuming that these forces would all work together to control healthcare costs was optimistic, but unrealistic. To some extent, the

265

programs worked, but they did not go far enough. New cost and use problems emerged to replace those that were corrected. A frustrating cyclical pattern emerges—costs rise; new strategies are introduced to control the cost; costs decline temporarily; and then costs rise again. The purchasers of health benefits have to keep constant pressure on insurers, HMOs, third party administrators, and other managers of healthcare to keep this cost cycle under control.

Why did initial cost-containment programs fail to keep costs under control? The reasons are complex, but among the most important are the following:

- Patients have not had complete information about medical services and have been unable to judge the effectiveness of alternative treatment programs.
- There has been significant elasticity in the demand for health services. Providers have stimulated the use of health services, particularly for elective procedures, testing, and new technologies.
- Standards have been lacking on the necessity and appropriateness of treatment.
- The price of care has not been controlled or negotiated except by a limited number of payers (for example, Medicare, Medicaid, HMOs, certain states, and some insurance companies and Blue Cross plans).

A more structured approach to managing healthcare costs was found in health maintenance organizations (HMOs). HMOs have managed costs by controlling all the key components—the scope of benefits, the fees paid to providers, access to healthcare services, and utilization of services.

While HMOs, particularly group models, offer the best potential for controlling costs, they require that the consumer receive all benefits through the HMO's providers. This "all-or-nothing" constraint helps to control costs but inhibits enrollment and consumer satisfaction. Some employees are not willing to trade "freedom of choice" for the lower overall cost that may be associated with the HMO.

The 1980s have been marked by an explosion of benefit plans that attempt to meld the cost advantages of HMOs with the freedom of choice found in traditional medical plans. Point-of-service products, such as preferred provider organizations (PPOs), exclusive provider organizations (EPOs), and open-ended HMOs, are a market response to the need to control healthcare costs and provide more freedom of choice than is provided by a traditional HMO model.

Point-of-service plans offer networks of primary care physicians, specialists, and hospitals. Unlike an HMO, a patient is not "locked in" to using specific providers. These plans encourage employees to use network providers but give employees the option of paying more out of pocket and using providers outside the network. The decision to use one of the network providers is made at the point of purchase. Essentially, the decision is a choice based on an employee's personal preference, income, and experience with the network providers.

MEDICAL PLAN DESIGN COMPONENTS

An understanding of how managed care plans are designed requires knowledge of the traditional elements of medical plan design. The following two sections review plan design components and demonstrate how those components are used in managed care plans.

A traditional medical plan includes components that can be structured in a variety of ways to influence the cost and use of services. As a first step, the overall scope of benefits is determined. Medical plans typically cover hospital room and board and ancillary care, physicians' fees, prescription drugs, and hospice and home healthcare. While a majority of expenses are covered by the medical plan, some plans may explicitly exclude expenses for routine medical exams, experimental procedures, cosmetic procedures, or services rendered in an unlicensed facility.

Also, a medical plan stipulates how the provider's allowable charges will be determined. Allowable charges may be based on fee schedules or negotiated rates. Thus, the benefits paid by the plan may be less than the charges submitted by the provider. (However, it should be noted that some providers agree to accept the allowed amount as payment in full and do not bill the patient for the balance.)

Once the allowable charges are determined and accepted as eligible expenses covered by the plan, the benefit design provisions are applied. These provisions might include the following:

- *Deductibles* A flat dollar amount (for example, $200) paid by the individual before benefits are paid. The amount is deducted from the covered charges. Any other cost-sharing requirements are calculated only after the deductible has been met.
- *Coinsurance* A percentage (for example, 80 percent) of covered charges paid by the benefit plan. Any remaining charges are paid by the individual up to an out-of-pocket maximum.
- *Copayments* A flat dollar amount (for example, $5) that is paid directly to a provider at the time services are received. Copayments are frequently required for physician office visits or prescription drugs.
- *Out-of-pocket maximum* A dollar limit (for example, $2000) placed on the total amount of covered charges paid by an individual and a family. After a certain point, cost sharing ends and the plan pays for covered charges in full. The intent of this maximum

is to limit the employee's liability and prevent a catastrophic expense.

- *Per confinement deductible*   A flat dollar amount (for example, $300) applied to each hospital confinement, including outpatient surgery. This form of a deductible is not intended to discourage individuals from receiving preventive care. Recently, this form of deductible has been used as a way of introducing greater cost sharing into the first dollar coverage provided by HMOs. Also, the deductible is fairly easy to communicate and only affects those persons who use services.
- *Percent-of-pay cost sharing*   A percentage of an employee's salary (for example, 1 percent) determines the premium contribution, deductible, or coinsurance. In addition, the out-of-pocket maximum can be capped as a percentage of pay (for example, 4 percent). Again, percentages could vary depending on whether services are rendered in-network or out-of-network. This approach presents some administrative difficulties and requires considerable accuracy on the part of the claims administrator. A clear advantage to this approach is that it is viewed positively by lower income employees as an equity issue. Cost sharing becomes more closely tied to economic means. Conversely, highly compensated employees may see the logic but resent the outcome.
- *Annual and lifetime maximums*   A fixed limit on benefits received during a 12-month period or over an individual's lifetime. Examples of annual benefit limits are $1000 for dental benefits, $500 for outpatient psychiatric care, and $500 for podiatric care. Limits may be stated as a total dollar amount (for example, $10,000) or number (for example, two inpatient chemical dependency admissions, 20 outpatient mental health visits). Common lifetime limits are $500,000 to $1 million. Specific lifetime limits have been applied to mental health and substance abuse. The trend was to increase lifetime limits as a goodwill gesture and to reassure employees that catastrophic expenses would be covered. Limits, such as $1 million, often were set with the expectation that they would never be reached. Technological advances have made it possible to surpass these catastrophic limits, thereby requiring employers to decide whether to enforce or raise the limit.
- *Penalty provisions*   Reductions in benefits for failure to comply with plan requirements (for example, a $1000 penalty for failure to have a hospital admission precertified and a 50 percent reduction in coverage of a surgeon's fee for failure to obtain a second opinion).
- *Incentives*   Increases in benefits for complying with plan requirements (for example, increasing benefits from 80 to 100 percent for preadmission testing and waiving a deductible for calling the utilization review organization) or as a means of encouraging

preventive care (for example, 100 percent coverage for well-baby care). While the "carrot" may be more appealing to employees than the "stick," incentives will increase costs and should be used cautiously.

A hypothetical example of how design features are applied to a surgeon's bill is shown in Table 1. In this example, the plan has a $200 per person deductible ($600 per family), 80-20 percent coinsurance, and an out-of-pocket limit of $2000.

Table 2 shows what happens when the surgeon's bill has been paid and is followed by a hospital bill of $15,000.

An obvious net effect of these design features is to shift costs to employees. The objective of cost sharing is to influence an individual's use of health services, improve awareness of healthcare costs, and reduce the rate at which costs increase. Some of the early managed care plans assumed that cost sharing would not be necessary, but experience indicates that cost sharing is important, even in the most well-managed environment. Cost sharing not only influences utilization but also creates incentives to use specific providers.

APPROACHES TO MANAGED CARE PLAN DESIGN

Initially, the definition of managed care was quite broad. A typical definition was "any employer plan intervention into an individual's selection of healthcare providers and use of services." As a result, the approaches to plan design were varied and wide-ranging. HMOs, PPOs, EPOs, and even utilization review (UR) programs all fit that broad definition. One way to picture the range of approaches is on a spectrum of loose to tight controls over access to healthcare services (see Figure 1).

TABLE 1   Applying Design Features to a Surgeon's Bill

Surgeon's submitted charge		$2000
Paid by employer plan		
Plan's allowable charge	1800	
Less: Employee's deductible	200	
Net allowable charge	$1600	
Total paid by employer plan (80%)		$1280
Paid by employee		
Amount not included in plan's allowable charge		
($2000 − $1800)	200	
Employee's deductible	200	
Employee's coinsurance (20%; $1600 − $1280)	320	
Total paid by employee		720
		$2000

TABLE 2   Applying Design Features to a Hospital Bill

Hospital submitted charge			$15,000
Paid by employer plan			
Plan's allowable charge		$15,000	
Less: Employee's deductible (already met)		0	
Net allowable charge		15,000	
Employer plan coinsurance (80%)		12,000	
Employee's coinsurance (20%)	$3,000		
Less: Maximum payable by employee			
(see below)	1280		
Portion of employee coinsurance payable			
by employer plan		1,720	
Total paid by employer plan			$13,720
Paid by employee			
Deductible (already met)		0	
Employee's out-of-pocket maximum		2,000	
Less: Amount paid by employee to			
surgeon (see Table 1)		720	
Total paid by employee			1,280
			$15,000

As managed care plans have evolved, a more focused definition has emerged. Generally, managed care plans are those which control cost and use of services. Theoretically, an HMO represents complete control. A point-of-service benefit plan, such as a PPO or open-ended HMO, offers less control than a pure HMO, but it is an attractive alternative to the lock-in aspect of HMOs. Key characteristics of the most effective managed care plans include the following:

- The cost, use, and appropriateness of services rendered by network providers are tightly controlled. Providers are selected on the basis of their ability to provide cost-effective care. Practice patterns are monitored, and specialist referrals are screened by the network's management. Some HMOs and point-of-service plans set targets for how much use should occur in- and out-of-network.

Unmanaged—Weak Control							Managed—Tight Control
Fee for Service	Fee for Service with UR	PPO without UR	EPO without UR	PPO with UR	EPO with UR	Open-Ended HMO	IPA HMO	Group-Model HMO

Figure 1   *Spectrum of managed care plans.*

- Benefit design provisions encourage use of network benefits. In an HMO, benefits are restricted to HMO providers and approved emergency care. In a point-of-service plan, network benefits generally parallel those of an HMO and require minimal cost sharing, while out-of-network benefits require cost sharing that is significant enough to encourage network use. For example, coinsurance for out-of-network care may be set at 20 percent less than network benefits and large deductibles may apply (for example, $500 or 1 percent of pay).
- Utilization controls are placed on both in-network and out-of-network services. The controls may be more visible to the employee using out-of-network services. HMOs, for example, manage utilization within their own organization and do not require an employee to call for precertification or obtain a second opinion. An employee will still have to comply with traditional utilization review requirements for using out-of-network benefits.
- A gatekeeper physician controls access to the network and is paid on a capitated or discounted fee-for-service basis. The physician's compensation may be tied to goals of what percent of services are provided in-network for his or her patients.
- If all or a majority of the employer's medical plans are administered by one carrier, the experience from all the plans is pooled. Pooled experience is preferable as it allows an employer to establish prices for medical plans based on each plan's benefit value. Typically, a plan's cost is based on experience and reflects the demographics of, and use by, the enrolled population. Costs can fluctuate widely depending on who enrolls in a particular plan. If all the costs for an employer's various plans (for example, traditional HMO or open-ended HMO) are pooled, the price of each plan can be established based on actuarial value rather than unique experience. This rating method helps smooth trends over the long term.

Structural Relationship Between In- and Out-of-Network Benefits

Benefits for network providers need to be greater than for nonnetwork providers by an appreciable margin (for example, at least 10 percent, but preferably 20 percent). The difference must be wide enough to encourage use of the network, but it should not be viewed as highly punitive or economically harmful. In both PPO and open-ended HMO arrangements, a large difference in coinsurance is important as a means of ensuring that patients will use the preferred providers thereby justifying the negotiated discount.

A caution in adopting generous coinsurance for network benefits is that 100 percent coverage will lead to cost increases because it encourages utilization. Modest cost sharing discourages some people from using services unless they really need care. If an employer has an 80 percent comprehensive plan benefit and adopts a 100 percent benefit as an incentive for individuals to use in-network services, it is a virtual certainty that overall plan costs will rise as a result of increases in utilization. Provider discounts will not be substantial enough to offset the rise in utilization. The discount must be large enough to offset increases in both benefits and utilization. For example, suppose an employer offers a comprehensive plan with 20 percent coinsurance and introduces a point-of-service plan that has 100 percent coverage of in-network benefits. In this case, the benefits paid will increase (from 80 to 100 percent), overall utilization will increase, and administrative expenses to support this more complex plan will increase. A 10 to 15 percent provider rate discount will not offset those increases.

Out-of-network benefits should be designed to mirror comprehensive plan benefits, using both coinsurance and deductibles. Ideally, cost sharing is set at a level that discourages unnecessary services but is not so high that it discourages employees from receiving necessary care. The only time more punitive out-of-network benefits may be acceptable is if an employer is located in an area where virtually all care could be rendered by the network providers—allowing exceptions only for persons traveling out-of-area or having a life-threatening emergency. In this case, a high deductible (for example, 1 percent of pay or $1000 per person) and high coinsurance (for example, 70 percent) may be acceptable.

Some employers will implement a managed care program and concurrently eliminate all competing HMOs to ensure that *all* claims are in the same risk pool. Those employers with HMO participation prior to managed care implementation are most likely to consider seriously 100 percent benefits for in-network services to parallel the prior program. These employers view the positive employee relations aspect of this approach as critical. An alternative approach would be to offer 100 percent reimbursement for in-network services for the first year or two of the managed care program but slowly begin to coinsure those services.

Within the overall managed care design, employers may want to consider using exclusive provisions whereby certain benefits are paid only if services are received in the network. This approach might be appropriate for procedures or treatments that are frequently used, are high cost, or present a risk unless performed in a specific setting. Organ transplants, mental healthcare, chemical dependency, heart surgery, and high-risk obstetrical deliveries are some examples.

Exclusive provisions also may be used to encourage use of primary care within the network by providing coverage only if the benefits are received in-network. The thought behind this approach is that if primary care is delivered in-network, there is a greater likelihood that specialty care will be referred in-network rather than self-directed by the patient to a provider outside the network. The primary care gatekeeper physician will recommend a specialist who also belongs to the network. Unless the patient dislikes the specialist or has a strong relationship with an out-of-network specialist, the odds are in favor of the patient staying with the network referral.

An alternative to exclusive provisions is to reduce dramatically the allowed benefit for out-of-network benefits. However, some states (such as Massachusetts) preclude an insured plan from reducing benefits below a 20 percent differential or restricting an individual's freedom of provider choice.

Open-Ended HMO Benefit Design

An HMO is well-suited to provide in-network benefits, since physicians are preselected for their ability to provide efficient health services. Also, utilization controls generally are built into the operating structure of an HMO. On the downside, consistency of benefits may be affected if a state or federally qualified HMO is used as the in-network provider; some states have unique mandates on the level of coverage that must be provided. Some HMOs have avoided this constraint by setting up two corporations — one qualified and another nonqualified. The nonqualified organization handles the design approaches required by major employers and those employers seeking lower cost HMO benefits. Also, carriers may avoid these restrictions by offering fully self-funded programs.

Network benefits for an open-ended HMO generally parallel those of a traditional HMO. Copayments of $5 to $10 may be set for network physician office visits while visits to nonnetwork physicians may be subject to an overall deductible (for example, $200) and paid at the out-of-network coinsurance level. A sample design of employee cost sharing in an open-ended HMO is shown in Table 3.

To ensure an effective level of cost sharing, out-of-network benefits can be structured as a comprehensive medical plan with annual deductibles and 80 percent employer and 20 percent employee coin-

TABLE 3 Employee Cost Sharing in an Open-Ended HMO

	IN-NETWORK	OUT-OF-NETWORK
Deductible	0	$500 per individual
Physician office copay	$10	20 percent
Coinsurance for hospital and other care	0	20 percent
Prescription drugs	$5	20 percent
Out-of-pocket maximum	N/A	$2000 per individual

surance. The advantage of this benefit design is that employees who live in areas that do not have a network can have a comprehensive benefit plan. These employees may resent the richer benefits available to employees who can use the network, but they still have a reasonable benefit.

An employer who wants to lower the out-of-network coinsurance to 70 percent or less should consider whether all employees have access to network providers. If so, the lower out-of-network benefit will provide a further incentive to use network providers. If there are access problems, the employer may want to retain a comprehensive plan with 80 percent coinsurance as an option.

Employers are moving toward sharing more costs with employees for HMO benefits. For example, the HMO level of benefit might include a per hospital confinement deductible (for example, $300 to $500), increased office visit copayments (for example, $15), increased prescription drug copayments (for example, $7), and greater cost sharing for hospital admissions and specialty referral services (for example, 20 percent). The net result of this design could be to create two levels of HMO benefits: a high option and a low option. These two levels of HMO benefits could form the in-network benefit for high- and low-option point-of-service plans.

PPO Benefit Design

The design of a PPO is similar to an open-ended HMO in that there should be a strong economic incentive to use PPO providers. PPOs have greater design flexibility because cost sharing is largely stated in terms of percentage of cost. Typically, copayments for physician care are not used. Both physicians and hospitals have agreed to specific rates, and employees pay coinsurance on a percentage of the total rate.

PPOs have found that a 100 percent benefit encourages high utilization, and as a result, they are lowering the in-network coinsurance level to 90 percent or less. Another approach being used is the maintenance of high levels of coverage for primary and preventive care and the introduction of more cost sharing for specialist care. Multiple levels of cost sharing, however, may confuse employees. An example of having too many levels would be a PPO plan that covers well-child care at 100 percent, primary care at 90 percent, specialists at 80 percent, hospital care at 90 percent, home health or hospice care at 100 percent, and psychiatric benefits at 50 percent. A simple, straightforward PPO or HMO plan design may be more appealing and less confusing to employees.

A basic PPO design might look like Table 4. A more complex design with greater incentives to use the preferred providers may be structured as shown in Table 5. The objective of this approach is to require some cost sharing on services inside the network and more

TABLE 4   PPO Design

	IN-NETWORK	OUT-OF-NETWORK
Deductible	$200 per individual $600 per family	$200 per individual $600 per family
Coinsurance	90%	70%
Out-of-pocket maximum	$1000 per individual $2000 per family	$3000 per individual $6000 per family
Prescription drugs	$5	70%

stringent cost sharing on out-of-network services. The overall structure suggests that some cost sharing on in-network services may help control inappropriate utilization and increase consumer awareness of the overall cost of the services.

PROBLEMS WITH UNIFORMITY

Depending on an employer's geographic locations and HMO relationships, the goal of having uniform benefit plans administered by one organization may not be feasible or desirable. Minor inconsistencies in plan design can occur even when benefits are managed by one carrier. For example, most states mandate benefits for insured plans. Also, there are instances, such as Pennsylvania law, where a carrier cannot force an employee to sign up for a gatekeeper physician. Such laws create the need for unique benefits to conform to each state's laws.

Another issue related to uniformity is that some carriers insist that benefit plans offered by any other carrier be discontinued and replaced with their own HMO and point-of-service products. The carrier's objectives are quite clear: gain control over the total population; eliminate HMOs that compete for market share; and request fully insured contracts as a means of improving cashflow and profit mar-

TABLE 5   PPO with More Complex Design

	IN-NETWORK	OUT-OF-NETWORK
Deductible	$250 per individual $750 per family	$500 per individual $1500 per family
Coinsurance	90%	70%
Out-of-pocket maximum	$1000 per individual $2000 per family	$3000 per individual $6000 per family
Prescription drugs	$5	70%

gin. However, in doing so, an employer may face the risk of canceling contracts with HMOs that are providing excellent care. In some instances, it may be advisable to retain certain local HMOs rather than accept the carrier's local product. The local HMO or PPO would be used to provide an exclusive benefit plan and to serve as the in-network provider in a point-of-service product. A third party or the carrier responsible for managing the other benefit plans could administer the out-of-network benefits.

MANAGED MENTAL HEALTHCARE

Increasingly, employers are looking at alternatives for providing managed mental healthcare. For some employers, mental health and chemical dependency rank among the most frequently used and costly components of medical benefits—with rates rising as much as 50 percent each year. The increases in cost and utilization are influenced by the increase in the number of hospital beds, treatment centers, and individual providers. In addition, some utilization review firms have had difficulty in establishing criteria for lengths of stay and appropriateness of admissions. How much care is needed and who the appropriate provider would be are difficult to judge. Further, providers have not been evaluated on their ability to have a positive impact on the outcome of treatment. Success rates in treatment, particularly for chemical dependency, are not widely available. These factors combined with a loss of the stigma associated with mental health treatment and enhanced benefits provided in medical plans have lead to unprecedented growth in such medical costs.

In response to this dilemma, some employers are using the exclusive benefit approach discussed earlier. Others are choosing to carve mental health and chemical dependency benefits out of all the various medical plans offered to employees and to assign one organization to serve as the gatekeeper for care. The organization is responsible for the following:

- Initial assessment of the patient's needs
- Referral to an appropriate provider
- Certifying the need for inpatient care
- Reviewing emergency admissions within 24 hours to determine the appropriate course of treatment and the need for hospitalization

In effect, the organization is like an HMO. The employee must pass through this gatekeeper to receive benefits. Otherwise, the patient bears full liability for treatment. Currently, few organizations are capable of providing this service. Employee assistance programs (EAPs), HMOs, PPOs, organized groups of mental health providers, or UR firms may eventually have the expertise to perform this function.

MANAGED CARE PLANS AND FLEXIBLE COMPENSATION

Some employers are under the impression that they have to make a choice between managed care and flexible compensation. This is not an either/or decision. The two concepts are compatible.

As a matter of review, the concept of flexible compensation involves providing employees with choices as to the form of their compensation—taxable cash, nontaxable benefits, and taxable benefits. A full flexible compensation program allows employees to choose how they will use employer contributions and their own salary to purchase benefits. A flexible program defines the employer's cost while also providing employees with meaningful choices for spending benefit dollars. Benefit choice-making recognizes that employees have individual needs that reflect their age, income, family status, and personal need. In other words, one size does *not* fit all.

An employer may offer one or several medical plans under a flexible program. The key issue is whether one medical plan can meet the needs of all employees and still control medical plan costs, particularly if employees are located in different locations. An employer may decide to offer more than one medical plan for the following reasons:

- Choice among medical plans responds to work force diversity. Employees have diverse needs and demographic characteristics. A member of a two-wage-earner family, for example, who has coverage through the spouse's employer may not need as much (or any) coverage as someone who has only one source of medical coverage. Lower income employees may want more first dollar coverage, while highly compensated employees can assume more risk for unanticipated expenses. For example, consider an employee who earns $20,000 and needs family coverage versus a single employee who earns $60,000. The former may want more first dollar coverage, such as that offered by an HMO, while the latter can economically afford to accept the greater risk associated with using coinsurance and deductibles. Further, an individual's economic and healthcare needs will change over time based on earnings, family status, and personal health.
- A pure HMO offers a less costly alternative to the point-of-service product. Employees who are satisfied with HMO coverage should be allowed to continue to elect that choice and spend their remaining benefit dollars on other benefits.
- Managed care plans are not available in all geographic locations. A major insurance carrier may have a presence in some, but not all, of an employer's key locations. Local HMOs might be retained to fill the gaps on a short-term basis. Alternatively, a local HMO may be judged superior to a carrier's HMO, outweighing the advantage of using one carrier to provide all benefits.
- New approaches to healthcare cost management will continue to

be developed. A benefit structure that provides a variety of options allows employers to introduce new approaches without totally replacing existing benefits. New options can be tested on an experimental basis without placing the entire program at risk. Some employees will be willing to try approaches that restrict their healthcare benefits, while others will want to retain freedom of choice in their use of healthcare services.

Managed care plans fit well within the overall philosophy of flexible compensation—particularly if employees are offered the chance to select among plans. A variety of medical options can be designed to (1) offer choices among provider delivery systems, (2) vary the degree of freedom of choice, and (3) introduce cost-sharing alternatives. An employer might, for example, offer the following benefit choices:

Option 1: No coverage (if the individual demonstrates proof of other coverage) This option is designed to minimize duplicative coverage by discouraging enrollment by employees who have coverage through a spouse's employer.

Option 2: Traditional HMO benefit plan All care received from HMO providers; no coverage outside the HMO; minimal cost sharing (for example, $5 copay on office visits, $3 copay on prescription drugs).

Option 3: Low-option HMO benefit plan All benefits received from HMO providers; no coverage outside the HMO; increased cost sharing for primary care services (for example, $10 copay); higher cost sharing for specialist care (for example, 20 percent); and cost sharing for hospital admissions (for example, 20 percent and $300 per confinement).

Option 4: Point-of-service plan In-network benefits similar to the high-option HMO plan and out-of-network benefits comparable to a traditional comprehensive plan (for example, $300 deductible per individual, 20 percent coinsurance, $1200 out-of-pocket maximum).

Option 5: Low-option point-of-service plan Network benefits similar to the low-option HMO, and out-of-network benefits require higher cost sharing (for example, $500 deductible, 20 percent coinsurance, $2500 out-of-pocket maximum).

Similarly, combinations of low and high options can be designed for PPOs.

The objective of a flexible approach is to provide a range of economic and delivery system choices. Further, a flexible program provides different levels of cost sharing so that ideally an employee may choose a plan that reflects the individual's financial ability to budget and self-insure the economic risk of uncovered expenses.

PRICING MANAGED CARE PLANS

The price for a managed care plan may be based on actual cost or actuarial value. A plan's actual cost reflects the recent claims experience of that specific plan. The actuarial value represents the value of each option as if all employees participate in that option. A value is established based on the amount of cost sharing required. Using an actuarial value method maintains an actuarially sound relationship among different plan options and results in less rate volatility from year to year. Each plan's cost is set in relationship to one plan.

Basing prices on actual costs or "experience-rating" each option typically results in a more dramatic spreading of costs between the higher and the lower benefit options. Depending on the level of employer subsidy for each option, the higher benefit options can soon become too costly for most employees.

For example, an employer can offer the following options:

Plan 1   An HMO

Plan 2   An open-ended HMO in which the in-network design is the same as Plan 1 (for example, $5 copay, 100 percent) and out-of-network benefits require a $200 deductible and 20 percent coinsurance

Plan 3   An open-ended HMO in which the in-network design has more cost sharing than Plan 1 (for example, $300 per confinement deductible, $10 copay) and the out-of-network benefits have a $500 deductible and 70 percent coinsurance

Plan 2 is higher in value than Plan 1 because it offers the identical benefits in-network and allows for out-of-network use. The HMO provides rich benefits in-network but covers no expenses outside its own network. Plan 3 may be the same or lower in value than the pure HMO benefit. If arbitrary prices are assigned to these plans, the relationship might look like the following:

PLAN	PRICE
Plan 1: HMO	$1600
Plan 2: High open-ended HMO	$2000
Plan 3: Low open-ended HMO	$1400

No matter what unique, one-time events affect claim experience, the relationship of these plans is permanently set so that plans 1 and 3 are more attractive than plan 2, the most expensive plan.

Under the actuarial valuation method, a low-option plan, for example, might cost the employer $1000 per year but could be priced at $1500. Each employee electing this option will in effect save the employer $500. This savings, however, might be offset by employee participation in options that cost the employer more than the employee pays for the plan.

Generally, however, employers that tend to encourage employees to select plans requiring more cost sharing (higher deductibles and copayments) will see some savings that result from both better pricing strategies and the more efficient use of services by employees.

One requirement for effective plan design that emerges from this discussion is that employers need more flexibility to pool the experience of their medical plans and to price each plan based on its value to the employee. This means that HMOs, PPOs, and insurers will have to be flexible enough so that employers can charge employees on the basis of plan design value. An employee should be able to select a plan based on cost sharing, perceived quality and extent of the provider network, and freedom of choice of provider. Both qualitative and quantitative measures need to be considered in setting prices that reflect benefit values.

FUTURE TRENDS

Gaining control over provider prices, appropriateness of utilization, and cost sharing are the first steps in managing care. What lies beyond the concept of getting employees to use managed healthcare systems? Many employers will decide to manage the healthcare risks of both prospective and current employees more aggressively. Premiums or deductibles may be based on an employee's willingness to undergo health screening and the actual results of the tests. For example, an employer plan may have a $1000 deductible which could be waived in specific increments if the employee agrees to a health screening that indicates he or she does not smoke and maintains acceptable weight, cholesterol, and blood pressure levels. Family members may also be included in such a screening effort. At a risk of being controversial, some employers may feel they have no choice but to aggressively control the health of their employees.

Cost Containment Starts with the Employee Benefit Book

RONALD H. WOHL, President

In Plain English, Gaithersburg, Maryland

Communication is the greatest problem facing employers who want to reduce healthcare costs. Why? Because no healthcare cost reduction program, no matter how simple or extensive it is, will be effective unless it is successfully communicated to employees.

The simplest form of healthcare management—explaining how the health plan works, that is, employee rights and obligations, the plan's terms and conditions, and healthcare coverage—depends on adequate, accurate, and timely communication to employees. Not only is this information recommended, it is strictly required by law to be in the summary plan description—the employee benefit book. Yet, this book generally represents the poorest effort to communicate on the part of most employers.

In order for employers to reduce unnecessary health plan costs, employees must understand three concepts: (1) the plan provides adequate protection, (2) the rising cost of healthcare imperils their employer's ability to offer the same or better coverage, and (3) their individual actions affect healthcare costs. An understanding of these concepts depends on the employer's credibility in the eyes of the employee and on the employer's ability to explain the healthcare plan in language the employees can understand and believe.

To get these concepts across successfully, the employer or plan administrator must be able to translate highly complex insurance, legal, financial, and healthcare terminology into terms that are readily understandable by the target audience. Bear in mind, that this audience includes not only the company's employees, but the employees' families as well as lawyers, doctors, accountants, insurance sales peoples, the plan's administrative personnel, hospital admitting staff, government regulators, the press, and maybe a judge and jury. Translations of this information must overcome a number of technical problems, not the least of which is choosing language that can be understood by the average employee.

An employee will be most concerned about the benefit plan when he or she, or a family member, has a health problem. After talking to coworkers and supervisors, the employee may look at the benefit book for an answer. If the answer is not clear, readily accessible, and quickly understood, the employee will put the booklet down and possibly never refer to it again.

The booklet must answer the employee's questions accurately and in a clear and logical fashion. Otherwise, the booklet and the employer lose credibility. Then, no matter what kind of cost containment or management techniques are employed, the booklet and all its terms, provisions, instructions, and value are lost to that employee. One of the most important ways to determine which questions employees will ask and which order they ask them in is to get into the employee's shoes and visualize what information is important and when. Questions raised about benefits start with general inquiries on the scope of the benefit program; for example, who is eligible, how much does it cost, can dependents be covered, what is covered, and how can benefits be obtained. Once these general questions are answered, the booklet should branch to specific questions about each subcategory of benefits; for example, surgery, emergency care, hospitalization, and testing. Far-reaching cost management practices, such as usual, reasonable and customary fees, precertification review, case management, deductible copayments, preventive care, wellness programs, and out-of-pocket limits, must be explained prior to discussions of each benefit they affect. Then, each benefit and subcategory of benefits must refer to these practices to emphasize their importance in the reader's mind. Finally, information on claims, coordination of benefits, continuation of coverage after termination, and plan administration should be addressed in a clear and logical fashion. The table of contents should reflect this structure and guide the reader quickly to the appropriate information.

If the booklet describing the plan fails, the employee will be unable to find or to use the information properly, and the basis for consistent plan administration will be lost. The employee will seek answers from the benefits office staff, who will have to explain, patiently, what the booklet failed to do. If staff members resort to policy answers instead of using the language and procedure in the booklet as the basis for their response to employee questions, they will confuse the employee and show that the company lacks confidence in the booklet. It will also be a sign to the employee that the booklet is not a valid reflection of the plan. For example, a complicated discussion of conversion privileges or Consolidated Omnibus Budget Reconciliation Act of 1986 (COBRA) will confuse the reader and may cause someone who actually is eligible to delay applying for coverage, or perhaps not apply at all, and then sue to regain coverage. The resulting litigation and "bad will" can affect employee confidence in the plan and in all company communications.

The old axioms apply to healthcare cost containment as well: "get back to basics" in communications between the employer and the employee. After all, "when all else fails, read the instructions." The following nagging questions must be answered:

Can employees read and understand the information? Is it written in a style and level appropriate to the reader?

Are reader handicaps considered? For example, some employees may be immigrants who do not understand English well or use it at all; others may be functionally illiterate, dyslexic, blind, or visually handicapped, or deaf employees who have only elementary reading skills. These groups may each consist of only a small number of employees, but together these employees may constitute a significant population in the company.

Will the employees want to read the booklet, and if they do read it, will they believe what is written in it? Negative publicity, rumors of bad plan experiences, or impending financial problems or layoffs will color the way employees view all management communications, including the benefit booklet. Employees appreciate and deserve the truth no matter how unsettling it may be.

Will the benefit plan and the cost-containment features be administered according to what is written in the benefit book?

Once these questions are answered affirmatively, the benefit book will itself be a powerful cost-management program and the basis for all future cost-containment programs as well.

CASE STUDY

Allied-Signal: Health Care Connection Program

JOSEPH W. DUVA, Corporate Director,
Employee Benefits

Allied-Signal, Morristown, New Jersey

Allied-Signal implemented a managed healthcare plan, called Health Care Connection Plan, for its salaried and nonunion hourly employees in 1988. The plan is administered by CIGNA and is being phased in over 3 years since CIGNA provider networks were not available at all company operations at the inception of the plan. It now covers approximately 110,000 employees and dependents in 22 healthcare networks across the country.

In 1987, company healthcare costs for employees, dependents, and retirees increased by 39 percent. Projections indicated that costs would go from $355 million in 1987 to $614 million in 1990 unless significant plan changes were made. The projection assumed an annual increase of 20 percent for 3 years. Projected premium increases are currently running from 20 to 26 percent based on an insurance company's book of business, so the 20 percent trend may be a conservative estimate for fee-for-service indemnity plans.

Allied-Signal also reviewed the balance sheet and charge-to-earnings impact of the accounting changes proposed by the Financial Accounting Standards Board for retiree medical plans. The preliminary results of the study convinced management that it had to take immediate action to restructure retiree medical plans.

After studying all the factors driving healthcare costs and talking to many healthcare experts, it became clear that Allied-Signal could not afford fee-for-service indemnity plans in the future. These plans were not managing mental health and chemical dependency claims cost effectively nor were outpatient medical services being aggressively monitored.

In redesigning the medical benefits plan, Allied-Signal decided to encourage, rather than force, employees and their dependents to use the managed care network. As a result, participants were able to choose whether to use a network physician or an-

other doctor each time they required care. This is commonly called a "point-of-service" option.

If participants choose a network primary care physician, there is a $10 copayment for an office visit and a $5 copayment for prescription drugs. If they go to a nonnetwork physician, they are reimbursed at 80 percent after meeting a deductible of 1 percent of pay for the employee and 3 percent for the family. This gives employees a financial incentive to seek care from a network physician. However, they have the freedom to visit any doctor and pay more. Some 75.4 percent of employees are using the networks 95 to 100 percent of the time, but 12.5 percent of employees and dependents are only using the networks 0 to 5 percent of the time.

As an inducement to use the network, preventive care services are also provided. They include periodic physicals, eye examinations, hearing examinations, and health promotion or wellness information.

This design is the same for all salaried and nonunion hourly employees across the country where healthcare networks are available. Conceptually, this method provides the best of the fee-for-service (employee freedom of choice) and prepaid medicine (cost management) approaches.

Of 55,000 employees eligible for the program, 48,000 are enrolled in the plan. The remaining 7000 employees are basically scattered in rural areas across the country. The company provides local management with a number of alternatives for selecting a more cost-effective healthcare arrangement. They range from some type of local managed care plan, special arrangements with doctors and hospitals, in-house medical facilities, or a revised indemnity plan.

The company's financial experience for the first year indicates that actual costs are running substantially lower, as indicated by the 1988 and 1989 trends for managed care programs.

Based on the experience of developing the Allied-Signal program, employers should consider the following when implementing a corporate-sponsored managed care plan:

- Determine corporate healthcare objectives and how long it should take to reach them. Make sure the plan design, implementation strategy, and on-going plan management support these objectives.
- Identify the important criteria for evaluating and

selecting a healthcare manager; the financial arrangement; quality of the provider networks; geographic coincidence of employees' homes and physicians' offices; the program support needed from a healthcare vendor.

- Know what managed care is. It is a way for employers to better manage healthcare costs and quality, but it demands a high degree of corporate involvement and intervention.

- Good communications are extremely important because managed care requires that employees change their behavior and perceptions, as well as develop an understanding of why this type of change is necessary.

It is important that employees understand the business reasons for adopting such a program. Keep in mind, however, that a comprehensive communication effort does not guarantee employees will accept the program.

Employees consider healthcare coverage one of their most important employee benefits, and it is a sensitive and emotional issue. Therefore, it is important that the communication program be ongoing and that employees and their dependents be continually updated on the benefits and requirements of the health plan. Accordingly, employers must continue to tell the story to ensure that employees understand the seriousness of the issue.

- By adopting a corporate-sponsored care plan, the company becomes a pioneer. Although managed care is gaining in popularity, the number of plans in operation is still small. It means breaking new ground. Much can go wrong and Murphy's Law will surely apply to a concept this new and complex.

- The program works well when there is a good partnership between local company management and the health plan administrator. Where this does not occur, corporate management must take the necessary action to bridge the gap and fix the problems as quickly as possible. The biggest challenge to making managed care work is management itself. If all levels of management buy in and support the program, implementation is less difficult.

There are a number of different approaches to implementing managed healthcare plans, and each of them has certain advantages.

- *Nationwide basis* One overall healthcare manager uses its own networks throughout the country and/or subcontracts with other networks to cover all eligible employees within an established timeframe.

- *Regional basis* A healthcare manager with its own network is chosen for each geographic region. The manager may be authorized to subcontract with other networks in the area if this makes good business sense to all parties.

- *Location-by-location basis* A healthcare manager is selected by actual location site. This requires that a number of different healthcare managers be monitored.

- *Independent company network* Some employers and business coalitions are developing their own networks independent of provider or insurance company networks.

Each company interested in managed care must decide on the proper approach, based on its business objective, corporate culture, and the speed with which it wants to implement the program.

CASE STUDY

Southern California Edison: Good Health Rebate and Preventive Health Account

MARY SCHMITZ, Ph.D., MANAGER

Corporate Health Services, Southern California Edison Company, Rosemead, California

Southern California Edison (SCE) is a public utility that provides electricity to a 50,000-square-mile territory throughout southern California. The company has approximately 17,000 employees and 5000 retirees. SCE is a self-insured medical plan employer and covers approximately 55,000 lives. Employees and their dependents can choose healthcare coverage through HealthFlex, the company's self-insured employee plan, or through one of eight health maintenance organizations. HealthFlex participants can receive medical services at a reduced rate from any of SCE's eight in-house healthcare centers (staffed by company doctors and nurses) or from a preferred-provider network established by the company; services received from any other provider may be covered but at a higher cost to the participant.

The Good Health Rebate and Preventive Health Account programs are integral parts of HealthFlex. These are annual programs designed to improve the general health of employees and their spouses and to contribute to a reduction in company healthcare costs by offering financial incentives to those who participate. SCE incorporated the two programs into HealthFlex in order to offer a unique incentive for good health and to emphasize the connection between disease prevention and cost savings.

Participants in the Good Health Rebate program can receive a $10 per person rebate off the cost of their monthly healthcare contribution if they undergo a special health screening, and

- They meet acceptable guidelines for five risk factors.

or

- They have elevated risks but choose to seek medical advice for risk-factor reduction.

The Preventive Health Account program provides a "credit account" of up to $100 per year per participant to cover many preventive health procedures and programs not covered by HealthFlex.

HOW THE GOOD HEALTH REBATE WORKS

Under the program, screening appointments are available before work hours, during lunch, and on weekends. (Screenings are not offered after work because participants must fast for 10 hours prior to the tests in order to get accurate blood sugar level readings.) Screenings are held at company-operated healthcare centers and at special facilities set up at other SCE sites. The $10 screening cost for the employee and spouse can be charged to the Preventive Health Account.

Participants in the rebate program must be re-screened each year to qualify for the annual rebate. The program measures five modifiable risk factors during the 15-minute screening: body weight (using the Body Mass Index), blood pressure, cholesterol, blood sugar, and carbon monoxide (smoking). Acceptable levels for passing the screening are based on national scientific guidelines and expert recommendations.

SCE's Health Care Department maintains close management control over all aspects of the program. All administrative functions, laboratory analyses, and some screenings are handled by SCE personnel. Other screenings are conducted by a contracted vendor.

The Health Care Department notifies participants of their screening results for each risk factor. Individuals must pass all five risk factors in order to qualify for the rebate. However, a participant can also qualify by becoming certified by a physician who completes a form stating that the participant has sought medical advice to reduce any elevated risk factor indicated by the screening. Participants who qualify for the rebate through certification are asked to have their physician complete a recertification form after 6 months stating that they have continued appropriate participation in treatment; risk factor reduction is not required. If this form is not completed, the rebate is discontinued for the remainder of the year.

THE PREVENTIVE HEALTH ACCOUNT

The Preventive Health Account is a companion program to the Good Health Rebate and encourages continued preventive activities. This special "credit account" coordinates with the rebate program by covering the cost of screenings and providing funds to offset the cost of participation in a risk-reduction program or preventive medical procedures.

The Preventive Health Account also pays for participation in company-approved health education activities such as weight loss and smoking cessation programs, routine physical exams, immunizations, and other approved preventive procedures not covered under HealthFlex, up to the $100 per person annual maximum.

GOOD HEALTH REBATE INITIAL RESULTS

Nearly 11,000 employees and spouses, or 52 percent of the eligible population, were tested in Good Health Rebate screenings during the program's first year. About 60 percent of the participants passed all five risk factors. An additional 20 percent qualified through physician certification. Approximately one-fourth of those tested were sent a follow-up letter stating that although they passed, their borderline readings merited further review by a physician.

Table 1 shows the percentage of people who did not pass the screening for each risk factor and indicates the percentage of people who chose to qualify for the rebate through doctor certification.

These initial results indicate that eligible employees and spouses with visible risk factors, that is, weight and smoking, are choosing not to be screened. Communications need to be developed

TABLE 1

	% NOT PASSED	% NOT PASSED/ DR. CERTIFIED
Weight	13	8
Blood pressure	5	5
Cholesterol	6	9
Blood sugar	0.3	0.5
Carbon monoxide	4	1

that appeal directly to this group, emphasizing their ability to receive the rebate through physician certification.

The Health Care Department is conducting a major evaluation of these programs. This includes an assessment of employee satisfaction with the screening process; identified risk prevalence compared to national norms; the number of newly discovered risks; employees' perception of the company's concern about their health; a thorough cost-effectiveness analysis; annual comparisons of changes in health risks correlated with absenteeism, healthcare utilization and costs; and Preventive Health Account usage characteristics and volume.

Without a comparable control group, it will not be possible to establish a direct, causal relationship between SCE's prevention programs and healthcare costs. However, the evaluation team will use SCE's internal integrated database to facilitate tracking of all correlational data on an annual and year-to-year basis.

CHAPTER THIRTEEN

Pricing, Risk, and Reimbursement

PRICING, RISK, AND ACTUARIAL ANALYSIS

DAVID V. AXENE, F.S.A., M.A.A.A., Principal and Consulting Actuary

Milliman & Robertson, Inc., Seattle, Washington

As the managed healthcare marketplace has developed, so the role of the actuary has changed. No longer is the actuary just a rating specialist needed to satisfy certain regulators; the actuary is becoming an increasingly important part of the healthcare management team. Actuaries are specialists in understanding and quantifying critical risk issues faced by a managed healthcare plan. The newly developing healthcare models with their increased sophistication require sophisticated actuarial approaches.

An actuary might be asked to evaluate the financial impact of a revised provider reimbursement strategy and perhaps predict the likely outcomes of the new approach. This type of analysis requires a blending of actuarial science with more traditional behavioral science (that is, how will the provider react) and basic control theory (that is, how does a plan keep the provider reacting the right way). Actuaries that can adapt to the rapidly changing environment are an invaluable asset to plan management.

Actuarial analysis falls into three different areas based on the user's perspective: (1) plan or carrier, (2) provider, and (3) plan sponsor. This chapter discusses each perspective and the types of analysis that should be considered.

THE PLAN OR CARRIER PERSPECTIVE

As managed healthcare programs continue to develop and expand, it is harder to differentiate between HMOs, PPOs, and carriers. Each is intensively involved in developing products that compete with their own plans and those of others. HMOs are trying to increase their market penetration with indemnity opt-out products, while at the same time insurers are developing HMO look-alike products. HMOs are developing point-of-service products to compete with PPO products. Carriers and PPOs are developing EPOs to compete with HMOs. Traditional distinctions are quickly becoming blurred. Perhaps the best way to differentiate between programs is by quantifying the program's degree and/or type of healthcare management (that is, utilization controls or provider incentives) since common labels no longer accurately define what the plan is.

For example, the utilization management programs in both PPOs and HMOs have achieved such varying degrees of effectiveness, as measured in terms of overall utilization and cost reductions, that it is almost impossible to predict which is more cost efficient. HMOs have generally achieved much more cost-effective systems, but this is not the case in many areas of the country. In some communities, HMO products have the best price, even when they provide richer benefits. In others, HMOs still tend to be unaffordable without major benefit reductions.

A key area for actuarial analysis is the assessment of how successful a healthcare management program is. This can be measured by using an actuarial cost model (that is, utilization, cost per unit, and claims cost assumptions). Using this methodology, an actuary can consistently and accurately compare two completely different systems to determine their relative effectiveness. After the models have been appropriately modified to put them on consistent bases, the relative efficiencies become obvious. An example is discussed at the end of the chapter (see Table 14).

When a plan or carrier considers a new product, the type and extent of actuarial analysis needed depends heavily on the product type and the number of options included. If the product is a replacement product (that is, a single medical plan and one that is intended to continue a sole-source product with no or very limited alternatives), the plan or carrier has an improved risk position since the likelihood of adverse selection is decreased. The current multiple-company multiple-benefit-plan environment has tended to bias results to the disadvantage of the carrier and in turn of the plan sponsor (that is, employer). The actuary must consider this effect and make it part of the actuarial assumptions.

On the other hand, if the product is a nonreplacement product (that is, one of several HMO and carrier options offered to the employees of a group), the potential for increased adverse selection must be considered and reflected in the actuarial analysis. Adverse selection against at least one option is a certainty. The only uncertainty is which option will be selected against.

Even when the replacement versus nonreplacement issue is decided, other packaging approaches affect the actuarial analysis. In the case of a stand-alone product with an annual open enrollment period, the assumed risk differs from a single program that internally offers multiple choices or the more current point-of-service multiple-option products. Enrollees tend to choose what is best for them at the time of choice. The actual decision and the permitted frequency of this decision determine the risk.

No longer can the actuary use conventional actuarial approaches to estimate the anticipated use rate and cost of services. The actuary must consider when, where, and why the services will be pursued. This requires that the population be segmented into those who are willing to use the managed care system all of the time, most of the time, some of the time, and never. Only when this distribution of enrollees is known can the actuary have any hope of accurately projecting or anticipating the healthcare cost. The actuary can help predict likely patterns of enrollee choices and also conduct retrospective analyses summarizing prior enrollee choice patterns.

Widely differing demographic distributions (that is, age and sex, health status, family size mix) are anticipated in each of these categories. Since demographic characteristics are key determinators of actual utilization and cost characteristics, the projected assumptions will vary by each type of projected population. In addition, the local competitive situation will determine the actual mix of enrollees.

A generic actuarial pricing model can be used to develop actuarial assumptions for any of the above options. This model requires some basic information.

1. *Community normative utilization and cost-per-service characteristics* This information can be expressed in a format similar to that shown in Table 1. Anticipated utilization and charge levels are shown for each type of service being considered. The utilization and cost-per-service assumptions are determined for a specific demographic mix. Each utilization rate reflects a composite of utilization rates for each demographic cohort. Generally, the anticipated labor force demographic mix (that is, employees, spouses, and children) is used. To the extent that the underlying demographic mix changes, each of the actuarial assumptions would also change.

2. *Impact of an ultimately managed delivery system* This can be described in the same format as presented in Table 1, except that it reflects the impact of the healthcare management system and anticipated provider contracting. Utilization rates for inpatient services might be reduced to the extent that the utilization

TABLE 1   Generic Unmanaged System — Actuarial Cost Model, Anytown, U.S.A.

	Per Capita Assumptions		
TYPE OF SERVICE	ANNUAL UTILIZATION PER 1000	AVERAGE COST PER SERVICE	PER CAPITA MONTHLY CLAIM COST
INPATIENT HOSPITAL			
Nonmaternity			
Medical	197 days	$617.85	$10.14
Surgical	224 days	740.17	13.82
Psychiatric	53 days	402.23	1.78
Alcohol and/or drugs	30 days	198.40	0.50
SNF/ECF	8 days	143.49	0.13
Maternity			
Mother	63 days	522.76	2.74
Well newborn	63 days	260.40	1.37
Nondelivery	9 days	613.60	0.46
Subtotal	584 days	$635.14	$30.91
OUTPATIENT HOSPITAL			
Emergency hospital	195 cases	$ 87.64	$ 1.42
Outpatient surgery	45 cases	560.72	2.10
Radiology	90 cases	118.41	0.89
Pathology	114 cases	28.97	0.28
Maternity	7 cases	201.24	0.12
Subtotal	451 cases	$127.98	$4.81
PHYSICIAN			
Inpatient surgery			
Primary surgeon	59 procedures	$868.00	$ 4.27
Assistant	9 procedures	292.95	0.22
Anesthesia	39 procedures	302.91	0.98
Outpatient surgery			
OP facility	83 procedures	248.50	1.72
Office	238 procedures	64.58	1.28
Anesthesia	25 procedures	184.38	0.38
Inpatient visits	349 visits	47.18	1.37
Extended care visits	4 visits	55.80	0.02
Emergency room visits	158 visits	47.27	0.62
Office visits	2,943 visits	28.95	7.10
Home visits	1 visit	53.57	0.00
Critical care	4 procedures	83.70	0.03
Consultation	89 consults	88.17	0.65
Therapeutic injections	103 procedures	14.25	0.12

TABLE 1 Generic Unmanaged System — Actuarial Cost Model, Anytown, U.S.A. *(Continued)*

TYPE OF SERVICE	Per Capita Assumptions		
	ANNUAL UTILIZATION PER 1000	AVERAGE COST PER SERVICE	PER CAPITA MONTHLY CLAIM COST
PHYSICIAN *(Continued)*			
Allergy tests	17 procedures	44.64	0.06
Allergy immunotherapy	199 procedures	11.72	0.19
Physical medicine	235 visits	28.16	0.55
Cardiovascular	94 procedures	86.66	0.68
Diagnostic testing	51 procedures	55.80	0.24
Dialysis	2 procedures	223.20	0.04
Chiropractor	228 visits	25.34	0.48
Radiology	552 procedures	44.69	2.06
Pathology	1,568 procedures	15.04	1.97
Immunizations	229 procedures	12.88	0.25
Well baby	131 exams	33.76	0.37
Vision exams	209 exams	62.85	1.09
Speech exams	4 exams	55.80	0.02
Hearing exams	81 exams	24.13	0.16
Physical exams	161 exams	123.07	1.65
Podiatrist	45 visits	40.83	0.15
Outpatient psychiatric	277 visits	81.04	1.87
Outpatient alcohol and drug	24 visits	65.95	0.13
Maternity			
Deliveries	21 procedures	1186.48	2.08
Nondeliveries	11 procedures	401.76	0.34
Subtotal	8,243 procedures	$ 48.29	$33.17
OTHER			
Prescription drugs	4,333 scripts	$ 17.10	$ 6.28
Home health or PDN	17 visits	96.72	0.14
Ambulance	9 runs	209.25	0.16
Durable medical equipment	20 units	111.60	0.19
Prosthetics	3 units	297.60	0.07
Eyeglasses or contact lenses	125 services	84.19	0.88
Subtotal	4,507 services	$ 20.55	$ 7.72
Total	13,785 services	$ 66.69	76.61

TABLE 2   Generic Managed System — 20 percent Provider Discounts Actuarial Cost Model, Anytown, U.S.A.

	Per Capita Assumptions		
TYPE OF SERVICE	ANNUAL UTILIZATION PER 1000	AVERAGE COST PER SERVICE	PER CAPITA MONTHLY CLAIM COST
INPATIENT HOSPITAL			
Nonmaternity			
Medical	77 days	$543.71	$ 3.49
Surgical	87 days	651.35	4.72
Psychiatric	21 days	353.96	0.62
Alcohol and/or drugs	12 days	174.59	0.17
SNF/ECF	3 days	126.27	0.03
Maternity			
Mother	53 days	434.94	1.92
Well newborn	53 days	216.65	0.96
Nondelivery	7 days	510.68	0.30
Subtotal	260 days	$563.54	$12.21
OUTPATIENT HOSPITAL			
Emergency hospital	127 cases	$ 70.11	$ 0.74
Outpatient surgery	52 cases	448.58	1.94
Radiology	104 cases	94.73	0.82
Pathology	132 cases	23.18	0.25
Maternity	7 cases	160.99	0.09
Subtotal	422 cases	$109.19	$ 3.84
PHYSICIAN			
Inpatient surgery			
Primary surgeon	45 procedures	$861.05	$ 3.23
Assistant	7 procedures	290.61	0.17
Anesthesia	29 procedures	300.49	0.73
Outpatient surgery			
OP facility	99 procedures	244.52	2.02
Office	249 procedures	55.80	1.16
Anesthesia	35 procedures	181.43	0.53
Inpatient visits	268 visits	40.76	0.91
Extended care visits	2 visits	48.21	0.01
Emergency room visits	103 visits	37.82	0.32
Office visits	3,384 visits	23.16	6.53
Home visits	1 visit	42.85	0.00
Critical care	5 procedures	66.96	0.03
Consultation	102 consults	70.54	0.60
Therapeutic injections	119 procedures	11.40	0.06

**TABLE 2   Generic Managed System — 20 percent Provider Discounts
Actuarial Cost Model, Anytown, U.S.A.** *(Continued)*

TYPE OF SERVICE	Per Capita Assumptions		
	ANNUAL UTILIZATION PER 1000	AVERAGE COST PER SERVICE	PER CAPITA MONTHLY CLAIM COST
PHYSICIAN (*Continued*)			
Allergy tests	19 procedures	35.71	0.06
Allergy immunotherapy	229 procedures	9.37	0.18
Physical medicine	271 visits	22.53	0.51
Cardiovascular	108 procedures	69.53	0.62
Diagnostic testing	58 procedures	44.64	0.22
Dialysis	3 procedures	178.56	0.04
Chiropractor	262 visits	20.27	0.44
Radiology	635 procedures	35.75	1.89
Pathology	1,803 procedures	12.03	1.81
Immunizations	263 procedures	10.30	0.23
Well baby	151 exams	27.01	0.34
Vision exams	240 exams	50.28	1.01
Speech exams	5 exams	44.64	0.02
Hearing exams	94 exams	19.31	0.15
Physical exams	185 exams	98.45	1.52
Podiatrist	52 visits	32.66	0.14
Outpatient psychiatric	319 visits	64.83	1.72
Outpatient alcohol and drug	28 visits	52.76	0.12
Maternity			
Deliveries	21 procedures	949.19	1.66
Nondeliveries	11 procedures	321.41	0.29
Subtotal	9,205 procedures	$ 38.22	$29.32
OTHER			
Prescription drugs	4,983 scripts	$13.92	$5.78
Home health or PDN	19 visits	77.38	0.12
Ambulance	10 runs	167.40	0.14
Durable medical equipment	23 units	89.28	0.17
Prosthetics	4 units	238.08	0.08
Eyeglasses or contact lenses	144 services	67.35	0.81
Subtotal	5,183 services	$ 16.44	$ 7.10
Total	15,070 services	$ 41.78	$52.47

review system eliminates unnecessary admissions and shortens the length of stay. Other utilization rates will likely increase as more services are provided in an ambulatory setting. Table 2 presents a hypothetical version of this.

Except for regional cost differentials, this model will ideally be uniform in all areas of the country since it should reflect the absolute best provider practice patterns. This assumes that no one geographic area has a worse average health status than another. To the extent that the model reflects the best that could be done, a provider in Seattle should have the same practice style as a provider in Houston or in Boston. Regional differences do exist now, but many of them can be ascribed to differences in training or comfort levels of the provider rather than to differences in the health status of the region.

3. *Impact of proposed delivery system*   This model presents the impact of the actual or the proposed healthcare management model. If the results of Tables 1 and 2 are considered as extremes along the continuum of healthcare management scenarios, the model will fall somewhere between them, depending on the degree of healthcare management. The results of actual provider charge level negotiation and acceptance of utilization control protocols would be included in this model. The utilization assumptions would also reflect the provider reimbursement system (that is, incentive mechanisms) to be implemented within the program. All factors affecting the rate or cost of consumed healthcare services must be considered.

4. *Distribution of enrollment*   It is very important to accurately anticipate the distribution of enrollment by type of benefit option, including the anticipated demographic mix and health-status mix. With this information it is possible to develop individual actuarial models for each one. The key categories are:

- Those using the managed system for all conditions
- Those using the managed system for most conditions
- Those using the managed system for some conditions
- Those not using the managed system but still signing up for the system (that is, using the swing option only)
- Those not consuming any healthcare services but still willing to sign up for the system
- Those choosing another option and using healthcare services
- Those choosing another option and not using healthcare services at all

The actual distribution of enrollees with respect to these options will vary from one network to the other, especially with changes in the local competitive situation. For example, in a community where managed healthcare plans are able to continue profitable operation with rates much below indemnity rates, the managed care plan will often be the employer's plan of choice. In this environment, enrollee cost sharing will decrease the probability that the unmanaged healthcare product will be chosen and lead to much higher managed care plan penetration. In a community where the managed care prices tend to be much higher than the indemnity prices, a much different scenario will develop.

For example, in a city like Los Angeles, where managed care plans have been quite attractive from a premium point of view, as many as 75 to 85 percent of employees may be willing to sign up for managed care plans, especially when the indemnity option is the most expensive. On the other hand, in an environment where the typical indemnity option is much cheaper than a managed care plan, it would be unreasonable to expect more than 30 to 40 percent to sign up for the managed care option.

5. *Development of cost models*   With the above information, the actuary can then develop composite cost models for each enrollment category. Table 3 presents an illustrative distribution of members by demographic type and their choice of plan. This example is consistent with a multiple-option replacement product in an area where managed care plans are favorably priced compared to indemnity plans and the swing option has a 40 percent benefit difference for out-of-network care.

Two examples that show how this generic approach can be used to develop actuarial cost models follow. The first example develops a stand-alone traditional HMO product design (Tables 4 and 5). The second shows the development of a 40 percent differential opt-out

TABLE 3   Distribution of Demographic and Cost Characteristics (40 percent Benefit Differential)*

	DISTRIBUTION OF CONTRACTS,† %	DISTRIBUTION OF MEMBERS,‡ %	MEMBERS PER CONTRACT§	COST RATIO,¶ %
Managed care only	58	68	2.73	94
No preference	15	15	2.29	107
Traditional providers	20	14	1.65	148
No services	7	3	1.11	0
	100	100	2.33	100

*Enrollees subject to a 40% benefit penalty or differential when using a nonnetwork provider.
†Contractholders or employees.
‡Members include dependent spouse and children.
§Overall average size of contract or family size.
¶Relative cost per member in choice category. Note high cost of indemnity or traditional plan (that is, adverse selection). Based on composite demographics, health status, and contract size for each choice.

TABLE 4   Traditional HMO Cost Model
(Based on Table 2)

TYPE OF SERVICE	Per Capita Assumption			COPAY AMOUNT	VALUE OF COPAY	PER CAPITA MONTHLY BENEFITS COST
	ANNUAL UTILIZATION PER 1000	AVERAGE COST PER SERVICE	PER CAPITA MONTHLY CLAIM COST			
INPATIENT HOSPITAL						
Nonmaternity:						
Medical	77 days	$543.71	$3.49		$0.00	3.49
Surgical	87 days	651.35	4.72		0.00	4.72
Psychiatric	21 days	353.96	0.62		0.00	0.62
Alcohol and/or						
drugs	12 days	174.59	0.17		0.00	0.17
SNF/ECF	3 days	126.27	0.03		0.00	0.03
Maternity:						
Mother	53 days	434.94	1.92		0.00	1.92
Well newborn	53 days	216.65	0.96		0.00	0.96
Nondelivery	7 days	510.68	0.30		0.00	0.30
Subtotal	260 days	$563.54	$12.21		$0.00	$12.21
OUTPATIENT HOSPITAL						
Emergency hospital	127 cases	$ 70.11	$ 0.74	$25.00/case	$0.26	$0.48
Outpatient surgery	52 cases	448.58	1.94		0.00	1.94
Radiology	104 cases	94.73	0.82		0.00	0.82
Pathology	132 cases	23.18	0.25		0.00	0.25
Maternity	7 cases	160.99	0.09		0.00	0.09
Subtotal	422 cases	$109.19	$3.84		$0.26	$3.58
PHYSICIAN						
Inpatient surgery						
Primary surgeon	45 procedures	$861.05	$ 3.23		$0.00	$3.23
Assistant	7 procedures	290.61	0.17		0.00	0.17
Anesthesia	29 procedures	300.49	0.73		0.00	0.73
Outpatient surgery						
OP facility	99 procedures	244.52	2.02		0.00	2.02
Office	249 procedures	55.80	1.16		0.00	1.16
Anesthesia	35 procedures	181.43	0.53		0.00	0.53
Inpatient visits	268 visits	40.76	0.91			
Extended care visits	2 visits	48.21	0.01		0.00	0.01
Emergency room visits	103 visits	37.82	0.32		0.00	0.32
Office visits	3,384 visits	23.16	6.53	$5.00/visit	1.41	5.12
Home visits	1 visit	42.85	0.00	$5.00/visit	0.00	0.00
Critical care	5 procedures	66.96	0.03		0.00	0.03
Consultation	102 consults	70.54	0.60		0.00	0.06

TABLE 4   Traditional HMO Cost Model *(Continued)*
(Based on Table 2)

TYPE OF SERVICE	Per Capita Assumption			COPAY AMOUNT	VALUE OF COPAY	PER CAPITA MONTHLY BENEFITS COST
	ANNUAL UTILIZATION PER 1000	AVERAGE COST PER SERVICE	PER CAPITA MONTHLY CLAIM COST			
PHYSICIAN *(Continued)*						
Therapeutic injections	119 procedures	11.40	0.06		0.00	0.11
Allergy tests	19 procedures	35.71	0.06	$5.00/procedure	0.01	0.05
Allergy immunotherapy	229 procedures	9.37	0.18		0.00	0.18
Physical medicine	271 visits	22.53	0.51		0.00	0.51
Cardiovascular	108 procedures	69.53	0.62		0.00	0.62
Diagnostic testing	58 procedures	44.64	0.22		0.00	0.22
Dialysis	3 procedures	178.56	0.04		0.00	0.04
Chiropractor	262 visits	20.27	0.44	$5.00/visit	0.11	0.33
Radiology	635 procedures	35.75	1.89		0.00	1.89
Pathology	1,803 procedures	12.03	1.81		0.00	1.81
Immunizations	263 procedures	10.30	0.23		0.00	0.23
Well baby	151 exams	27.01	0.34		0.00	0.34
Vision exams	240 exams	50.28	1.01		0.00	1.01
Speech exams	5 exams	44.64	0.02		0.00	0.02
Hearing exams	94 exams	19.31	0.15		0.00	0.15
Physical exams	185 exams	98.45	1.52	$5.00/exam	0.08	1.44
Podiatrist	52 visits	32.66	0.14		0.00	0.14
Outpatient psychiatric	319 visits	64.83	1.72	50%	0.86	0.86
Outpatient alcohol and drug	28 visits	52.76	0.12	50%	0.06	0.06
Maternity						
Deliveries	21 procedures	949.19	1.66		0.00	1.66
Nondeliveries	11 procedures	321.41	0.29		0.00	0.29
Subtotal	9,205 procedures	$ 38.22	$29.32		2.53	$26.79
OTHER						
Prescription drugs	4,983 scripts	$13.92	$ 5.78	$5.00/script	$2.08	$3.70
Home health or PDN	19 visits	77.38	0.12		0.00	0.12
Ambulance	10 runs	167.40	0.14		0.00	0.14
Durable medical equipment	23 units	89.28	0.17		0.00	0.17
Prosthetics	4 units	238.08	0.08		0.00	0.08
Eyeglasses or contact lenses	144 services	67.35	0.81		0.00	0.81
Subtotal	5,183 services	$ 16.44	$ 7.10		$2.08	$5.02
Total	15,070 services	$ 41.78	52.47		$4.87	$47.60

TABLE 5   Standard HMO Development

Healthcare cost	$52.47*
Value of copays	−4.87*
Benefit cost	$47.60*
Claim cost ratio	×0.94†
Adjusted benefit cost	$44.74

*From Table 2.
†From Table 3; reflects anticipated cost or risk level after selection or choices.

product where a limited indemnity package has been added as a rider to an existing HMO product (Table 6). In this plan, members can at the time of service elect to go to any provider outside the system subject to a 40 percent benefit penalty. Table 4 differs from Table 2 only to the extent that copays, deductibles, and benefit restrictions need to be identified. For example, Table 4 shows a $5 office visit copay with a value of $1.41. The $1.41 was calculated as follows:

Number of office visits per 1000 members	3384
Copay revenue per visit	×$5
Annual copay revenue	$16,920
	÷12
Monthly copay revenue	$1,410
	÷1000
Value of copay per member	$1.41

TABLE 6   Opt-Out Product Development

	MANAGED CARE PLAN		OPT-OUT PLAN
Healthcare cost	$52.47[a]		$76.61[b]
Value of copays	−4.87[c]		−30.64[d]
Benefit cost	$47.60		$45.97
Claim ratio	×0.94[e]		×1.48[e]
Adjusted benefit cost	$44.74		$68.04
Assumed distribution	62%		38%
Composite benefit cost		$53.59[f]	
Managed care cost		44.74[g]	
Opt-out cost		$ 8.85[h]	

[a]From Table 2.
[b]From Table 1, since unmanaged system is used.
[c]From Table 4.
[d]Set at 40% of cost to reflect 40% benefit differential or penalty.
[e]From Table 3.
[f](0.62 × $44.74) + (0.38 × $68.04) = $53.59.
[g]From Table 5.
[h]Cost to add opt-out option.

The value of the copay is subtracted from the claims cost to determine a net benefit cost (that is, the far right column). Overall totals are shown at the bottom.

Table 6 shows how an opt-out product could be added to the HMO product developed in Table 5. Not only does the in-network price need to be developed, but the price for the opt-out portion does too. Such an analysis must be done with care since the results can be misleading. As shown in Table 6, the HMO cost is $44.74 and the cost of adding the rider appears to be $8.85. However, out-of-network expenses will much greater than $8.85. The 62 percent to 38 percent distribution means that 38 percent of the claims will be for $68.04, which will be paid to out-of-system providers. This represents over 48 percent of the total healthcare dollars paid out by the plan, not the 16 percent net increase over the composite cost. In-plan provider budgets and reimbursement systems need to be adjusted to reflect the true cost of adding an opt-out product.

In order for a plan to optimize its performance, it is very important that its managed healthcare system be evaluated on a regular basis. This evaluation should include at least an assessment of the provider network (that is, reimbursement strategy, incentives, and provider risk protection), extent of adverse selection, and stability of controlling mechanisms.

Providers, especially those involved in primary care, are an obvious focus for healthcare management since they control the quantity of services provided. A complete analysis would include expected rates of use in addition to actual rates of use. This type of review is quite complex since each variable needs to be quantified with a high degree of accuracy. The evaluation process can be subject to considerable subjectivity unless the evaluators are very careful. Actuaries perform an integral part of this analysis since their skills are very helpful in evaluating the provider network, especially those related to risk analysis.

Reimbursement strategy analysis can be broken down into several components, the most obvious of which is provider reimbursement levels. The plan must assure that provider reimbursement levels are consistent with the underlying actuarial assumptions used to set premium rates. Another way of saying this is that the actuarial analysis should reflect the rates agreed on by the provider negotiating teams; that is, an across-the-board 20 percent discount from community norms should not be used unless a real 20 percent discount was negotiated.

Presumably the initial negotiating objectives were set so that a competitively priced program could be maintained. Unfortunately, these objectives are too often completely ignored until it is too late to develop a plan.

One of the best ways to monitor the effectiveness of provider negotiations is to translate provider reimbursement levels into easy-to-use measures (for example, relative value conversion factors). Starting with a reasonable measure of relative values (that is, California relative value units or McGraw-Hill relative values), it is possible to readily translate provider fee levels into a standard.

Table 7 shows a simple illustration of how this might be done for surgical procedures. The procedures identified in this sample fee schedule are the most common ones used by physicians. A similar analysis should be completed for each type of service (that is, medi-

TABLE 7 Surgical Relative Value Conversion Factors

Procedure Codes			UNIT		FEE ×	UNIT VALUE ×	CONVERSION
RVS-1974	CPT-4	FEE*	VALUE	WEIGHT†	WEIGHT	WEIGHT	FACTOR‡
NONOBSTETRIC SURGERY							
10040	10040	$ 42.00	0.20	65.31	$ 2,743.02	13.06	$210.00
12011	12011	97.00	0.55	3.05	295.85	1.68	176.36
19120	19120	569.00	2.90	1.05	597.45	3.05	196.21
30520	30520	2118.00	7.70	0.66	1,397.88	5.08	275.06
33515	33511	4012.00	32.00	0.11	441.32	3.52	125.38
40200	45378	669.00	4.20	0.16	107.04	0.67	159.29
44950	44950	1070.00	5.80	1.29	1,380.30	7.48	184.48
47600	47600	1482.00	8.20	0.32	474.24	2.62	180.73
54150	54150	133.00	0.40	3.76	500.08	1.50	332.50
55250	55250	389.00	2.10	1.97	766.33	4.14	185.24
57452	57452	107.00	0.55	1.16	124.12	0.64	194.55
58100	58100	101.00	0.45	1.52	153.52	0.68	224.44
58120	58120	547.00	2.70	0.92	503.24	2.48	202.59
58150	58150	2023.00	10.00	2.31	4,673.13	23.10	202.30
58260	58260	1811.00	9.90	1.79	3,241.69	17.72	182.93
58265	58265	2202.00	10.50	0.32	704.64	3.36	209.71
58920	58920	68.00	7.50	0.08	93.44	0.60	155.73
58980	58990	3.80	0.32	0.00	0.00	0.00	
58982	58982	1120.00	4.60	1.58	1,769.60	7.27	243.48
63030	63030	3075.00	13.50	0.29	891.75	3.91	227.78
64721	64721	868.00	5.00	0.37	321.16	1.85	173.60
Subtotal				88.34	$21,179.80	104.43	$202.82
OBSTETRIC SURGERY							
59400	59400	$1857.00	6.10	7.41	$13,760.37	45.20	$304.43
59500	59500	1123.00	7.90	1.65	1,852.95	13.04	142.15
59501	59501	2346.00	9.60	1.76	4,128.96	16.90	244.38
59521	59521	2232.00	9.60	0.24	535.68	2.30	232.50
59862	59840	598.00	3.70	0.60	358.80	2.22	161.62
Subtotal				11.66	$20,636.76	79.66	$259.07

*Actual provider fee per fee survey.
†Based on likely distribution of procedures.
‡(Fee × weight) ÷ (unit value − weight).

cine, anesthesia, radiology, pathology). This type of cursory analysis could be used initially to measure the level of fees in the community, or it can be used to develop assumptions for actuarial pricing. When dealing with different specialties, specialty-specific procedure groupings must be used. Table 8 shows a sample of the more common orthopedic procedures. The analysis would then follow a pattern similar to that shown in Table 7, except that the specialty-specific average conversion factor calculations would be different because new unit values and weights would be required to develop composites.

Observed reimbursement levels are only one measure of the reimbursement strategy. Although physician charge levels constitute a major part of the total reimbursement, they are not enough to characterize completely a plan's reimbursement system. The actual reimbursement method must be analyzed. Some critical questions that should be raised include:

- Which percentile should be used as the maximum fee level (50th, 70th, 90th)?
- Should a discount apply to all providers, or is the percentile cap enough (for example, 90 percent of all charges should not exceed 90 percent of the 85th percentile)?
- Should the plan use provider withholds? If so, at what level? Should they be increased? Should they vary with the individual provider's performance?
- Should the plan use capitation reimbursement in any form? Who should and should not be capitated (primary care only, specialists)?
- Will the reimbursement method optimally affect the quantity of healthcare being provided to patients (fee-for-service motivates more services, capitation fewer)? Is quality of care hampered?
- Are providers receiving adequate income? Are they receiving too much? What is the local competitive situation? Is the reimbursement consistent with other plans that have similar provider risk-sharing methods? Has the contract with the provider affected charge levels (for example, have there been unexpected increases)?

Table 9 shows a sample analysis of provider fee levels which demonstrates how percentile analysis can be quantified in terms of easy-to-understand implications. This analysis needs to be completed both for the community at large and for network providers. The 60th percentile of one will not be the same in the other. They will also have differing values. This type of analysis will help to quantify the negotiated fee schedule in terms of a standard (that is, a distribution of fees). It is common to express this in terms of percentiles. The impact on claims cost is defined by the methodology of Table 9.

TABLE 8   Physician Fee Survey—Orthopedics

CODES	PROCEDURE DESCRIPTION	CHARGES*	PAYER A PAYMENT†	PAYER B PAYMENT‡
22700	Lumbar spine fusion; anterior interbody fusion	————	————	————
23350	Injection procedure for shoulder arthrography	————	————	————
73040	Arthroscopy, shoulder	————	————	————
23600	Treatment of closed humeral fracture without manipulation	————	————	————
23605	Treatment of closed humeral fracture with manipulation	————	————	————
23610	Treatment of open humeral fracture	————	————	————
27130	Arthroscopy (total hip replacement), simple	————	————	————
29870	Arthroscopy knee, diagnostic	————	————	————
29871	Arthroscopy knee, surgical debridement with cartilage shaving and/or drilling and/or resection of reactive synovium	————	————	————
27447	Arthroplasty, knee, plateau, and condyle medial and lateral (total knee replacement)	————	————	————
27487	Secondary reconstruction for total knee arthroplasty	————	————	————
28290	Hallux valgus correction (silver type)	————	————	————
28298	Hallux valgus correction by phalanx osteotomy	————	————	————
29065	Shoulder to hand (long arm) cast application	————	————	————
29075	Elbow to finger (short arm) cast application	————	————	————
29085	Hand to lower forearm (guantlet) cast application	————	————	————
29345	Thighs to toes (long leg) cast application	————	————	————
29355	Thighs to toes (long leg) cast application, walker type	————	————	————
29365	Thigh to ankle (cylinder) cast application	————	————	————

The adequacy of the provider incentives needs to be assessed as much as the level of reimbursement. A slight change in incentives can actually lower the cost of reimbursement, thereby leading to lower plan cost and eventually lower premium rates.

Provider catastrophic risk protection is also an important part of this analysis. Many plans have a series of provider incentives that are based on the the extent of referral services and hospital inpatient care provided during the contract period. In many cases one individual with excessive claims during a single period can have a significant adverse effect on the provider's income. Therefore, it will be very important for a plan to go out of its way to dampen the impact of these catastrophic claims or "shock losses." The use of specific stop-loss protection is one of the best ways to accomplish this, especially under incentive programs. One proven technique combines a deductible with coinsurance up to a very high level (for example, a $5000 deductible for hospital and referral claims, with 90 percent

TABLE 8 Physician Fee Survey—Orthopedics *(Continued)*

CODES	PROCEDURE DESCRIPTION	CHARGES*	PAYER A PAYMENT†	PAYER B PAYMENT‡
29405	Knees to toes (short leg) cast application	_____	_____	_____
29425	Knees to toes (short leg) cast application, walker type	_____	_____	_____
29435	Patellar tendon bearing cast application	_____	_____	_____
29440	Adding walker to previously applied cast	_____	_____	_____
22200	Osteotomy of spine for correction of fixed deformity, lumbar	_____	_____	_____
22201	Osteotomy of spine for correction of fixed deformity, thoracic or cervical	_____	_____	_____
22206	Osteotomy of spine for correction of scoliosis	_____	_____	_____
22370	Open treatment and fusion, posterolateral and anterolateral approach with ileal or other autogenous bone grafts for fracture; lumber	_____	_____	_____
22379	Harrington rod technique	_____	_____	_____
22560	Arthrodesis with diskectomy, lumbar or thoracic, posterior posterolateral or posterior interbody approach	_____	_____	_____
97014	Physical medicine; electrical stimulation	_____	_____	_____
73560	Radiologic examination knee, anteroposterior and lateral views	_____	_____	_____
28675	Treatment open interphalangeal joint dislocation with uncomplicated soft tissue closure	_____	_____	_____

*Charges to Payer A, self-pay, and commercially insured patient (exclude Medicare or Medicaid).
†Payment made to physician for the service rendered (may be lower than billed charge).
‡Payment made by Payer B, which is net of any withhold in effect.

protection up to a total claim of $25,000 and 100 percent protection in excess of $25,000). Claim probability distributions can be used to evaluate this type of risk sharing. Table 10 summarizes a sample claim probability distribution and shows how it could be used to calculate a claim cost for a high deductible. Using the values in Table 10, the value of the protection described above is $4.47 or 32 percent of the total cost of $14.05 [that is, $(0.90 \times 4.78) + (0.10 \times 1.65) = 4.47$].

Adverse selection is a popular topic among plans with financial struggles, but one issue that is rarely discussed is the extent of adverse selection by provider. To the extent that providers are also experiencing adverse selection, this may actually become the most severe issue for a plan. The plan needs to consider ways to analyze adverse selection to determine what biases, if any, exist among providers.

One of the best ways to analyze the extent of adverse selection is to first review total member experience by primary care provider. For

TABLE 9   Impact of Maximum Fee Levels

(1) CHARGE PERCENTILE	(2) AVERAGE PERCENTILE CHARGE RELATIVE TO MEAN	(3) MIDPOINT OF RANGE RELATIVE TO MEAN	(4) DISTRIBUTION IN RANGE	(5) (3) × (4)	(6) SUM OF (5) FOR PERCENTILES LESS THAN OR EQUAL TO (1)	(7) ADJUSTMENT FACTOR REFLECTING CUT OFF AT PERCENTILE IN (1)
No limit	1.50	1.45	0.05	0.073	1.000	1.000
95th	1.40	1.35	0.05	0.068	0.927	0.997
90th	1.30	1.28	0.05	0.064	0.859	0.989
85th	1.25	1.23	0.05	0.062	0.795	0.983
80th	1.20	1.18	0.05	0.059	0.733	0.973
75th	1.15	1.14	0.05	0.057	0.674	0.962
70th	1.12	1.11	0.05	0.056	0.617	0.953*
65th	1.09	1.08	0.05	0.054	0.561	0.943
60th	1.06	1.05	0.05	0.053	0.507	0.931
55th	1.03	1.02	0.05	0.051	0.454	0.918
50th†	1.00	0.99	0.05	0.050	0.403	0.903
45th	0.97	0.94	0.05	0.047	0.353	0.887
40th and less	0.90	0.77	0.40	0.306	0.306	0.846
			1.00	1.000		

*Calculated as follows: $0.953 = 0.617 + (0.30)(1.12)$.
†For this example the 50th percentile is 1.00. This is not a necessary condition for the distribution.

example, for all members assigned to each primary care provider, accumulate all claims regardless of the ultimate provider. The relative cost of care on a per person per month basis can then be determined. To the extent that one or more providers are attracting patients with severe conditions, adverse selection is occurring. This comparison needs to be made after appropriate adjustments are made to normalize risk factors. For example, an adjustment to reflect actual age and sex mix is mandatory. Comparisons across similar specialties are valuable. This type of analysis must be adjusted by all key risk variables to minimize measurable differences. The results must be adjusted by demographic, benefit plan, and health status (where available) variables to normalize results by experience pool.

The provider reimbursement system is a form of a feedback loop control theory application. Control theory is used in other industries as a mechanism for controlling the outcome of a system based on monitoring of outcomes. As applied in the healthcare industry, this mechanism can be used to monitor provider practice patterns and motivate providers to practice a more cost-effective, yet high quality

TABLE 10 Calculation of Claims Cost at High Deductibles

(1) ANNUAL FREQUENCY	(2) TOTAL ANNUAL CLAIM	(3) ANNUAL COST OF CLAIM	(4) PROBABILITY THAT CLAIMS ARE GREATER THAN OR EQUAL TO (2)	(5) ANNUAL COST OF CLAIMS GREATER THAN OR EQUAL TO (2)	(6) CALENDAR-YEAR DEDUCTIBLE	(7) ANNUAL CLAIM COST	(8) MONTHLY CLAIM COST
0.95061783	0.00	0.00	1.00000000	168.59	0	168.59	14.05
0.01870937	1,107.39	20.72	0.04938217	168.59	5,000	57.38*	4.78
0.00235034	1,283.44	3.02	0.03067280	147.87	25,000	19.76	1.65
0.00299492	1,435.72	4.30	0.02832246	144.85	100,000	4.54†	0.38
0.00543235	1,595.24	8.67	0.02532754	140.55			
0.00279484	2,106.56	5.89	0.01989519	131.88			
0.00558969	2,972.85	16.62	0.01710035	125.99			
0.00326331	3,920.49	12.79	0.01151066	109.37			
0.00228138	4,250.87	9.70	0.00824735	96.58			
0.00114069	4,709.02	5.37	0.00596597	86.88			
0.00044228	5,773.41	2.55	0.00482528	81.51			
0.00090433	7,051.68	6.38	0.00438300	78.96			
0.00087358	8,662.91	7.57	0.00347867	72.58			
0.00066892	10,660.73	7.13	0.00260509	65.01			
0.00026112	13,072.32	3.41	0.00193617	57.88			
0.00060122	15,404.14	9.26	0.00167505	54.47			
0.00019068	19,496.77	3.72	0.00107383	45.21			
0.00024655	23,611.47	5.82	0.00088315	41.49			
0.00016856	28,570.78	4.82	0.00063660	35.67			
0.00014075	35,061.45	4.93	0.00046804	30.85			
0.00009723	42,998.62	4.18	0.00032729	25.92			
0.00007959	52,693.60	4.19	0.00023006	21.74			
0.00003993	65,941.44	2.63	0.00015047	17.55			
0.00003661	81,787.75	2.99	0.00011054	14.92			
0.00003147	100,432.39	3.16	0.00007393	11.93			
0.00002545	116,116.56	2.96	0.00004246	8.77			
0.00000363	155,865.87	0.57	0.00001701	5.81			
0.00001030	343,681.07	3.54	0.00001338	5.24			
0.00000308	553,317.75	1.70	0.00000308	1.70			

*Calculated as follows: 57.38 = 81.51 (Col.5) − 5000 (Col. 6) × 0.00482528 (Col. 4).
†Calculated as follows: 4.54 = 11.93 (Col. 5) − 100,000 (Col. 6) × 0.00007393 (Col. 4).

form of healthcare. Actuarial analysis can apply known feedback mathematical concepts to the healthcare environment. This is a state-of-the-art application that actuarial science is currently developing.

The packaging of the managed healthcare plan product (that is, PPO versus HMO versus point-of-service product) affects the actuarial method because different products require different assumptions. The generic actuarial approach suggested earlier does not change with new packaging approaches. Rather, certain parameters and assumptions are set to values that do not have an impact on rates or costs for certain product packages. For example, the required premium rates for a stand-alone managed care product (that is, HMO) need to be based on assumptions about individual employees. They rarely would include an assumption as to the number of individuals that would choose the plan if they had the freedom to go out of the network at will. The stand-alone HMO product does not permit people to opt out of the network, so it does not directly apply. On the other hand, an open-access managed care product is heavily dependent on these assumptions and would need to be based on realistic assumptions about employee choices. For these two extremes, the general methodology is the same, but there are far-reaching differences in actual calculations.

The actuarial analysis is affected by whether the product is marketed as an optional product or as a replacement product. Radically different demographic mixes are obtained under these differing approaches, and the actuarial assumptions must reflect the anticipated results. As shown in Table 3, the relative cost levels under the conditions of this example show more than 50 percent differences between the managed care and traditional categories.

The extent of provider, plan, and plan-sponsor risk-sharing also affects the actuarial assumptions. For example, the plan's appropriate or reasonable or equitable profit margin depends on the level of risk assumed by the plan. When very large withholds are negotiated with providers, much of the risk has been transferred to the providers. An equitable profit objective for the plan would be much less than in a situation where the withholds do not exist or are very small. In community-rated plans, the higher level of plan risk often require a greater margin than a plan that pursues only an experience-rated route. Often community-rated plans enroll many smaller groups with higher risk levels. Larger groups are usually experience-rated since their costs are more stable and predictive. The experience-rated route transfers considerable risk to the employer, thus reducing the plan's risk.

There are several ways of evaluating these risk-sharing mechanisms, but one of the most useful is based on actuarial risk principles. Table 11 summarizes an illustrative distribution of claims which will

TABLE 11   Illustrative Distribution of Claims

PERCENT OF MEAN	DISTRIBUTION	AVERAGE OF RANGE	ACTUARIAL VALUE	DISTRIBUTION ≥ VALUE	ACTUARIAL VALUE ≥ VALUE
>50%	0.04	40%	0.0160	1.00	1.0000
50–59	0.07	55	0.0385	0.96	0.9840
60–69	0.08	65	0.0520	0.89	0.9455
70–79	0.09	75	0.0675	0.81	0.8935
80–89	0.10	85	0.0850	0.72	0.8260
90–99	0.12	95	0.1140	0.62	0.7410
100–109	0.12	105	0.1260	0.50	0.6270
110–119	0.10	115	0.1150	0.38	0.5010
120–129	0.09	125	0.1125	0.28	0.3860
130–139	0.08	135	0.1080	0.19	0.2735
140–149	0.07	145	0.1015	0.11	0.1655
150+	0.04	160	0.0640	0.04	0.0640
	1.00		1.0000		

be used to demonstrate an evaluation of risk sharing. A symmetrical distribution has been presented for ease of presentation. Actual distributions will likely be asymmetrical. The first three columns characterize the distribution. The remaining columns have been generated to speed up calculations. They are computational aids. The "Actuarial Value" column is the product of the "Distribution" column and the "Average of Range" column. The "Distribution≥Value" column is the back-sum of the "Distribution" column. (If Distribution at Value $t = D_t$, then the back-sum of Distribution at Value $t = \Sigma_\infty^t D_t$.) The "Actuarial Value≥Value" column is the back-sum of the "Actuarial Value" column.

Figure 1 presents a graphical illustration of the aggregate claim distribution shown in Table 11. Two vertical lines have been added to help explain the risk characteristics. Line A identifies the mean or average level of claims (that is, claims=1.00). In this symmetrical illustration, this line also identifies the mode and median. Line B is to the right of line A and corresponds to a level of claims equivalent to the mean plus a 15 percent margin.

As various risk-transfer mechanisms are considered, Table 11 and Figure 1 will become very helpful for understanding their impact on pricing and margins. In Figure 1, there is a 50:50 chance that actual results will be greater or less than line A. As margins are added (that is, line B) there is a greater chance that the actual results will not exceed line B (that is, the sum of the mean and an explicit margin). For example, according to Table 11, there is less than a 38 percent

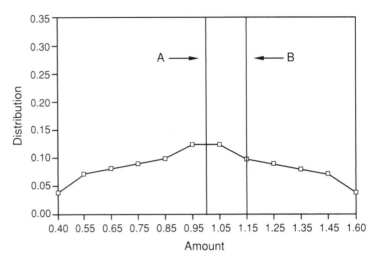

Figure 1

chance that actual claims will exceed B (that is, 115 percent of A). The greater the margin, the greater the chance that assumptions will be adequate, assuming they are based on line B (that is, the value with a margin).

In the very simple case, a plan that sets its underlying claim cost assumptions at a level corresponding to line A should expect no margin at all (that is, break-even) over the long term. Assuming that the projected claims distribution is realistic, the good years will offset the bad years and the actual cost, over the long term, will approach the mean of the distribution, or line A. Only if margins are added to the underlying claims cost assumptions will the plan ever have a chance to make a profit over the long term. The specific inclusion of margins in either the claims cost assumptions or the expense load are the most common ways to include margins to build up profits.

Provider withholds also help change the financial impact of the underlying claims distribution. In those years when actual claims are less than or equal to the assumed level of claims, the entire withhold is returned to the provider. In these years (that is, left of line A) the distribution of claims remains unchanged. In those years when actual claims exceed the assumed level of claims, the withhold is used to help reduce the amount of claims paid by the plan. For example, in the case a 20 percent withhold of claims, the actual payout to providers will be 80 percent of claims. This clearly changes the payout pattern and the financial impact on the plan and the providers.

Table 12 uses a model that assumes a 20 percent withhold on all claims. Table 12 shows that approximately 50 percent of the with-

TABLE 12 Development of Forfeited Withholds, Adjusted Amounts, and Adjusted Gain (Loss)

DISTRIBUTION	AMOUNT	20% WITHHOLD	Allocated Withhold RETURNED	Allocated Withhold FORFEITED	ADJUSTED AMOUNT	Gain (Loss) INITIAL	Gain (Loss) ADJUSTED
0.04	0.40	0.08	0.08	0.00	0.40	0.60	0.60
0.07	0.55	0.11	0.11	0.00	0.55	0.45	0.45
0.08	0.65	0.13	0.13	0.00	0.65	0.35	0.35
0.09	0.75	0.15	0.15	0.00	0.75	0.25	0.25
0.10	0.85	0.17	0.17	0.00	0.85	0.15	0.15
0.12	0.95	0.19	0.19	0.00	0.95	0.05	0.05
0.12	1.05	0.21	0.16	0.05	1.00	(0.05)	0.00
0.10	1.15	0.23	0.08	0.15	1.00	(0.15)	0.00
0.09	1.25	0.25	0.00	0.25	1.00	(0.25)	0.00
0.08	1.35	0.27	0.00	0.27	1.08	(0.35)	(0.08)
0.07	1.45	0.29	0.00	0.29	1.16	(0.45)	(0.16)
0.04	1.60	0.32	0.00	0.32	1.28	(0.60)	(0.28)
1.00	1.00	0.200	0.102	0.098	0.902	0.000	0.098

hold in this example is forfeited, reducing claims outgo, and creating a gain to the plan. This is a change in risk.

Figure 2 characterizes the change in risk. Line A still is equal to the initial mean of the distribution. According to Table 12 (that is, the "Adjusted Amount" column), the new mean net of withholds is actually reduced. Line C is set at a point equal to 1÷(1 − withhold %) (that is, for a 20 percent withhold this would be 125 percent of the mean).

Figure 2

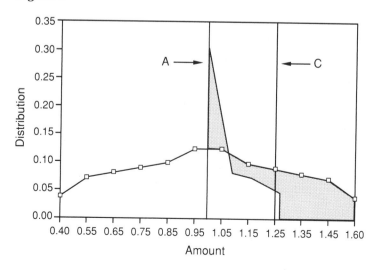

To the left of line A (that is, claims ≤ 1.00) the results are just like the original situation. For claims initially falling between line A and line C, the plan is subject to no risk, since the withholds are used to absorb the excess claims. (Note the spike at 1.00.) Note the shaded area where the initial distribution is changed. Under this scenario, providers are reimbursed subject to their withholds. The plan is subject to losses but at the net-of-withhold level. Figure 2 shows that the maximum loss is reduced and the overall risk (that is, the chance that claims will be greater than the calculated mean) is also reduced under a withhold scenario.

Table 12 shows the allocation of withholds between values returned and values forfeited. The withhold has significantly dampened the plan's risk. This suggests a potential reduction in desired margins from those commonly found in a no-withhold environment. Established actuarial risk theory calculations can be completed to determine what portion of the risk has been transferred to the physicians, thus quantifying the amount of reduced margin. This is described in the next few paragraphs.

Table 12 can be used to evaluate the financial impact of withholds on the claims distribution. Assuming a 20 percent withhold, the actuarial value of costs in all years with claims in excess of 125 percent of the mean is reduced to 80 percent of the initial value (see "Adjusted Amount" column). Between 100 and 125 percent, withholds are returned to the extent that the claims do not exceed 100 percent, and below 100 percent the entire withhold is returned so the initial claim value is a correct representation of the claims amount.

This can be used to determine what portion of the gains in the good years (that is, events to the left of line A) should be shared with the providers as a form of a reward for positive performance. This type of risk balancing helps to assure long-term provider relations. Table 12 showed that the introduction of a 25 percent withhold on all claims creates almost a 10 percent gain to the plan (that is, 9.8 percent). This occurs by transferring risk to providers. From the provider's perspective, he or she accepted a 10 percent loss (that is, discount).

A good solution to this inequity is to offer a percentage of gains to the providers to offset the risk transfer. Table 13 splits out the gains and losses to help calculate this risk. For example, establishing a provider incentive of 77.32 percent of gains balances the risk sharing (that is, 77.32 percent of 0.127 equals 0.098). At this point the plan's risk is balanced with that of the providers'. This type of illustration can be used to encourage providers to accept bigger withhold levels. The larger the withhold, the larger the share in gains. Fortunately, it also reduces plan risk.

Similar analyses can be completed to determine the magnitude of

TABLE 13   Actuarial Value of Gains and Losses

	Gain			Loss	
DISTRIBUTION	INITIAL	ADJUSTED	ADJUSTED WITH INCENTIVE*	INITIAL	ADJUSTED
0.04	0.60	0.60	0.14	0.00	0.00
0.07	0.45	0.45	0.10	0.00	0.00
0.08	0.35	0.35	0.08	0.00	0.00
0.09	0.25	0.25	0.06	0.00	0.00
0.10	0.15	0.15	0.03	0.00	0.00
0.12	0.05	0.05	0.01	0.00	0.00
0.12	0.00	0.00	0.00	(0.05)	0.00
0.10	0.00	0.00	0.00	(0.15)	0.00
0.09	0.00	0.00	0.00	(0.25)	0.00
0.08	0.00	0.00	0.00	(0.35)	(0.08)
0.07	0.00	0.00	0.00	(0.45)	(0.16)
0.04	0.00	0.00	0.00	(0.60)	(0.28)
1.00	0.127	0.127	0.029	(0.127)	(0.029)

Actuarial value of net gain (loss):
- Initial: $0.127 - 0.127 = 0.000$
- Adjusted: $0.127 - 0.029 = 0.098$
- Adjusted with incentive: $0.029 - 0.029 = 0.000$

*Incentive set at 77.32% of gain.

risk transfer in the case of experience rating, plan reinsurance, adverse selection, and various packaging schemes, including risk sharing between joint venture partners in a multiple-option product.

The actuary must also consider benefit levels when pricing the plan. This includes more than a mere evaluation of the copays. There is a much more important element which anticipates underlying levels of utilization based on the ultimate plan design. For example, a no-copay office visit program will have much higher office visit utilization than a $5 office visit copay plan. In the case of the $0-copay program, the plan tends to attract more higher-than-normal users in a multiple-plan environment. Potential members evaluate what is in their best interest. As the member balances the financial impacts of the more favorable copay, there is a tendency for those needing more services to choose the plan with the richest benefit. In addition to these potential selection patterns, the lack of a financial barrier tends to increase the utilization levels.

Recent Rand studies demonstrate a strong correlation between copay levels and rate of use of benefits. The plan will attract higher-than-normal users in a multiple-plan-selection environment. Once patients have selected a plan, they tend to use the plan more because of the lack of a financial barrier. This not only affects the number of office visits and related lab and x-ray procedures but has an even greater impact on prescription drug claims.

There often is also a "domino"-type effect between the prescription drug and office visit plan design. The higher the prescription drug copay, the lower the office visit utilization, and vice versa. In fact, there is demonstrated actuarial evidence to show that a plan with no prescription drug benefit can achieve perhaps the most favorable utilization, assuming the market will accept this product. This has been used quite successfully with TEFRA Medicare Risk Contracts as a method of passive underwriting. Plans that have developed Medicare Risk Contract programs without a prescription drug benefit tend not to attract the patients requiring extensive prescriptions. Since the TEFRA contracts prohibit the selection of healthier risks, this approach helps dissuade prospective members from joining the plan if they need extensive prescriptions.

Careful plan design is an important ingredient in the actuarial process for avoiding especially unstable product designs. One of the actuary's roles is to advise management on the soundness of the plan design. This input should be balanced with that from marketing and other departments not clearly versed in the financial implications of certain plan design decisions.

Market analysis is an important aspect of a plan's operations, but too often it is neglected. The actuary's input can be very helpful in this phase to assure reliable comparisons of competing plan rates and benefits. First of all, the comparison should try to neutralize any obvious differences. No matter how consistent the benefit plan appears, there are often differences in benefits that have meaningful financial differences. For example, identical substance abuse benefits might be offered with the exception of a lifetime limit in one plan and no lifetime limit in the other. A significant financial difference could result, especially if the plan has been experiencing a recidivism problem.

The actuary can help evaluate these differences between competing plans in order to develop more meaningful comparisons. One approach that has proved very helpful is to translate the benefits of the competing plans to the plan's internal plan structure. In other words, summarize all plans in terms of a single plan, preferably the one that the plan is most familiar with. Use the titles from local plan benefits to describe the competition. This will likely present the local plan in the most favorable manner possible without appearing biased. Another meaningful alternative is to derive the value of all copays, deductibles, and benefit limitations and add them back to the plan cost to determine a total cost of healthcare for comparison purposes. The cost of one system can then be accurately compared to another since coverages are common (that is, "apples versus apples").

This last approach shows how efficient each plan's delivery system is if rates reflect actual costs. This approach can readily become part of a marketing department's sales pitch to help explain the effectiveness of their plan, assuming this is something they want to communicate to the public. An example of how this might be done is shown in Table 14, which is based on the following assumptions.

1. Indemnity rates are set at a 90 percent loss ratio
2. Managed care rates are set at an 80 percent loss ratio
3. Indemnity benefits: $100 deductible, 80-20 percent coinsurance, no well care benefits, 50 percent psychiatric and substance abuse, no durable medical equipment, no lenses or contacts
4. Managed care plan: Table 4 benefits
5. Same time period
6. Indemnity providers: 5 percent discount from PPO contracting results
7. Managed care providers: 20 percent discount from PPO contracting results
8. Employer contribution: 80 percent of indemnity option.

TABLE 14 Actuarial Analysis of Plan Cost

	INDEMNITY PLAN	MANAGED CARE PLAN
EMPLOYER ANALYSIS		
Rate	$55.15	$59.50
Value of deductible	6.25	0.00
Value of copays	0.00	4.87
Value of coinsurance	10.53	0.00
Value of excluded benefits	6.70	0.00
Adjusted rate	78.63	64.37
Employer contribution	$44.12	$44.12
EMPLOYEE ANALYSIS		
Payroll deduction	$11.03	$15.38
Value of deductible	6.25	0.00
Value of copays	0.00	4.87
Value of coinsurance	10.53	0.00
Value of excluded benefits	6.70	0.00
Adjusted employee cost	$34.51	$20.25

The adjusted rate shows which plan is the best deal for the employer. Table 14 shows that the managed care plan is the best even with a higher rate. The adjusted employee cost shows which plan has the most value to the employee. Both of these comparisons are based on actuarial averages.

THE PROVIDER PERSPECTIVE

For several years, providers tended to be the unsophisticated partner in managed healthcare plans. This is quickly changing, as more and more providers have been part of a program that has not met their objectives. The financial pressures on the provider community have been greater than anyone would have anticipated. Some of this pressure is necessary, but the overreaction of providers to the actions of managed care plans now is becoming a detriment to those plans. It is harder and harder to negotiate the much needed concessions from the provider community.

To complicate matters, the provider community has developed a sophisticated lobbyist activity that is further restricting the actions of managed care plans. Today, plans must be very careful to communicate the appropriate information or they might find themselves in a lengthy and very expensive litigation. The providers are interested in four critical factors: discount, risk transfer, utilization controls, and provider incentives.

Early negotiation efforts focused on provider discounts (that is, a percent off billed charges). Various fee schedules and reimbursement methods were developed that made the extent of the discount less obvious, but the discounts were significant. For example, a plan might negotiate a primary care capitation arrangement with providers that is based on overall results of many providers, and perhaps bearing almost no relationship to the provider's fee structure. Some providers understood the results, but far too many others blindly accepted proposals leading to serious financial difficulties in their practices. The "volume" argument (that is, the managed care plan will increase their patient volume) was widely espoused and accepted, but satisfactory results were rarely delivered.

Far too many physician groups blindly accepted IPA capitation programs. For example, any IPA might accept capitation payments from a managed care plan, yet pay each member of the IPA on a fee-for-service basis. The plan's total payment to the IPA might be capped, yet the IPA's payments to each provider is based on the number of actual patient visits. In many cases this leads to 100 percent discounts as the IPA runs out of funds—often the result of inadequate provider utilization controls (that is, a lack of healthcare management).

Too much risk has been transferred to providers without adequate explanation or analysis by either party. To the extent that the capitation payments are inappropriate, they should be adjusted to reflect more realistic utilization levels. To the extent that providers do not manage care efficiently, the plan should effectively transfer the risk to the providers. The managed care plan has almost as many problems with this aspect of managing risk as the IPA since it is likely that the plan will lose its network unless something is changed to more appropriately compensate the providers.

As providers assess proposed managed care contracts, they must consider how they will achieve the required utilization levels. It is not appropriate to portray a panacea situation where providers will be assured of significant financial success just by participating in the program. Healthcare management is an active process, not a passive one. It requires real effort on the part of plans and providers. Before a provider accepts a contract from a managed healthcare plan, he or she should make certain that the plan is a "managed care plan." Discounts and incentives will not be enough. Signing up only the good providers will not work either. The providers and the plan have to create a joint effort to control the consumption of healthcare services. Each individual provider is concerned about his or her own fiscal viability. Poorly negotiated contracts can eventually create a serious financial problem for the provider. Only the provider can effectively control the consumption of healthcare services, although others will try to restrict the scope of treatment. Most medical schools fail to teach providers how to deliver healthcare in a cost-effective manner. Much time is spent on procedural and diagnostic techniques, but there is very little emphasis on how those techniques affect the cost of healthcare.

A fairly simple concept, but a difficult exercise to complete, is the evaluation of potential income streams under the proposed provider contract. Providers should make this type of actuarial evaluation. Several questions that they should ask include:

- What is the effective discount on my billed charges?
- Is the amount of risk I am assuming under this contract reasonable (that is, does my compensation reflect this)?
- Will the incentive payments offset any portion of the negotiated discount?
- Will this plan succeed? Do I need them or do they need me?
- Is the contract clearly laid out so there will not be any misunderstandings or problems in the future?

As the provider reviews the contract, he or she should identify whether a bias exists and in what direction. For example, a provider might propose healthcare budgets that will be used to determine provider incentive payments. The budgets might be skewed to favor the providers or a subset of providers, or perhaps to favor the plan.

Their proposal will likely be different than that of the managed care plan but should be used as input to establish a fair compromise. For example, the providers might want to establish a target utilization level for incentive payments that exceeds that proposed by the managed care plan. The higher the target, the easier it is to qualify for incentive payments, and the higher the cost of the program. These biases are difficult to deal with. Such an assessment should be completed very early in the process. Many plans try to build in a favorable bias to protect themselves, while others do not. It is important for providers to understand the ground rules before getting involved.

One fairly common bias that providers need to be cognizant of relates to the portion of health cost savings they are entitled to in favorable years. This bias is the easiest one to assess. For example, providers that accept withholds but do not share in the savings are clearly biased against. Savings might be defined as the difference between anticipated healthcare costs (that is, say, for referral and hospital utilization) and those actually incurred. Those willing to accept a withhold are assuming a major portion of risk, even though they control much of the consumption of services. This risk assumption can be materially offset by creating a bonus for providers based on a portion of savings. Once a savings pool is determined, the providers might be paid on a pro rata basis. The sharing of savings is one way of equalizing the risk sharing. It is difficult to implement one without the other.

The bottom-line success of a managed care plan will be heavily dependent on controlling provider behavior. Even in a plan plagued with adverse selection, the plan can continue reasonably successful operations if providers are working toward a common goal. It is unlikely that the plan can continue to attract severely adverse populations forever. The more managed its operations, the more likely it will become a financial success.

As a result, it is mandatory to integrate the financial controls with the providers' practice patterns. Individual providers need to be held accountable for appropriate provider behavior. Provider practice patterns vary widely, even within similar communities.

The primary care model presents one of the most effective ways for evaluating a provider's practice style. In a primary care network model, each member is assigned to a primary care physician. Each member also has a premium rate or anticipated healthcare budget that is based on various risk characteristics (that is, age, sex, and health status). This direct tie between the budget for the individual patient and the individual primary care physician is critical in managing patient care. Without the direct tie, a managed care plan is restricted to profiling approaches which are not very effective. The direct tie provides a succinct methodology where actual claims can be compared to anticipated budgets so that relative provider performance can be measured. Assuming the budgets are reasonable, this provides a straightforward method for establishing provider incentive payments or bonuses.

Under some capitation programs, there may be a tendency on the part of providers to underserve the assigned population in order to maximize their bonus payments. Thus, the utilization control system should have checks and balances that limit access to care while assuring that patients are getting quality care.

From the provider's perspective it is very important that the system be financially balanced; that is, the provider must be sure that the system will, over the long run, provide a reasonable incentive to manage healthcare. Actuarial analysis can validate the plan's claims that the system is balanced. The following example demonstrates how an incentive system might be evaluated.

The providers must assure themselves that the proposed managed care system will enable them to practice appropriate healthcare. The managed care plan's utilization review (UR) system may present some difficulties to certain providers. Assuming the system is appropriately controlling the levels of healthcare, some providers may choose not to participate because the system is too rigid. UR systems are hard to transfer from one area of the country to the next. Systems that are readily transferred without local physician interaction are perhaps not as stringent as they should be. The UR system should be designed to minimize unnecessary care. The more providers that are affected, the more effective the system will be. Once presented with facts, most providers are willing to admit that their practice standards could be improved. Much inappropriate care is a result of the provider's lack of definite practice standards.

THE PLAN-SPONSOR PERSPECTIVE

Employers purchase the vast majority of all healthcare coverage. In recent years, employers have become increasingly concerned about the ability of the insurance community to control the cost of healthcare, and the managed care community has not been spared from these concerns. As the employer considers healthcare issues, the risk issues related to various plans should also be assessed.

Risk transfer is perhaps the most important factor for the employer to evaluate. There are several risks that the employer faces when providing a healthcare reimbursement program. The employer should first identify the risks faced and then evaluate how undesirable risks can be transferred to the healthcare company or managed care plan. Some of the key risks include:

- Affordable and stable costs
- Charges reflecting real costs

- Minimal administrative expenses
- Lowest possible healthcare costs for desired healthcare program
- Catastrophic risk

To the extent that an employer wants to transfer risk to a carrier, most carriers are willing to assume the risk for a price. Especially during inflationary times, employers want to keep the cost of programs affordable and stable, avoiding an unpredictably large rate increase. Rate guarantees might be available to protect the employer. The more that rates reflect an employer's actual experience, the greater the chance that rates will deviate from one period to the next. When rates reflect the aggregate experience of several employers, overall experience and rates tend to be more stable, assuming that the underlying grouping of employers is somewhat stable. As the employer moves from "pool rates" to "experience rates," the employer's risk from potential claims fluctuation increases, but the chance that premium rates will exceed claim levels decreases.

The employer can transfer the financial risk for catastrophic claims through pooling charges and/or stop-loss reinsurance, both of which help the employer stabilize healthcare costs. Each requires some type of actuarial analysis for appropriate evaluation.

The employer needs to understand the renewal underwriting process. This might begin with a better understanding of how the industry generally completes this type of analysis. Actuarial analysis includes experience analysis, which is an integral part of the underwriting process. The actuary can help the employer understand. One of the key components that must be validated is the estimation of outstanding claim liabilities or incurred-but-not-reported claim liabilities (IBNR). Other assumptions required to project future claim levels include trend, demographic mix, benefit changes, and credibility formulas, which can all be enhanced by actuarial input or analysis.

As more and more of the employer risk is retained internally (that is, self-funding), the need for stabilization or risk reserves increases. When the risk is totally transferred to a managed care plan or carrier, the experience of a large number of employer groups is combined to minimize the carrier's risk. A single group's contribution to the reserve margins is inadequate for the single group when considered by itself. As a result, the individual group must seriously consider the buildup of stabilization reserves when they are building their own reserves in a self-funded environment. To appropriately establish these levels, actuarial analysis is required. As part of a feasibility study or other analysis to help the employer understand the risks of their benefit plan, the actuary's analysis is very important.

The employer must be sure that the benefit plan is meeting both the employer's objectives and the needs or objectives of the employees. Each employee group is unique, but there are many common factors that can be predicted based on the demographic and socioeconomic characteristics of the population. This should be expanded using survey methods and focus groups. Many times actuarial analysis of this data can provide valuable information.

BALANCING OF PERSPECTIVES

Since each perspective is so important and cannot be ignored, it is important to maintain a reasonable balance between each one. Actuarial analysis is required to understand all the perspectives; however, it is probably almost impossible to maintain a reasonable balance. A recently developed concept, the "healthcare umbrella," appears to be a valuable tool in this balancing act. The concept is very simple. From a plan point of view, all of the plans are financially integrated to appear almost as one to the employer. Each plan continues to act independently unless there are key financial links between each plan. The actual premium for each plan is highly dependent on actual experience. Sophisticated risk-sharing mechanisms are established to assure that plans are treated equitably, thus minimizing the chance of windfalls from shadow pricing. Within each plan, providers have a greater chance of being treated more equitably since the plan is getting reasonable income. From the employer perspective, all healthcare costs are effectively bundled under one organization, which helps them better coordinate the total program. As a result, the employee ends up with a reasonably priced program where out-of-pocket costs make more sense and the likelihood of continued programs is very high.

This partnership approach appropriately integrates all of the plans so their performance can be evaluated. The risk-sharing mechanisms help minimize the severe impact of adverse selection and protect the plans that have, for one reason or another, been selected against. Instead of excess funds becoming windfalls to one plan or another, they are used to help subsidize the underpriced options.

Actuarial analysis is required to establish appropriate allocations of revenues and costs. This process works quite effectively in multiple-option programs and is perhaps the only way that such programs can continue. The current free-for-all approach will self-destruct if not put in check. The umbrella concept helps to accomplish this.

CONCLUSIONS

Managed care perhaps creates the best opportunity for corporate America and other sponsors of benefits to provide healthcare benefits. The long-term viability of these benefit schemes is doubtful unless adequate analysis precedes their implementation. Actuarial analysis is critical to protect every interest involved in the system.

Many of the failures to date can be attributed to an inadequate understanding of the business. Actuarial analysis helps to enhance this understanding and provide input for current operations and strategic planning for the future. When one perspective is ignored or inadvertently damaged, the system tends to fall apart. The partnership concept inherently needed by the system must be developed to assure the long-term viability of managed care. The "healthcare umbrella" is one of several approaches that attempt to create viable partnerships. As long as some employees and dependents can totally opt out of a managed care program, it is unlikely that the employer-provided employee benefit system can successfully continue in a fragmented environment.

CASE STUDY

Heritage National Healthplan: Developing a Health Plan for Smaller Communities

G. MICHAEL HAMMES, President
Heritage National Healthplan, Davenport, Iowa

In 1985, Deere & Company formed a managed care subsidiary called Heritage National Healthplan. It was an outgrowth of earlier Deere involvements in self-funding healthcare for employees; starting an internal healthcare department; and funding the initial operation of the Quad-City Health Plan and the Cedar Valley Health Plan in Waterloo, Iowa. Deere felt that its 150 years of manufacturing and supplying equipment for rural America might also be helpful in developing a healthcare plan for that same marketplace.

There were basic philosophies tied to the development of Heritage that made the new company unique. Deere wanted to ensure that its own corporate image of strong management and quality product was carried over to its healthcare subsidiary. In its initial development and operation, Heritage attempted to use management expertise hand in hand with quality initiatives to distinguish it from other managed care providers.

Its approach was to offer healthcare products in

smaller communities, where its philosophy of limited financial risk for providers, combined with strong local physician involvement, seemed most acceptable. An open-panel IPA-model health plan seemed to appeal more to physicians in smaller communities, where local involvement and control were major issues. Inclusion of most physicians within a community and Heritage's ability to relate to local needs and concerns of medical providers was an essential element to long-term success. This is in contrast to larger cities, where a greater physician population with fewer patients fosters competition among providers and makes the need for patients from a prepaid plan more of a reality. Many times the physicians in smaller communities have full practices and thus do not need additional patients.

In addition to strong local physician ties, Heritage also has reduced the potential for a major financial loss on the part of the doctors. This approach was taken because most of these communities had a limited number of managed care participants. Smaller, nonmetropolitan areas usually had some form of managed care but typically did not have the same level of competition seen in the larger cities. There was a definite need to put physicians at risk for their services, but the risk sharing was limited to a loss of 20 percent of approved fees and charges. The 20 percent figure was used because it still represents a significant factor considering that the first portion of any loss in the Physician Fund is charged to the doctors.

The participating doctor is usually a member of an individual physician association (IPA). A monthly capitation is paid by Heritage to the IPA Physician Fund, which then pays the individual doctors. Reimbursement is made on a fee-for-service basis, with 10 percent withheld from an approved fee schedule. The withhold can be increased to 20 percent if the financial results warrant. In the event of a loss, the doctors lose their withhold first; thus the majority of the initial risk is borne by the doctors, even though it is limited to 20 percent.

The other part of the risk arrangement limits the amount of liability doctors have for insufficient hospital funding. Heritage took the approach of establishing prospective contracts with participating hospital providers. It then works with the IPAs to develop strict protocols which eliminate inappropri-

ate hospitalization by using hospital admission pre-certification, inpatient concurrent review, and home health arrangements. While doctors as a whole (the IPA) are not held liable for hospital deficits, individual physicians are held financially accountable for admissions or lengths of stay that are inappropriate based on the review process managed by the IPA. For many Heritage IPAs this combination of factors has produced hospital admission rates and days confined that are consistent with national HMO averages.

The Heritage philosophy of working together with doctors, using limited risk arrangements, and preserving the traditional fee-for-service approach is attractive to doctors in smaller communities. They have an appreciation for the ability of a health plan to relate to local needs and concerns. Establishing local offices with operations managers and local staff dedicated to working with the physicians through their quality assurance activities helps to promote the "partnership" concept. This approach is also used in working with enrollees who have problems or complaints through local member services personnel. Employers appreciate the local attention and have access to data detailing their company utilization.

Finally, Heritage has the ability to provide usable data reports to physicians that allow them to evaluate medical services rendered by their peers to Plan enrollees. These reports, which contain procedure- and diagnosis-specific information, compare physicians and show utilization trends that help to analyze care provided. Comparing data among IPAs and showing aberrant practice patterns has allowed doctors, through peer review committees, to work with their peers to then modify poor practice patterns.

Solving the myriad of healthcare problems is a complex task requiring a long-term commitment from all parties. The Heritage approach—establishing a relationship with employers through data sharing, cost control, and member service; working together with doctors to approach problems and concerns on a local level; developing financial arrangements with providers that address inappropriate reimbursement mechanisms; providing all parties with information to evaluate results—combines the characteristics that make managed care a viable, attractive alternative for rural America.

AV-Med Health Plan of Florida: The Physician Incentive Bonus Plan Based on Quality of Care

JEROME BELOFF, M.D., Vice President and Chief Medical Officer

AV-Med Health Plan of Florida, Miami, Florida

Incentives have been used for years to change physicians' behavior. The financial incentive in most instances has been based on some form of cost saving. In the past 2 years, the HMO industry has gone through a violent shakeout where the more successful healthcare plans have focused on providing consistent quality of care rather than low-cost premiums. The use of lowered premiums as a strategy for building membership has bankrupted many plans.

The AV-Med Health Plan, an IPA-model HMO with 200,000 members and 3000 physicians, has concentrated its effort on the quality of its physicians and hospitals. It has purposely not been competitive with low-premium providers. Marketing emphasis has been on demonstrating a sophisticated quality assurance program for continual monitoring of care in hospitals, physicians' offices, nursing homes, home care, and ancillary services.

In keeping with this emphasis, it initiated an incentive bonus plan weighted toward quality of care provided, that is, primary care physicians who deliver high quality and patient-satisfying care. The bonus is based on three objective measures: (1) patient satisfaction surveys, (2) quality of care measures, and (3) cost effectiveness.

METHODS

Patient satisfaction surveys are conducted annually for all primary care physicians. On joining the plan, members select a primary care physician who is their case manager for all healthcare services, including consultation referrals. Primary care physicians (PCPs) are family practioners, internists, and pediatricians. To conduct the survey, 20 randomly selected panel members receive a telephone questionnaire involving aspects of physician access, communication issues, outcome of care results, and satisfaction with the quality of care provided. A final question asks the member to rate the degree of satisfaction on a scale of 1 to 10 where 10 is very satisfied and 1 is dissatisfied. Quality of care is further measured from surveys of hospital records compared to peer standards, office record reviews, quality assessment survey results done four or more times per year, complaint log reviews, and a measure of panel members requesting transfer to another PCP.

Cost effectiveness is scored on a comparative basis of cost per member per month (PMPM), age, and intensity of service related to peers of like panel composition. Medical cost profiles, which are sent monthly to the physicians, compare the composite of cost PMPM of their panel to the median cost of their peers. Peer comparisons are made separately for the three primary care groups, that is, comparing internists to internists. Cost-effective physicians are generally high scorers in both quality of care and patient satisfaction surveys. Each physician has a composite score from the three measures described above.[*]

The upper 75 percent of each group received bonus awards which ranged from 3 to 15 percent of their annual capitation income. An award pool of 10 percent of total system payments to primary care physicians was set aside. The dollar amount allocated to each of the practioner groups was based on each group's capitation percentage of the total amount available for awards. In 1988, $400,000 was distributed as bonus awards.

Those physicians in the lowest 25 percent of the score distribution received no bonus awards. The lowest 10 percent were apprised of their poor showing and were considered for possible termination.

DISCUSSION

The incentive bonus plan was approved for implementation by the board of directors of AV-MED Associates, Inc., the medical policy setting group of the

---

[*] A z-score distribution is established for each of the three primary care groups, with 0 as the median and 3 standard deviations above and below. These scores were then transformed to a *t*-distribution with a mean of 70 and a standard deviation of 10. This provided a sort for each primary care group of the highest and lowest scores.

IPA. In 1988, the first year that the program was implemented, the plan was received with a very positive response. Previous withholding of 10 percent of the capitation payments was discontinued and a net capitation amount was provided on a patient age–related basis for this bonus program.

Details of the patient satisfaction survey question-naire are presented in Attachment A. The detailed description of the cost analysis for each physician is found in Attachment B. Development of more specific and objective measures of quality of care is in process. The goal is to find outcome measures for which objective and quantitative scores can be assigned.

ATTACHMENT A

AV-MED HEALTH PLAN PATIENT SATISFACTION SURVEY

Hello, my name is _____ with AV-MED Health Plan. We are conducting a survey of current AV-MED members and we would like to include you among the persons who get to express their views.

01. How long have you been an AV-MED member? (*Do not read list*)

    Less than 1 year 1
    1 year but less than 2 years. 2
    2 years but less than 4 years 3
    4 years but less than 6 years 4
    6 years or more 5
    Don't know . . . . Y
    Not an AV-MED member. . . . . .terminate

02. What was the main reason you selected AV-MED?

    Reason 1. 1
    Reason 2. 2
    Reason 3. 3
    Reason 4. 4
    Reason 5. 5
    Reason 6. 6

03. When you first joined AV-MED, would you say that it cost less than, about the same as, or more than other similar types of medical coverage?

    Less than 1
    About the same. 2
    More than 3
    Don't know . . . . Y

04.   Before you joined AV-MED, what kind of medical insurance did you carry? Was it . . . ?
(*read list*)

     Blue Cross/Blue Shield 1
     Indemnity or traditional insurance 2
     PPO (Preferred Provider Organization 3
     HMO (Health Maintenance Organization 4
     Medicare/Medicaid 5
     Other, specify————————————————————— 6
     None 7
     Don't know 8

04b.   If HMO mentioned in Q.8, ask: What is the HMO's name?

_____

05.   How long have you been a patient of Dr.——————————?

     Less than 1 year 1
     1 year but less than 2 years 2
     2 years but less than 4 years 3
     4 years but less than 8 years 4
     8 years but less than 12 years 5
     12 years or more 6
     Not a patient of that doctor X

05b.   If not a patient of Dr.———————————, ask: What is the name of the physician you
currently use?

_____

06.   Approximately how many times have you seen this physician since you selected
him/her?————————————

07.   Since you joined AV-MED, would you say that you see a physician more than, about the
same as, or less than you did before you joined our program?

     More than 1
     About the same 2
     Less than 3
     Don't know . . . . Y

08.   What was the main reason you selected this physician?

     Reason 1 1
     Reason 2 2
     Reason 3 3
     Reason 4 4

09. Did you have a primary care physician before you joined AV-MED?

Yes.............................. continue 1
No .... Skip to Q.12......................... 2
Don't know .... Skip to Q.12......................... 3

10. Did you have to change your physician when you joined AV-MED?

Yes.............................. Continue 1
No .... Skip to Q.12......................... 2

11. Would you describe your current physician as better than, about the same as, or worse than your former physician?

Better than.. 1
About the same.. 2
Worse than 3
Don't know .... Y

12. Now, I'm going to read a series of statements concerning the quality of doctor's care you have received under AV-MED. For each statement, please indicate whether your experience was excellent, good, fair, unacceptable, or whether the statement doesn't apply to you.

(*Begin with item checked and continue until all items asked.*)

		Exc.	Good	Fair	UA	DA
[ ]	Your ability to obtain adequate follow-up of a problem or test result is	1	2	3	4	Y
[ ]	The explanation given to you about medical tests and procedures is	1	2	3	4	Y
[ ]	The friendliness and courtesy shown to you by your doctor is	1	2	3	4	Y
[ ]	The personal interest in you and your medical problems shown by your doctor is	1	2	3	4	Y
[ ]	The respect shown to you and the attention to your privacy by doctors is	1	2	3	4	Y
[ ]	The amount of time you have with doctors during a visit is	1	2	3	4	Y
[ ]	The thoroughness of examinations and the accuracy of diagnosis is	1	2	3	4	Y
[ ]	The apparent skill, experience and training of your physician is	1	2	3	4	Y
[ ]	The physician's explanation regarding prescribed medication is	1	2	3	4	Y

13. On a scale of 1 to 10, with 10 being excellent and 1 being very poor, how would you rate the overall quality of care given by your physician?

Exc.   Very poor   DK
10   9   8   7   6   5   4   3   2   1   Y

14. What could your physician do to improve the quality of care you receive? (*Probe*)

_____

15. Now, I'm going to read a series of statements concerning the quality of the medical staff's care you have received under AV-MED. For each statement, please indicate whether your experience was excellent, good, fair, unacceptable, or whether the statement doesn't apply to you.

    (*Begin with item checked and continue until all items asked.*)

		Exc.	Good	Fair	UA	DA
[ ]	The friendliness and courtesy shown to you by staff members is	.1	.2	.3	.4	.Y
[ ]	The amount of time you have with staff members during a visit is	.1	.2	.3	.4	.Y
[ ]	The apparent skill and professionalism of the medical staff is	.1	.2	.3	.4	.Y

16. On a scale of 1 to 10, with 10 being excellent and 1 being very poor, how would you rate the overall quality of care given by your physician's medical staff?

Exc.   Very poor   DK
10   9   8   7   6   5   4   3   2   1   Y

17. The following statements concern the overall medical care you have received under AV-MED. For each statement, please indicate whether your experience was excellent, good, fair, unacceptable, or whether the statement doesn't apply to you.

    (*Begin with item checked and continue until all items asked.*)

		Exc.	Good	Fair	UA	DA
[ ]	The emergency medical care is	.1	.2	.3	.4	.Y
[ ]	The overall thoroughness of the medical treatment you receive is	.1	.2	.3	.4	.Y

18. On a scale of 1 to 10, with 10 being excellent and 1 being very poor, how would you rate the overall quality of care given by AV-MED?

Exc.   Very poor   DK
10   9   8   7   6   5   4   3   2   1   Y

19. In your opinion, what could be done to improve the quality of medical care you receive? (*Probe*)

_____

20. The following statements concern the timeliness with which you have received service under AV-MED. For each statement, please indicate whether your experience was excellent, good, fair, unacceptable, or whether the statement doesn't apply to you.

(*Begin with item checked and continue until all items asked.*)

		Exc.	Good	Fair	UA	DA
[ ]	Your ability to make contact with the physician during office hours is	1	2	3	4	Y
[ ]	Your ability to make contact with the physician when the office is closed is	1	2	3	4	Y
[ ]	The length of time you must wait between making an appointment and the day of your visit is	1	2	3	4	Y
[ ]	The promptness by which you are taken to an examination room from the time you arrive is	1	2	3	4	Y
[ ]	Your ability to get to see a specialist by referral is	1	2	3	4	Y

21. On a scale of 1 to 10, with 10 being excellent and 1 being very poor, how would you rate the convenience of your doctor's office from your home or place of work?

```
Exc.                 Very poor    DK
10  9  8  7  6  5  4  3  2  1      Y
```

22. Using the same scale, from 1 to 10, how would you rate the physical appearance of your doctor's office?

```
Exc.                 Very poor    DK
10  9  8  7  6  5  4  3  2  1      Y
```

23. Again, using the same scale, how would you rate your overall health?

```
Exc.                 Very poor    DK
10  9  8  7  6  5  4  3  2  1      Y
```

24. In the future, would you definitely recommend, AV-MED, probably not recommend, or definitely not recommend AV-MED to others?

Definitely recommend 1
Probably recommend 2

Probably not recommend. 3
Definitely not recommend 4
Don't know . . . . Y

25. Do you intend to leave AV-MED for another program at the next opportunity to do so?

Yes. . . . . continue 1
No . . . . Skip to Q.26. 2
Don't know . . . . .Skip to Q.26. 3

25b. What would be your most important reason for leaving AV-MED?

_____

26. What, if anything, do you particularly like about your physician, his/her office staff, or his/her office procedures? (*Probe*)

_____

27. What, if anything, do you particularly dislike about your physician, his/her office staff, or his/her office procedures? Anything else? (*Probe*)

_____

Now, I have just a few questions for classification purposes only.

28. Which of the following categories includes your age? (*Read list*)

18–24. 1
25–34. 2
35–44. 3
45–54. 4
55–64. 5
65 or older. 6
Refused . . . . Y

29. Which of the following categories best describes your ethnic background? (*Read list*)

Black. 1
Hispanic. 2
White. 3
Asian 4
Other 5
Refused . . . . Y

30. What is the last grade of school you completed? (*Read list*)

Less than eighth grade. 1
Some high school 2

High school graduate 3
Some college or technical school 4
College graduate 5
Postgraduate work 6
Refused . . . . Y

31. If you are employed outside the home, what is your occupation?

Blue collar 1
White collar 2
Managerial professional 3
Not employed 4
Don't know/refused . . . . Y

32. (*Record sex of respondent.*)

Male 1
Female 2

That concludes our survey. Thank you very much for your participation.

Name ─────────────────────────────────────

Physician's name: Dr. ──────────────────────────

Phone number ───────────────────────────────

Interviewer number ──────────────────────────(-)

ATTACHMENT B
MEDICAL EXPENSE REPORT

The Medical Expense Report is an instrument for measuring and comparing the effectiveness of capitated primary care physicians in containing the cost of medical services for patients in their HMO panel.

Notes

A. The identified medical expenses for panel patients for service dates during the period of the report are presented both as a total dollar amount and as a cost per member per month (PMPM).

B. An adjustment to the demonstrated PMPM cost is made to reflect the percentage of high-cost patients in the physician's panel, to the extent that this is different than the percentage for all

physicians. Thus, if the panel includes a *greater* than average number of high-cost patients, the adjusted cost PMPM is *less* than the unadjusted cost. This adjustment is calculated independently for each age group, and the overall adjustment is a weighted average for all age groups in the panel.

C. Comparison is made with the average PMPM cost for all capitated primary care physicians. This is determined independently for each age group, and the comparison PMPM cost represents the weighted average of all age groups in the physician's panel.

D. The cost containment comparison is based on a peer group average for a hypothetical patient panel that matches the physician's panel in terms of age group characteristics and percentage of high-cost patients.

Frequency

For the primary care physicians (or groups) with a patient panel size of 100 or more, individual reports are provided monthly. Primary care physicians with smaller panels are pooled and, for the purposes of this report, are considered to be one large primary care group. The reports are cumulative, and follow a 2-month lag to increase completeness of claims payment. Thus, the report made in December of each year demonstrates the experience for the previous fiscal year, October–September.

AV-MED Health Plan
Medical Expense Report
for Capitated Physicians

Physician's name: Dr. X   <u>285</u> members assigned

Physician's I.D.: 9999   <u>3802</u> member months Y-T-D

Medical Expenses	Y.T.D Amounts
1. Payments to primary physician (PCP)	
Copayments ($5 per office visit)	3,365.00
Capitation payments	26,523.95
Fee-for-service payments	25.00
	29,913.95
2. Other medical expenses for panel patients*	
Physician consultants	86,646.68
Hospital inpatient costs	64,640.68
Hospital outpatient costs	35,350.65
(includes ER, diagnostic centers, prescription drugs, ambulance, ambulatory surgery)	186,638.01
Total amount	216,551.96
Total amount PMPM	56.95
Intensity adjustment amount PMPM ±	(1.35)
Physician's adjusted expense PMPM	55.60
Age adjusted peer group average PMPM	58.14
Cost containment, favorable (unfavorable) to peer group PMPM	2.54
Percentage	4.37%

*Note: Excludes maternity claims, neonatal claims, claims over stop-loss $7500 per member per year.

CHAPTER FOURTEEN

Reimbursement Methodologies

APPROPRIATE REIMBURSEMENT METHODOLOGIES FOR MANAGED CARE SYSTEMS

MARIKA K. GORDON, M.A., Healthcare Consultant
Los Angeles, California

RANDALL P. HERMAN, F.S.A., Principal
Deloitte & Touche, Minneapolis, Minnesota

The medical service needs of large populations can be predicted with fair accuracy when the demographics of the group are known. The way in which services are utilized by such populations is within the control of the healthcare providers. Cost-effective providers utilize services judiciously, gauging quantity and intensity of care to the medical service requirements of the patient.

The methodology used by insurers to reimburse providers has significant impact on the efficiency of medical practice patterns. It is a primary objective of managed care programs to create meaningful incentives for providers to practice cost effectively.

The viable model of managed care is best viewed as an integrated system—dependent for its effective operations on the cooperative efforts of employer, insurer, provider, and consumer. By transferring appropriate financial risk to providers for the management of patient care, insurers can confine their liability and curtail the escalation of healthcare premiums. Employers can design and implement health benefit plans which meet their corporate objectives and the diverse needs of their employees around cost-effective provider networks.

Despite what appear as many different health insurance plan options, there are only two basic alternatives which underlie managed care packaging: care is either available only through a predefined provider network or from an appropriately licensed provider selected by the patient. Variations or combinations of these two alternatives comprise the spectrum of alternatives. For illustrative purposes, a plan can be depicted as a donut (HMO, PPO, fee-for-service plan), or a slice of pie—a multiple-option point-of-purchase product.

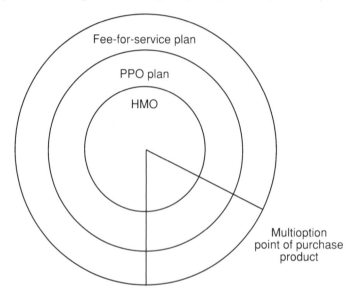

The predictability of who will select each option is what differentiates the pricing, reimbursement, and risk-sharing methods which fit the different plan combinations. This is calculated in terms of numbers and of demographic and health-risk characteristics and how those who select the plan will elect to move between network options and noncontracted providers of choice.

Effective provider compensation arrangements must reflect the decisions which the plan design allows members to make and those which members are most likely to exercise. In situations where member experience proves to be substantially different than was predicted by the insurer, all segments of the managed care system will suffer financially. Conversely, where the utilization and cost of services has been accurately projected, positive financial performance can result for all parties.

Managed healthcare systems are driven by financial incentives which direct the behavior of insurer, provider, employer, and consumer. When the measure of risk which is borne by each segment corresponds to the level of control each has over the quantity and source of services needed, the system can exert measurable impact on the aggregate cost of healthcare.

HISTORICAL OVERVIEW

When first conceived, health insurance was purchased for the purpose of averting catastrophic liabilities which, in the traditional cash payment system, presented major financial risk to consumers. By the 1950s the responsibility for payment of health insurance premiums shifted from individuals to their employers and the scope of covered services and related costs broadened. The increased liability of the insurer was passed along to the employer through continually escalating premiums.

Insurers initially sought to institute measures to curtail provider charges in order to maintain profitability and to keep premiums in line. The Blue Cross plans, as early as the 1930s, were the first to negotiate discounts with hospitals in exchange for the volume of business they covered. The Blue Shield plans began to extend this same philosophy to physicians. Such reimbursement arrangements failed to have an effect on the variation of fees among providers or on the appropriateness of charges for the rendered services.

Consequently, by the 1950s, insurers started to refine their definitions of covered services by creating classification systems of diagnoses and procedures which were linked to "usual, customary, and reasonable" ranges determined on the basis of provider charges and practice patterns in the region. Although these efforts had little effect on the nature or duration of services provided, they did serve to establish limitations on the amounts which insurers would pay and on copayments for which consumers were obligated.

Along a parallel track, as early as 1930, the concept of HMOs was being explored as a vehicle for containing aggregate healthcare expenditures. Founded on the premise that the service needs of large population groups are predictable, HMOs aligned a complementary network of providers to take care of their patients and compensated caregivers through fixed price contracts or salaries. HMOs could offer a wider range of services at predetermined premiums by defining appropriate medical practice criteria, enforcing their application through effective utilization controls, and eliminating the financial incentives of the fee-for-service system.

With the passage of the federal HMO law in 1974, HMOs could compete effectively with most insured plans by offering immediate savings to employers on premiums and by reducing administrative costs through the elimination of claims forms. With care management tools and favorable financial arrangements with their select providers, HMOs held the promise of also controlling future premium increases.

The acceptability of the original staff and group HMO models was limited because consumers were reluctant to exchange their freedom of choice of providers for an extension of benefits. In response, many variations of the HMO theme have evolved in the course of the last 10 years which, to a greater or lesser extent, aim to control costs through the management of service utilization and provider compensation. These emerging alternative delivery systems (IPA-type HMOs and PPOs) have sought to apply HMO techniques to the fee-for-service sector by devising reimbursement methods which would instill HMO incentives into the practices of independent professional and institutional providers.

Provider Experience

In many of the more developed HMO and PPO markets, such as California and Minnesota, the initial period of resistance by providers to contract with any form of alternative delivery system was followed by a period of experimentation. During the late 1970s and early 1980s, many physicians and hospitals signed all HMO and PPO contracts which came their way. They believed that the potentially limited enrollment from any one contract represented an insignificant portion of the total business yet served as a hedge against possible loss of market share. Although more patients could mean more money, it did not always mean that revenues were sufficient to cover expenses, much less result in profits.

These providers often learned, too late, that some of these arrangements yielded disastrous financial results. Problems commonly encountered under contractual reimbursement included:

- Inadequate payment rates due to poor actuarial assumptions.
- Additional administrative expenses resulting from duties such as filling out referral authorization forms, collecting copayments, suppressing normal billing routines, and negotiating and settling contracts. The performance of such extra duties required additional staff and, often, extra legal or consulting costs. These expenses frequently doubled or tripled the administrative costs normally associated with fee-for-service billing.
- Insufficient clarity of contracts regarding responsibilities, settlement terms, stop-loss arrangements, and payment rates.
- Additional patient volume promised by HMOs and PPOs did not materialize, and providers saw existing patients shift from fee-for-service to contracted reimbursement.

Many providers now have a track record of experience in managing HMO and PPO patient care and related finances. Desirable network providers are more selective about the terms they will accept and the nature of risk they will assume. Financial promises are compared to actual experience. Enrollment is evaluated in terms of new patients and conversion of existing patients. Contracts which have not afforded sufficient volume or revenue are not being renewed under the same terms, or at all.

At the same time, insurers are also scrutinizing their experience with providers. The popularity of specific providers is no longer sufficient for membership in the network if their utilization experience is unmanageable. HMOs and PPOs which have developed sophisticated service tracking capabilities can now identify individual providers whose practice patterns deviate from community norms. HMOs and PPOs are also taking measures to validate discounted fees against usual customary charges. Armed with this information, they can take action to counsel; effect modification; and, if necessary, terminate agreements.

The current environment is one of increased sophistication on the part of providers of healthcare; buyers of healthcare (employers and government); and insurers, HMOs, and PPOs who provide the interface between those two groups. An understanding of the complexities and incentives behind the various provider compensation strategies is essential for the buyers and providers of healthcare services.

The systems used by managed care plans to pay providers of medical services are driven by the need to manage costs and to limit the financial risk of adverse claims experience. Provider payment systems used by payers differ according to the type of service being purchased (hospital, physician, ancillary) and by the form of the plan being sponsored (group HMO, IPA HMO, PPO).

BASIC PHYSICIAN PAYMENT SYSTEMS

Physicians play a key role in the delivery of medical services. They not only control utilization of their own services but also direct the use of most other healthcare services. Managed care physician payment methods should be designed to reduce the cost of physician services as well as to contain the utilization of hospital and other medical services.

Managed care payment systems should also be designed to reduce or eliminate some of the inappropriate incentives to increase services and charges which exist in the traditional fee-for-service system and to reduce the losses an HMO or PPO might experience as a result of adverse experience. This is accomplished primarily by passing a portion of the risk to physicians.

In order to control costs, a reasonable goal of an HMO or PPO payment system should be to reward the low-cost physician and penalize the high-cost physician. The reward or punishment could be in the form of a higher or lower relative payment (that is, higher and lower percentage of charges) or higher or lower actual payment (that is, higher or lower total dollars paid).

The following basic physician payment systems contain an increasing level of risk transfer to physicians.

1. Discounted fees
2. Capped fee schedule
3. Capped fee schedule with withhold
4. Primary care capitation
5. Full capitation

Each system results in progressively more risk being passed on to the physician. The more risk passed to the physician, the greater the potential gain to the physician from reduced medical care usage and the greater the potential loss due to excessive usage of services.

Discounted Fees   Perhaps the most straightforward method of reducing costs is the discounted fee approach, where physicians agree to accept a percentage reduction from their fees as payment in full. This method is used by HMOs and PPOs to pay for primary care and specialty services.

For example, Table 1 summarizes the annual payments made by the ABC HMO to each of three physicians under a contract paying a 15 percent discount from charges. Each physician provides services for an identical group of 1000 HMO members. Assuming that the physicians are providing services to an identical group of 1000 HMO members, the differences in costs and utilization are associated with differences in charge level and practice patterns rather than with differences in the patient base. The low-cost physician has lower charge levels and fewer office visits and performs fewer tests than the high-cost physician. Under this system, the high-cost physician experiences the same percent recovery as the other physicians and receives the largest payment from the HMO.

With discounted fee reimbursement, each physician experiences the same recovery from charges, regardless of charge level or number of services performed. Therefore, there is no economic incentive to control charge increases or utilization. For this reason, this type of reimbursement is losing popularity among HMOs and PPOs.

TABLE 1   Annual Experience of 1000 HMO Members
15% Discount Contract

	LOW-COST PHYSICIAN	MEDIUM-COST PHYSICIAN	HIGH-COST PHYSICIAN
Primary care services			
Office visits	4000 at $25 each	4000 at $35 each	4500 at $35 each
Laboratory tests	3000 at $10 each	4000 at $12 each	6000 at $15 each
Total charges	$130,000	$188,000	$248,000
HMO payment	$111,000	$160,000	$211,000
Charges recovered	85%	85%	85%

Capped Fee Schedule

A more common approach utilized by PPOs and HMOs is the capped fee schedule. Here a maximum allowable fee (or fee cap) is determined for each procedure, and a physician will be paid charges up to the maximum amount.

For example, if ABC HMO uses a capped fee schedule approach with a $30 per visit maximum fee for office visits and a $10 per test maximum fee for laboratory tests, then the recovery from charges will differ by physician, depending upon each physician's own charge level. This is shown in Table 2.

The high-cost physician experiences the lowest recovery as a result of high charges. The high-cost physician still receives the greatest patient revenues from the HMO since he or she performed more services than the other physicians.

The advantage of capped fee schedule payments compared to discounted charges is twofold: First, they help limit the impact of fee increases by physicians, and second, they are more equitable in that physicians with higher fees realize greater discounts than those with low fees. Since reimbursement is based on the number of services performed and excessive hospital or referral services result in no financial impact, this system does not motivate physicians to limit the services they perform, their use of hospitals, or other medical services they order.

Capped Fee Schedule with Withholds

A common variation of the capped fee schedule approach, primarily employed by IPA-model HMOs, is to withhold a percentage of payment (typically 15 to 20 percent) and to pay back the withheld funds if certain performance goals are met. These goals often relate to the

TABLE 2 Annual Experience of 1000 HMO Members
Capped Fee Schedule

	LOW-COST PHYSICIAN	MEDIUM-COST PHYSICIAN	HIGH-COST PHYSICIAN
Primary care charges	$130,000	$188,000	$248,000
HMO payment			
Office visits	4,000	4,000	4,500
Payment per visit	× $25	× $30	× $30
Office visit payment	$100,000	$120,000	$135,000
Laboratory tests	3,000	4,000	6,000
Payment per test	× $10	× $10	× $10
Laboratory test payment	$ 30,000	$ 40,000	$ 60,000
Total HMO payments	$130,000	$160,000	$195,000
Recovery			
Capped fee schedule	100%	85%	79%
Discounted charges	85%	85%	85%

use of referral and hospital services by the individual physician. Incentives are created to control the use of all medical services through the use of withholds.

Withholds are not commonly used by PPOs since members often have open access to physicians outside of the PPO panel, limiting the PPO physician's control over use and ability to meet performance goals.

For example, suppose the ABC HMO uses the same capped fees shown in Table 2 but also uses a 20 percent withhold which is applied to pay for any referral or hospital costs exceeding $40 per member per month (PMPM). If referral and hospital costs are less than $40 PMPM, then the withhold is returned. Table 3 shows the resulting HMO payment under this contract, assuming the referral and hospital costs of the low-, medium-, and high-cost physicians were $39, $41, and $48 per member per month, respectively.

The low-cost physician was refunded all of the withhold because referral and hospital costs were less than the goal. The medium-cost physician received some of the withhold because funds remained after payment of the shortfall in the referral and hospital pool. The high-cost physician received no withhold return because referral and hospital costs far exceeded the budget.

This payment method has all the advantages of the capped fee schedule and generally creates an incentive not to overuse services since excessive utilization may reduce withhold returns. However, where a physician does not expect to get a withhold return (usually

TABLE 3   Annual Experience of 1000 HMO Members
Capped Fee Schedule with 20% Withhold

	LOW-COST PHYSICIAN	MEDIUM-COST PHYSICIAN	HIGH-COST PHYSICIAN
Primary care charges	$ 130,000	$ 188,000	$ 248,000
HMO payment			
Withhold amount	26,000	32,000	39,000
Referral and hospital pool	480,000	480,000	480,000
Actual costs	−468,000	−492,000	−576,000
Referral gain (loss)	$ 12,000	$(12,000)	$(96,000)
Withhold returned	26,000	20,000	0
Payment after withhold	104,000	128,000	156,000
Total HMO payments	$130,000	$148,000	$156,000
Recovery			
Capped fee with withholds	100%	79%	63%
Capped fees	100%	85%	79%
Discounted charges	85%	85%	85%

based on past experience), the incentive impact of the withhold may be limited. The physician may view the withhold as a discount and increase the use of services in order to increase compensation.

Primary Care Capitation

Capitation systems feature a payment to the physician of a fixed monthly amount per member (or per capita, hence the name). The capitation payment is made to the provider whether or not services are rendered.

The services covered by capitation payment systems vary. Under a full capitation approach, the physician is at risk for all medical services, including referral services and hospitalization. A more limited capitation approach is commonly used for primary care reimbursement by IPA model HMOs or for specialty services such as mental health or vision care.

Under primary care capitation, the primary care physician is capitated for a fixed list of services. The physician receives the same payment regardless of the number of covered services performed, which creates an incentive to control the use of these services.

For example, suppose ABC HMO pays primary care physicians a primary care capitation rate of $13.25 per member per month, with a withhold of 20 percent of the capitation. As with the previous example, withhold funds are applied against referral and hospital costs exceeding $40 per member per month. The withhold will be returned if referral and hospital costs are less than $40 per member per month. Table 4 shows the resulting payment under this contract compared to the contracts previously examined.

TABLE 4 Annual Experience of 1000 HMO Members
Primary Care Capitation with 20% Withhold

	LOW-COST PHYSICIAN	MEDIUM-COST PHYSICIAN	HIGH-COST PHYSICIAN
Primary care charges	$130,000	$188,000	$248,000
HMO payment			
Capitation after withhold	$127,000	$127,000	$127,000
Withhold amount	32,000	32,000	32,000
Referral gain or loss (from Table 3)	12,000	(12,000)	(96,000)
Withhold returned	32,000	20,000	0
Total HMO payments	$159,000	$147,000	$127,000
Recovery			
Primary care capitation	122%	78%	51%
Capped fees with withhold	100%	79%	63%
Capped fees, no withhold	100%	85%	79%
Discount charges	85%	85%	85%

With primary care capitation and a withhold, the low-cost physician actually recovers more than charges. The low-cost physician also receives greater payment from the HMO than the high-cost physician on a total dollar basis. Unlike previous models, the number of services performed does not positively affect reimbursement.

Capitation systems eliminate traditional fee-for-service incentives to increase charges for covered services and to overutilize such services since payment will be the same regardless of the cost or frequency of services used. In addition, capitation systems can be designed to transfer much of the financial risk of claims fluctuation to the capitated provider.

Case Study 1 in the Appendix illustrates the design of several primary care capitation arrangements and affords a comparative analysis of the financial impact of each scenario considering the demographics of the population to be served and the circumstances of the contracting providers. It highlights the critical issues which must be considered in evaluating risk-based agreements, and it demonstrates how financial performance can be affected by these factors.

Full Capitation
The full capitation system creates the most dramatic financial incentives to control the cost of medical services. Under full capitation, a physician would receive a capitation rate covering all medical services, including hospital and referral services. Typically, the actual payments for hospital and referral services would be made by the HMO and deducted from the capitation.

For example, suppose ABC HMO uses a full capitation approach with a capitation rate of $53.25. The primary care physicians will receive whatever funds are left over from the capitation pool after referral and hospital claims are paid. Table 5 illustrates the experience of each physician under this approach.

The high-cost physician recovers only 25 percent of charges, probably not even covering expenses. Clearly, full capitation rewards the low-cost physician and penalizes the high-cost physician.

Full capitation is not commonly used to reimburse individual physicians. Group practices or hospital and physician joint ventures are more typically fully capitated in states which permit this form of risk transfer.

Impact of Physician Payment Strategies on HMO Finances
The basic physician payment systems just outlined create different financial incentives for providers to control costs. The effectiveness of these incentives relies on the nature of the financial risks which are transferred from the HMO to the providers.

Passing risk to physicians also reduces the financial risk to the HMO, the risks of both negative and positive utilization and cost experience.

TABLE 5   Annual Experience of 1000 HMO Members
Full Capitation

	LOW-COST PHYSICIAN	MEDIUM-COST PHYSICIAN	HIGH-COST PHYSICIAN
Full primary care charges	$130,000	$188,000	$248,000
Capitation amount before deductions	$639,000	$639,000	$639,000
Referral and hospital costs	−468,000	−492,000	−576,000
Remainder paid to primary care physician	$171,000	$147,000	$ 63,000
Recovery			
Full capitation	132%	78%	25%
Primary care capitation	122%	78%	51%
Capped fees, with withhold	100%	79%	63%
Capped fees, no withhold	100%	85%	79%
Discounted fees	85%	85%	85%

Under capitation, the HMO pays a fixed budgeted amount without regard to actual claims experience. If claims exceed budget, the capitated physicians absorb the loss. Under the other forms of payment, the physicians may absorb risk up to the amount of withholds, which can also dramatically reduce losses to the HMO.

For example, suppose ABC HMO had budgeted medical costs of $53.25 PMPM (that is, the full capitation rate). Table 6 shows the experience of ABC HMO compared to budget if the HMO contracted only with the three primary care physicians used previously. Table 6 clearly shows that the HMO has limited its losses by passing risk on to the physicians. Where no withholds were available, the HMO experienced the greatest losses. With withholds, the losses were partially absorbed. With full capitation, there was no loss.

Passing financial risk to providers also means reducing the possible gains to the HMO if experience is more favorable than expected. Had

TABLE 6   Total Annual Experience of ABC HMO
(in $1000)

	PRIMARY CARE	REFERRAL AND HOSPITAL	TOTAL	BUDGET	GAIN (LOSS)
Discounted fees	$482	$1536	$2018	$1917	$(101)
Capped fee schedule	485	1536	2021	1917	(104)
Capped fee schedule with 20% withhold	434	1536	1970	1917	(53)
Primary care capitation with 20% withhold	433	1536	1969	1917	(52)
Full capitation	381	1536	1917	1917	0

claims been significantly below budget, the HMO would have experienced the greatest gains if providers had not been capitated.

The gain or loss experience of the HMO is affected by the accuracy of budget projections. The budgeted amounts for physician, hospital, and referral services would usually be set by the HMO based on actuarial projections of usage and cost per service. The accuracy of these projections is vital to the HMO which does not use full capitation. HMOs using capitation and withholds have a decreasing interest in the accuracy of the actuarial projections because providers absorb the losses due to claims exceeding projections. As a result of competitive market conditions, HMOs which capitate providers often create budgets based on the desired premium rate levels rather than the actual expectation of costs and utilization. Consequently, the appropriateness of the risk transfer from HMO to providers must be judiciously evaluated.

BASIC HOSPITAL SERVICE PAYMENT STRATEGIES

Outside of the managed care environment, hospitals, like physicians, have traditionally been paid on a fee-for-service basis. Hospitals charge patients for the services used during a hospital stay. The majority of these charges are related to diagnostic testing, supplies, operating room fees, and other ancillary services which supplement the basic room and board costs. In recent years, the increase in charges for ancillary services has far outpaced the growth of room and board fees. According to the Equicor hospital surveys, daily ancillary costs rose 17 percent during the 1985–1987 period, versus 8 percent for daily room and board costs. The rapid rise in ancillary service costs is due to an increase in the number and the intensity of services ordered by physicians as well as a general increase in the level of charges.

The fee-for-service payment system promotes increases in charges and in the usage of ancillary services since hospital payments are directly tied to charges. Furthermore, hospitals prosper with increased admissions and lengths of stay. The design of HMO and PPO payment systems is intended to eliminate incentives to increase charge levels and usage of services.

The basic types of payment strategies used by HMOs and PPOs create cost-containment incentives by removing charges from the payment basis and passing the financial risk for excessive utilization to the hospitals. The primary payment strategies used by HMOs and PPOs are:

1. Discounted charges
2. Per diems
3. Per stay
4. Capitation

These strategies result in progressively greater risk transfer from the HMO or PPO to the hospital. The various payment systems afford differing rewards and penalties for hospitals depending upon the hospitals' charge level, frequency of admissions, and length of stays. HMO and PPO payment system designs strive to reward hospitals which control costs and usage of services. Conversely, they penalize facilities which are not successful in meeting these objectives.

Discount from Charges

Unlike the case of physician services, discounted charge-based payment is still popular with PPOs and HMOs as a hospital reimbursement method. This is probably because there is little standardization in the services billed by hospitals; therefore, a maximum allowable fee by service cannot be easily developed. Also, since many Blue Cross–Blue Shield plans have reimbursed hospitals on the basis of discounted charges, the process is already familiar to the institutions. Simply discounting the charges for hospital services, however, does not reward low-cost hospitals or penalize high-cost hospitals.

By way of example, Table 7 illustrates the financial experience of three hospitals, each providing services to 1000 members of the ABC HMO at a 15 percent discount from charges. The first hospital is low cost from several perspectives. As a result of either lower charges or lower ancillary costs, the hospital has lower costs per day than its competitors. The hospital is also low cost since it has shorter lengths of stay and fewer admissions per 1000 HMO members. In contrast, the high-cost hospital has high charges, high admission rates, and longer lengths of stay.

The discount from charges reimbursement method does not reward the low-cost hospital with payment of a higher percentage of charges nor penalize the high-cost hospital, which, in fact, derives the greatest revenue.

TABLE 7 Annual Experience of 1000 HMO Members
Discount from Charges Contract

	LOW-COST HOSPITAL	MEDIUM-COST HOSPITAL	HIGH-COST HOSPITAL
Number of patients	70	80	90
Length of stay	4.0	4.0	5.0
Days of care	280	320	450
Charges per day	$500	$600	$800
Charges per patient	$2000	$2400	$4000
Total hospital charges	$140,000	$192,000	$360,000
HMO payments (15% discount)	$119,000	$163,000	$306,000
Recovery, discounted charges	85%	85%	85%

Per Diem Reimbursement

The most common form of reimbursement used by HMOs and PPOs is per diem payments. Under this arrangement, a hospital is paid a fixed amount per day regardless of the amount of ancillary services provided. While this method creates an incentive to reduce utilization of ancillary services, an incentive to increase length of stay still exists since the hospital is paid more for longer stays.

For example, suppose the ABC HMO pays hospitals a per diem rate of $550 per day. Table 8 shows the payment and recovery of charges each hospital experiences. In this case, the low-cost hospital is rewarded by recovering more than charges. But under this system the high-cost hospital still receives more total income since payment can be increased by extending the length of patient stays.

Per Stay Reimbursement

Many payers have begun using per stay contracts. With these contracts, a hospital will be paid a fixed amount per stay regardless of the length of stay. This type of contract creates the incentive to contain the use of ancillary services and the length of stay.

For example, suppose the ABC HMO pays each hospital a rate of $2300 per stay. Table 9 shows the resulting payment for each hospital. With per-stay contracting, the high-cost hospital receives lower payment from the HMO than under a per diem contract because of the longer than average length of stay. But because the hospital experiences more admissions, the total revenue is in fact higher.

In actuality, since physicians are responsible for admitting and discharging patients, a hospital may have little control over the frequency of admissions and the length of stay of patients. Therefore, hospitals will often be reluctant to enter into contracts which require the assumption of risk for control of the length of patient stays. Alternatively, facilities will curb length of stay through aggressive utilization review programs in order to derive maximum financial benefit from per stay contracts.

TABLE 8   Annual Experience of 1000 HMO Members
Per Diem Hospital Contract

	LOW-COST HOSPITAL	MEDIUM-COST HOSPITAL	HIGH-COST HOSPITAL
Total hospital charges	$140,000	$192,000	$360,000
Hospital days	280	320	450
Per diem rate	×550	×550	×550
HMO payment	$154,000	$176,000	$247,500
Recovery			
Per diems	110%	92%	69%
Discounted charges	85%	85%	85%

TABLE 9   Annual Experience of 1000 HMO Members
Per-Stay Contract Rates

	LOW-COST HOSPITAL	MEDIUM-COST HOSPITAL	HIGH-COST HOSPITAL
Total hospital charges	$140,000	$192,000	$360,000
Number of admissions	70	80	90
Per stay amount	×2,300	×2,300	×2,300
HMO payment	$161,000	$184,000	$207,000
Recovery			
Per stay	115%	96%	58%
Per diem	110%	92%	69%
Discounted charges	85%	85%	85%

Per stay contracting is not favored by some HMOs and PPOs since the cost advantages of length of stay reductions accrue to the provider instead of the plan. On the other hand, if per stay rates can be negotiated at favorable terms, such contracts allow an HMO or PPO to focus utilization review efforts on preadmission screening rather than on concurrent review, resulting in savings to the HMO or PPO on utilization review costs.

Capitation Payments

Many group- and some staff-model HMOs pay hospitals on a capitation basis. The capitation may cover all hospital services regardless of where services are rendered or just cover the services rendered by the contracting facility. Capitation reimbursement creates a significant incentive for the hospital to reduce the frequency of admissions as well as the length of stay and usage of ancillary services.

For example, suppose the ABC HMO pays each hospital a fixed payment of $14.67 per member per month, regardless of the services performed. Table 10 illustrates that the high-cost hospital receives the same total payment as the low-cost hospital and that the recovery is much less than under the other reimbursement methods.

The key to success in a hospital capitation contract is limiting admissions and length of stay. Because physicians have greater control over these factors than hospitals do, such arrangements are typically utilized only in situations where the hospital has a very close working relationship with the physicians. Consequently, capitation payments for hospitals are not common for either HMOs or PPOs.

Case Study 2 in the Appendix illustrates the rationale of one hospital for assuming increased risk in accepting capitation payments from a contracting HMO. The study reviews the initial experience

TABLE 10   Annual Experience of 1000 HMO Members
Hospital Capitation Contract

	LOW-COST HOSPITAL	MEDIUM-COST HOSPITAL	HIGH-COST HOSPITAL
Total hospital charges	$140,000	$192,000	$360,000
Member months	12,000	12,000	12,000
Capitation rate	×14.67	×14.67	×14.67
HMO payment	$176,000	$176,000	$176,000
Recovery			
Capitation contract	126%	92%	49%
Per stay	115%	96%	58%
Per diem	110%	92%	69%
Discounted charges	85%	85%	85%

under the contract, highlights the critical issues in the contents and interpretation of contract terms as well as in the providers' capabilities in contract management. The analysis addresses the impact of these factors on the providers' financial performance and pinpoints remedies which were instituted to improve profitability of the arrangement.

Impact of Hospital Payment Strategies on HMO and PPO Finances

The basic hospital payment strategies used by HMOs and PPOs transfer various levels of risk to hospitals, thereby reducing the financial risk of the plans.

Table 11 shows the gain and loss to ABC HMO, assuming a hospital services budget equal to $14.67 PMPM. Moving from discounted charges to capitation payments, reimbursement to the hospital is minimized and the losses to the HMO decrease. This is because the actual cost per service and the frequencies of admission and lengths

TABLE 11   Experience of ABC HMO
Combined Three-Hospital Experience

	BUDGET HOSPITAL PAYMENT	ACTUAL PAYMENT	GAIN (LOSS)
15% discount	$528,000	$588,000	$(60,000)
Per diem	528,000	578,000	(50,000)
Per stay	528,000	552,000	(24,000)
Capitation	528,000	528,000	0

of stays were higher than budgeted. If experience had been better than budgeted, the HMO would have experienced gains under the noncapitated system. In practice, the gains or losses in the hospital services budget would also affect the physician reimbursement to the extent that risk sharing is being used.

ANCILLARY SERVICES PAYMENT SYSTEMS

As much as one-third of healthcare expenditures do not fall under the categories of hospital inpatient or physician services. These types of services include hospital outpatient care, such as same-day surgery and diagnostic testing, as well as prescription drugs, vision care, durable medical equipment, and prosthetic devices.

HMOs and PPOs have developed a number of unique contracting and reimbursement approaches for these services. As with physician and inpatient hospital payment methods, these approaches are designed to create appropriate cost-containment incentives by transferring financial risk to the direct providers of services.

Hospital Outpatient Services

Ambulatory or same-day surgery as an alternative to hospitalization has become increasingly popular as a cost-containment measure. Traditionally, managed care payers have used a discounted charge basis to pay for these services since costs varied widely depending upon the procedures performed and there was no commonly used system for categorizing different types of surgical claims. Also, hospital outpatient services were often viewed by HMOs and PPOs as minor compared to inpatient services; therefore, complicated payment strategies were not pursued.

Relatively low discounts (typically 5 to 20 percent, compared to 25 percent or more for inpatient services) and annual charge increases of 15 percent or more by many hospitals have resulted in dramatic increases in hospital outpatient surgery costs. As a result, the payment for an outpatient surgery may now exceed the payment for an overnight surgical stay.

To correct this problem, some HMOs and PPOs have adjusted payments to pay the lesser of the discounted charges or the surgical per diem. Another common approach is to establish a separate same-day surgery per diem.

More and more intensive surgical procedures are performed on an outpatient basis with an accompanying increase in time and use of ancillary services. This is forcing some HMOs to adopt surgery rates based on the procedure performed. Many of these systems follow the Medicare reimbursement method for ambulatory surgery centers, which features six procedure groupings based on the intensity of the service performed. The groupings cover thousands of procedures

TABLE 12   Medicare Ambulatory Surgical Center 1988 Rates

PAYMENT GROUP	RATE	PROCEDURE CODE	EXAMPLE
1	$250	23655	Treatment of closed shoulder dislocation
2	310	20005	Incision of soft tissue abscesses
3	380	19160	Mastectomy, partial
4	460	19180	Mastectomy, simple, complete
5	500	30420	Rhinoplasty, primary; including major septal repair
6	620	30450	Rhinoplasty, secondary; major revision

Source: *Federal Register* 8/18/88 (53 FR 31468).

which Medicare has determined are appropriately provided in an outpatient setting. Table 12 shows the 1988 rates for selected procedures falling in each category of service.

This system has the advantage of moving away from charge-based payments. Since 1987, hospitals have been required to code outpatient surgery by procedure code, so this type of payment system will likely continue to gain popularity with HMOs and PPOs.

Procedure-based payment for hospital outpatient and diagnostic laboratory and radiology procedures is also becoming more common. Here the shift has been slower since standard coding practices, such as a Medicare surgical procedure payment system, are not used by hospitals. Discounted charges are still the most commonly employed payment method for PPOs and HMOs.

Prescription Drugs

Discount arrangements for prescription drugs are common. Typically, contracts separate the payment into two components: the average wholesale price (AWP) of the medication and a dispensing fee. Generally, the AWP will be discounted 5 to 10 percent and a fixed dispensing fee will be negotiated. Often the fixed dispensing fee will be $2.50 to $4.00 per prescription and set at the Medicaid dispensing fee allowance.

There are specialty prescription drug claims services which will administer prescription drug benefits and may also assume the risk on a capitated basis. One of the major advantages of using such a service is to reduce the cost of the large volume of small claims to be processed for prescriptions. Many major pharmacy chains ease administration by processing prescription drug benefits and billing the managed care plan monthly.

A common cost-containment approach for prescription drug coverage is the use of a formulary. Under a formulary approach, the only drugs covered are those on an approved list. Participating physicians agree to limit prescriptions to the specified list. With this approach, only generic drugs will be listed when such drugs are available. Significant savings can be experienced under such programs.

Other prescription drug cost-containment measures used by HMOs and PPOs include:

- Mail-order drug programs, where "maintenance" type drugs can be obtained in bulk through the mail
- Direct discount from drug companies, where an HMO or PPO provides to the drug company a summary of payments made to pharmacies for specific drugs and the drug companies pay an amount directly to the HMO or PPO for the value of the discount negotiated
- Maximum allowable cost programs, where the benefit is limited to the generic cost and the patient must pay the difference between brand and generic costs if a brand drug is prescribed
- Exclusions of specific types of drugs, such as fertility drugs, nicotine gum for stop-smoking programs, and cough or cold medications

Mental Health and Chemical Dependency

Mental health and chemical dependency costs have increased annually at 20 percent or more in some HMOs and health plans. These costs commonly account for 10 to 20 percent of medical expenses in many groups. This increase is partly supply-driven, with a rapid increase in for-profit treatment programs. Managing these costs has become increasingly important for HMOs and PPOs.

To better manage these costs, HMOs and PPOs often limit the number of mental health and chemical dependency providers used. HMOs and PPOs will negotiate discount payment rates on a per visit, per day, or per treatment program basis.

Another common approach is to pay a specialty mental health or chemical dependency group a capitation rate to provide all psychiatric and substance abuse services. These third parties often provide services for several HMOs and PPOs in a particular market. They reduce costs through the use of salaried or contracted physicians and counselors and by obtaining significant discounts from area psychiatric and substance abuse rehabilitation facilities. Since payment is on a capitation basis, a strong incentive exists for these specialty services providers to refrain from overtreating patients.

ADJUSTING REIMBURSEMENT FOR APPROPRIATE RISK

Managed care plans have made a number of adjustments to the basic hospital and physician payment strategies which result in increasingly complicated payment systems. These adjustments have been made in order to limit specific risks, that is, risks which are not controllable by the provider or are not considered appropriate risks to transfer. In general, these adjustments are designed to address the following risks:

- *Demographic risks* related to the attributes of patients who choose a specific provider
- *Catastrophic risks* related to the experience of several large, complex, unforeseen cases
- *Other noncontrollable risks,* such as out-of-area services

The reasoning behind payment adjustments is to decrease risks inherent in the basic payment strategies which are either uncontrollable by providers or excessive for individual providers.

Demographic Risk

The use of health care services by a group of people will vary depending upon the demographic makeup of the group. For example, young men generally use relatively few hospital or physician services. Young women generally use more services, primarily related to maternity care. All people use more services as they age, with increased use of cardiac services and cancer treatment. Also, regardless of age or sex, the use of healthcare services will be higher in a group which has a history of chronic illness compared to a group of people with no such prior experience.

Hospitals and physicians have little control over the demographic characteristics of the members enrolled in an HMO; therefore, they are often reluctant to accept payment systems which do not make adjustments for the demographic characteristics of the patients assigned for treatment.

The following are examples of adjustments made to basic payment systems in order to reduce the demographic risk to the providers:

- *Hospital per diems which vary by type of service* Most per diem payment systems have rates that vary by type of service. For example, a typical contract would include at least the following categories:

Medical	$ 500
Surgical	550
Intensive care unit	1100
Obstetric	650
Mental health and chemical dependency	250

By using per diem categories, the payments to a hospital can be adjusted to reflect the nature of the patients seen and the services provided.

- *Age and sex capitation payments* It is common for both physician and hospital capitation rates to vary by age and sex to reflect the varying patterns of use which correlate with these factors. Table 13 shows a typical age and sex schedule for primary care, referral, and hospital services.
- *Diagnosis or severity of illness adjusted hospital rates* Some hospital payment systems vary the payment by the diagnosis or severity of illness of the patients using the facility. By adjusting for diagnosis or severity, the payment system can more accurately reflect the controllable service needs of the patients rather than be affected by the uncontrollable risks relating to patient case mix. For example, a per stay system based on Diagnostic Related Groups (DRGs) might pay the following amounts shown in Table 14 for a sample of DRGs.

Payment adjustments for patient demographics are generally not needed for the discount from charges or fee schedule approaches because the provider reimbursement is based on the volume and intensity of services rendered.

Catastrophic Risk Physicians and hospitals under risk-based reimbursement arrangements often seek protection for the costs of treating patients with catastrophic illnesses. Protection from catastrophic claims stabilizes experience, reducing claims fluctuations and avoiding the situation where the experience of one patient can wipe out any hope of

TABLE 13   Example of Age and Sex Capitation Rates

Age Band	Demographics		Primary Care		Referral		Hospital	
	MALE	FEMALE	MALE	FEMALE	MALE	FEMALE	MALE	FEMALE
<1	1.0%	1.0%	$32.00	$32.00	$ 7.56	$ 7.56	$22.17	$22.17
1	0.9	0.9	13.00	13.00	6.64	6.64	12.07	12.07
2–5	3.5	3.5	6.25	6.25	7.12	7.12	11.37	11.37
6–19	11.7	11.7	5.56	5.56	8.90	8.90	8.78	8.78
20–44	24.0	28.6	6.56	10.78	13.85	20.05	18.48	33.68
45–54	4.2	4.4	8.77	14.58	19.76	25.48	39.81	38.75
55–64	2.3	2.1	13.14	16.71	28.96	32.12	59.70	49.56
65 +	0.1	0.1	15.93	17.79	41.06	40.68	90.03	64.89

TABLE 14   Example of Per Stay Contract Using Diagnostic Related Groups

DRG NUMBER	DESCRIPTION	RATE PER CASE
21	Viral meningitis	$ 1,853
60	Tonsillectomy and/or adenoidectomy (only ages 0–17)	1,260
107	Coronary bypass without cardiac catheterization	18,614
373	Vaginal delivery without complications	1,493

recovering a withhold or experiencing a favorable risk-sharing gain. The following are common examples of payment adjustments made to protect against catastrophic risks.

- Physician capitations are commonly supplemented by fee-for-service type payments for patients whose physician service costs exceed an annual amount. For example, an HMO might pay 90 percent of all primary care charges exceeding $5000 in a year for patients covered under a primary care capitation system.
- When amounts withheld from physicians are paid back based on the hospital or referral service usage of that physician's members, the referral and hospital cost for individual members which exceed a predetermined amount will commonly be excluded when comparing the physician's experience against performance goals. For example, once patients incur $100,000 in claims, the entire referral and hospital pool of a physician could be wiped out. An HMO might limit the charges against the pool to $10,000 per patient to reduce the catastrophic risk.
- Per stay hospital contracts commonly have an "outlier" provision, allowing per diem payments to supplement per stay payments should a patient's length of stay exceed a fixed number of days. For example, the PPO paying the DRG rates shown in Table 14 might also include per diem payments for each day that exceeds a long-stay threshold (See Table 15). In this case, the per diem is calculated as 75 percent of the average per diem, based on the rate per case from Table 13 and the average length of stay (ALOS) from Table 14.

The adjustments to the payment system for catastrophic risks put a plan in the position of "reinsuring" catastrophic risk. For this reason, many plans attempt to coordinate the protection extended to providers with stop-loss reinsurance coverage obtained from an outside carrier.

TABLE 15 Example of Per Stay Contract Using Diagnostic Related Groups with Outlier Provision

DRG NUMBER	DESCRIPTION	ALOS	LONG-STAY THRESHOLD	PER DIEM
21	Viral meningitis	4.1	11	$ 339
60	Tonsillectomy and/or adenoidectomy (only ages 0–17)	1.3	2	727
107	Coronary bypass without cardiac catheterization	10.0	21	1396
373	Vaginal delivery without complications	2.7	5	415

When this is done, the HMO or PPO must be careful to use consistent descriptions of the stop-loss coverage between the provider contract and the reinsurance contract. Otherwise, it is possible that the HMO's obligations to providers may differ from amounts which may be collected from the reinsurer. For example, stop-loss provisions in provider contracts may call for reimbursement of *charges* greater than a fixed amount. Most reinsurance contracts, however, will reimburse HMOs only at *cost* to the plan after the application of discounts. The discrepancy between the contract terms may result in unanticipated expenses to the plan and create grounds for controversy between the plan and its providers.

Risk Adjustments for Noncontrollable Services

A number of other adjustments are commonly made to payment systems, particularly capitation or withhold systems, to reduce provider risk for services which the provider cannot directly control. Examples of these adjustments are:

- Removal from provider capitation rates or performance goals of "out-of-plan" services provided to members enrolled in an open HMO plan. Open HMO plans are similar to PPOs in that patients may self-refer outside of the provider network if they pay additional copayments or deductibles. If withhold returns are based on referral and hospital performance goals, charges for services rendered outside of the HMO network will not be deducted from the risk pool.
- Exclusion from hospital capitations of services which cannot be performed within the facility is common. When this is done, no deductions will be made from the capitation rate for services provided by other facilities.
- Removal of mental health, chemical dependency, and vision and hearing care coverage from capitated performance goals. Many providers do not feel that they can adequately control these services.

Considering the Financial Impact of Transferring Risk

The provider payment strategies of managed care plans transfer financial risk to create economic incentives to control costs and service usage. Without adjustment, these systems can, however, transfer risk to providers which in fact they are not in the position to control. For this reason, a payment system may be adjusted to shift demographic, catastrophic, and other uncontrollable aspects of risk from the provider back to the managed care plan.

In that managed care plans are insurance companies, they must maintain financial reserves sufficient to cover potential adverse experiences in the utilization and cost of healthcare services. Many plans have moved away from fee-for-service based systems specifically to reduce the risk to their capital by transferring risk to the providers who direct patient care.

By accepting risk, however, providers are in some ways acting as small specialized insurance companies. Since fluctuations in the experience of small groups of patients cannot be predicted with accuracy, the insurance risk for uncontrollable and catastrophic claims can be better absorbed by the plan than its providers.

The application of adjustment factors to the basic provider reimbursement systems can facilitate the transfer of appropriate risk to providers while leaving the plan responsible to fund adverse deviations beyond the control of such providers. In implementing such payment adjustments or developing new provider reimbursement systems, plans must carefully assess the potential risks reverting to the plans and ensure that sufficient funds have been set aside to offset potential adverse experience.

REIMBURSEMENT RISK MANAGEMENT FACTORS

Payers—whether insurer, HMO, or an intermediary PPO or IPA—relate provider reimbursement to appropriateness of care measurements. The process of applying measurement standards is carried out through the broad utilization review function. The focus of such programs is primarily threefold:

1. Determine necessity of service and, thereby, eliminate unwarranted procedures.
2. Identify least intensive setting (inpatient or outpatient; acute or intensive) or source (primary or specialty) for delivery of required care.
3. Prescribe parameters for expected duration of service.

The criteria by which appropriateness of care is measured is an integral element of the managed care process and is one which cycles through the total system. Prospectively, targeted service utilization is established in order to project the anticipated cost of care and, thus, the premiums for insurance products. In conjunction with actual service delivery, standardized utilization functions are invoked to determine the appropriateness of care to the patient's condition. Retrospectively, similar criteria are applied to measure conformity among provider practice patterns and to evaluate efficiency of performance relative to the projected utilization objectives. Thus, in managed care systems where the utilization standards actually reflect the practice patterns of the provider community, the cost of care can be predicted with reasonable accuracy and reimbursement strategies can be developed accordingly.

In actuality, however, providers who have traditionally considered healthcare as a service rather than as a business and who were accustomed to being reimbursed on the basis of actual charges are poorly positioned to assess their true unit cost and to determine their required operating margins under managed care programs. Without accurate data on the cost of providing direct services and covering overhead and related administrative expenses, providers are frequently hard pressed to evaluate whether case pricing, discounting, or capitation at levels proposed by payers can be profitable.

The potential profitability of alternative reimbursement strategies is also affected by factors beyond the control of providers. In negotiating discounts and other means of preferential treatment, plans will bargain based on the volume of business they control. The plan's general presence in the marketplace, however, will not necessarily result in significantly more business for the providers because existing members may be reluctant to switch providers and the plan's marketing efforts may not be focused in the providers' locality. Locking in the plan's business also does not necessarily guarantee profitable business, even when volume is generated, if the actual patient mix differs from projections as a result of the plan's particular marketing thrust. Further, as many tertiary facilities have found, the providers may end up treating the patients they would normally have received but would, under contract, be serving at reduced charges. Finally, in cases where multiple institutions have been contracted, patients may be directed through the plan's prior authorization process to the least costly facility. Thus, the hospital which succeeded in negotiating what appeared to be a better deal may not realize the anticipated volume and may experience adverse selection in terms of the severity of cases which are authorized.

Many of the shared-risk arrangements adopted by managed care plans incorporate provisions which tie reimbursement to performance targets. In signing such contracts, the providers are agreeing to meet or improve upon the plan's goals. Whether the plan's targets are realistic in specific, local markets depends on the compatibility of the actuarial assumptions with the practice patterns of the providers, cost of services, and the demographic composition of the plan's members in the providers' locale.

In selecting among health insurance options and in electing preferred providers within the chosen programs, consumer decisions will be driven by familiarity and perceived reputation of network care givers and by attitudes about the relative importance and value of healthcare access. Insurers must, therefore, work closely with employers to understand both corporate goals and employee characteristics in order to increase the predictability of service utilization. Similarly, insurers must recognize the philosophical leanings of contracting providers, including their attitudes about managed care and utilization review, their commitment to existing referral patterns, and their relative position in the medical community.

For providers and payers to assess the impact of these factors on the development and evaluation of appropriate reimbursement strategies and the effective operation of risk-based contracts, they must have access to reliable data. There is a continual need to track membership service utilization and costs in order to match actual experience against projected targets—prospectively, concurrently, and retrospectively. It is on the basis of such comparisons that the managed care model can be developed, evaluated, and revised to better support the objectives of consumers, employers, providers, and insurers.

Case Study 3 in the Appendix provides an effective illustration of the many factors which influence the behavior of all segments of the managed care system. It places into a larger context, the implementation issues related to some of the reimbursement strategies previously discussed. It highlights the effect of the behaviors and attitudes of insurer, purchaser, and consumer on the financial experience of providers and the viability of the managed care system.

FUTURE OUTLOOK   The experiences of the past 5 years are driving the health insurance system in new directions. More employers are now taking an active part in designing cost-effective benefit programs. As a result of these prevailing market forces, the distinctions between traditionally diverse products, delivery systems, and reimbursement methods are blurring. HMOs are experimenting with open networks, diverse provider reimbursement arrangements, and new forms of product design and experience-based premium rating. Traditional insurers are directing more of their business toward contracted providers. Consumers are making economic decisions to opt for obtaining services through managed care networks and generally finding that quality of care is not compromised.

As the philosophical and behavioral commitment of a significant portion of employers, providers, insurers, and consumers to the concept of managed care is growing, the necessity for redefining the terms of their interaction has increased. The evolving market forces and prevailing economic issues are pressing toward the establishment of long-term marriages between the sectors in place of passing relationships. The foundation for these marriages is in the potential economic incentives available to all parties, which affect how services are used, from where they are received, and how they are financed through a managed healthcare system.

The view of managed care programs as integrated systems recognizes the critical role of insurer, provider, employer, and consumer in shaping the effectiveness of the managed care process. It facilitates an understanding of the financial incentives which drive the system. It affords the flexibility to redefine the parameters of the total arrangement and its component elements based on experience to better adapt to the environmental changes and the longer-term objectives of healthcare cost containment.

APPENDIX

Case Study 1 — Hospital Capitation Contract

In 1987, a medium-sized hospital, which was part of a regional hospital chain, entered into a capitation arrangement with its largest physician group and a closely affiliated HMO. Prior to 1987, the hospital provided services on a per diem basis. The hospital agreed to this arrangement in order to:

- Maintain the existing business of the physician group
- Pick up the substantial amount of the group's referrals, which were going outside of the hospital system
- Direct the outpatient services previously going to vendors not affiliated with the hospital system to affiliated vendors
- Improve cashflow through monthly up-front capitation, since the HMO had a history of slow claims payments

The physician group wanted the capitation arrangement to improve its ability to budget costs because it was on a full capitation arrangement with the HMO.

The 1987 capitation rate was arrived at through a negotiation process where only limited experience data were provided by the physician group and the HMO.

The capitation arrangement called for a fixed monthly payment of $20.16 per member per month, which covered inpatient and certain outpatient services. At year end there was to be a financial settlement based on the inpatient days per 1000 experience of the group. If the days per 1000 exceeded a target of 280, the hospital would receive additional payments from the physicians. If the days per 1000 were less than 280, the physician group would receive additional payments from the hospital.

The financial experience of the hospital is summarized in Table 16. The 1987 experience was substantially worse than recoveries under the 1986 agreement. Furthermore, this poor performance occurred in spite of the fact that the total days per thousand was less than the target utilization.

The poor performance under the contract was primarily a result of the large volume of service sent outside the hospital system for which payments were made at rates much higher than the rate levels assumed in the calculated capitation. While out-of-system services were expected, since the hospital system could not provide some tertiary services, the majority of services performed outside of the hospital system could have been performed inside. Since there was no financial incentive for the physician group to move services into the system, the physicians were unable or unwilling to change their admitting patterns. Also contributing to the loss were outpatient services volumes which exceeded expectations and claims processing errors made by the HMO, resulting in overpayments (which were later resolved).

For 1988 and subsequent years, significant changes were made to the capitation arrangement.

1. The capitation was modified to only cover services provided by a specific list of affiliated hospitals and vendors. This created a strong incentive for the group to move patients into the hospital system.
2. The capitation rate was recalculated based on actual experience with an expectation of a service shift to affiliated facilities.
3. The days per 1000 targets were adjusted to cover only services provided within the hospital system. The adjustment was based on a per diem rate which gave increased revenue to the hospital if either utilization was higher than expected or more services were shifted in than anticipated.

TABLE 16   1987 Experience under Hospital Capitations
(in 1000s)

	SERVICES WITHIN HOSPITAL SYSTEM	SERVICES OUTSIDE HOSPITAL SYSTEM	TOTAL
Charges for services rendered			
Inpatient	$1205	$1114	$2319
Outpatient	456	357	813
Total	$1661	$1471	$3132
Payments under agreement	$952	$1138	$2090
Discount from charges	43%	23%	
Days per thousand	178	96	274

4. Outpatient risk sharing was established based on a target PMPM pool, with discounted fee-for-service payments made in the event that the pool was depleted.

With these modifications the hospital saw a substantial shift of services into affiliated facilities, which was both desired and expected. Furthermore, since facilities outside the system were not covered by the capitation, no deductions were made by the HMO and no claims overpayments occurred.

From the physician group perspective, the new contract provided greater incentives for utilizing facilities within the system and increased the providers' financial risk for patients sent outside of the system. Consequently, if all covered services were shifted into the system, there was little financial risk to the physician group.

Case Study 2— Comparing Primary Care Capitation Rates

Primary care physician payment systems used by HMOs have become much more complex than in the past. These payment systems have been redesigned to create incentives for primary care physicians to control the usage of referral and hospital services. This case study shows the analysis of three primary care capitation proposals made to a group of primary care physicians in a large midwest urban area.

The primary care proposals were from three IPA model HMOs. The proposed arrangements are consistent with the types of primary care capitation arrangements which are used in many areas of the country. The programs feature

- Age and sex distinct capitation rates and referral and hospital performance goals
- Withholds on primary care capitation payments
- Specific lists of capitated services with fee-for-service payments for non-capitated services
- Surplus and loss sharing for referral and/or hospital services

The three primary care proposals were evaluated to determine which offered the greatest reimbursement potential and the least financial risk to physicians. The steps performed in evaluating the proposals were as follows:

1. Age and sex population figures for the area HMO population were applied to the age and sex capitation rates and pooling rates to determine the average per member per month capitation rates and performance goals.
2. Noncovered services were evaluated to determine the fee-for-service revenue to be received by the primary care physician outside the capitation.
3. Referral and hospital goals were evaluated in light of the expected experience to determine the likelihood of withhold returns and surplus distribution.

The calculation of the average PMPM capitation is shown in Table 17 for HMO A. Similar analyses were performed on the other HMOs, as well.

TABLE 17   Calculation of HMO A Average Capitation and Pooling Rates

AGE BAND	Demographics MALE	Demographics FEMALE	Primary Care MALE	Primary Care FEMALE	Referral MALE	Referral FEMALE	Hospital MALE	Hospital FEMALE
0–1	1.9%	1.9%	$31.64	$31.64	$21.15	$21.15	$22.17	$22.17
2–4	2.8	2.8	13.63	13.63	7.53	7.53	12.07	12.07
5–19	12.5	12.5	7.43	7.43	7.53	7.53	11.37	11.37
20–29	11.4	15.4	7.09	10.72	12.41	33.31	8.58	8.58
30–39	9.6	10.0	8.78	11.82	15.66	30.10	18.48	43.68
40–49	5.3	5.7	11.04	13.17	21.97	27.66	39.81	38.75
50–59	3.6	3.6	13.96	15.31	31.73	32.14	59.70	49.56
60–69	0.7	0.5	16.78	17.23	49.43	39.66	90.03	64.89
Average	100%		$10.90		$19.75		$22.01	

Each primary care arrangement covered different services. Other services provided by primary care physicians which were not covered under the capitation were reimbursed on a fee-for-service basis. For example, HMO A excluded office surgery, radiology, and immunization serum costs. HMO B excluded only immunization serum costs, and HMO C excluded office surgery, laboratory tests, radiology, and the complete cost of immunizations, both administrative and serum costs. Table 18 shows the per member per month value of the services paid fee-for-service by the HMO. The utilization of services and cost per service developed in Table 18 are based on actuarial assumptions specific to the physician groups.

The third step in the analysis was to estimate the experience of the referral and hospital pools in order to determine potential withhold return and

TABLE 18   Cost of Primary Care Services Paid Fee-for-Service

TYPE OF SERVICE	HMO A UNITS PER 1000	HMO A COST PER UNIT	HMO A PMPM	HMO B UNITS PER 1000	HMO B COST PER UNIT	HMO B PMPM	HMO C UNITS PER 1000	HMO C COST PER UNIT	HMO C PMPM
Office surgery	78	$82.00	$0.53	Capitated		$0.00	78	$82.00	$0.53
Inpatient visit	Capitated		0.00	Capitated		0.00	Capitated		0.00
Office visits	Capitated		0.00	Capitated		0.00	Capitated		0.00
Periodic exams	Capitated		0.00	Capitated		0.00	Capitated		0.00
Well baby	Capitated		0.00	Capitated		0.00	Capitated		0.00
Pathology	Capitated		0.00	Capitated		0.00	675	9.71	0.55
Radiology	78	29.36	0.19	Capitated		0.00	78	29.36	0.19
Immunizations	304	13.19	0.33	304	$13.19	0.33	304	17.58	0.45
Miscellaneous services	Capitated		0.00	Capitated		0.00	Capitated		0.00
			$1.05			$0.33			$1.72

surplus distribution. The HMO A primary care capitation was not subject to withholds. Surpluses in the referral services pool were shared 50 percent by primary care physicians and 50 percent by HMO A. HMO B had a 20 percent withhold on primary care capitation. Half of the gains or losses in the hospital pool and all of the gains or losses in the referral pool were the responsibility of the primary care physicians. HMO C also had a 20 percent withhold. All of the gains or losses in both the hospital and referral pools were the responsibility of the primary care physicians. In both HMO B and HMO C, the primary care physician's responsibility for losses was limited to the amount of withhold funds. In each of the arrangements, different services were covered in the referral pools. For example, HMO C excluded out-of-area hospital costs from the hospital pool, while these were included for HMO A and HMO B. HMO B excluded obstetrics-related referral and hospital costs, while these were included for the other two HMOs.

Table 19 shows the development of the PMPM referral and hospital services cost, reflecting the services which were at risk for each HMO arrangement.

The final step in the process was to combine the information developed in the first three steps. Table 20 shows the development of the payments to physicians before considering risk-sharing recoveries and the payments to physicians after considering expected risk-sharing recoveries.

Table 20 shows that the HMO B capitation, before considering withholds or risk-sharing recoveries, is the highest. When withholds are subtracted and fee-for-service revenue is added, HMO B has the lowest per member per month capitation rate. If hospital and referral experience is poor, the physician will receive the minimum payment shown in this section. Therefore, HMO B has the lowest minimum recovery of the three HMO arrangements.

Table 20 also shows the expected hospital and referral risk-sharing experience, given a set of standard assumptions. In this example, HMO A physicians do not receive any surplus because no surplus is generated in the pool. HMO B physicians receive back their withhold plus an additional surplus of $.76 per member per month. HMO C physicians receive back part of their withhold equal to the total withhold funds less a $1.03 deficit in the referral and hospital pool. When the risk-sharing recoveries are combined with the payments before risk-sharing, it can be seen that the reimbursement for HMO B is greater than that for the other two HMOs.

As a result of this analysis, the physicians could determine that the HMO B arrangement presented the greatest potential recovery, as the referral and hospital pool amounts developed by the HMO were sufficient to cover costs, but HMO B also had the lowest minimum recovery should hospital and referral utilization exceed the standard assumptions used in the analysis.

Case Study 3 — Impact of Managed Care Design and Implementation

In a large metropolitan area, a major insurance carrier developed and marketed a favorably priced, point-of-purchase product which permitted members to receive covered medical services from both in-network and nonnetwork providers, although coverage of nonnetwork provider services was at reduced benefit levels. The plan rapidly gained substantial market share as a

TABLE 19 Cost of Hospital and Referral Services

TYPE OF SERVICE	UNITS PER 1000	COST PER UNIT	PMPM	HMO A		HMO B		HMO C	
				HOSPITAL	REFERRAL	HOSPITAL	REFERRAL	HOSPITAL	REFERRAL
HOSPITAL INPATIENT									
Medical and surgical	170	$ 650.00	$ 9.21	$ 9.21	$0.00	$ 9.21	$0.00	$ 9.21	$0.00
ICU and CCU	30	1000.00	2.50	2.50	0.00	2.50	0.00	2.50	0.00
Maternity	67	700.00	3.91	3.91	0.00	0.00	0.00	3.91	0.00
Mental health and substance abuse	30	350.00	0.88	0.88	0.00	0.88	0.00	0.00	0.00
Extended care	10	150.00	0.13	0.13	0.00	0.13	0.00	0.13	0.00
Out of area	4	1000.00	0.33	0.33	0.00	0.33	0.00	0.00	0.00
	311		$16.96	$16.96	$0.00	$13.05	$0.00	$15.75	$0.00
HOSPITAL OUTPATIENT									
Emergency room	150	$100.00	$1.25	$1.25	$0.00	$1.25	$0.00	$1.25	$0.00
Lab and radiology	180	122.00	1.83	1.83	0.00	1.83	0.00	1.83	0.00
Surgery	40	600.00	2.00	2.00	0.00	2.00	0.00	2.00	0.00
Out of area			0.10	0.10	0.00	0.10	0.00	0.00	0.00
			$5.18	$5.18	$0.00	$5.18	$0.00	$5.08	$0.00
PRIMARY CARE SERVICES									
Office surgery	78	$82.00	$0.53	$0.00	$0.53	$0.00	$0.00	$0.00	$0.53
Inpatient visits	134	49.50	0.55	0.00	0.00	0.00	0.00	0.00	0.00
Office visits	2123	33.47	5.92	0.00	0.00	0.00	0.00	0.00	0.00
Periodic exams	155	70.22	0.91	0.00	0.00	0.00	0.00	0.00	0.00
Well baby	240	25.13	0.50	0.00	0.00	0.00	0.00	0.00	0.00
Pathology	675	9.71	0.55	0.00	0.00	0.00	0.00	0.00	0.55
Radiology	78	29.36	0.19	0.00	0.19	0.00	0.00	0.00	0.19
Immunizations	304	17.58	0.45	0.00	0.33	0.00	0.33	0.00	0.45
Miscellaneous	216	11.80	0.21	0.00	0.00	0.00	0.00	0.00	0.00
			$9.81	$0.00	$1.05	$0.00	$0.33	$0.00	$1.72

result of the carrier's reputation and the price of the product, which was below most other indemnity plans.

When originally priced, several plan designs were developed which incorporated different levels of financial incentives for members to use the contracted network of providers. Deductibles ranged from $100 to $500 with family maximums ranging between $300 to $1000. The most generous plan reimbursed services of nonnetwork providers at 80 percent. The most cost-effective design reimbursed services of network providers at 80 percent and reimbursed services of providers without contracts at 50 percent. Projections of membership by product type were generated considering the expected demand for the products given the various plan designs.

In anticipation of the volume of business, the carrier was able to negotiate favorable per diems from quality hospitals. These hospitals and institutions

TABLE 19   Cost of Hospital and Referral Services (*Continued*)

TYPE OF SERVICE	UNITS PER 1000	COST PER UNIT	PMPM	HMO A HOSPITAL	HMO A REFERRAL	HMO B HOSPITAL	HMO B REFERRAL	HMO C HOSPITAL	HMO C REFERRAL
REFERRAL SERVICES									
Surgery procedures									
1. Inpatient	60	$681.53	$3.41	$0.00	$3.41	$0.00	$3.41	$0.00	$3.41
2. Outpatient	65	319.77	1.73	0.00	1.73	0.00	1.73	0.00	1.73
3. Office	122	127.73	1.30	0.00	1.30	0.00	1.30	0.00	1.30
4. Anesthesia	65	265.60	1.44	0.00	1.44	0.00	1.44	0.00	1.44
5. Assistant	10	303.62	0.25	0.00	0.25	0.00	0.25	0.00	0.25
Obstetrics	24	1650.00	3.30	0.00	3.30	0.00	0.00	0.00	3.30
Inpatient visit	84	55.78	0.39	0.00	0.39	0.00	0.39	0.00	0.39
Office visits	757	39.68	2.50	0.00	2.50	0.00	2.50	0.00	2.50
Consults	90	93.25	0.70	0.00	0.70	0.00	0.70	0.00	0.70
Emergency room	150	53.90	0.67	0.00	0.67	0.00	0.67	0.00	0.67
Therapy	145	26.95	0.33	0.00	0.33	0.00	0.33	0.00	0.33
Mental health	155	36.10	0.47	0.00	0.47	0.00	0.00	0.00	0.47
Substance abuse	30	36.10	0.09	0.00	0.09	0.00	0.00	0.00	0.09
Pathology	1685	14.60	2.05	0.00	2.05	0.00	2.05	0.00	2.05
Radiology	472	47.36	1.86	0.00	1.86	0.00	1.86	0.00	1.86
Immunizations and injections	46	24.10	0.09	0.00	0.09	0.00	0.09	0.00	0.09
Miscellaneous services	309	28.31	0.73	0.00	0.73	0.00	0.73	0.00	0.73
Out of area			0.22	0.00	0.22	0.00	0.22	0.00	0.22
			$21.53	$0.00	$21.53	$0.00	$17.67	$0.00	$21.53
OTHER SERVICES									
Home health	15	$80.00	$0.10	$0.10	$0.00	$0.10	$0.00	$0.10	$0.00
Ambulance	10	150.00	0.13	0.13	0.00	0.13	0.00	0.13	0.00
Appliances/DME	18	110.00	0.17	0.17	0.00	0.17	0.00	0.17	0.00
			$0.40	$0.40	$0.00	$0.40	$0.00	$0.40	$0.00
Grand total			$53.88	$22.54	$22.58	$18.63	$18.00	$21.23	$23.25

feared the loss of patients if they did not contract with the carrier and also anticipated increased patient demand as a result of becoming a network hospital. For the same reasons, the carrier was also able to contract, on a capitated basis, with physicians organized in IPAs around each of the hospitals. The physician panels afforded patients access to primary care and most specialty physicians, even though the number of network providers varied greatly among the IPAs.

The carrier was a new entrant in the local managed care market and had limited administrative and systems capabilities for conducting rigorous utilization review and experience tracking. This affected its ability to channel members, monitor service demand, and advise providers of their financial status during the contract year.

TABLE 20 Primary Care Payment per Member per Month

	HMO A	HMO B	HMO C
Payment before risk-sharing recovery			
Capitation rate	$10.90	$11.40	$10.80
Withhold	− 0	−2.28	−2.16
Capitation less withhold	10.90	9.12	8.64
Fee-for-service	+1.05	+0.33	+1.72
Total	$11.95	$9.45	$10.36
Risk-sharing recovery			
Hospital pool	$22.01	$19.85	$22.60
Hospital claims	−22.54	−18.63	−21.23
Surplus (deficit)	(0.53)	1.22	1.37
Physician share	✕ 0	✕.50	✕1.00
Hospital gain (Loss)	0	0.61	1.37
Referral pool	19.75	18.15	20.85
Referral claims	−22.58	−18.00	23.25
Surplus (deficit)	(2.83)	0.15	(2.40)
✕Physician share	✕.50	✕1.00	✕1.00
Physician gain (loss)	(1.42)	0.15	(2.40)
Total gain (loss)	(1.42)	0.76	(1.03)
Recovery to physician	$0	$3.04	$1.13
Payment after recoveries	$11.95	$12.49	$11.49

The first year's experience was as follows:

- The product which actually sold in the market provided traditional 80 percent coverage for use of noncontracted providers. To encourage in-network usage, coverage of services rendered by network providers was increased to 90 percent. These benefit differentials were not perceived as penalizing consumer decisions to seek care from noncontracted providers. The product appealed to purchasers who were cautious in moving employees from traditional insurance to restrictive managed care for fear of an employee perception of "benefit take-aways."
- Significantly different levels of in-network utilization were experienced among participating IPAs. In most cases, the full-service IPAs with many participating physicians had more favorable experiences. This suggested that the plan design incentives were not particularly effective in steering patients to alternative providers and served primarily to cement relationships which already existed with panel physicians.
- The out-of-network utilization among IPAs was generally very significant, in some instances as much as 70 percent, and substantially higher than assumed when the shared-risk agreements negotiated between the carrier and the physicians were formulated.

- The capitation payment to the IPAs failed to cover sufficiently the cost of care rendered to members that used the network. Furthermore, it did not offset the amounts charged against the accounts of the physicians whose patients were receiving care from nonpanel providers.
- Physicians were dissatisfied with receiving the short end of the stick and began to exert pressure on their affiliated institutions to rectify their losses.
- Physicians told patients about their resentment of the financial arrangement under which they were to treat members.
- Members complained to their employers and to the carrier about the unacceptability of provider attitudes.

When it came time for the settlement of risk-sharing between the carriers and the providers, and negotiations for contract renewals, four predictable reactions occurred.

1. *Providers* contested the proposed settlements citing failure on the part of the carrier to channel patients into the network and to adjust for the transfer of risk accordingly. The carrier was unable to produce sufficient evidence to the contrary and, in some cases, redefined the risk of the adverse experience and refunded portions of withheld amounts in the interest of continuing relationships with the providers. Some IPAs subsequently negotiated more favorable arrangements for the following year, while others terminated their contracts.
2. The *carrier's* anticipated profits were not realized. Utilization and cost experience did not sufficiently correspond with projected results despite having negotiated favorable contracts. The carrier's primary product was redesigned and repriced based on experience. The risk sharing with providers was revamped to reflect the level of financial risk which providers could support.
3. Most *employers* received substantial premium increases or elected the option of purchasing coverage which had more forceful incentives for network utilization. Certain employers who were expected to continue to have adverse experience were canceled. Some employers increased their efforts to encourage acceptance of managed care through employee education and redesign of company health benefit contribution strategies.
4. Some *consumers* who had negative experiences during the prior year elected other coverage when options were offered. Others who were satisfied with the plan continued their coverage even under increased financial risk for out-of-network usage. The impact of consumer dissatisfaction was sufficient, however, to prevent significant growth in aggregate membership. Despite the carrier's success in enrolling new members, prior subscribers and groups were disenrolling in virtually equal numbers.

This case study underlines the importance of understanding local markets in order to develop appropriate products, premium rates, and reimbursement approaches. It illustrates the influence of product and delivery system design on the utilization and cost of healthcare services. It clearly emphasizes the imperative to determine, with reasonable accuracy, the level of risk which is appropriate under prevailing circumstances, for both insurer and provider to assume and transfer.

Further, the case study demonstrates the very critical need of supporting managed care systems with comprehensive and timely information systems for projecting and measuring utilization and cost of services. Perhaps most important, it demonstrates the interrelationships between the roles of insurer, provider, employer, and consumer in the repercussions of behaviors and attitudes which shape the effectiveness of the managed care process.

POINT OF VIEW

Physician Payment Structures

PAUL B. GINSBURG, Ph.D., Executive Director
Physician Payment Review Commission, Washington, D.C.

The largest purchaser of "unmanaged" care, the Medicare program, has embarked on a serious attempt to change the structure of physician payment. The objectives are to remove distortions in incentives to physicians and to increase the "equity" of the payment structure. In addition, it is contemplating a formal tie between fee increases over time and the rate of growth in expenditures. Managed care is likely to be affected by these policies in a number of ways.

Payment reform is motivated by the conclusion that the "market" for physician services does not deliver what is usually expected of markets, that is, prices that reflect consumer preferences and provider costs

and provide incentives to allocate resources efficiently. As a result of the availability of extensive health insurance and the fact that consumers (patients) make important purchasing decisions when they are sick and worried, the pattern of payment is distorted. Technical procedures are overpaid in relation to visits and consultations when they are compared by the time and effort that goes into them. The geographic pattern of payment bears little relation to variations in practice costs. This gives physicians the wrong incentives concerning practice style, specialty choice, and locational choice. Many physicians consider the pattern to be highly inequitable.

An effort to change the structure of Medicare payments to physicians has been underway since the mid-1980s. Congress mandated a study of relative values and created the Physician Payment Review Commission in 1986. In 1987, on the advice of the Commission, it reduced payments for 12 major procedures determined to be relatively overvalued in

Medicare and exempted primary care services from general fee constraints.

In 1989, the Commission recommended a Medicare Fee Schedule based primarily on estimates of costs. Results from the study by William Hsiao of Harvard University, when revised and expanded, would be an important component of estimates of the physician input. The Commission devised a different method for integrating practice costs into the relative value scale. Payments would vary geographically on the basis of estimates of practice costs (for example, rent and salaries) but not on the basis of differences in costs of living.

To provide collective incentives for physicians to slow the increase in volume of services, updates in fees would be based on how growth in Medicare expenditures compare to a target. While this mechanism would not affect the incentives of individual physicians, the medical community would have incentives to improve peer review and develop and disseminate practice guidelines. These administrative and educational mechanisms would slow increases in expenditures by reducing services deemed inappropriate.

If these payment reforms come to pass, how will managed care be affected? For one thing, the knowledge generated—how current fees compare to costs and what services are effective—will be put to use in managed care systems. Also, the success of these reforms in the "unmanaged" sector will affect the relative attractiveness of managed care to patients and providers.

POINT OF VIEW

Managed Care Contracts Affect Hospital Bond Ratings

Nancy Rubini, Vice President, Health Care Finance Group

Standard & Poor's Corporation, New York, New York

Managed care contracts have assumed an increasingly larger role in Standard and Poor's hospital bond rating analysis. Since the enactment of Medicare's Prospective Payment System (PPS), virtually all acute care hospitals have faced severe cuts in reimbursement and declining admissions. In an effort to fill empty beds, many hospitals quickly entered into HMO contracts that proved to be a financial drain after a year or so. Increased HMO penetration in many cities created further incentives for hospitals to serve the growing HMO population. A variety of industry pressures, including unprofitable HMO contracts, have resulted in an unprecedented number of downgradings on debt issued by private nonprofit hospitals. Lower ratings signal increased credit risk and can mean higher interest rates for a hospital's future debt issues. As a result of managed care activity, S & P expanded its analysis of HMO contracts in assigning new credit ratings and reviewing more than 1000 existing ratings.

S & P's hospital credit analysis includes a review of operations, medical staff characteristics, the local economy, competition, and both historic and projected financial statements. Reimbursement details are analyzed with an emphasis on revenue composition. The average community hospital receives about 40 percent of its revenues from Medicare and about 6 to 8 percent from Medicaid, with the remainder coming from Blue Cross, commercial insurers, and HMOs and PPOs. In the early 1980s it was unusual to see a hospital with more than a few percent, if any, of revenues derived from alternative delivery systems like HMOs. Today, the percent has risen dramatically. In some cities where S & P maintains debt ratings on local hospitals, HMO and PPO revenues are accounting for a third of the revenues, and occasionally more.

Managed care contracts become a rating factor when the HMO or PPO has a strong market presence in the the hospital's service area or when the contribution to revenues is significant. Rating implications are positive when the contract both enhances the hospital's market share and improves profitability. Increased admissions alone are not necessarily a positive rating factor. The marginal revenue gained from an extra admission can vary depending on the hospital's cost structure and terms of the contract. The most common form of contract has been one where the hospital offers discounts on charges. Discounts range from a few percent to 30 percent or 40 percent

in some cases. S & P has noted many cases where the increased managed care patients reduced income since the discounted price failed to cover both fixed and variable costs. In these cases, HMO and PPO patients helped stabilize or even increased admissions but the benefit to the bottom line never materialized. In certain capitated contracts, hospitals lost money because the actual acuity level of HMO patients exceeded expectations and the hospital was left covering expensive resources.

In the future, contracts with HMOs and PPOs may become more favorable to the hospital. By trial and error hospitals have become more familiar with the contracting process and more accurate in pricing their services. Limits on length of contract and defined levels of maximum exposure to cost and acuity risk are now demanded by many hospitals. Their negotiating position should improve in cities where utilization declines are stabilizing and where managed care plans are competing among themselves for providers and enrollees. In some markets, hospitals have joined together, in both formal and informal alliances, to negotiate with HMOs as a group, often commanding better prices for their services. It is likely that discounting or other contractual arrangements with health plans will continue to occur as long as managed care grows in popularity and hospitals have excess capacity. At the same time, it is certain that hospitals will become more aggressive in protecting themselves from accepting too much risk in such contracts.

CASE STUDY

Florida Gulf Coast Health Coalition: Employer Analysis Pro Forma

FRANK M. BROCATO, Executive Director

RICHARD G. TRAPP, Chairman — PPO Task Force

CHARLES L. SCALIA, Project Manager
Florida Gulf Coast Health Coalition, Tampa, Florida

In late 1983 when the Florida Gulf Coast Health Coalition was in its developmental phase, the employer community identified premium increases ranging from 30 to 300 percent a year as their number one problem.

The proposed solution to this problem was based on the premise that the Coalition, as a consolidated group, would be able to achieve more and have a greater impact than any single employer acting on their own. Developing an employer-controlled preferred provider organization was one of the "group purchase" actions taken to prove that the premise was in fact valid.

The first step was to collect paid hospital claims data from employers in order to track where the companies' employees were historically going for healthcare. This was done to properly evaluate the charge value differentials among local providers. Case mix adjusted charge data were collected using DRG severity weights to adjust for provider comparability regardless of the level of services.

The collection of these data allowed the Coalition staff and membership to objectively select hospitals which had the greatest utilization by the majority of Coalition member employees and their dependents. The database study highlighted 25 hospitals out of 50 within a six-county area, which accounted for 92 percent of the employers' admissions. Based on utilization and case mix adjusted charge data, 12 of those 25 hospitals were then selected through a request for proposal process to become PPO providers.

The charge differential, adjusted for severity, provided a tool for accurately evaluating the value of services rendered for charges received. Case mix adjusted charges were then used in negotiating discounts at proposed hospitals. Charges varied from a low of $2400 per admission to a high of $6200 after severity was taken into account. This case mix adjusting procedure allowed several tertiary hospitals with high severity case loads and high unadjusted charges to come closer to the community norm, while some moderate to low severity case providers moved from the norm to become the higher-cost hospitals for care.

Request for proposals were then distributed to 85 hospitals, insurers, hospital management companies, and PPO administrators. Prospective administrators had to demonstrate that the PPO could:

1. Be "multicarrier friendly." Simply put, employers needed to continue letting their insurer or TPA process and pay claims, while using the PPO's negotiated provider discounts.

2. Collect claims data on a multicarrier basis.

3. Cover service-related malpractice law suits within sufficient limits that they could cover both the Coalition and employers.

4. Offer and monitor outpatient, mental health, substance abuse, and physician office services.

Out of the 85 requests for proposals, 55 bids were returned; of those bids, 40 were from preferred providers and 15 were from PPO administrators. Florida Health Network (referred to as American Health Network outside of Florida) was selected to administer the PPO under the supervision of the Coalition.

During the vendor evaluative phase, employers questioned the capacity of the PPO to generate adequate net savings. It quickly became obvious that the real problem with perceived PPO performance was not one of outcome, but rather the level at which financial incentives were being set to encourage in-network participation by employees and dependents.

Employers were all too often setting employee PPO financial incentives at too high a percentage. The question then became one of how to calculate what the financial incentive should be for each employer before arbitrarily setting the incentive at 10 or 20 percent above regular benefit levels. This could result in little or no savings at year's end.

The question of how to determine financial incentives was addressed by designing an employer rate

369

of return on investment pro forma which projected the break-even point which the incentive should not pass.

Take employer A as an example. Data were captured on the number of admissions and total dollars spent at each of the preferred hospitals (historically) over a 12-month period. The employer's historical admissions and average charge per admission were then compared to the Coalition's average. An average weighted discount was computed by multiplying the discounts at those preferred hospitals by the utilization rate (for example, the average *unweighted* "arithmetic" discount was 15 percent, while the average weighted discount, by utilization, per hospital among PPO hospitals for employer A was only 8.1 percent). Had employer A used the unweighted arithmetic average, 6.9 percent more in incentives would have been given than the hospitals gave in discounts. The end result may have been catastrophic for employer A, based on normal statistical averaging.

Employer A set the employee financial incentive below 8 percent and used stop-loss and utilization review savings to offset any increase in claims from higher than expected PPO use, thus, realizing a savings rather than a potential loss.

This pro forma, prepared prior to entering the PPO, projected an average 15 percent net savings per employer, which included both hospital discounts and utilization review savings. After 12 months of operation, the average employer realized an actual savings of between 14 to 15 percent of paid claims. The accuracy of pro forma projections has been consistently close to actual PPO results.

Another major indicator derived from the pro forma was the level of historical utilization within the PPO hospitals versus non-PPO hospitals. This indicated which hospitals the employees and their dependents used prior to the PPO marketing efforts. It also suggested the level of education necessary to get employees and dependents to use PPO hospitals. For example, based on 3 years' trend data, the Coalition was able to select highly used and cost-effective hospitals, which resulted in employer A having over 80 percent of its admissions at PPO hospitals. Only 20 percent of the employee base needed to be educated about PPO hospitals. Based on historical utilization patterns, this meant that employer A would immediately realize discounts on 80 percent of their admissions with little employee education.

If the results had shown only a 40 percent PPO utilization, then further employee education would be essential. In this situation potential savings due to employee shifts to more cost-effective PPO hospitals would be even greater.

PPO hospital costs *after discounts* (based on case mix adjusted charges per admissions) were predominately ranked in the lower fourth quadrant, that is, they were the best buy for services rendered.

The PPO network has grown from 4900 to approximately 22,000 employees in a six-county area with minimal marketing to date. As a result of this success, the Coalition designed and implemented an employee assistance program which was custom designed for and by its members. Dental and vision care are currently being evaluated as still other designed care products.

CHAPTER FIFTEEN

Utilization Review Techniques

IN PURSUIT OF VALUE: AMERICAN UTILIZATION MANAGEMENT AT THE FIFTEEN-YEAR MARK

ARNOLD MILSTEIN, M.D., Managing Director
LINDA BERGTHOLD, Ph.D., Senior Consultant
LESLIE SELBOVITZ, M.D., Principal
National Medical Audit, William M. Mercer, Inc., San Francisco, California

Curbing unnecessary utilization of healthcare services has been a cornerstone of America's 15-year-old broad effort to control healthcare costs. The lion's share of these efforts has been focused on eliminating unnecessary hospital days. This focus was fueled by relentless significant increases in overall healthcare costs and by specific empirical evidence indicating that circa 1980, roughly 40 percent of hospital days in America's fee-for-service system were not of value in improving patient health status.[1] Efforts to control ambulatory services have been comparatively sparse and have not been carefully evaluated.

By 1980, all Medicare hospitalizations and many Medicaid hospitalizations were subject to substantial utilization control efforts. By 1989, the same was true of the majority of hospitalizations covered by employee health insurance plans.

During the 1980s, the perceived importance and difficulty of fully successful utilization management (UM) has increased. This growth is attributable to three factors. First, physician unit price constraints, which are now commonplace in American cost management programs, cause utilization to increase.[2] Thus, even if preexisting utilization levels were optimum, the current cost management climate would be expected to create a new problem which requires utilization management. Second, the weight of available evidence suggests that utilization can be responsive to management. Third, evaluations of utilization review (UR) programs have suggested substantial variation in their effectiveness.[3]

This chapter (1) reviews primary methods of UM, (2) outlines the primary barriers which successful UM programs must hurdle, and (3) predicts changes in the next generation of UM. Since scientifically based assessment of UM is in an embryonic state, the foundations of this chapter encompass expert opinion and nonrefereed evaluation reports in addition to published research.

METHODS OF UTILIZATION MANAGEMENT

UM can be defined as deliberate action to induce a more economical mix of treatment inputs without sacrificing health outcomes. There are many interventions that fit this definition: the way in which providers are selected to be part of a delivery system, the education of providers in cost-effective treatment methods, economic incentives or sanctions to induce provider use of more cost-effective treatment, utilization review of inpatient and outpatient care, individual claim review, comparative profiles of physician utilization practices and costs across multiple patients. and patient-directed techniques aimed at curbing unnecessary service demand.

Provider Selection

One pathway to efficient utilization is to select physicians with efficient utilization practices and then induce preferential use of these physicians. Both health maintenance organizations (HMOs) and preferred provider organizations (PPOs), or preferred provider arrangements (PPAs) significantly rely on this UM method. One national PPO manager has estimated that excluding inefficient physicians via analysis of claims data reduced his plan's annual per enrollee healthcare costs by about 10 percent.

The analysts of one of the most widely described HMO failures, SAFECO/United Healthcare, cite flaws in initial physician selection as a substantial contributor to ultimate plan failure. Another closely related shortcoming was failure to use provisional physician membership status to facilitate postselection management of practice habits. "High utilizers" who were full members proved more difficult to subsequently terminate.[4]

A frequent barrier to careful physician selection procedures is the inaccessibility of meaningful data about individual physician performance and the expense of obtaining and reviewing it when it is potentially available. To gauge physician utilization practices, claims data, hospital discharge data, or actual medical records can be reviewed. Except for hospitals and large claims payers with substantial physician-specific databases on past utilization practices, obtaining this information before program start-up is often considered prohibitively time-consuming and expensive.

Compounding this cost barrier to meaningful provider selection has been uncertainty about whether historically inefficient physicians can be readily induced to practice efficiently via threat of termination from the PPO or HMO, utilization review, or other methods of utilization management. As a result, many start-up efforts have limited their provider selection efforts to elimination of an extremely small subset of physicians who previously have been sanctioned by a hospital, government-sponsored peer review organization, or state medical licensing board.

Provider Education

Educating physicians in the most cost-effective treatment techniques represents another possible method of utilization management. Until recently, physicians have been largely ignorant of the costs of medical care. In a series of studies in the late 1970s, physicians were surveyed about their knowledge of the costs of specific medical procedures. Their knowledge of costs was surprisingly low. In one study, community physicians estimated only 14 percent of medical costs correctly, and physicians in one teaching hospital estimated only 50 percent of costs correctly.[5] As recently as 1977, only 34 percent of American medical schools had cost-containment education programs for medical students or residents, and the effectiveness of these programs has been subject to considerable skepticism.

A number of studies have examined whether education can alter physician behavior by providing general information on medical costs or desirable utilization practices.[6,7] In one early study in 1971, an educational program reduced the rate of increase in the cost of laboratory testing for several months. Later studies found the decreases to be temporary, with a return to baseline after the program was terminated. When researchers at a university hospital attempted to control the use of medical resources by educating physicians about costs, their results achieved only modest reductions in the use of services and had no effects on overall hospitalization costs.[8] Their recommendations included several elements that can apply to any attempt to educate physicians: cost savings must be coupled with demonstrations of adequate quality of care for patients, the visible support of clinical authority figures is critical, practicing physicians must be actively involved in patient care decision making, and concrete evidence of excessive ordering of services must be presented to physicians.

A composite of research findings and practical implementation experiences yields the following general conclusion about education as a tool of UM. Education might have temporary effects, but without a continuing program, administrative support, and direct or indirect economic incentives, physicians lapse into prior practice habits. This conclusion is consistent with the principle of general behavior modification that newly learned behavior requires reinforcement or it will die out.

Provider Economic Incentives

Within the HMO industry, there is a wide diversity of opinion on the subject of using provider economic incentives to reduce unnecessary utilization. Incentive structures are similarly diverse. Careful empirical analysis of the effect of varying arrangements is in a very early stage. In addition, the cofactor of physician organizational structure —IPA fee-for-service, group practice, or staff model—has major implications for the applicability and effect of various incentive structures.

One of the lessons drawn from the SAFECO experience was that financial incentives of less than 10 percent of cumulative charges were not enough to change the behavior of physicians in a fee-for-service system. United Healthcare's physician gatekeepers were required to manage the care of all patients in their caseload, cosign all bills before they were paid by the plan, and share in financial risk for their patients' total medical care costs.[9] Although the plan did well during its first 2 years, it began to lose money in the third and fourth year, resulting in the plan's termination in 1982. Physicians could only lose a maximum of 10 percent of their fee-for-service charges, and that amount was deemed not enough to change behavior. Some estimate that a contingency of 20 percent or more would be the minimum necessary to change behavior. An obvious, but largely unexplored, cofactor in such incentive fee-for-service reimbursement is the percentage of physician caseload affected by the incentive arrangement and the resulting overall economic impact on individual physicians. As the percentage of the physician's *total* income which is affected by the incentive arrangement increases, the size of the incentive required to affect behavior decreases. The interaction of these two variables has not been systematically explored.

In most staff-model HMOs, physicians work on a fixed salary and receive equal bonuses if collective utilization by all physicians is kept below targeted levels for the year. A common concern about this approach by staff-model HMO medical managers is that when all bonuses are equal, individual physician behavior is too weakly affected, because individual practice variations are not linked directly to the incentive structure.

Is it necessary to have both incentives *and* penalties to alter provider behavior? Some studies have shown that financial penalties add very little to overall reductions in cost, beyond the contributions of data profiling and feedback.[10] A recent comprehensive empirical study[11] of incentives across multiple HMOs quantified the impact of different incentives and practice settings and separated effects on inpatient utilization from effects on outpatient utilization. For inpatient utilization, capitation was associated with a 7.5 percent reduction. This was comparable to reductions inherently associated with the group practice setting (9.6 percent reduction) and for-profit HMO setting (8.2 percent) and was substantially lower than the reduction associated with physicians who were paid on fixed salaries (13.1 percent). While this study did not examine the effect of various incentives on total outpatient utilization, it did examine their effect on primary care office visits. Incentives tied to individual physician performance or placing physicians at risk for deficits in the HMO's hospital referral withhold fund were associated with 10.5 and 8.1 percent reductions, respectively, in the frequency of primary care visits.

There is strong anecdotal evidence that physicians will respond to economic incentives if they are well constructed, large enough to get their attention, and directly related to their own behavior. In a large urban HMO participating in a Medicare risk contract, both the hospitals and physicians were capitated, with a goal of keeping hospital days per 1000 under 1850, which was more than 25 percent below local Medicare fee-for-service averages. For each day saved, the hospitals and doctors shared equally in the savings. This steep physician incentive structure was based on the logic that physicians can control admissions to the hospital substantially by taking more care in outpatient management and will have a strong motivation to do so if they share significantly in the resulting savings. For a Medicare population of 100,000 patients, this IPA-HMO was able to maintain hospital days per 1000 below 900 during the first 2 years without detectibly jeopardizing patient safety or patient satisfaction.[12] These extraordinary results are credited to strong economic incentives, clear linkages to specific physician behavior, and rigorous independent quality of care monitoring.

Equal in importance to concerns about the adequacy of provider economic incentives for economical utilization are concerns about excessive incentives and resulting jeopardy to adequacy of care. While causally linking overly potent economic incentives with insufficient services is frequently difficult, most HMO managers rate this danger as real and have adopted a variety of control measures. These measures include limiting the size of performance-based incentives to a maximum of 20 percent of base compensation or fee-for-service charges, expanding the unit of performance measurement from single physicians to small groups of physicians, and expanding evaluation criteria to include the results of patient satisfaction surveys and quality of care assessment.

Utilization Review

The essence of utilization review is the use of independent professionals to scrutinize and curb unnecessary services, usually before they are provided. Primarily directed at hospital bed use, UR has been the mainstay of most efforts to manage utilization. It encompasses preservice, concurrent, and retrospective review; second opinion consultation; and case management. Since the content and process of UR programs is widely known, this discussion focuses on factors associated with UR program success.

INGREDIENTS IN SUCCESSFUL UR As a complex interaction in a complex system, the number of variables on which good UR outcomes hinge is large. Based on experience at the National Medical Audit unit of William M. Mercer Inc., which consists of over 300 UR program performance evaluations, six components of UR programs seem most highly associated with their effectiveness:

1. *Reviewer knowledge* UR programs generally rely on nurses as frontline reviewers, who, in turn, refer questionable utilization to physician advisers. Mismatches in medical knowledge between review staff and attending physicians can account for a significant number of inappropriate approvals. Matching the previous clinical experience of the reviewer to the clinical area of the case under review seems to be important for purposes of both knowledge and credibility. For example, a pediatrician may not have the knowledge to fully recognize overutilization by an orthopedist or the credibility to induce a different approach, especially for more subtle forms of overutilization. While a pediatrician reviewer may be effective in persuading an orthopedist of the reasonableness of a 4-day, rather than a 5-day, stay for an uncomplicated lumbar laminectomy, he or she is less likely to induce a 3-day stay.

2. *Reviewer courage* Reviewer courage is important because attending physicians frequently experience UR as an unjustified dilution of their professional autonomy and may react hostilely to the assertion that their utilization practices may not be cost-effective. In this context, it takes special courage not only to question but to persist in encouraging change. Many reviewers are not comfortable with the level of measured confrontation that is critical to reviewer efficacy. As a result, they may inap-

propriately retreat in response to minimal physician resistance. While diplomacy and discretion are essential to maximum reviewer efficacy, reflexive retreat can significantly weaken UR program results.

3. *System integrity* For a UR program to work effectively, it must be free of major loopholes. For example, as recently as 1988, most UR programs did not examine the medical necessity of proposed elective surgeries. Thus, unjustified surgeries were approved if the surgery required at least one night of postoperative hospitalization.

Another aspect of system integrity is the ability of telephone-based UR systems to curb exaggerations by the attending physician of the severity of a patient's condition. Fully effective UR systems have developed inoffensive methods to minimize such distortions.

4. *Rigor of standards* Explicit in the written screening criteria and implicit in the physician adviser decisions of every UR program are utilization standards that can be classified in relation to three levels of rigor.

- Level 1 is the loosest, most inefficient level, representing the most extravagant forms of fee-for-service practice and obliviousness to considerations of cost effectiveness. This level is typically associated with over 700 annual hospital days per 1000 covered lives in a group health plan for active employees with average enrollee demographics.
- Level 2 is consistent with adherence to "average" or "prevailing" utilization practices and reflects elimination of the most deviant types of overutilization. Level 2 standards are found in many UR programs, and their use is consistent with 450 to 550 annual hospital days per 1000.
- Level 3 represents the most efficient practices compatible with patient safety and is embodied by the most successful HMOs. The result is 200 to 350 annual hospital days per 1000. This approach makes much greater use of practices such as morning admission for surgeries that require subsequent overnight hospitalization, outpatient settings for selected complex surgeries, and early discharges, often with home care, than programs with level 1 or 2 standards. Table 1 illustrates differences between level 2 and level 3 standards. The standards of American UR programs generally fall at widely disparate points along the spectrum between level 2 and level 3.

5. *Physician hostility* Telling a professional "how to practice" may risk offense to professional pride and spark hostility. The most effective UR programs train their reviewers in techniques

TABLE 1   Comparison of Two Levels of Stringency of UR Standards*

	LEVEL 2	LEVEL 3
Necessity of admission		
Routine approval of overnight stay following cardiac catheterization	Yes	No
Necessity of preoperative hospitalization		
Routine approval of preoperative stay for abdominal hysterectomy	Yes	No
Target length of stay		
Single level lumbar laminectomy	5 days	2–3 days
Elective cholecystectomy	5 days	2–3 days

*These examples assume absence of significant comorbidities or treatment complications.

that prevent or minimize such hostility. Such techniques include close familiarity with previously conveyed clinical information and sensitivity to the attending physician's time constraints. For example, using the attending physician to confirm patient identifying information is a patent waste of physician time and, accordingly, highly provocative.

6. *Supportive benefit plan design*   In order to be fully effective, a UR program must be supported by the underlying benefit plan. For example, many patients cannot be discharged from the hospital on the earliest possible date if home health benefits or psychiatric residential homes are not covered, and employees will continue nonessential use of emergency rooms if plan incentives do not discourage such utilization. Even the best functioning UR systems cannot be fully effective if plan enrollees are not well-educated about the importance of early notification of the UR system prior to elective hospitalization and not given financial incentives to do so.

THE QUESTION OF IMPACT   Quantification of the impact of UR programs is in a relatively embryonic state. Scientifically rigorous research has provided limited evidence on the cost effectiveness of utilization review. Most UR impact studies have been anecdotal and have not accounted for important confounding variables. For example, a mandatory second opinion program introduced at Owens-Illinois in 1983 was reported to have achieved cost savings of more than $4 for each $1 it cost to operate the program.[13] However, a detailed description of the methodology for calculating savings was not published, so the results could not be adequately evaluated. An especially problematic omission in this and most other UR impact studies is the failure to account for the cost of services which substitute for the services which UR has curbed.

The results of a widely discussed national UR evaluation study of over 200 insured groups, published in two rigorously refereed scientific journals, concluded that private utilization review programs appear to be effective in reducing hospital use and decreasing overall medical expenditures.[14,15] The study controlled for a variety of potentially confounding variables, such as employee characteristics, healthcare market factors, benefit plan features, and naturally occurring trends toward lower utilization. UR reduced admissions by 13 percent, inpatient days by 11 percent, hospital room and board expenditures by 7 percent, hospital ancillary service expenditures by 9 percent, and total medical expenditures by 6 percent. When the researchers analyzed employee groups with relatively high admission rates before UR was introduced, they discovered even larger reductions: a 34 percent reduction in patient days and a 30 percent reduction in hospital expenditures. The savings-to-cost ratio of UR for this high utilizing group was approximately 8 to 1. Although the study's methodology has been criticized for failing to take into account price escalation and its lack of generalizability to all UR systems, its findings constitute the most sophisticated corroboration of a general consensus among employers, carriers, and HMOs that UR can be highly cost-effective.

Individual Claim Review

In order to curb payment for unnecessary service, Medicare Part B carriers and Medicaid programs began in the early 1970s to review physician and other outpatient service individual claims after the service was performed but before payment was made. More recently, several software-based claims screening systems have been piloted and tested in HMO, PPO, and indemnity plan settings. The best known of these are based on a set of hard copy screens, marketed under the name *Patterns of Treatment* and originally developed for outpatient physician Medicaid claims in California.[16] Metropolitan Life, which transformed these screens into a software program, has reported that 75 percent of screen failures are associated with only 5 percent of physicians. Metropolitan targets their ambulatory utilization review program at this 5 percent and reports that such selective review produces minimal employee disruption and a savings-to-expense ratio of about 4:1.[17] Metropolitan had not yet publicly released detailed information on the magnitude of savings as a percentage of total outpatient claims or, more important, on the basis of the savings calculation.

Another utilization management company has used *Patterns of Treatment* screens in IPA-HMO settings. They estimate that 20 percent of outpatient dollar billings are screened into the "questionable" category and 50 percent of the questioned services are ultimately denied reimbursement based on a subsequent medical record review or failure to submit medical records for review. Of questioned physician visits, less than 1 percent are defended by the physician who delivered the care. Of questioned procedures, 20 to 25 percent are defended by the treating physician. Of these, the attending physician prevails in roughly 20 percent of the cases.[18] As in the case of the Metropolitan results, these findings have been orally reported and should be regarded with substantial caution.

UR firms have developed screens other than *Patterns of Treatment* in order to assess the medical necessity of individual outpatient claims. CAPP CARE, a national managed care firm based in southern California, uses proprietary physician claims screens that CAPP CARE calls "patterns of practice." CAPP CARE sends out 300 to 400 letters a month to physicians to let them know that CAPP CARE's utilization standards have been exceeded. They report that physicians are highly responsive and that very few follow-up letters are necessary. Overall, 3 percent of claims dollars are recovered by CAPP CARE's aberrant practice review.[19] Like Metropolitan, CAPP CARE also uses its screens in its initial PPO physician selection process and for multipatient claims data profiling.

One area where claims screens can provide a unique, even life-saving, benefit is in the management of prescription drug utilization. With 7 percent of all hospital admissions (and 23 percent of admissions for the elderly) alleged to be related in some way to drug interactions, managing prescription drug usage may become a high priority, as employers search for ways to reduce cost and maintain quality. At least one vendor, Value Health, Inc., has created a software program that uses claims data or prescription drug card utilization data to identify potential misuse of multiple drugs. Through these two sources of data, employers or carriers can identify all the drugs used by a patient, flag those that might produce both short- or long-term negative interactions, and notify the providers involved of these potential problems. In Value Health's 9 million life program, 20,000 warning letters are sent to providers each month, and in 50 percent of the cases, medication is changed as a result of feeding back this information to physicians.[20] Since this program is quite new, there is no adequate way to evaluate its effectiveness in reducing costs.

Multipatient Data Profiling

Using utilization and cost profiles of past physician performance across multiple patients in order to influence current physician performance is an essential component of comprehensive utilization management. Such profiling programs were implemented first on a large scale by PSROs in the late 1970s. These profiles focused on inpatient length of stay and did not appear to be associated with substantial impact.[21] With the advent of Medicare's prospective payment system in 1983, hospitals began profiling, by DRG, the average length of stay and charges for hospitalizations managed by their medical staff members. More refined profiling systems, such as Medisgroups and Severity of Illness Index, were subsequently introduced to improve the validity of interphysician comparisons by better controlling for severity of illness. Since these more refined profiling systems require custom data collection via full hospital record review, they are considerably more expensive to implement than profiling systems based on routinely collected data. The cost effectiveness of these more expensive profiling approaches is currently under investigation by public and private sector organizations.

Small area analysis[22] represents another important use of inpatient data profiling in order to influence physician practices. To date, the essence of this technique has been population-based comparisons of admission rates, by DRG, across small geographic areas. Its unique contribution as a utilization management tool is its ability to identify excessive rates of hospital *admission*, rather than excessive lengths of stay. Small area analysis by Wennberg and others resulted in physician behavior change when physicians were provided with profiles of geographic variations in hospital admission rates and elective surgical admission rates in particular. In one of the earliest studies to measure the effect of collective regional data profiles on physician behavior, Wennberg and his colleagues demonstrated a 40 percent decline in tonsillectomies in Vermont during a 4-year feedback program to physicians.[23]

Systems of aggregating multipatient claims or encounter data for *outpatient* care and then making interphysician comparisons were developed primarily by the HMO industry in the early 1980s. Many computerized profiling programs were developed and, while considered effective, were criticized for failing to account sufficiently for case mix. New outpatient case mix adjustment systems, such as AVGs, are now being pilot tested as a means of correcting this analytic flaw.

The question of how to achieve the most impact from conveyance of multipatient profiles to physicians with excessive utilization practices remains an area dominated by opinion rather than systematic investigation. Showing physicians how their practices compare to average patterns for a geographic area and/or specialty is generally believed to be more influential in changing physician practice patterns than general education in what constitutes desired practices. The simple distribution of comparative practice profiles, without conclusive value judgments, has been reported to change physician attitudes and induce more parsimonious utilization practices among physicians shown to be "high utilizers."

One authoritative source on HMO utilization management emphasizes the power of medical record review by physician peers to reinforce the impact of an aberrant data profile. Its power comes from its ability to penetrate counterarguments about sicker-than-average patients and the "smoking gun" quality of direct medical record evidence. When implemented with physician participation and an orientation toward education, the peer chart review can significantly reinforce the impact of data profiles.[24]

Patient-Based Techniques

Most utilization management effort has concentrated on controlling physicians, because decisions by physicians determine the bulk of medical care expenses. Education and incentives inducing patients to seek medical care only when appropriate is another important element of UM. Using cost sharing by patients to dampen service demand is a widely invoked strategy. A Rand study in the early 1980s provided convincing evidence that patient cost sharing can dramatically reduce utilization.[25] However, later findings indicated that the blunt tool of cost sharing was indiscriminate and resulted in reductions of *both* necessary and unnecessary care.[26]

A later controlled study at the Group Health Cooperative of Puget Sound examined the impact of more moderate economic disincentives on ambulatory visits in a group-model HMO. The study found that a $5 per visit copayment reduced ambulatory visits by 8.2 percent. This statistically significant reduction was greater for primary care visits than for specialist visits and among heavy users than among average patients.[27]

Education, rather than cost sharing, appears to offer more promise as a tool to selectively reduce *inappropriate* utilization. Several studies strongly suggest that written materials emphasizing self-care can significantly reduce ambulatory utilization.[28] A study of medical care utilization in a Rhode Island HMO found that the use of educational materials on the proper role of self-care reduced total ambulatory care utilization by an average of 17 percent in the experimental group. An inexpensive system of written communication was found to reduce the number of outpatient visits for the common cold by 40 percent in the experimental group of another study. Even the elderly, whom many researchers assume are more reluctant to change their habits and less likely to benefit from education programs, have been found to reduce their utilization of emergency rooms after the introduction of educational programs.[29] Unfortunately, none of these studies examined the critical question of whether the prevented services were predominantly unnecessary.

SIX GENERIC BARRIERS TO OPTIMAL UTILIZATION MANAGEMENT

Fifteen years of American UM efforts have revealed a variety of generic barriers. Efforts to improve the performance of UM programs must effectively cope with these common problems. Among the six most significant such problems are: (1) lack of effective execution, (2) absence of a gold standard, (3) claims data limitations, (4) medical records limitations, (5) professional autonomy, and (6) balance billing.

1. *Lack of effective execution* Skill in execution can profoundly affect net program yield. In one comparison by National Medical Audit of two UR firms serving the same population, net return on investment differed by more than 300 percent. In 1987, a major U.S. retailer was able to reduce hospital utilization by more than 10 percent by implementing a better executed UR program.[30] The previously described cofactors of reviewer knowledge, reviewer courage, system integrity, and physician hostility constitute the core of superior execution. As healthcare costs continue to outpace inflation, employers and carriers are likely to push their UR organizations to improve program execution substantially.

2. *Absence of a gold standard* The absence of a research-based "gold standard" for optimally efficient medical practice will continue to thwart UM for at least the next decade. This problem not only impedes physician's willingness to modify their practices but also creates liability risks for "leading-edge" UR organizations. Aggravating this problem are malpractice standards hinged to "customary practices" and the daunting task of integrating individual patient values into the determination of "optimum" utilization standards. On a higher level of aggregation, UM is also frustrated by the absence of methods to generate a population-based gold standard for utilization. For example, given a set of population characteristics (age, sex, geography, and morbidity levels), it is not yet possible to estimate with confidence the numbers of hospital days and ambulatory visits that would constitute the most economical route to good health outcomes. Accordingly, an employer who is told that a UR program has reduced hospital days per 1000 enrollees by 25 percent to 375 days, does not know whether "fat" in the form of excess utilization has been fully eliminated or whether a substantial amount remains. The absence of such a standard has stimulated both public and private research efforts that should yield a better reference point for gauging and improving the effectiveness of UM in the 1990s.

3. *Claims data limitations* Managing and evaluating programs to control utilization requires access to high quality claims data. Claims data are usually originated by provider billing clerks

and then key-entered by bill processing personnel working for carriers or independent claims administration companies. Although mundane in nature, errors and omissions in this information chain jeopardize meaningful data analysis. For example, studies of the accuracy of diagnoses on hospital bills consistently have documented error rates in excess of 20 percent, with even higher error rates on physician bills.

Data quality limitations are likely to be resolved in several ways: providers and claims processors will need to make a much heavier investment in quality control of bill data; paperless transactions between providers and payers will increase; and significantly greater use by employers and carriers of preferred provider arrangements, utilization review programs, and legislative initiatives will increase both the accuracy and range of information provided by doctors and hospitals.

4. *Medical record limitations* Though medical record review is a mainstay of current utilization management, imperfections in medical records pose considerable problems. Not all pertinent evidence is recorded in the record, and some recording is incorrect. Research has shown some significant variance between the medical record and videotaped "reality." In addition, outpatient physician records are notoriously spotty in the level of detail they provide. Unless and until there is more uniformity in the maintenance of complete medical records, this source of information will continue to be an imperfect basis for UM.

5. *Professional autonomy* One of the most powerful norms of any profession is the perceived right of its practitioners to make individual decisions without outside control. As UM systems encroach on this norm, increasing physician hostility, whether latent or overt, will inhibit UM staff. While training and careful selection of UR staff can reduce the magnitude of this problem, most UR staff sacrifice a degree of effectiveness in order to minimize the risk of overt physician hostility.

6. *Balance billing* In most indemnity plans, physicians "balance bill" the patient for services which have not been approved as medically necessary. In the absence of PPO or HMO contracts with physicians or hospitals to the contrary, balance billing thwarts most efforts at postservice utilization review and a small but significant fraction of preservice utilization review.

In summary, barriers to optimal utilization management are multiple. They include failures of knowledge, will, and authority. Successful UM programs generally have recognized these problems and developed explicit strategies to minimize their impact.

UTILIZATION MANAGEMENT: THE NEXT GENERATION

Utilization management is a highly complex process unfolding in a sector characterized by rapid change. For this reason, anticipating its next evolutionary forms is fraught with uncertainty. Based on current successes and failures, three primary changes seem likely.

- *Changes in sponsorship* Purchasers and health plan sponsors are aggressively seeking to transfer the financial risk for unnecessary services to providers through bundled reimbursement (for example, Medicare's DRG-based hospital payment system) and capitation contracts. As this transfer occurs, the primary sponsorship of UM will shift from purchasers to providers. In addition, purchasers increasingly will require independent monitoring of quality of care.
- *Changes in scope* UM will be applied increasingly to categories of service other than hospital bed utilization. Physician services, home healthcare, and chiropractic services will be more extensively managed. Much of this review will be conducted by specialized managed care companies or subunits of comprehensive managed care companies. These specialized units will focus on the review of service categories such as mental health, high-risk pregnancies, catastrophic cases, chiropractic services, and podiatry.

  The impact of these more focused efforts may be even greater than that of first-generation nonspecialized UM programs. Ford Motor Company's specialized UM program for podiatry reduced the number of annual podiatric interventions per 1000 Ford employees in Detroit from 160 to 6. Program managers estimate that roughly one-third of Detroit's podiatrists relocated elsewhere after the program was initiated.[31] A company specializing in UM of surgical indications was able to dissuade 10 percent of proposed elective procedures in a large pilot project by AEtna in Texas.[32] With some studies indicating that 20 to 40 percent of laboratory testing in hospitals is unnecessary or inappropriate,[33] these and other ancillary services are likely to draw new utilization management efforts in the 1990s.
- *Changes in methods* The need for good data will drive both purchasers and providers to develop more sophisticated data collection systems, better ways of identifying over- and underutilization problems, faster compilation and analysis of data, and more reliable profiles of providers whose behavior lies substantially outside the norms of efficient practice. UM standards will be rooted in a better-developed body of scientific evidence. This, in turn, will allow UM decisions to be made more confidently and accepted more readily by physicians and patients. The ability of review staff to influence physician behavior will be enhanced by more sophisticated knowledge of methods and training in the

"science" of persuasion. In short, utilization management staff will know more, feel more confident about what they know, and be more persuasive in their dealings with physicians.

Utilization management is at the vortex of what many observers have deemed a revolution in American healthcare. By opting for utilization management, the majority of payers have adopted a once heretical view that determinations of what generally accepted services would be of value to particular patients cannot be fully entrusted to the treating physician. Early implementation of utilization control methods has been highly imperfect, as pioneers struggled to understand the complex system in which their efforts were embedded and heavily relied on available resources, like claims data, which were often designed for other purposes.

A 15-year-old implementation process has generated a much better understanding of the most imposing barriers to success and more refined solutions. As this process continues, the central objective of assuring health service value will be increasingly well served.

REFERENCES

1. Willard Manning, A. Liebowitz, G. Goldberg, W. H. Rogers, and J. P. Newhouse, "A Controlled Trial of the Effect of a Prepaid Group Practice on Use of Services," *New England Journal of Medicine* **310**(23): 1505–1510, June 7, 1984.

2. Thomas H. Rice, "The Impact of Changing Medicare Reimbursement Rates on Physician-Induced Demand," *Medical Care* **21**(8): 803–815 (August 8, 1983).

3. Arnold Milstein, Marvis Oehm, and Geraldine Alpert, "Gauging the Performance of Utilization Review," *Business and Health* 10–12, (February, 1987).

4. Stephen Moore, Diane Martin, and William Richardson, "Does the Primary Care Gatekeeper Control the Costs of Health Care?" *New England Journal of Medicine* **309**(22): 1400–1404 (December 1, 1983).

5. John Eisenberg and Sankey Williams, "Cost Containment and Changing Physicians' Practice Behavior: Can the Fox Learn to Guard the Chicken Coop?" *Journal of American Medical Association* **246**(19): 2195–2201 (November 13, 1981).

6. Steven Schroeder, L. L. P. Meyers, S. J. McPhee, J.A. Showstack, D. W. Simborg, and S. A. Chapman, "The Failure of Physician Education as a Cost Containment Strategy: Report of a Prospective Controlled Trial at a University Hospital," *JAMA* **252**(2): 225–230 (1984).

7. A. R. Martin, M. A. Wolf, L. A. Thibodeau, V. Dzau, and E. Braunwold, "A Trial of Two Strategies to Modify the Test-Ordering Behavior of Medical Residents," *New England Journal of Medicine* **303**: 1330–1336 (1980).

8. Stephen J. McPhee, Susan A. Chapman, Lois P. Myers, Steven A. Schroeder, and Janice K. Leong, "Lessons for Teaching Cost Containment," *Journal of Medical Education* **59**: 722–729 (September 1984).

9. Moore, op. cit.

10. J. D. Restuccia, S. M. C. Payne, and C. H. Welge, "Reducing Inappropriate Use of Inpatient Medical/Surgical and Pediatric Services," Report on HCFA Contract No. 18-C-98317/1-02 (Boston, Mass.): Health Care Research Unit, University Hospital, 1986; D. K. Freeborn, D. Baer, M. R. Greenlick, and J. W. Bailey, "Determinants of Medical Care Utilization: Physician's Use of Laboratory Services," *American Journal of Public Health* **62**: 846–853 (1972).

11. Alan L. Hillman, M. Pauly, and J. Kerstein, "How Do Financial Incentives Affect Physicians' Clinical Decisions and the Financial Performance of HMOs?" *New England Journal of Medicine* **321**(2): 86–92 (July 13, 1989).

12. Facts quoted by Dr. Tom Mayer, formerly with FHP, a Medicare Risk Contract HMO, and currently with National Medical Audit, Los Angeles, California (December 1988).

13. Richard T. Hanley and Jacquelyn T. Ayers, "Second Opinion: A Tool to Save Money, Improve Care," *Business and Health*, March 1985, as quoted in *Medical Benefits* 1 (March 31, 1985).

14. Paul Feldstein, T. Wickizer, and J. R. C. Wheeler, "The Effects of Utilization Review Programs on Healthcare Use and Expenditures," *New England Journal of Medicine* **318**(20): 1310–1314 (May 19, 1988).

15. Thomas Wickizer, J. Wheeler, and P. Feldstein, "Does UR Reduce Unnecessary Hospital Care and Contain Costs?," *Medical Care* **27**(6): 632–645 (June 1989).

16. "Patterns of Treatment" was created by Dr. Donald Harrington of Concurrent Review Technology, Inc., and adapted for use by Metropolitan Life's Ambulatory Utilization Review program in 1988.

17. Memo to Group Field Personnel from Anthony Treni, vice president, Metropolitan Life, 1989.

18. Interview with Alex Swedlow, Mercer/NMA, December 1988, based on information conveyed by Michael Spinharney, a representative of Utilization Management Systems.

19. Interview with Ed Zalta, president of CAPP CARE, December 1988.

20. Interview with Rick Lee, vice president, Value Health, Inc., December 1988.

21. Nancy Adler and Arnold Milstein, "Evaluating the Impact of Physician Peer Review: Factors Associated with Successful PSROs," *American Journal of Public Health* **73**(10): 1182–1185, October 1983.

22. John Wennberg and A. Gittelsohn, "Variations in Medical Care Among Small Areas," *Scientific American* **246**(4): 120–134 (April 1982).

23. John Wennberg, L. Blowers, R. Parker, and A. Gittelsohn, "Changes in Tonsillectomy Rates Associated with Feedback and Review," *Pediatrics* **59**(6): 821–826 (June 1977); also see John Wennberg and A. Gittelsohn, "Small Area Variations in Healthcare Delivery," *Science* **182**: 1102–1108 (1973).

24. Interview with Richard Cooper, former vice president of Health America, December 12, 1988.

25. Joseph F. Newhouse, W. G. Manning, C. N. Morris et al., "Some Interim Results from a Controlled Trial of Cost Sharing in Health Insurance," *New England Journal of Medicine* **305:** 1501–1507 (1981).

26. Albert Siu, F. A. Sonnenberg, W. G. Manning, et al., "Inappropriate Use of Hospitals in a Randomized Trial of Health Insurance Plans," *New England Journal of Medicine* **315**(20): 1259–1266 (November 13, 1986).

27. Daniel Cherkin, L. Grothaus, and E. Wagner, "The Effect of Office Visit Co-Payments on Utilization in a Health Maintenance Organization," *Medical Care* **27**(11): 1036–1045 (November 1989).

28. Donald Vickery, Howard Kalmer, Debra Lowry et al., "Effect of a Self-Care Education Program on Medical Visits," *Journal of the American Medical Association* **250**(21): 2952–2956 (2 December 1983).

29. Telephone call to Blue Cross of California regarding results from their HealthTrac plan for seniors, November 1988.

30. Payer data from two Mercer/NMA clients.

31. Linda Demkovich, "Controlling Healthcare Costs at General Motors," *Health Affairs* **5:** 58–67 (Fall 1986).

32. Interview with Rick Lee of Value Health.

33. John Eisenberg, S. Williams, L. Garner, R. Viale, and H. Smits, "Computer-Based Audit to Detect and Correct Overutilization of Laboratory Tests" *Medical Care* **15:** 915–921 (November 1977).

CAPP CARE: *Utilization Review of Ambulatory Services*

NIGEL ROBERTS, M.D., Project Director,
Medicare Demonstration
ED ZALTA, M.D., Chief Executive Officer
CAPP CARE, Fountain Valley, California

CAPP CARE is a utilization management company and a preferred provider organization. It undertook an extensive review of its ambulatory services in 1988 in order to quantify the extent of billing errors by physicians, payers, and patients. The results illustrate the need for a comprehensive utilization review program to monitor the appropriateness of ambulatory services.

The review covered 2 million line items on claims from physicians for services in 1988. These items totaled approximately $214 million: $79 million was for physicians' office services and $135 million was for services rendered in hospitals or other healthcare facilities. There were over 5000 surgical procedures which were billed above $500 and nearly 6500 hospital admissions.

CAPP CARE performed prospective, concurrent, retrospective, and ambulatory review services. The claims data were screened by the computer edits shown in Table 1. For the purposes of this case study, six categories of review were selected to illustrate the types of coding and billing abuses by physicians, errors of data entry by payers, and duplicate billing by patients (see Table 2).

PHYSICIANS

The principal categories of errors are discharge day codes, maternity and surgery package fees, and hospital visit codes.

Discharge Day Codes

These codes are appropriately used when the physician examines the patient, discusses the hospital stay, instructs the patient as to continuing care, and prepares the discharge records. This code must be used for the final day of a multiple stay in excess of 3 days. As such a hospital visit carrying a Physician's Cur-

TABLE 1   Categories of Ambulatory Review

VOLUME AND INTENSITY OF SERVICE

Practice patterns
  Upcoding of office visits
  Frequency of consultations
  Frequency of x-rays and ultrasound
  Frequency of laboratory tests
  Frequency of injections
  Frequency of referrals
  Frequency of visits by diagnosis
Misuse of procedure and service codes
  Misuse of new patient codes
  Misuse of anesthesia times
  Misuse of hospital discharge codes
  Misuse of phlebotomy codes
  Misuse of breast cysts excision codes
  Misuse of medical service codes by mental health
    professionals
  Misuse of office visit codes for physical therapy
Billing errors
  Hospital and office visits during follow-up period
  Surgery charges without hospitalization
  Anesthesia charges without surgery
Fragmentation
  Surgery package fee
  Maternity package fee
  Exploratory laparotomy
  Extended anesthesia times
Quality issues
  Readmissions within 31 days
  Caesarean section rate
  Failed outpatient therapy

CONTRACT COMPLIANCE

Noncompliance issues
  Failure to obtain prior authorization
  Admission to noncontracted facility
  Billing for archaic procedures
  Billing for assistant surgeons in absence of
    medical need
  Billing for cosmetic procedures and experimental
    procedure
  Unnecessary hospitalization
  Data entry by payers

TABLE 2   Miscodings, Frequency, and Cost of Ambulatory Services in 1988

CATEGORY	TOTAL	NUMBER OF MISCODINGS	FREQUENCY	SAVINGS
Discharge day codes	868	74	8%	$ 780
Maternity package fee	1087	208	13	220,000
Surgery package fee	4253	663	16	317,000
Hospital visit without facility charge	5131	317	6	37,000
New patient code (90020)	6680	921	13	59,000
Surgery charge without facility charge	5340	2004	37	850,000
Total				$1,483,780

rent Procedural Terminology (CPT) code of 90292 commands a higher reimbursement than does a routine hospital visit. In the cohort of claims studied during 1988, this code was used 868 times and was found to be in error 74 times. The most common reasons cited by physicians were that their offices failed to comprehend the code. Savings from these 74 instances would have totaled $780; however, the cost of obtaining refunds and attributing them to the individual payer was greater.

Maternity Package Fees
Unbundling maternity package fees accounted for a 19 percent billing error rate and resulted in the overpayment of approximately $220,000 during the study period. As specified in the CPT manual, the maternity package fee includes antepartum care, delivery, and postpartum care. The manual is quite specific about the definition of each component of care.

Surgery Package Fees
Surgery fees, or global surgical fees, are the reimbursement method for the majority of surgical procedures. These global fees include the preoperative evaluation of the patient, all hospital visits, and a specified length of time following the surgery as an outpatient. There was a billing error in which the surgical fee was unbundled in 16 percent of all surgical bills. The errors amounted to overpayment of $317,000.

Charges for Hospital Visits in the Absence of Hospital Claims
In 6 percent of all claims for acute hospital care, there were errors which amounted to overpayments of $37,000. The most frequent findings were that the physicians charged emergency room visits as hospi-

tal visits and that there were bills for hospital visits after the patient had been discharged.

PAYERS
Transpositions of numbers during data entry result in miscodings. There were 6680 new patient codes (CPT # 90020) submitted during 1988; 1177 were not new patients as defined by the CPT guidelines. In 256 (21 percent) of the miscoded visits, the payer data entry had entered 90200 (an initial hospital visit) and not 90020 (a new patient visit, comprehensive service). However, there were 921 incorrect new patient codes, of which 270 were multiple infractions. The misuse of the "new patient" code caused overpayment of $59,000.

PATIENTS
The computer program that is used has edits for the payment of claims from physicians for surgical procedures normally performed in an acute care facility or free-standing outpatient surgical center in the absence of claims for facility charge. There were 1060 such instances. Fewer than 3 percent of these claims were errors in coding and billing for canceled surgery and transposition errors by the payers. The majority of errors were due to patients who submitted claims to multiple payers without indicating the existence of other coverage. Coordination of benefit agreements preclude the collection of more than the billed amount for services.

Employer demands for prompt payment of all medical claims prevent payers from holding claims for surgical procedures until a facility charge is received. This sets up the milieu for double payment, which often will result in the patient receiving substantially more than the total amount charged. The patient pays the physician in full and keeps the remainder. In this way the benefit design, which may call for a copayment by the patient as a method for reducing unnecessary services, is circumvented, and it actually encourages the patient to have medical services. Had there been a method by which coordination of benefits could be determined, the amount recovered would have been in excess of $850,000.

MODIFICATION OF PHYSICIAN BEHAVIOR

During 1988, there were 5531 instances of errors or misuse of procedure codes detected by the CAPP CARE edits. Only 571 of these were repeat infractions.

The CAPP CARE program identifies potential abuse of billing codes. The CAPP CARE program also identifies practice pattern anomalies, quality issues, and contract compliance (Table 1). Letters are generated individually on any aberration. There is also a newsletter that summarizes potential billing problems and summarizes the more frequently found aberrations. This newsletter is distributed to all CAPP CARE members.

As a result of this program, CAPP CARE physicians are asked to refund overpayments. In instances where overpayments were not refunded, physicians resigned from the PPO.

It appears that the screening process and the ongoing education of the CAPP CARE physicians is successful in not only reducing billing errors and mis-

codings, but also in reducing the intensity of the office visit.

When the CAPP CARE contracted providers (that is, PPO members) were compared to the non-CAPP CARE members, there was a reduction in intensity of service determined by the charge per encounter. The charge for a CAPP CARE member averaged $102 and that for the non-CAPP CARE member averaged $122.

This difference in the intensity of service would amount to a saving of $17.5 million if there had been a reduction of $20 per visit for the 876,210 physician encounters by non-CAPP CARE physicians. The $20 difference per visit appears to be due to a reduction in the ancillary tests ordered at the time of the office visit. The total saved or potentially saved from these computerized reviews was in excess of $19 million or 8.9 percent of total physician claims.

In summary, errors and misuse of billing codes in claims submission to payers occur. They are not simply related to hospital billing practices but are common to providers, payers themselves, and patients.

The savings accruing to payers through review of ambulatory services is very significant. When added to the savings achieved by CAPP CARE for its payers through a 35 percent reduction in the frequency of use of hospital services, the total savings produced by a vertically integrated program of complete utilization management results in the development of a truly preferred provider network. It also significantly reduces the costs of healthcare services with savings-to-cost ratios exceeding 25:1.

CASE STUDY

Provider Selection

ED ZALTA, M.D., Chief Executive Officer

CAPP CARE, Fountain Valley, California

The task of selecting cost-effective quality-conscious providers to be members of a preferred provider organization (PPO) is not an easy one. It is, however, a process that must be undertaken if the PPO is to provide its users with a degree of certainty that the objective is quality care at reasonable cost. The selection process cannot be an arbitrary one. Nor can it rely on the "good old boy" methodology. Rather, definite criteria must be established and implemented during the selection process and maintained during the term of the agreement.

CAPP CARE has established uniform criteria for its selection process and membership retention. It attempts to assure objectivity while giving meaning to the term "preferred" in the phrase "preferred provider organization."

CAPP CARE maintains computerized data on every physician in the United States with a cross-reference to state license. The following biographical data are on file and updated quarterly: name, title, address, phone numbers, hospital affiliations, specialty, board certification, date of birth, and school of graduation. In addition, data on past disciplinary actions against providers by state licensing agencies, Medicare and Medicaid programs, or other disciplinary bodies are maintained and updated.

Using the extensive claims data files received from payers, CAPP CARE develops a practice profile on all providers, members and nonmembers, who have submitted claims. Claims data are run against screens which are designed to detect billing irregularities and noncompliance with contract provisions. The claims data are aggregated and totals compared to specialty specific standards designed to detect aberrations in volume (for example, x-rays, injections, and laboratory procedures) and intensity of services (for example, upcoding and CPT creep). Frequency percentages are calculated for each provider to determine the rate of injections, use of codes with higher reimbursements, laboratory tests, x-ray procedures, and visits. Computerized audit programs detect errors or misuse of new patient codes, consultation codes, upcodings, readmission rates, complication rates, unbundling of surgical services, errors in billing for hospital services, excessive referrals, duplicate billings, and variations in intensity of services.

Two categories of provider are typically excluded from a solicitation for membership and do not receive an application: providers not in active practice and those with known past disciplinary problems, coding irregularities, high volume and intensity percentages, hospital disciplinary actions, or drug or substance abuse records. In a "mature" market with a significant volume of payer pooled claims data, the percentages of M.D.s, D.O.s, and podiatrists excluded from membership typically exceeds 33 percent.

Providers solicited for membership undergo an additional level of review prior to acceptance. Each must maintain professional liability coverage and have an acceptable record of hospital staff privileges.

In spite of the rigorous selection process, monitoring providers and applying sanctions is essential. Some providers will ignore contractually agreed-upon cost-containment provisions of their contract. Others will be admitted to drug and substance abuse programs or disciplined by a federal or state agency. These providers must be granted due process and placed on probation; their membership may be terminated when warranted.

CAPP CARE's initial thrust is to educate participating providers in the appropriate use of codes to describe services. Advice is provided by a large staff of specially trained personnel through regular communication and on an individual basis. This program has not always been successful. During the past 4 years, over 2000 providers have been placed on probation because of their failure to follow the tenets of their contract. An additional 1238 providers have either resigned or been terminated because of noncompliance or aberrancies in the frequency and volume of services. This rate of attrition represents a 5 percent termination rate. This is a high percentage given the rigorous selection process and provides evidence that contract monitoring and review is essential in order to maintain a network of truly preferred providers.

Quality care is cost-effective. The selection and maintenance of high quality physicians who provide quality care will result in significant and immediate reductions in medical care costs and the higher costs of care resulting from technological advances will be made more affordable.

POINT OF VIEW

It Is Time for Science-Based Managed Care

ROBERT E. PATRICELLI, President and Chief Executive

Value Health, Inc., Avon, Connecticut

Managed care is in a grim horse race. It is a race to establish its own credibility in the face of continually rising healthcare costs and a race to achieve some success before the forces for a legislative solution gain ascendancy.

The principal techniques of managed care to date are in fact quite limited:

- Create networks of doctors and hospitals and seek unit price discounts from them in return for promises of increased patient volume

- Seek to put these networks at financial risk for excessive utilization through withholds or capitation

- Manage the setting or location of care toward less costly alternatives through techniques such as hospital preadmission certification, continued stay review, discharge planning, and case management.

These three techniques represent most of the managed care techniques. Have they worked? Only in a limited way. Some of what has been achieved is cost shifting—from those who have discounts to those who do not, and from inpatient to outpatient cost centers. Costs in managed care systems are rising more slowly than in unbridled fee-for-service and indemnity insurance, but not slowly enough. Hospital days per thousand in HMOs have bottomed out and

outpatient visits and procedures are climbing nationwide. So where does the industry go from here?

Managed care has not been managing utilization toward some vision of appropriate practice patterns. Financial risk and hospital stays have been managed, but tools have not been developed to help doctors determine what is the *right* care. The heart of the matter is the lack of consensus and outcomes-based data on what works and does not work in healthcare.

Next-generation utilization management will require evidence from patient outcomes as to what techniques work on both a risk-benefit and cost-benefit basis, and then a clear set of indications (patient descriptors) for the application of the techniques that do work. Available literature and the consensus of qualified physicians should be used as a starting point even where outcomes data are currently lacking.

Value Health researchers using the rigorous appropriateness methodology developed over 7 years in the Rand/UCLA Health Services Utilization Study have now created appropriateness standards for 35 high-cost inpatient and outpatient procedures. The RAND/UCLA study found that 16 to 32 percent of covered procedures were clearly inappropriate on grounds that their risks outweigh their benefits. Reducing the number of such procedures achieves both cost containment and quality improvement.

Networks, financial incentives, and hospital preadmission certification are here to stay, but it is time to move to a second-generation science-based form of managed care. These techniques will use clinical standards and protocols which can serve both as practice guidelines for physicians and as review criteria for managed care organizations. No one should repeat past mistakes by overpromising what such a standards-based system can achieve, but it is time to begin.

Physician Utilization Profiling: The Key to Managing Ambulatory Utilization

KEVIN F. O'GRADY, M.D., M.S.P.H., Executive Director

Center for Consumer Healthcare Information, Santa Ana, California

Services delivered to ambulatory patients account for a rapidly rising proportion of healthcare expenses. The reasons for this are many: new technologies, changing attitudes among physicians and patients, benefit incentives for outpatient treatment, inpatient utilization review, and reimbursement incentives faced by providers. Until recently, insurers and employers tended to view outpatient services as a preferred alternative to inpatient care and too small a target for utilization management. However, the rapid increase in ambulatory costs has focused widespread attention on methods of managing ambulatory utilization.

Most of this attention has centered on precertification and prepayment review. Utilization review firms are beginning to review outpatient surgical services. Software packages that screen individual claims against various criteria are on the market. However, despite expected technical improvements in these methods, it is already clear that both of these approaches have significant limitations for ambulatory utilization management (UM). Consequently, many within the field are coming to believe that an effective and efficient ambulatory UM program will rest on a cornerstone of retrospective analysis of physician-specific utilization data.

Retrospective analysis of physician utilization data —retrospective profiling as it is often called — is not a new technique. However, the growth in ambulatory services makes it an increasingly important UM tool, and one with strategic implications for health plans and claims administrators. The reasons why physician profiling is the key to ambulatory UM and the requirements for its effective use are outlined below.

WHY PHYSICIAN PROFILING

To understand the logic in support of physician profiling, it is helpful to examine the content of ambulatory healthcare. For the purposes of this discussion, ambulatory services are defined as all noninpatient care. In employed populations, ambulatory services account for between 40 and 50 percent of total benefit payments. The numbers in Table 1 are taken from the experience of a major employer and illustrate a typical breakdown of ambulatory costs.

For outpatient surgery, the average payment per episode in this data set was under $300 in 1989 dollars. This figure reflects a mix of procedures of varying costs, as well as the fact that the insurer does not pay 100 percent of most expenses. For most outpatient surgical procedures performed in a hospital setting, the average would be much higher. For the other categories in Table 1, the average payment per service was under $100 (although if these services could be grouped into "episodes" the average payment in some cases would exceed $100, but not by much).

Precertification and Ambulatory Care

With these figures in mind, the economics of precertifying ambulatory care can be considered. Based on 1989 market prices for UR services, employers currently pay $150 to $200 per inpatient admission reviewed. Outpatient review might be less costly than inpatient review because the continued stay review function is eliminated. However, outpatient review might have added costs because of a need for more in-depth scrutiny of treatment indications in comparison to current practices for inpatient review.

TABLE 1   Breakdown of Expenditures for Noninpatient Care
Typical Privately Insured Population

Outpatient surgery (MD and facility costs)	28%
Diagnostic services (laboratory and radiology)	25
Emergency room services	5
Other physician services	39
Miscellaneous	3
Total	100

Even with the optimistic assumption that the cost for outpatient review could be cut to $75 to $100 per case, it is clear that routine prior review will never be cost-effective for most ambulatory care, with the possible exception of those outpatient surgical procedures which cost at least $1500 to $2000. Even if it is shown to be cost-effective for some outpatient surgeries, the point of the data in Table 1 is that this subset will probably represent no more than about 10 percent of ambulatory expenses.

Automated Prepayment Review Systems

Many claims processing systems have for some time incorporated "edit" modules which check claims for acceptable procedures, logically incompatible combinations of data items within a single claim, and other medical policy factors. However, the actual benefit derived from such systems has been limited. First, many insurers have lacked the resources to keep these systems current with changing medical practice and billing patterns. Second, a distressingly large proportion of claims which fail these screens do so because of data quality as opposed to utilization or billing problems. The review effort results in better data but no cost savings. Third, pressures for claim turnaround have often induced carriers to quietly "turn off" these edit modules to avoid the claim review burden they generate.

Recently, several proprietary claim review software products have appeared on the market. In itself, this is a welcome development because the focused attention of firms who make this their business will almost certainly result in improvements over services offered by claims processing system vendors, for whom this has never been a priority, and modules developed internally by carriers. Several services screen surgical claims for billing irregularities such as "unbundling," impermissible procedure combinations, and outmoded procedures. Early experience with these products seems to suggest that they may result in meaningful savings. However, their effectiveness with respect to outpatient claims is not yet known. Also, they address only the one-fourth of ambulatory care costs due to surgery.

Other services take a more comprehensive approach, reviewing all or almost all classes of ambulatory services. These services check the logical compatibility of various data on a single claim, for example, the appropriateness of a given procedure for the listed diagnosis. Prior claims on the same patient are also reviewed to check whether the patient has received the service more often than allowed by frequency criteria which are linked to the patient's diagnosis.

Versions of such automated review services have existed for several years, but it is only recently that the quality of claims data has been adequate to lead major payers to test such systems. Because the leading products are proprietary, reliable information on their actual performance is difficult to acquire. Based on their design, it seems that these systems should be successful in identifying (1) upcoding of some physician service codes, (2) overutilization of services subject to overly frequent use in a single patient, and (3) selected data quality problems.

However, full implementation of these products would almost certainly result in a mountain of "false positives," that is, claims which fail the edits but for which no overutilization or billing abuse has actually occurred. Furthermore, edit systems which are based on review of claims for a single patient will always miss a high proportion of overutilization. Unnecessary repetitive testing on a single patient arguably accounts for much less excess utilization than do single unnecessary tests on many patients. But if a frequency criterion based on the experience of a single patient is set at one per period, all this overutilization will be missed. If the criterion is set at zero, every claim must be reviewed offline.

Advantages of Retrospective Physician Profiling

Because retrospective profiling involves computerized analysis of many claims, it avoids the high cost of case-by-case prior review which inevitably restricts the latter to a small segment of ambulatory care. It also sidesteps the expensive and difficult process of developing medical criteria for such review. With utilization profiling, the reviewing organization can essentially say, "Look, doctor, compared to your peers who treat similar patients, your patients have test X 60 percent more often. We don't want to argue about whether patient Jones or patient Smith really needed that test. The issue is why your overall utilization pattern is so different from that of your colleagues."

In comparison to prepayment review systems, retrospective profiling offers the opportunity for both higher sensitivity (it will miss fewer "true positives") and higher specificity (it will flag fewer "false positives"). Why is this true? Retrospective profiling examines utilization patterns by physician, not by patient. It is inherently more sensitive because if the upper reasonable limit for the frequency of test X is 0.65 per patient, it can detect patterns which exceed this limit but which do not exceed 1.0, in contrast to prepayment systems which review frequencies per patient. It is more specific because it can take into account the treatment of other patients in deciding whether to respond to an unusual combination of data on a single claim.

Retrospective profiling's opportunity for more accurate identification of utilization problems means a potentially more efficient review process, both in terms of administrative time as well as the time which providers expend in complying with review activities.

RETROSPECTIVE PROFILING AS A UTILIZATION MANAGEMENT TOOL

In highlighting the advantages of retrospective profiling, it is important to keep in mind that retrospective profiling by itself is not a utilization management program. The role of profiling is to provide the information needed to appropriately target other management controls. Without specific interventions linked to profile results, data analysis is a sterile exercise.

Some of the ways in which retrospective profile data can be used to manage utilization are outlined below. The discussion here is directed principally toward the use of physician data to manage ambulatory utilization, although the use of hospital and other facility data raises similar issues.

Education

Utilization and cost data have been given to physicians in a number of controlled and uncontrolled experiments. Although a few studies have shown an impact from information feedback, the preponderance of evidence indicates that information not linked to incentives is ineffective in influencing physician behavior.

However, feedback of utilization data to physicians can be valuable in winning physician support for UM efforts based on utilization data. The greater the potential impact of the incentives or sanctions contemplated, the more important it is that physicians are comfortable with the data and analyses employed. Consequently, prior to implementing other profiling-based UM efforts, a period in which data are shared solely as an informational step should be strongly considered.

Provider-Focused Prior and Prepayment Review

One way in which the cost-effectiveness of both prior and prepayment review can be dramatically improved is to focus these efforts on the subset of physicians identified through retrospective analysis as having aberrant utilization patterns. Physicians would greatly prefer to avoid the burden of compliance associated with such review processes, as well as the potential loss or delay in reimbursement. Merely establishing the option of invoking physician-specific review in contracts can significantly improve physician cooperation with UM efforts and increase the incentive to avoid practices which may trigger sanctions.

Selective review can find considerable support among physicians if it is presented as an alternative to more extensive generalized review. One way to structure selective review is to exempt providers with favorable patterns from review requirements. This approach has been tried with hospitals but is more politically difficult to implement and administer for physician review requirements.

Like most UM methods, provider-focused review is subject to challenge by affected physicians through legal and regulatory channels. Sound data demonstrating the justification for imposing selective review can be very important in defending such challenges.

Selection and Deselection of Contracted Providers

The use of physician utilization profile data to establish panels of truly "selected" physicians is conceptually most appealing. However, the reality is that most organizations do not have the time, data, or market flexibility to construct their panels in this manner. Of greater practical importance is the use of profile data to "deselect" already enrolled physicians.

The effectiveness of deselecting physicians as a UM tool depends upon many factors, most important of which is the value which physicians place on panel membership. This in turn depends on the competitiveness of the physician marketplace, the market share of the health plan, and the plan's coverage for use of out-of-network providers. Even if panel membership is highly valued, the ability to use deselection to influence behavior may be constrained by provider contract language or state laws and regulations. Lastly, deselection can realistically be invoked only in fairly extreme situations and is thus not an appropriate lever with which to influence most utilization issues.

Nevertheless, any effective UM plan must include as an option deselection based on utilization experience and must demonstrate to physicians that this option will be used when needed.

Audit for Financial Recovery

Most large payers review provider payment and utilization data to identify suspected instances of fraud or gross abuse. The results of these analyses are used to direct audits of medical records which seek to determine whether the billed services were actually delivered and were medically necessary. If a problem is documented, financial recovery may be sought from the provider or criminal prosecution may be initiated.

While such programs are often important deterrents to fraud, they are not very effective in preventing many overutilization problems. First, the audit process is expensive; thus audit activity is restricted to a relatively small number of cases. Second, the process typically involves attorneys and sometimes state regulators. Courts and regulators are often poorly informed about utilization management concerns and tend to be more sympathetic to physicians than to insurance companies or other corporate entities.

Financial Incentives and Disincentives

Potentially the most effective lever on physician-controlled utilization is the use of financial incentives or disincentives linked to their individual practice patterns. Experience with individual-based physician incentives has been limited primarily to primary care providers within HMO settings because of the need for relatively large and homogeneous patient panels upon which to spread risk. Physicians have generally been wary of such arrangements because of their basic risk-aversion and because of limited confidence in the data and management of many HMOs.

Nevertheless, in a setting in which a health insurer or health plan had high quality data covering a substantial proportion of the patients of the physicians with whom it dealt, there is an opportunity for physician acceptance of individual incentives linked to utilization. To be both acceptable and effective, such a program would have to be carefully designed and would require better data and analytic techniques than have been available to date.

Some would argue that, ultimately, the best approach to managing utilization among nonsalaried physicians will be through use of a case-based reimbursement system, for example, ambulatory visit

groups (AVGs). Like incentive arrangements, AVGs are a way of shifting more risk to the physician. Although the use of global-billing codes which define larger packages of services under a single fee will continue to expand, a widespread move to AVGs is unlikely anytime soon. However, the use of incentives linked to profile results could accomplish much the same objective as AVGs and may be easier to experiment with.

REQUIREMENTS FOR EFFECTIVE PHYSICIAN PROFILING

Data Quality

Effective physician profiling requires a high quality database, in terms of both its accuracy and its completeness. Some of the more important data requirements include the following:

- Each procedure performed must be coded and should be linked to at least one diagnosis coded in 5-digit ICD-9-CM.
- The ability to identify the specific physician who provided the service is critical. In some settings, physicians bill under common provider numbers. This practice is outdated and should be replaced by a requirement for unique provider identifiers.
- Data items needed to establish linkage between claims should be present. These items include enrollee name, age, and sex (or better yet, a unique number); the date, type, and location of service; and provider identifying data.
- A database for provider specialty should be available if this information is not captured on each claim.
- Clear identification of financial adjustment data is needed to avoid double-counting of services and to permit accurate analysis of physician payment.
- Data items that may be important for some analytic applications include an indicator for whether the patient was referred; identification of the physician who ordered the service; and the patient's zip code (for use as a proxy for socioeconomic class).

In the past, poor quality data have been a major impediment to effective profiling systems. Recently, some claims payers have improved their data to the point where the rate-limiting step is no longer data quality but an understanding of what to do with the data.

Data Volume

There are many reasons why utilization management can be most effective when the UM organization sees a substantial volume of a physician's practice. This is especially true for retrospective review. More data means:

- More statistically valid comparisons
- The opportunity for more sophisticated analyses which adjust for important variations in the types of clinical conditions treated by individual physicians
- The ability to define better-matched physician peer groups
- Shorter intervals required to develop a meaningful volume of data, thus permitting a shorter analysis-intervention-reassessment cycle

In addition to the above, just having enough dollars at stake in a physician relationship can improve the ability to cost justify the process of review and information feedback, as well as the physician's responsiveness to the program.

Analytic Considerations

Some sophistication in the choice of analytic techniques will be required to produce meaningful comparisons among physicians that will correctly identify true utilization problems and that will be accepted by physicians. The more important analytic issues include those below.

- *Volume-independent measures.* The measures upon which physicians are compared should be relatively uninfluenced by the number of patients they see. Physicians who see more patients will order more tests and do more procedures, and should not be penalized for this. Measures should incorporate an appropriately chosen denominator to adjust for patient volume.
- *Ordered as opposed to performed services.* Many utilization problems will only be detected if the services which are ordered by a physician but performed by someone else (or by the same physician under a different billing number) are considered. This can be accomplished most easily if an "ordering physician" data element is available but is possible even without this.

- *Peer grouping.* Physician comparisons should be specialty-specific. This is an imperfect but good first-order adjuster for patient variation among physicians. Issues such as whether family practitioners should be grouped with internists can only be answered in the context of data availability and specific analyses planned.
- *Geographic variation.* How should geographic variation be treated? For most medical services, sound reasons for geographic variation have never been demonstrated. However, a practical problem often arises when a large urban area is involved. Physicians located in lower socioeconomic areas sometimes have very different utilization patterns. Should these physicians be compared only among themselves?

  The answer to this depends on the type of utilization under review. For example, studies of hospital use have documented a greater resource intensity requirement for lower socioeconomic patients. Thus, it may be appropriate that such patients have longer inpatient stays or need more intense postdischarge follow-up. However, why should less affluent cardiac patients need more ECGs than other cardiac patients?
- *Clinical groupings used for defining denominators.* For some physician services, it may be important to measure utilization rates using a denominator that accurately reflects the population at risk for this service, as opposed to the total number of patients seen. For example, an internist with a special interest in pulmonary medicine may order more spirometric studies than other internists. Measuring spirometric studies per patient with a respiratory diagnosis will provide a more valid assessment of this physician's practice.
- *Adjusting for referral status.* Analogous to the above example, some physicians have a higher than average referral content to their practice. This can influence utilization for many services, and an ideal profiling system should be able to take this into consideration when appropriate.
- *Definitions of "overutilization."* There is no scientific basis for defining boundaries for "overutilization" or aberrancy. In practice, such definitions are inherently arbitrary, which does not mean that they are unreasonable. Commonly, statistical definitions are used, for example, two standard deviations from the mean. It is often appropriate to vary

the threshold depending on the action which results from its transgression.

- *Scoring systems.* Because retrospective profiling often employs multiple measures or comparisons of a physician's practice, some organizations are experimenting with scoring systems which combine separate performance measures into a single "score." Composite scores are more attention-getting and are sometimes needed for ranking purposes. There is no "correct" way to construct such scores. Factors that should be considered in deciding how to weight subscores in a composite score include the perceived validity of the subscore as a measure of a true utilization problem, the number of dollars at issue, and the statistical precision of the subscore.

- *Ad hoc query capabilities.* In analyzing large claims databases, computer and personnel costs are both lowered to the extent that analyses can be performed on a scheduled basis using standardized programs. Nevertheless, there is an inescapable requirement for access to ad hoc queries. Inappropriate or suspect results will always occur, requiring follow-up database queries and special analyses.

Personnel and Programmatic Requirements

An effective physician profiling program requires a cooperative effort from multiple operating units within a health insurer or health plan.

Claims and systems personnel must understand the requirements regarding data elements and data quality. They must help ensure that appropriate computing resources are available to the data analysis staff. Data analysts must be thoroughly familiar with the intricacies of working with claims databases and should have a reasonable grounding in statistics.

Analysts must have access to appropriate clinical consultants who can help them interpret the clinical and utilization significance of the data. Consultants who understand the relevant clinical, utilization, and cost issues, but who also speak "data analysis" are critical to a successful program, although they are not easy to come by.

Provider relations personnel should be intimately involved in the design of programs for communicating data results to physicians and for any sanctions that may be invoked as a result of data findings. The communication of data to physicians is a significant undertaking which requires careful planning. Staff must be able to explain the origin and implications of data findings to inquiring physicians. Contracting and PPO staff should likewise be involved in the design of profiling-related programs. They should understand the requirements for profiling data systems and the implications of profiling for provider contracting.

STRATEGIC IMPLICATIONS OF PHYSICIAN PROFILING

The significance of retrospective physician profiling in the management of ambulatory utilization has important implications for health insurers and health plans. First, and most obvious, is the need to upgrade data quality now. It takes several years to change required claims data elements, to communicate these changes to providers, and to achieve compliance. It takes even longer to develop a historical database of experience, to understand how to use these data, and to build confidence in the data among physicians.

Second, an explicit program is needed to build support among physicians and state regulators for programs which manage utilization through utilization profile data. The use of profile data for managing utilization is in essence a very "physician-friendly" proposition because of the potential for selectivity — only the "problem" physicians are affected while the conscientious physicians are left alone. This message should be conveyed to physician organizations, and physician involvement in creating clinically intelligent profiling techniques should be encouraged. Contracts with physicians should anticipate the use of profile data by establishing the right to take certain actions based on such data. In states in which regulators control utilization review and contracting practices, the rationale for using profile data should be shared with regulators on a proactive basis.

Lastly, the role of profiling data suggests that health insurers with larger market shares will have an important advantage. Depending on the physician's specialty, effective profiling requires data on 15 to 40 percent of his or her private-pay patients. Insurers or health plans who do not have this market share will have to find ways to participate in shared data or utilization management programs.

CHAPTER SIXTEEN

Design and Implementation of Quality Assurance

UTILIZATION REVIEW: CHANGING PERSPECTIVES

JOANNE LAMPREY, Senior Vice President
CHARLOTTE K. CORCORAN, Vice President
InterQual, Inc., North Hampton, New Hampshire

The healthcare environment has evolved from emphasizing access to care and providing services for all to expressing grave concerns about escalating healthcare costs and discussions of national health insurance and of rationing services.

In this environment of escalating costs and tighter controls on spending, utilization review activities have become a major part of everyday life. However, current utilization practices, focusing on obtaining or denying payment, still fail to contain costs and may compromise the quality of care.

The current process suggests that a change in perspective regarding utilization strategies is necessary. Providers must take a proactive stance to implement utilization programs which integrate quality and cost and address the needs of the patient population they serve.

Today's utilization review practices seem to focus on limiting access to healthcare through harassment of would-be patients, employees, physicians, and hospital utilization review staffs. Private review agencies are reporting profits while employees are victims of intense pretreatment scrutiny, the physician's office overhead has increased to meet prior authorization requirements, and hospital costs have escalated in part because of an increase in staff size needed to meet utilization review mandates. While these measures are attempts to reduce or control inpatient costs, they have in many instances become barriers to obtaining healthcare.

Insurers and businesses are still paying the highest amount for short-term acute care and denying payment for other less costly levels of care. Thus, there is no incentive for providers to develop alternate levels of care.

Utilization review programs must focus on utilization management that incorporates a case management approach. For case management to be effective, there must be alternate levels of care available and negotiated reimbursement rates for the various levels of care.

Hospitals need to view themselves as healthcare centers, not hospitals in the traditional sense. Healthcare centers offer many levels of care and create an environment most conducive to case management. Effective case management results in patients receiving tests, therapies, procedures, critical care, and general care in the least costly setting without compromising quality.

EXISTING UTILIZATION REVIEW METHODS

The current system—characterized by preadmission authorizations, second opinions, gatekeepers, and continued-stay review—continues to deny payment rather than manage resource use. Because of this policy, the potential also exists to deny needed benefits and care. Hospitals and physicians are expending too much time, energy, and money trying to be insurance agents. The average hospital responds to 45 to 50 private review agencies, all demanding that their requirements be met or reimbursement will be jeopardized. Regulations regarding admission, length-of-stay, and intensity of service are ambiguous at best; yet, most hospitals' utilization review programs try to keep abreast of the latest changes in the regulations and react to them. The system is designed to chase after reimbursement, not solve utilization problems.

Currently, the main question that is asked to determine appropriateness of the acute care setting is: "Is this patient receiving services that will be reimbursed?" Payment is equated with appropriate services or care and nonpayment with inappropriate services or care.

To determine the appropriateness of the acute care setting, providers should be asking the following questions:

- Does the patient require clinical services that can only be provided in the acute care setting?
- If not, are there alternatives available?

Instead, the current situation results in:

- Healthcare costs that are not being contained because services that could be provided at a nonacute level are still being provided in the acute care setting.
- Hospitals that are not maximizing reimbursement because they have not determined the clinical needs of their patient population and developed strategies to address these needs.
- Physicians who believe they are not being allowed to care for the patient as they deem appropriate. Physicians are being notified that the patient does not require a hospital level of service, but no alternatives are made available to the physician or the patient. For example, many patients are admitted to the hospital for some type of care or stabilization when they do not need a hospital level of care but do need some care. When physicians see these types of patients, they need to be able to provide some level of care and comfort, but the choices for reimbursed levels of care are few. Frequently patients are sent home even when there is no care-giver at home or they may be sent to the hospital only to have hospital payment denied because the care needs are not at the hospital level of care. The hospital then chastises the physician for being responsible for lost revenue. Would it not be better to respond to the physician with a "yes" (you may treat at this level) rather than a "no" (it is not covered)? Physicians whose patient population includes primarily the elderly and chronically ill are depicted as losers in the system. At the same time, physicians whose patient population does not fall into one of the categories under scrutiny, may be providing services of marginal benefit and quality without any consequences.
- Patients who are being denied access to care. Patients and families are angry because they are often informed that the benefits are being terminated because the acute care setting is not required, yet there are few if any alternatives to hospital care available. Patients are informed by physicians and nurses that they cannot be admitted to the hospital or cannot remain in the hospital because insurance will not pay for it. When insurance may not pay for the admission or hospital stay, there is a catch 22 for the physician who is primarily responsible for the clinical decision affecting the patient's welfare.
- There is a lack of correlation between cost and quality. Many hospitals continue to have separate utilization review and quality assurance programs. One individual is reviewing the medical record for appropriateness of hospital level of services, while others are collecting data regarding complications and undesirable outcomes. There is no attempt to study the relationship between the deficiencies in the quality of care and prolonged lengths of stay and higher costs.

The managed care industry needs to spend more time, money, and energy determining how to best serve legitimate patient care needs rather than constructing barriers that create confusion, increase the income to third party reviewers, and still increase the cost of healthcare while possibly eroding the quality of care for those needing it.

SHIFTING FROM UTILIZATION REVIEW TO UTILIZATION MANAGEMENT

Effective utilization management programs enable the provider to manage the allocation of resources to the benefit of the patient and the provider. The patient receives services which are medically necessary and delivered in the appropriate care setting, and the hospital and physician provide quality care and maximize reimbursement.

A suggestion would be to provide payment for alternatives to acute care; this would create the incentive for the development of the alternatives. Hospitals with low occupancy rates might be well served to reallocate beds for various alternate levels of care. Case management works extremely well if the various levels are made available on the hospital premises. Hospitals with higher occupancies may have to purchase or contract with alternate off-site facilities. However, it is more difficult to make case management effective if the levels of care are scattered in a 20- to 30-mile radius.

To achieve this goal, the utilization management program must identify and establish alternative levels of care, thus providing the requisite environment to enable effective case management. The first step in establishing a utilization management program is to define the levels of care and services needed. The following illustration depicts the hospital as the acute care center with the potential to provide many alternative levels of care (Figure 1).

Planning for alternate levels of care must be based on a sound database which identifies the needs of the community served by the hospital. The utilization management program developed by Inter-Qual, for example, stresses the importance of this first step.

The review methodology, which is based on the use of InterQual's intensity of service, severity of illness, appropriateness of services, and discharge criteria (ISD-A) enables hospitals to identify the number of days and types of nonacute care being delivered and to evaluate the over- and underutilization of existing services. Table 1 provides definitions of the more common levels of care. These nonacute days are referred to as variance days. Briefly, the review methodology includes the following:

- All patients are reviewed every day regardless of payment source.
- Every patient is reviewed for intensity of service, severity of illness, and discharge criteria.

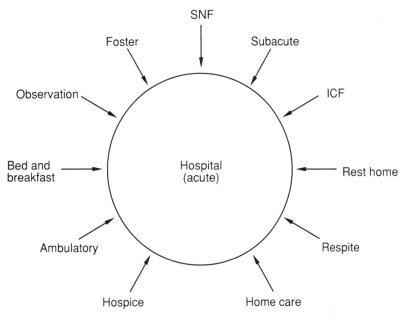

Figure 1 *Alternate levels of care.*

- Review coordinators work closely with and communicate daily with physician advisers.
- All patients not meeting criteria are referred to the physician adviser who is requested to consider the following questions:

  Does the patient clinically require the acute care setting?

  If not, what is the most appropriate level of care for this patient?

- All referrals to the physician adviser and the decision of the physician adviser are logged. Aggregation of these data produces a profile of variance days by number and levels of care required. The log is depicted in Figure 2.

Figures 3 to 6 illustrate the information obtained by four hospitals of varying size and location. The InterQual system frequently identifies 3000 to 4000 days of care per quarter that could have been provided in alternate levels of care.

The data displayed in Figure 3 were collected over a 3-month period. This 600-bed acute care hospital believed it had an active utilization review program in place. There was daily interface between the utilization review coordinators and physician advisers regarding patients not meeting professional review organization (PRO) criteria. Procedures for denial letters and termination of bene-

TABLE 1   Guidelines for Assigning Variance Days

Outpatient (OPT): Assigned to patients receiving therapeutic or diagnostic tests or procedures that do not require admission to the hospital.

Residence (RES): Assigned to patients whose clinical condition does not require admission to the hospital or an alternate level of care.

General Unit (GEU): Assigned to patients who are in a special care setting but could be transferred to a general care unit.

Delay (DEL): Assigned to patients when there is a delay in providing services which extends the hospital stay.

Skilled Nursing Facility (SNF): Assigned to patients who are not receiving hospital level of care but do require skilled care on an inpatient and daily basis.

Subacute level (SAL): Assigned to the chronically ill patient who requires continuous observation, evaluation, and supporting medical equipment but who has limited or no potential for improvement. The chronic ventilator patient is an example.

Intermediate care facility (ICF): Assigned to patients who do not receive care by a registered professional but who do require assistance in activities of daily living and continuous nonskilled care.

Home care (HoC): Assigned to patients who are home-bound and require one of the following:

- Skilled nursing care
- Respiratory, physical, or speech therapy
- Social services
- A homemaker or home health aide

Hospice (HOS): Assigned to patients who are terminally ill and may require:

- Skilled nursing care and other services such as IV analgesia or alimentary support
- Physical therapy

fits were in place and actively pursued. The facility was aware of the problems associated with the lack of skilled nursing or intermediate care beds but had not previously identified the extent of the problem. The days associated with the underutilization of outpatient, home health, and hospice services, and the overutilization of critical care units represented new information.

Figure 4 represents 6 months of data collection for a 300-bed acute care facility that was experiencing 95 to 100 percent occupancy despite an active utilization review program based on concurrent Diagnostic Related Group (DRG) assignments and medical record coding. There was a diligent effort on the part of the utilization review coordinators to respond to PRO denials and track actual versus expected reimbursement. However, there was limited activity focused on posthospital care. The data were presented to the administration and the utilization review committee, prompting reevaluation of the utilization process. The focus now is on early discharge

TABLE 1   Guidelines for Assigning Variance Days *(Continued)*

- Social services and pastoral care
- Rooming-in facilities for family members (if hospital)
- Bereavement counseling

Preadmission testing (PAT): Assigned to patients who can have preoperative diagnostic tests such as blood studies, radiology studies, or ECGs performed on an outpatient basis

Bed-and-breakfast (B&B): Assigned to patients who need lodging close to the hospital but do not require admission such as:

- Patients receiving daily outpatient therapies
- Patients requiring frequent transportation for long distances, and transportation is not available
- Patients receiving daily chemotherapy or radiation therapy but not requiring professional observation

Observation unit (OBS): Assigned to patients requiring close nursing observation for a limited period of time such as:

- Patients who had day surgery procedures and are not ready for discharge
- Patients receiving outpatient chemotherapy
- Patients requiring short-term observation to determine if admission is necessary
- Patients requiring observation to "play it safe"

Other (OTH): Assigned to patients requiring levels of care not described above such as:

- O_1—patients who require "respite" care (intermittent or continuous team support for patients with progressive diseases)
- O_2—patients in a rehabilitation unit
- O_3—patients who require adult day care services
- O_4—patients who no longer need intense service but who are not ready for discharge (transitional)

planning, and social service intervention meetings were held with a rehabilitation hospital in an attempt to reduce the rehabilitation variance days. Data are not yet available to evaluate the impact of the strategies.

Figure 5 represents data from a 250-bed acute care facility that was very concerned about the financial impact of the high number of retrospective payment denials related to inappropriate admissions. They thought the solution to the problem would be an observation unit. However, only 3 months of data indicated that this was probably not the solution to the problem since placing the patient in an observation unit addressed only 3 percent of the variance days. In response to these data, the hospital opened a preadmission testing center and converted six beds to a bed-and-breakfast unit.

The 750-bed tertiary care teaching hospital shown in Figure 6 has the advantage of a full year of data and has begun tracking the increasing and decreasing trends in variance days by alternate care settings. This graphic display illustrates the change in variance days

Figure 2 *Level of care log.*

IDENTIFICATION			QRC REFERRAL			PHYSICIAN REVIEWER DECISION						VARIANCE DATA													RESP PHYS	
							REFERRALS																			
							ADM		SUBS																	
REF NO	PATIENT IDENTIFIER	PAY SRC	DATE	CODE	QRC ID	PR ID	APP Y/N	VAR CODE	APP Y/N	VAR CODE	OPT	RES	GeU	DEL	SNF	SAL	ICF	HoC	HOS	PAT	B&B	OBS	OTH		ID	CAT

KEY:

REF NO	=	Reference Number
PAY SRC	=	Pay Source
QRC	=	Quality Review Coordinator/Nurse
ID	=	Identifier
PR	=	Physician Reviewer
ADM	=	Admission
SUBS	=	Subsequent
APP Y/N	=	Approve Yes/No

VAR	=	Variance
OPT	=	Outpatient
RES	=	Residence
GeU	=	General Unit
DEL	=	Delay
SNF	=	Skilled Nursing Facility
SAL	=	Sub-Acute Level
ICF	=	Intermediate Care Facility

HoC	=	Home Care
HOS	=	Hospice
PAT	=	Preadmission Testing
B&B	=	Bed & Breakfast
OBS	=	Observation
OTH	=	Other
RESP PHYS	=	Responsible Physician
CAT	=	Category

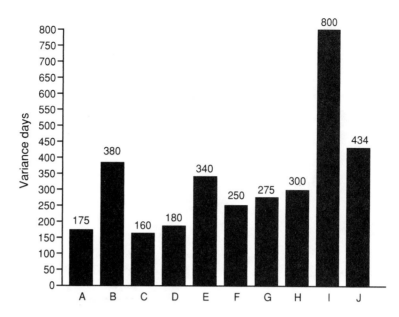

Figure 3 Facility A—variance days by alternate levels of care (three months). Total variance days: 3294. Key: A—Services could be performed on outpatient basis. B—Patient could be discharged home. C—Patient could be treated in a general unit. D—Same as C; bed not available. E—Delay in providing care or services. F—Intermediate-care-level bed not available. G—Care could be delivered by home health. H—Hospice level of care. I—Skilled nursing level of care. J—All others.

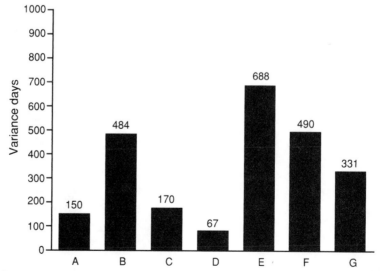

Figure 4 Facility B—variance days by alternate levels of care (six months). Total variance days: 2380. Key: A—Outpatient. B—Patient could be discharged home. C—Patient could be treated in a general unit, not critical care. D—Delay in services. E—Skilled nursing level of care. F—Patient could be transferred to a rehabilitation facility. G—All others.

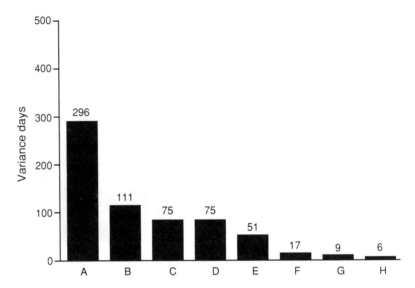

Figure 5 *Facility C—variance days by alternate levels of care (three months). Total variance days: 640. Key: A—Services could have been provided on an outpatient basis or preadmission testing. B—Skilled nursing level of care. C—Care could have been provided by home health. D—Patient could have been cared for in a general unit. E—Delay in service. F—Patient could have been observed for 24 hours. G—Hospice level of care. H—Rehabilitation level of care.*

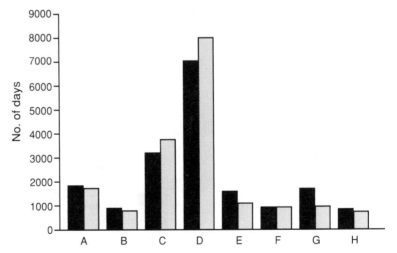

Figure 6 *Facility D—variance days by alternate levels of care (comparison of two 12-month periods). Total variance days: Prior year to date—17,654; year to date—17,593. Key: A—Outpatient testing. B—Patient could be discharged home. C—Skilled nursing care. D—Intermediate care level. E—Home health. F—Observation unit. G—Cooperative care. H—Other.*

for alternate care settings with greater than 500 variance days. This hospital continues to collect data but has not developed any alternate level of care strategies.

The second step is for the utilization review committee to analyze the variance data which indicate the levels of care required by the patient population, evaluate the current use of levels, and make recommendations regarding those levels of care that do not exist. Some of the more interesting information is obtained from data reflecting over- and underutilization of levels of care. Many hospitals have established levels of care with the intent of moving patients through the levels and maximizing reimbursement. The assumption cannot be made that because the levels of care exist, they are utilized effectively. Two of the more common examples are the overutilization of telemetry or progressive care units and the underutilization of preadmission testing programs, observation units, and outpatient services.

To address these problems requires an analysis of the systems supporting these levels of care and a profile of physicians utilizing these services. When hospitals and healthcare plans obtain data on individual physician practice patterns, they can provide feedback to physicians which identifies good performance as well as deficiencies. Physicians are more receptive to clinically based information and data which demonstrate practice patterns among peers than performance based on DRG or payment parameters.

The profile of variance days and physician-specific information places the provider in a position to move forward with a utilization plan incorporating case management. The utilization management flowchart outlines the steps to follow (Table 2).

Item 5 in the process flowchart (establishing a preadmission center) is a strategy common to many hospitals. However, most preadmission centers have been established without the benefit of variance data and planning for alternate care levels. The result is that the preadmission center accomplishes little more than obtaining information related to payment source and insurance authorizations for elective admissions. It may be viewed by the medical staff as one more source of harassment. The key to effectively utilizing a preadmission center is the availability of alternate levels of care. Without the ability to triage the patients to the appropriate levels of care, there are no options but to admit the patient, and the preadmission center cannot function at an optimal level.

The goal of the preadmission center is to evaluate the needs of the patient and plan necessary resources prior to admission, thus avoiding costly retrospective payment denials. The objectives of a preadmission center should include:

• Provision of a centralized location to coordinate all aspects of

TABLE 2   Utilization Management Flowchart

1. Identify variance days
   ↓
2. Profile variance data by number of days, levels of care, and practitioners
   ↓
3. Evaluate over- and underutilization of existing levels of care
   ↓
4. Establish alternate settings
   ↓
5. Establish preadmission center
   ↓
6. Case manage the admissions to the levels indicated by severity of illness and treatment plan
   ↓
7. Case manage inpatients to appropriate level indicated by severity of illness and treatment rendered
   ↓
8. Market utilization management program
   ↓
9. Negotiate reimbursement rates based on appropriate levels of care

preadmission evaluation and patient triaging to the appropriate level of care

- Coordination of patient admission, including preadmission diagnostic testing, preprocedure instructions, referrals to social services, and/or referrals for financial counseling
- Provision of a centralized location for communication to and from physicians and their offices, eliminating the necessity of many phone calls to arrange admission, diagnostic testing, and/or procedure scheduling.

An effective preadmission center facilitates the triaging of inpatients to appropriate levels of care as their needs change. What was once a reactive discharge planning process begun after the patient is admitted evolves into a proactive continuing care process begun in the preadmission phase.

An effective utilization management program, which focuses on providing care at the appropriate level, represents a more effective long-term strategy for the hospital to maximize reimbursement. Gains achieved by second-guessing or out maneuvering third party payers are short-lived at best.

Item 6 and 7 in the flowchart address case management. A complete case management program includes:

1. Preadmission approval

2. Preadmission planning (admission to the appropriate level for the severity of illness and the proposed treatment plan)

3. Preadmission testing:

Laboratory studies

ECGs

X-rays

4. Preadmission evaluation and referral:

History and physical

Anesthesia evaluation

Social service evaluation

Preoperative teaching for postoperative care

Physical therapy instruction for postoperative care

5. Case review after admission or transfer

6. Continuous case review to identify when patients can safely be moved to an alternate level of care

7. Patient care planning with nursing, social service, and discharge planners

8. Continuous interfacing with the attending physician

9. Follow-up after discharge from the healthcare center

10. Coordination of care providers and services postdischarge

FUTURE UTILIZATION MANAGEMENT PROGRAMS

Future utilization management programs will focus on effective case management concepts. Through case management, healthcare delivery is coordinated on behalf of the patient. Patient-centered case management requires direct contact with the patient by the case manager who assesses needs, coordinates care, and monitors services provided. In addition to assisting the patient, the case manager also works with the patient's family and significant others who may be directly involved in the patient's care or provide emotional support.

Virtually every major private insurer offers some type of medical case management. While healthcare providers such as HMOs maintain that they use medical case management, this usually refers to discharging patients from the hospital setting to another facility. Currently, the goals of case management programs are to obtain comparable or better patient care at lower costs than the hospital setting, coordinate care among the patient's family and providers, and evaluate the patient's benefit plan to cover medical services. The future should include complete case management at the hospital level in addition to the pre- and posthospital phases of care.

In addition, mechanisms for comprehensive and accurate monitoring of patient progress, especially in the posthospital and/or outpatient setting, must be developed. Since effective case management requires the optimal use of alternative levels of care, the ability to evaluate the appropriateness of the setting and the quality of services provided becomes a critical element. The ability to triage the patient to the most appropriate level of care becomes an obligation of the facility managing the case.

Finally, a good case management program will include physician selection. Physicians must be selected on the basis of sound utilization practices. Such variance data as discussed in Figures 3 to 6 will help facilities to identify practitioners who provide quality care and who use resources most efficiently. Data which display patterns of practice among peer groups should relate to over- and underutilization of existing services, mortality rates, and complications.

This information will enable hospitals to identify effective and efficient practitioners and provide valuable feedback to physicians. The purpose of the feedback is to present the physician with the opportunity to change her/his behavior when indicated by the data.

By establishing effective utilization management programs and by progressing to case management, hospitals will be in a position to negotiate with third party payers for preferred provider status, offer services that meet the needs of the patient population, and enable physicians to treat patients as they deem appropriate in the optimal level of care setting.

Severity Measurement Tools: Comments and Cautions

LISA I. IEZZONI, M.D., M.S., Director of Health Services Research

Health Policy Institute, Boston University, Boston, Massachusetts

The common thread linking many recent changes in the healthcare delivery system is the need for data. Current trends tout increasingly detailed clinical information for purposes ranging from payment to quality assessment to evaluation of medical technologies. This has fostered the growth of an entire industry whose goal is to collect and aggregate clinical data specifically to judge patient "severity." Examples of severity measures include the Acuity Index Method (AIM), the Acute Physiology and Chronic Health Evaluation (APACHE), the Computerized Severity Index (CSI), Disease Staging, and MedisGroups. Such systems offer new opportunities for understanding the relationships between patients' clinical status and a variety of outcomes of the healthcare delivery process. However, as with any new source of information, severity measurement tools have both strengths and limitations. Four cautions are important.

First, before selecting a severity measure, it is crucial to understand the goals of its intended use. A given measure will be better for certain purposes than for others, based largely on how it defines "severity" and how it was derived. For example, Disease Staging's Q-scale equates severity with increasing resource needs; the system was derived empirically using cost as the dependent variable on a database containing almost 7 million discharges. In contrast, APACHE aims to predict risk of imminent death in an intensive care unit population, while the CSI's goal is to suggest treatment complexity presented to physicians. Both measures were based largely upon clinical judgment, with empirical refinements using data gathered through early testing of the systems.

Second, the current severity measures focus exclusively on a single, acute care hospitalization as the unit of observation. None has an "episode of illness"

perspective. Few measures include information on underlying chronic disease, functional impairment, or factors considered by nursing assessments (for example, patient dependency). For example, MedisGroups collects information on patient histories of chronic ischemic heart disease and diabetes mellitus, but it does not include these findings in computing severity scores. Given the purposes of such measures, this emphasis on acute clinical derangements is reasonable, but it suggests that not all factors which could affect patient outcome are considered fully. This could be a limitation in acute care settings which treat many chronically ill patients and in post–acute care settings, which require appreciation of comorbidities and functional disability (for example, rehabilitation or chronic disease hospitals or outpatient care).

Third, with few exceptions, most of these measures are intended to be used in the aggregate to indicate average resource needs within a class of patients or to screen for quality shortfalls across groups of patients. The measures are not meant to predict outcomes at the individual patient level and are therefore not appropriate to dictate specific patient care decisions. A possible and somewhat controversial exception is APACHE, which has been used by some hospitals with scarce intensive care unit resources to allocate beds to patients who are most likely to benefit clinically.

Finally, systems which require primary data collection from the medical record offer useful strategies for reliable and consistent abstraction of a range of information. For example, MedisGroups provides a glossary which facilitates consistent interpretation of vague or idiosyncratic medical terminology. The accuracy of the data depends on the accuracy of medical record documentation, which is unfortunately often suspect. Nonetheless, these abstraction guidelines are extremely useful. However, most of the measures compute their severity rating using simple formulas, developed to predict particular patient outcomes. For example, APACHE simply adds the points assigned to acute physiologic derangements, and MedisGroups counts the number of clinical findings at different severity levels to assign its overall score. If other outcomes are of interest, it may be possible to use the individual clinical data elements to derive empirically an alternative to these current algorithms. The challenge in creating an empirically based measure is to produce one which is clinically meaningful.

Quality: No Magic Bullets

PHILIP NATHANSON, Vice President

Quality and Outcomes Management, UniHealth America, Burbank, California

Perhaps because of the amazing achievements of modern medicine, providers sometimes think there must be a specific high-tech solution for whatever care delivery problem presents itself. Pneumonia? Administer antibiotics and (possibly) steroids. Appendicitis? Perform an appendectomy. Better quality assurance? Buy some books, some software, some hardware, some consulting services, or perhaps all four.

In the case of quality assurance, though, many providers that have simply opted for a magic bullet—be it somebody's model total quality assurance (QA) package or a computerized severity of illness indexing system—are finding that there are no quick fixes. Before buying sophisticated QA tools or technology, providers must first be sure that their *culture and climate* are ready to accept an aggressive quality monitoring, management, and marketing program. Four essential elements must be in place:

- *Agreement on what quality is and how it should be monitored*   There must be a consensus statement setting forth what measurable aspects of quality— clinical outcomes, patient satisfaction, appropriateness, cost-effectiveness—will be monitored, and what monitoring methods will be used (occurrence screens, a patient opinion survey, physician practice pattern profiles). The medical staff in particular must have "bought in" on this statement.

- *A shared perception that management and professional staff are serious about dealing with quality problems*   If the provider has long-standing unresolved quality problems that "everybody knows about," or if those in the medical staff committee or QA leadership positions lack credibility with the medical staff, or if there are other signals that the provider is less than totally committed to high quality (for example, chronically understaffed nursing or ancillary departments; unwillingness to buy or replace equipment when physicians believe quality is at issue; refusal to deal with other clearly *provider*-related rather than caregiver-related quality problems), then these signals must be changed before the provider installs new quality assurance tools.

- *Open, honest, constructive communication*   Particularly in managed care settings, improving quality is a systems issue involving cooperation among many departments and caregivers. The provider's climate must discourage finger pointing and blame assignment, and facilitate cooperative approaches to performance improvement.

- *Enough of the right staff*   The QA staff is no place for clinical burn-outs, and there must be enough staff to allow performance analysis rather than simple compliance with outside regulatory, accreditation, or purchaser demands.

Providers that already have those elements in place in their approach to quality may indeed be in a position to benefit from sophisticated quality management programs and techniques. Others should concentrate their time, energy, and resources on putting the basics in place first.

St. Clair Hospital: The Quality Enhancement Process

CLARA JEAN ERSOZ, M.D., MSHA, Vice President, Medical Affairs
NANCY FORNEY, R.N., B.S.N., MBA, Director, Surgical Services
St. Clair Hospital, Pittsburgh, Pennsylvania

Quality of healthcare has become everybody's business. It is no longer sufficient to establish quality assurance programs to meet accreditation requirements. Hospitals and freestanding healthcare centers must begin to analyze and adopt a proactive model of quality enhancement that involves not just the medical staff but the whole organization.

The teachings of the industrial triumvirate of quality management, J. M. Juran,[1] E. W. Deming,[2] and Philip Crosby,[3] have direct applications to healthcare. Quality enhancement, whether it be product- or service-oriented, is a planned top-down and bottom-up phenomenon. Top management must have quality as its first priority and commitment. Quality must not be just a "buzzword," but an action plan that shows every employee that top management is committed to quality. "Added value" at each step in the process of production or of service delivery must be enhanced and reinforced. Immediate correction of recognized flaws in the process is mandatory. A manager must not let either flawed merchandise or flawed service reach the marketplace. One small lapse in attention to detail can send employees a strong message that management is not really committed to quality.

Employees must be involved in all aspects of planning for quality and understand that each employee has many customers within the organization. The major quality goal is to provide both internal and external customer satisfaction 100 percent of the time. Well-defined corporate values and a supportive corporate culture are essential ingredients in any quality enhancement initiative.

The Juran trilogy of quality planning, quality control, and quality improvement interlocks well with the Crosby model. Both models stress the importance of planning for quality. When a new product or service is identified or an existing one is being reviewed, the first step is to identify customers, both internal and external. Following identification of the customers who will use or purchase the product or service, customer requirements or needs are defined. Caution is necessary in determining needs. Needs may be considered as either stated or perceived. Perceived needs are particularly elusive and are prominent in a service sector such as healthcare. Needs (requirements) can be specified as primary, secondary, and even tertiary. Juran believes that the end point for the delineation of needs is that point at which the customer's needs "become known with such precision that no further subdivision is necessary." Crosby's definition of quality as "conformance to requirements" fits the Juran model well.

Once customer requirements have been identified, they must be translated into the appropriate "language" of the supplier or producer. Units of measure are then established, and the product or service design is optimized against these units. At this point a pilot project is often advisable to test the product or service. If the pilot is successful, production can begin. Performance is measured against predefined tolerances as defined by statistical quality control and the level of customer satisfaction with the product. Customer satisfaction with an industrial product is defined as "fitness for use."

In both the service and manufacturing sectors, one of the keys to quality is the culture of the organization and how well it supports the efforts of various groups of employees to work together. Each supplier group within an organization must be responsible for identifying its customers' needs with respect to allocation of resources, problem solving, decision making, and technical specifications. In any organization, employees and employee groups are both customers and suppliers in ever expanding circles. From the support parts of a healthcare organization to the production and provision frontline personnel, all groups within the organization are interrelated.

Crosby identifies four absolute definitions of quality:

1. There is conformance to requirements.
2. The system of quality is prevention.
3. The performance standard is zero defects.

4. The measurement of quality is the price of nonconformance.

The first two definitions relate to the planning function, and the second two relate to the measurement function. The price of nonconformance has been measured in industry for many years and has been estimated to account for a range of 2 to 25 percent of the cost of doing business. The price of nonconformance has not been well documented in healthcare, but with ever increasing cost constraints, hospitals must address this vital issue. The price of nonconformance in healthcare organizations relates both to issues of risk management and prevention of lawsuit, and to the lower cost of "getting it right the first time." The Juran total quality planning model is designed to assist the process of getting it right the first time.

Planning for quality is best considered as process control rather than as inspection for defects. In process control, the product or service is designed so that defects or barriers to quality are eliminated in the course of translating customer requirements into appropriate specifications. There should be no on-line retooling or shims to make the product conform to customer requirements. The product should conform by virtue of its design.

One of Crosby's requirements is a corporate commitment to a set of policies and values that meets the following standard: "The quality policy of this company is that we will deliver defect-free products and services to our customers both internal and external, on time."

Highly structured models of specification control and customer satisfaction measurements, however, have their limits. While these are certainly valuable tools in the development of both industrial and healthcare models for quality control and management, there is a danger to "listening too hard."[4] External and certainly internal customers may begin to express their requirements in the same old comfortable way, stifling the innovation necessary to move an organization forward. A well-advised strategy may be that in addition to listening to customers, try listening to your competitor's customers and industry visionaries to see where the industry is going.

In healthcare, the quality enhancement process must link customer expectations and satisfaction with standards of professional performance to ensure the provision of a satisfying, appropriate, and risk-free healthcare experience. A model which describes the total quality management process for healthcare (Figure 1) has been devised which integrates the key components of manufacturing models with the professional standards of healthcare.

The exterior aspect of the triangle describes the quality management process while the interior aspects of the triangle describe the basic concepts and design. Prior to planning or analyzing a healthcare service, a manager must identify the scope of care and services: the "what do we do?" and "who are our customers?" issues. Identification of the scope of care and services is identical to step 2 of the Joint Commission on Accreditation of Healthcare Organization's Ten-Step Model for Quality Assurance:

1. Assign responsibility.
2. Delineate scope of care.
3. Identify important aspects of care.
4. Identify indicators related to these aspects of care.
5. Establish thresholds for evaluation related to the indicators.
6. Collect and organize data.

Figure 1 *The total quality enhancement process.*

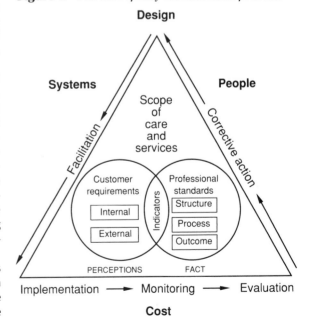

7. Evaluate care when thresholds for evaluation are reached.

8. Take actions to improve care.

9. Assess the effectiveness of the actions and document improvement.

10. Communicate relevant information to the organizationwide QA program.

Quality is defined as "meeting the requirements." Healthcare providers and managers must be concerned with meeting internal and external customer requirements as well as professional standards. Traditional quality assurance models did not usually acknowledge customers and their requirements. External customers include patients, physicians, purchasers, and third party payers who can easily go elsewhere if their requirements are not met. Internal customers are employees who depend on each other for goods and services. Internal customer dissatisfaction in a healthcare organization is frequently manifested by "turf" problems.

After customers and their requirements are identified and defined, the professionals involved in patient care in an organization are identified and their professional standards defined. Professional standards generally take three forms: structure, process, and outcome.[5] In the total quality management model, these have been placed inside the circle representing professional standards. The circles in the model are intertwined to indicate the overlapping relationships between customer requirements and professional standards.

Customer requirements and professional standards are then defined in terms of indicators. Indicators are measurable variables related to customer requirements and professional standards. The standard itself may serve as an indicator if it can be stated in measurable terms. Outcome indicators are often used as proxies to measure structure and process.

Returning to the exterior triangle part of the model, it must be stressed that the process of identifying customer requirements and professional standards is accomplished by design. Facilitation involves ensuring organizational support for providers and proofing the healthcare product before implementation whenever possible. The implementation phase is the phase where people provide services with a commitment to meet the established requirements. Throughout the implementation, the level of quality is monitored in terms of the indicators. The process of evaluation describes analysis of findings which indicate the level of conformance to professional standards and customer requirements and which may point to problems in design, facilitation, or implementation. Corrective action bridges the gap between the requirements and actual performance and reflects back to the design.

The model for healthcare total quality management acknowledges the importance of the context in which the process occurs, that is, the triad of people, systems, and cost. Systems should be user and customer friendly, and managers must know how to design them effectively. People are the most vital element of the system. Employees must have a clear understanding of what quality is, of its value to the healthcare organization, and of their role as both customer and supplier. In addition, the organization must value its employees. The cost of quality is an ever-present constraint to be considered throughout the process. The cost of quality includes the cost of conformance and nonconformance. Doing things right the first time will reduce costly errors and risk exposure. Nonconformance also risks the loss of future potential revenue.

Quality will be the survival tactic for hospitals for the 1990s. With decreased lengths of stay, limited resources, and increasing competition, there is an omnipresent challenge to manage healthcare quality. The most effective quality model for healthcare providers to adopt is one based on proven manufacturing models of quality control and which integrates professional standards.

REFERENCES

1. J. M. Juran, *Juran on Planning for Quality*. The Free Press, New York, 1988.

2. Thomas R. Gillem, "Deming's 14 Points and Hospital Quality: Responding to the Consumer's Demand for the Best Value Health Care," *J. Nurs. Qual. Assur.* **2:** 70–78 (1988).

3. Philip B. Crosby, *Quality Without Tears: The Art of Hassle-Free Management*. New American Library, Scarborough, Ontario, 1984.

4. Esther Dyson, "Don't Listen Too Hard," *Forbes* p. 12 (May 16, 1988).

5. Avedis Donobedian, *Explorations in Quality Assessment and Monitoring*, vols. I, II, and III. Health Administration Press, Ann Arbor, 1980, 1982, and 1985.

CHAPTER SEVENTEEN

Quality Control

ORGANIZATIONAL DYNAMICS OF QUALITY CONTROL

KATHLEEN JENNISON, M.D., Chief, Quality-of-Care Measurement
Harvard Community Health Plan, Brookline, Massachusetts

Dramatic increases in the cost and complexity of healthcare have created tremendous pressures to measure and improve the quality and efficiency of medical care. While the sophistication of medical technology is rising rapidly, the management of delivery systems lags far behind, particularly as it relates to quality.

The public has come to expect a guaranteed level of service and satisfaction as a consumer right. Payers make explicit demands for data on topics ranging from clinical outcomes to cost and utilization performance. There is increasing conflict between public expectations, payer expectations, and a rapidly evolving healthcare industry that lacks the vision and techniques to meet consumer demands for quality control. Furthermore, the demand for quality control appears on the rise, particularly for managed care systems.

Pressure has mounted on traditional quality assurance programs to document provider quality for two reasons: to establish the capacity to compare one provider to another and to provide a means of improving the process of delivering medical services. At the present time, the industry lacks a uniform philosophy and approach to measuring and managing quality.

From the perspective of quality management, there is room for radical change in the current approach to healthcare quality. The conventional medical paradigm about quality is misguided and fragmented. The approach is too narrow in its focus and methods to bring about the necessary advances in quality management for modern healthcare delivery systems.

This chapter begins with a brief description of the forces that are bringing healthcare quality under scrutiny. It then compares the conventional quality assessment and assurance approach to the paradigm of organizationwide quality management and improvement strategies under development in other industrial sectors and among innovative health organizations.

DEMAND FACTORS   The demand for quality control is based on five forces. First, cost containment and its potential negative impact on quality is the single most powerful force behind the current demand for medical quality control. Risk contracts, prospective payment, and capitated delivery models have the potential to create hazards for patients. Policies and procedures designed to reduce utilization and restrict access to care have contributed to the ever-increasing atmosphere of fear and apprehension about the quality of healthcare. Purchasers and payers now expect definitive information about the value, both in terms of cost and quality, of the services they are buying.

A second force operating to bring medicine under the microscope is increasing public awareness of the wide range of quality available within American medicine. Stories about bad medical care are now common topics for dinner party conversation and tabloid headlines. Health services researchers have conclusively shown that medical practice varies substantially across geographic regions, lending scientific credibility to the concern about variable quality. Patients as consumers expect more and more certainty about the basis for clinical decisions and the predicted outcomes of interventions. They increasingly approach their doctors with a feeling of distrust and inquisition, conscious that the physician's financial self-interest may conflict with their own expectations for service.

A third element is fierce competition within medical markets. As price competition begins to stabilize, providers left in the marketplace will be expected to document and display their competitive edge on quality. Although hospitals have had quality assurance systems for years, they were designed to respond to outside regulators and accreditation rather than to create corporatewide strategies for quality measurement and improvement. Managed care providers, exempt from many of the traditional quality assurance requirements, have competed to date largely on price and reputation of their providers. The current crisis of confidence about quality is forcing a fundamental change of focus for all healthcare organizations. Data on quality have become a consumer entitlement in medicine, like any marketplace, where an informed customer is a more satisfied customer.

Fourth, providers and suppliers now enter contractual price and service relationships, which creates highly integrated delivery systems and markets. The management of one clinical problem, such as PAP smear screening, may involve a number of service vendors ranging from contracted gynecologists to pathology laboratories. Responsibility for quality control is, therefore, less clear. Managed care systems necessitate sophisticated organizational strategies and techniques to survive as businesses and, at the same time, to meet the challenge of quality control for their services.

Finally, there is a commonly held belief that quality of medical care is directly related to expenditures. The transition from cost-based reimbursement to prospective payment has heightened the perceived conflict between quality and cost. Quality research and organizational efforts to assess or assure quality tend to be viewed by providers as annoying but necessary to meet the demands of regulators. Quality work is generally in response to external demands, not an integral and important part of an organization's management activities. This notion creates tension between increasing demands for well-documented high quality of care and the economic pressure to restrict the growth in the cost of that care.

CONVENTIONAL QUALITY ASSURANCE

Inherent in the predominant approach is a paradigm which presumes that quality is determined largely by the actions of individual physicians; therefore, identifying good and bad practitioners will highlight who needs to be better controlled or eliminated from delivery systems. Within this organizational paradigm, quality assurance is basically the search for performance outliers.

This notion originated at a time when physicians singularly controlled most of a patient's medical care. Today, physicians function within highly complex organizations. Patient care may include multiple specialists, laboratories, diagnostic technicians, and therapeutic products. The quality of these services involve complex information systems and technical expertise which include a receptionist or answering service, the laboratory and radiology services, the admitting office or benefits office, and the surgical nurse as well as the surgeon. It is naive to assume physicians can or should control the quality of each of these people, technologies, or organizational functions.

The role of physicians remains central to the patient and the success of medical care. However, a comprehensive, integrated approach to quality must encompass all aspects of the process of service delivery. When a patient calls a physician's office with abdominal pain, it is the entire treatment process (that is, responding to the call, completing and interpreting diagnostic tests, and designing the treatment plan for the problem) that determines the quality of care received by the patient, not just the actions of an individual physician. Malpractice litigation, perceived as a method of quality control, fosters the belief that quality can be assured by holding the individual practitioner culpable for all aspects of what is in actuality a highly complex system of many people and activities.

The current approach to quality management reflects three distinct personnel infrastructures within most medical delivery systems. First, there are physicians familiar with quality assessment, assurance, and, more recently, outcome-oriented health services research. The focus on physician performance has been directed at developing the means to distinguish good and bad providers, presumably with intent to reform, discipline, or remove low quality practitioners. Second, nursing personnel and their quality assurance activities are involved; they may or may not be integrated with the physician work force. Third, all other service and management functions are performed by a large nonclinical work force. The approach by nonphysician management has been to apply traditional business methods such as management-by-objective and operations audits to hospital and managed care settings.

The conventional approach to healthcare quality management generally segregates clinical and nonclinical activities into two distinct domains, each with different philosophies, methods, and organizational applications. Quality assessment and assurance, the two-step approach developed to control physician and nurse quality, functions separately from the management and quality control of the service industry itself.

Quality assessment defines and measures quality of clinical care and focuses almost exclusively on physician functions and activities. It generally defines quality to consist of a technical component (accuracy and effectiveness of diagnosis and treatment) and an interpersonal component (the caring function). Its application involves identifying targets or indicators, setting standards for acceptable performance, and comparing provider performance to specified standards.

Assessment is performed using inspection techniques such as retrospective medical audit or chart review and, more recently, payer claims database analyses are used to identify providers for more intensive review. Audits conducted by physician or nurse reviewers compare performance of clinical activities recorded in the medical record to criteria or protocols. In an effort to streamline these efforts, indicators such as surgical complications, hospital readmissions or transfers, and mortality rates are used to identify potentially low quality providers for more intensive review. Because of the need to generate comparative provider data, severity-of-illness systems have been designed that make comparisons theoretically possible. Two of the most wide-ranging examples to date are the comprehensive screening activities of the peer review organizations and the mortality statistics produced by the Health Care Financing Administration which compare hospital outcomes to empirical norms.

Assurance is the theoretical second step in the process of quality control. While much is known about physician behavior and cost containment, very little is understood about changing physician practices in relation to quality. Most assurance programs simply consist of educating the professional about good clinical practice. A more successful approach is feedback of information to providers concerning their performance in comparison to others over time. In general, most assurance programs assume surveillance of physicians will create an incentive to conform to a minimum acceptable standard. It suggests that by informing physicians of their shortcomings, they will correct the deficiencies. In a worst-case scenario, an incompetent or greedy physician will be identified and then kept from participating in a health plan.

MODERN QUALITY IMPROVEMENT THEORY

The current crisis in American healthcare stems, in part, from a lack of confidence in the conventional approach to quality assurance. The time has come for a shift in the approach to healthcare quality. The situation calls for a quality management strategy consistent with today's complex healthcare organizations. Industrial approaches to quality improvement provide the relevant principles and techniques to make the necessary organizational changes in managed care organizations.

The central purpose of quality improvement management theory (QI) is to create organizations with a clear vision of what constitutes quality for their "customers," and how every individual working for them contributes to continually improving the quality in their daily work. It is a multidisciplinary approach with a highly developed philosophy of management and organizational change, drawing on systems engineering, organizational development, psychology, and applied statistics. QI is a composite of scientific and managerial techniques to study and continually improve the quality of services.

Several principles in the quality improvement approach are germane to the challenge facing healthcare managers. The most important and most divergent from current quality assurance approaches is the emphasis on system analysis and process improvement. Process improvement as a concept refers to a scientific approach to studying and improving the way small tasks are performed. Examples of processes are triaging a patient in the emergency room, performing and interpreting a cardiogram on a patient scheduled for general anesthesia, or booking appointments for acute visits. Work is composed of small, interrelated processes. The quality of these processes and their outcomes determines the quality and efficiency of organizations. By careful study of problems in quality, industrial statisticians have discovered that defects in performance are usually built directly into work processes. Poor quality can only rarely be attributed to an individual or their intentions. Generally, poor performance indicates low quality process design.

This lesson applies to medical care as well as to any other technical or complex activity. A patient interfaces with many individuals, not just with an individual physician, in the course of his or her care. While the role of the physician's knowledge and judgment remains central, there are many points in the continuum of service delivery which are beyond the control of the clinician. Every person in an organization is part of a system of work processes which depend on many different individuals and functions for their successful completion. If a physician cannot get access to a patient's medical record, her or his ability to practice may be qualitatively compromised. If an answering service fails to page a physician in a timely and accurate manner with a patient call, the physician may not respond appropriately. If laboratory technicians do not recognize their role in the quality of care to patients, laboratory specimens may not be handled properly. QI assumes that over time individuals are interdependent in the delivery of complex services.

Consider the process of managing a bleeding patient. It involves numerous clinicians, laboratories, technicians, and information systems. Defects can occur at any step: the decision to triage, the drawing and transporting of blood samples, or the decision to operate. Medicine, like all service industries, is an interwoven network of processes, each interdependent on another. A process can be as large as performing an operation or as small as collecting clean voided urine samples. The general strategy of process improvement is to study and improve the design of individual processes, including their resultant outcomes. According to quality experts from other labor-intensive services, process improvement is the only way to keep pace with the rapidly changing technology and environment.

A second relevant principle from QI is that in order for an organization to achieve high quality service or production, everyone working in the organization must know who their customers are and understand their needs and expectations. "Customer" is a generic term referring to dependency in relationships. The customer is the person who depends on a supplier for a product or service. A managed healthcare organization's customers include patients and their families, clinicians, other staff, internal departments, employer groups, payers, and regulators. The customers of a specialist are both the patients and the referring physicians. The customers of a benefits manager might be employer groups, individual members, and the marketing department. Each customer has particular needs and expectations which define quality for them. Knowledge of the customer needs and expectations in explicit, measurable terms is a prerequisite for designing processes that can satisfy them. It is therefore a critical prerequisite for developing a quality improvement program within an organization.

Does everyone working in healthcare organizations today know who their customers are? Do they really understand the relationship between what they do in their daily work and their customers' definition of quality? Probably not. Managed care organizations and hospitals often function with very vague charters to serve the public. It is unusual to find these mission statements translated into operational definitions for every employee and professional. It is even more unusual to find internal measurement and management programs which track and report on improvements based on operational definitions.

A third lesson from QI sheds light on where to direct scarce time and resources for quality assurance. Medicine is currently investing heavily in surveillance and inspection as means to ensure quality. Identifying and comparing clinical outcomes or mortality rates is critically important to answering questions about the effectiveness of clinical interventions. Unfortunately, effectiveness research will not answer healthcare managers' questions about how to maximize the quality and efficiency of work processes within organizations. Knowing which medication is most effective or when a particular procedure is indicated does not address the complex question of how to design the process of service delivery to reduce errors and poor quality.

Without an organizational culture and strategy to support the efforts of the individual to do her or his job well, measuring outcomes and reporting incidents of poor quality functions like an inspection system. Quality work can easily become a hunt for outliers. Medicine is falling into traps other industries have learned to avoid. "Inspection never put an ounce of quality into anything," a favorite QI saying, is really a hard lesson learned from years of investing financially and organizationally in inspection systems. Quality management experts emphasize preventing the costs of poor quality by building quality into the process of providing services. They refer to the importance of analyzing how a service is provided in order to reduce inherent waste, rework, complexity, and unnecessary errors in delivery of service.

Consider the following example of low quality of care leading to a poor clinical outcome. A physician caring for a young diabetic undergoing eye surgery ordered only one postoperative blood sugar. The recovery room staff failed to draw the blood sugar. Later in the day, the nursing staff misinterpreted the symptoms of high blood sugar and treated the patient for eye pain. The patient was found nearly comatose 6 hours later and transferred to intensive care. No one involved in the care of the patient had poor intentions or was incompetent. Tracking intensive care unit transfers would simply identify the frequency of bad outcomes. The more critical question for the organization is to design a process for caring for postsurgical patients that protects the patient and staff against such unfortunate events.

Consider another example. A patient is admitted for the diagnosis of chest pain. The diagnosis is unclear and a work-up is ordered to rule out myocardial infarction, angina, and esophageal reflux. Twenty-four hours later the patient is diagnosed as having had a myocardial infarction, and the physician writes an order to cancel the barium swallow. An error in transmitting the cancellation occurs and transport takes the patient to the laboratory for the test the next day. The patient suffers recurrent ischemia, goes into pulmonary edema, and dies. A malpractice action is filed against the physician and the hospital for negligent care.

No one in these examples intended to harm the patients. They did not want to perform their duties poorly. But the design of certain work processes failed both the providers and the patients, and the result was poor quality. Had the employees and professionals of these organizations been trained in quality improvement, they would have an approach and scientific skills to improve these processes and prevent the costs of poor quality care.

A fourth principle from QI relates to how organizations view professionals and employees. It makes two basic assumptions about everyone working within the service delivery system: (1) Most people are doing their best most of the time and (2) people generally would like to take pride in their performance and therefore want the opportunity to do the best job possible. People need to know their performance and intentions are respected. This places the responsibility on leaders and managers to analyze how processes are designed in order to create the opportunity for workers to do their jobs well.

Conventional management theory tends to assume that if people would just do their jobs correctly, there would be few problems and high quality. Individuals are generally blamed for defects and poor outcomes rather than the design of the processes they work in. QI notes that fearful and defensive workers are not loyal to their organizations and their performance deteriorates. They spend most of their time and energy defending themselves rather than asking the question, "How can the design of an activity be improved so that we can have better outcomes with this process?" In the example of the diabetic, conventional quality assurance might tend to look for the culprit, the person or persons who made the mistakes. They, in turn, would mount their defenses, probably blaming one another for this unfortunate series of errors. A quality improvement expert would offer a different approach. Assuming that no one intended to harm the patient and everyone wanted to avoid the outcome, how could the process of care have been different? How could it be designed so as to prevent such an outcome? Most of the time it is the process design, not the worker, that is responsible.

Consider another example of a woman with a breast lump referred for mammography. The process begins with the physician's request, followed by the secretary scheduling the test, the patient complying with the test appointment, the technician performing the test, the radiologist interpreting the mammogram, and, finally, the radiologist communicating back to the patient and the referring physician. There are multiple points along the process which may be sources of error, including the physician's examination skill and judgment at the time of the original evaluation. Assuming the physician intends to identify every suspicious lump, there are still multiple other points in the process where errors or delays can occur. QI takes the focus off the intentions and competence of the individual and puts it on the design and execution of the process. Free from the doubt and defensiveness generated by the conventional approach, individuals are far more likely to participate in efforts to improve the quality of services within their organization.

A fifth principle of QI provides a vision of how organizations might function in the QI model. Improvement work becomes a part of everyone's daily effort. Quality is not just something to justify, defend, or inspect for. Everyone should think about how to build it into what they do. Quality work is not something that is avoided and resisted; it becomes a favored aspect of work because it is in everyone's self-interest to improve their own quality and efficiency. A quality organization rewards its people for their efforts to improve. Rather than being viewed as external and extraneous to their "real" work, the time and resources needed for quality improvement efforts become a routine aspect of the workplace. Quality services are the outgrowth of methodical efforts by everyone in an organization applying a scientific approach to solving problems. Furthermore, quality planning and design must be approached with the same degree of attention to detail and method as the annual budget. Most employees are aware of the annual budget process in healthcare organizations. How many are informed of the organization's quality planning process? If they are aware of an organizational strategy for quality, how many see it as a program to help them do their job better? Organizations that embrace quality improvement put their quality planning and improvement program at the top of their priority list and their employees participate in it regularly.

Within this approach, improvement is viewed as a process itself. In contrast to the conventional paradigm which tends to orient people around meeting a standard of "good enough," QI redirects the approach to an orientation of continual effort and makes continual improvement over time a fundamental element in an organization's work life. Service quality can never be good enough; it can always be improved. Measurement and improvement are components of a continuous, interdependent cycle based on operational experiments. Measurement in this context is no longer an end in itself; it is a means toward the goal of improvement. The cycle, known as the Shewhart cycle, begins with the planning of the process change or intervention. The second and third steps of the cycle involve carrying out the intervention on a small scale and measuring its effect on the process function and its outcomes. The final step is to act based on the information learned, either by abandoning the change, adopting the change, or revising it and running through the cycle again. Policy and procedure changes are instituted based on knowledge learned from operational experiments, not on intuition or speculation.

A sixth important principle of QI addresses the role of management in complex service organizations. Conventional management approaches encourage the notion that a good manager is one who instinctively knows the solution to problems. A good manager is expected to solve problems and to tell workers how to do their jobs correctly. QI has a different vision of good management. QI emphasizes the necessity of involving the workers in a particular process in its design and improvement. This management tenet is not based on simply being fair, it is based on experience within organizations and what has been found to be successful. QI relies on cross-functional project teams assigned to study and improve specific work processes. Project teams, not to be confused with quality circles, are groups of individuals selected because of their knowledge and responsibility for a process being considered for improvement. Team projects have proved to be critically important to QI successes in various industries and organizations and are one of the major vehicles for organizational change.

Healthcare organizations are changing at an extraordinary rate. Unfortunately, much of this change is being driven by external forces rather than internal planning and design. Cost concerns are driving the development of quality programs akin to the inspection systems of other industries. This approach failed in manufacturing and other service industries and is destined to fail in healthcare. Quality improvement strategies and techniques can provide healthcare managers with the skills they need to effectively address quality issues within their organizations.

Hospital Corporation of America: The Hospitalwide Quality Improvement Process

THOMAS R. GILLEM, Director of Quality Education and Communications

Hospital Corporation of America, Nashville, Tennessee

In 1986, Hospital Corporation of America (HCA) began translating for the healthcare industry the concepts of continuous quality improvement that have been used for decades in many industries worldwide, most notably in Japan. Organizationwide quality improvement has been demonstrated to be the most cost-effective way to increase quality and productivity and, at the same time, to reduce total costs. HCA is convinced that continuous, systematic improvement in the delivery of health services is the answer to providing quality medical care.

Initiating the Hospitalwide Quality Improvement Process (HQIP) in a hospital or healthcare organization begins with a commitment from an administrator or chief executive officer who understands that continuous quality improvement is not just another management program. The top leader must know that the responsibility for quality is so important to the long-term welfare of the organization that it cannot be assigned to a person or a committee where inspection after the fact, such as occurs with traditional quality assurance activities, is the mainstay. It cannot be delegated to subordinates who perceive quality improvement as simply something else they have to do. Continuous quality improvement requires a CEO who sends a clear signal to everyone below that the organization is going to be managed in a new way that uses proven methods and insights.

Continuous quality improvement is not business as usual. A healthcare organization involved in HQIP is a place where the definition of quality is clear and measurable, and relates to the organization's mission. All employees there know the purpose of the organization, the way that their customers judge quality, the way quality is measured, their roles in improving quality, and the tools necessary to measure and improve quality. The HQIP organization is a place where everyone knows who their customers are, both internal customers (their fellow employees) and external customers (patients, doctors, payers, boards, and the community).

Impatient managers who expect to see the HQIP implemented instantly throughout their facilities and who expect to reap huge, immediate benefits will almost surely be disappointed. Continuous quality improvement is a long-term process. Over time, HQIP leads to an organizational transformation, from traditional turf protection to a new custom of team spirit and cooperation. It applies the scientific method to the management of hospitals. Instead of using gut feelings to make decisions, leaders involved in the HQIP understand that all processes vary, and they use graphically displayed data to make decisions in a systematic manner.

HQIP forces managers and their employees to stop looking only at results and to concentrate instead on the innumerable processes that comprise a hospital. To improve results, management and employees work together to decrease variation in the processes; this makes them more reliable and predictable. HQIP introduces a common language for continuous improvement that allows employees from the various disciplines to work together more productively. It requires patience and constancy of purpose to accomplish because learning the new concepts and becoming proficient in the use of improvement tools and techniques can be painstakingly slow.

Continuous improvement begins by understanding how customers judge quality, how processes work, and how the variation in the processes can lead to wise management action. An integral part of HQIP is the need for hospital leaders to obtain accurate and reliable information about how their external customers judge the quality of their hospital's services. Efforts to measure hospital quality in the past have relied almost entirely on internal quality assessments made by professionals who operate the system, with little regard for the perceptions of the hospital's customers. Traditional patient satisfaction surveys used by hospitals typically fall short in providing the information necessary to direct real improvements in quality.

To provide appropriate feedback on hospital quality, a family of customer judgment systems called Hospital Quality Trends are being developed to gather accurate and reliable data for hospital leaders. The Hospital Quality Trends: Patient Judgment System (HQT Patients) required more than a year to plan, pilot, and implement. It was designed by a team that included hospital administrators, nurses, physicians, and specialists in health services research from the Quality Resource Group at Hospital Corporation of America, the Rand Corporation, and the Harvard School of Public Health. Leaders in scores of hospitals began using information from HQT Patients during 1988. HQT Physicians, which measures a hospital's quality as rated by the medical staff, was first offered in early 1989. Other surveys in the HQT series measure how employees feel about the hospital as a place to work, as a place to receive care and service, and as an institution involved in HQIP, and how people in communities and on hospital boards view the facility's quality improvement efforts and market strategy.

For hospitals involved in continuous quality improvement, three major underpinnings form the basis of their transformation: quality improvement policy, quality improvement teams, and quality improvement in daily work life.

Quality improvement policy is the mission statement, quality definition, and guidelines that explicitly state the organization's intentions concerning continuous quality improvement. Over time, that policy simply becomes *the* organizational policy—the way the hospital is managed—and every employee knows it.

Quality improvement teams are the most visible manifestation of the HQIP initiation. Teams should be organized to tackle the chronic causes of poor quality by improving the processes in hospitals; they should not replace the day-to-day decision making of management. Everything that happens in a hospital, or in any organization, is the result of a process. To improve the quality of services, ways must be found to improve the operation of processes. A team usually consists of five to eight people who have knowledge about and regular contact with the process being improved. In a team's regular meetings, an established strategy for improvement is followed to understand who owns, or controls, the process being improved; how it currently works; how waste, re-

work, and needless complexity can be eliminated; how to gather appropriate data to assist in the improvement; and how to change the process and hold the gains.

In hospitals already undergoing the HQIP transformation, teams have been organized to improve myriad processes. For example, quality improvement teams have been formed to minimize the turnaround time in the operating room, speed up the distribution of medications, decrease reliance on agency nurses, better meet patient expectations for food delivery systems, decrease the registration time for outpatients, decrease the waste associated with dispensing intravenous medications, and eliminate billing errors. As a hospital's transformation matures, employees begin working together more effectively regardless of whether they are on a quality improvement team.

The third underpinning, quality improvement in daily work life, simply translates into meaningful personal work for employees as the transformation proceeds. The value added to an organization is limitless when the lines on an organization chart are no longer barriers to working together and when employees know that their knowledge about their workplace is a valued asset to the organization.

A quality improvement transformation will likely take years, perhaps as long as a decade, in any healthcare organization, but the alternative is to continue business as usual. While hospital leaders are waiting to decide if they should take the first steps in hospitalwide quality improvement, a basic shift in the medical paradigm is under way. Traditionally, healthcare delivered in a scientific and caring manner was perceived as the accepted standard. In recent years, however, concerns about costs and medical competence have brought new pressures on the healthcare industry. Like auto makers, electronics manufacturers, and countless other businesses, hospitals are faced with more and more consumers who demand that quality products and services be provided at the best value possible. In healthcare, the pressure is coming from both individuals and third party payers.

HQIP will be critical to hospitals in the years ahead. As pressures mount to keep spiraling healthcare costs in check, the hospitals that survive will be the facilities that meet the needs and expectations of their customers by continuously improving everything they do.

CASE STUDY

Quality Control in the Delivery of Healthcare in the State of Vermont

HENRY M. TUFO, M.D., President
Given Health Care Center, Burlington, Vermont

HAMILTON E. DAVIS, Chairman
Vermont Hospital Data Council, Waterbury, Vermont

In the years after World War II, the Japanese have built the world's finest automobile industry from a base of rubble. Never in history has anyone produced a stream of such high quality products at such low prices. This industry was peculiarly Japanese in many ways, but the intellectual base on which its quality programs were constructed was, in fact, American. The intellectual discipline known as "quality control" was developed in America and ignored. It came to fruition half a globe away.

Quality theory is not magic. It is powerful mainly because it accords so well with the way most human beings function best: they want to do well; they need quick feedback of reliable information about the outcome of their efforts; and they need to observe and measure regularly, and strive continuously to do better.

The congruence between this intellectually rich discipline and all human endeavor renders it suitable for use in the delivery of medical care. At first glance, there appears to be little resemblance between manufacturing and the delivery of medical care. In fact, the underlying principles are the same. Indeed, it is doubtful that American medicine can achieve a high degree of quality control any other way.

A model that illustrates these principles is called the Juran trilogy.[1] Its three steps are:

1. *Design* This phase involves determining the consumer's needs—whether for a carburetor that functions flawlessly for 200,000 miles or a controlled blood pressure without side effects—and then establishing a process to produce it. The "need" and the process to meet it generate specifications and requirements.

2. *Quality control* The process established during the design phase must be monitored to determine whether the requirements are being met, that is, is the product acceptable? (Monitoring here means both running the process and measuring the output.) All processes produce variance in output to some extent; monitoring will tell whether the normal or "common variance" is acceptable. In other words, the product always meets the requirements despite the variance. If the product is not always acceptable, the process must be adjusted. Monitoring may also disclose "special variance," an occasional spike in the outcome that should not flow from the process. The spike indicates that something beyond the established process is at work; it must be eliminated.

3. *Quality improvement* Measuring and monitoring should go on regularly. Based on the quick feedback of this information, the process can be fine-tuned in order to reduce common variance, thereby reducing errors, waste, and unnecessary cost.

Moreover, continuous attention to the process itself and to the outcomes is likely to lead to significant improvements in that process over time—breakthroughs that produce quantum reductions in errors and marked decreases in cost.

The Juran trilogy is shown graphically in Figure 1. Once such a system is in place, several things quickly become clear. One is the definition of quality, often a maddening enigma. Quality is constant conformance to requirements. A specific, repeatable process must be in place; otherwise an assessment of quality is impossible. Requirements must be clearly set forth. Everything must be visible and explicit; otherwise there will be no way to track down and eliminate defects. All of these steps are vital in industrial quality control.

The evidence that this system is a powerful one fills our highways and parking lots every day. The question for health policymakers and physicians is whether it can be applied to the delivery of medical care. Fifteen years of clinical experience at a faculty-based group practice at the University of Vermont indicates that it can.[2,3] On the basis of that experience a coalition of providers and other healthcare players in Vermont has come together to design and implement a statewide quality assurance system. The

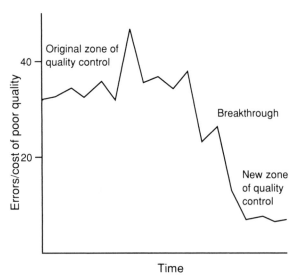

Figure 1   *The Juran trilogy.*

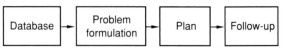

Figure 3   *Problem-oriented system.*

statewide system is the result of a marriage between the Juran model and the problem-oriented medical delivery system pioneered in the early 1970s by Dr. Lawrence Weed.[4]

The key issue here is the establishment of a process for care that can be controlled. Medical care has typically depended on an implicit process that is shown schematically in Figure 2. But there are no rules for controlling or monitoring this system. Physicians take shortcuts; they sometimes follow different treatment therapies; they occasionally forget to capture vital information; they very often do not write everything down in a way that would expose their reasoning and render visible the overall process.

Therefore, when "errors" in outcome appear it is impossible to go back and repair the process with any degree of reliability. This is the reason why quality control efforts in the past have had little effect on patient care and virtually no effect on medical costs.

Weed attacked the problem by designing an explicit process known as the problem-oriented medical record, which is shown schematically in Figure 3.

Figure 2   *Traditional process.*

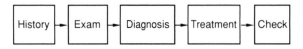

Within each of the four steps, rules were created to ensure that the patient moved from step to step only after each step was complete and explicit. The system works as follows:

- *Database*   Predefine the historical information and the clinical data to be gathered for each patient in order to be sure that all problems, as well as the main or presenting problem, can be ascertained. Failures at this step cause significant errors. In a major clinical practice 30 percent of database items were found to be erroneous or missing altogether.[5] Close monitoring and adjustment of the data-gathering process to assure that it was reliably collected and effectively displayed reduced errors to 2 percent within 6 months.

- *Problem formulation*   Define the major problem as it is understood from the database, but list all other important problems as well. There is no point in curing the major problem only to have the patient succumb to a secondary one.

- *Plan*   Establish a written goal for the treatment, and then set forth specific plans to meet it. Account for each active problem in the process.

- *Follow-up*   Record all actions taken, organized by title and numbered problem, in order to have a continuous record of the care given and the results obtained.

This organizing principle was of enormous importance to medicine. At its heart was Weed's understanding that the way professionals collect, organize, and analyze information is the central activity in a knowledge-based industry. Two examples of how these methodologies can be applied to the delivery of healthcare follow.

EXAMPLE ONE — GALL BLADDER SURGERY

Patient A enters the hospital for elective gall bladder surgery. The physician has selected this treatment course based on a history of pain in the right side, fever, and the indication in an ultrasound study of the presence of gall stones.

In an implicit process—the way much of medicine works today—the physician would begin the surgery and then use professional experience and a manual examination of the common bile duct to decide whether stones are likely to be present and, if they are, to explore the duct and remove them. This approach has been shown in the literature to miss stones about 20 percent of the time. In terms of the Juran trilogy (Figure 1) this would be shown as the original zone of quality control with a 20 percent error rate or common variance.

This error rate might be reduced incrementally over time by refinements in the common process, but in fact, there has now been developed a new common process that involves taking an intraoperative cholangiogram (an x-ray with contrast material) to determine if stones are present and then removing them. The error rate of this improved procedure is 1 to 5 percent, a huge improvement or breakthrough.

Further improvement will probably require improved techniques of reading the intraoperative x-rays, or better methods of contrasting the stones, or conceivably some entirely new way to cope with this disease. In any case, such a new breakthrough would produce a further sharp reduction in error rates and in associated costs.

This advance in gall bladder therapy may not seem remarkable, but the unfortunate fact is that while some medical communities will immediately use it and continue to push for improvements, others will not or will do so only slowly. A uniform quality control system will markedly advance the promulgation of such improvements across the system.

EXAMPLE TWO—CAROTID ENDARTERECTOMY

Patient B enters the hospital after the physician diagnoses a carotid artery occlusion, that is, a blockage of the major artery through the neck to the brain. Recent studies by the Rand Corporation have shown that some 65 percent of procedures to repair this condition are inappropriate. The procedure is therefore a major candidate for the application of quality control efforts. It might work in the following way.

The initial clinical finding here is most typically a loss of function or sensation reported by the patient. The physician in this example has heard a noise in the neck and has concluded there is a carotid blockage. The physician confirms the blockage with an x-ray of the artery and orders surgery in order to prevent a stroke. During surgery, the patient suffers an acute myocardial infarction (a heart attack) and dies.

The same case in the proposed system would undergo a very different process. At the outset, the physician would follow a specific history, gathering any clinical data protocol aimed at subsuming the current literature and experience in this disease. This ensures that the vital data are gathered the same way in every case.

For example, instead of moving only on the basis of dizziness, as often happens, the physician would do a neurological study to determine whether the patient has suffered episodes of loss of vision, sensation, or motor control in a way that coincided with loss of function in the section of the brain served by the blocked artery.

If there is no such evidence, there should be no surgery. Even if the blockage is present, the literature shows that in the absence of the correlating symptoms there is only 1 chance in a 1000 that the patient will have a stroke, and that risk is not decreased by surgery.

If the appropriate symptoms are present, then the physician needs to test the degree of blockage. The literature shows that surgery is not indicated unless at least one vessel is at least 70 percent blocked.

If all indications for surgery continue to be positive, then the protocols would call for still another assessment of problems with the heart. The fact that the patient died from a heart attack during surgery on an entirely different area of the body is a "spike" in the Juran trilogy—a result that should not flow from the process at all and must be eliminated, as far as possible.

The physician should therefore add to the database any evidence of significant coronary artery disease; this would include a determination of whether the patient has had a heart attack or angina and an ECG to test for previous silent heart attack. If any of these tests are positive, the physician should do an exercise thallium study of the heart to see if significant blockage exists.

Only if these tests are made and weighed should surgery go forward. In Juran terms, the common variance is now in the neighborhood of 65 percent, which is clearly an unacceptable level. This failure rate would include surgeries that could not be justified on the basis of the neurological findings plus the residual variation from the procedure itself. The

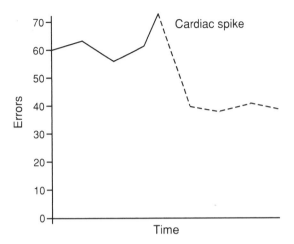

Figure 4 *Juran diagram for carotid endarterectomy.*

heart attack rate of 3 to 5 percent would be superimposed on that variation and should be eliminated. The Juran diagram would look as shown in Figure 4. It is not yet known what the common variance would be once these improvements were made.

When the Juran trilogy is combined with the Weed problem-oriented method and is converted to a linear expression of the movement of a patient through the system, it resembles Figure 5.

The potential power of fusing the discipline of industrial quality assurance to the delivery of medical care is enormous. It is also clear, however, that the difficulties are formidable. There are unexplored limitations in the construction of automobiles, but they are relatively small in number and have only a minor impact on the overall process.

In medicine, there are many unexplored limitations. The interactions among the known and unknown variables are many. It is difficult to establish disease protocols because of interactions among problems. The amount of sheer information relevant to each symptom and disease, and disease combination is already impossible to memorize—and it is growing exponentially. This growth lies at the root of the move toward specialization in medical practice. And the patient's own desires and participation in treatment vary widely.

In an important sense, these alarming parameters argue in favor of moving toward a fused industrial quality medical delivery approach. This conviction is based on principles that rise directly out of the complexity of the medical quality problem. They are:

1. An explicit system with rules for information handling that can be shared by all physicians and patients must be installed. Without this, there can be no feedback and no quality control.

2. The computer must be used not only as a memory tool but as a processing tool. Facts, and the relationships between the facts, are proliferating beyond the power of human memory.

3. Information must be accessible to patients and physicians and organized in such a way that they can use it.

The extent to which quality can truly be measured in the medical care delivery system depends on the extent to which these principles can be set in place. The synthesis of industrial quality methods and the

Figure 5 *A proposed care delivery system.*

Treatment phase

Two-phase intake protocol	Problem formulation	Treatment protocol	Plan	Weed process action	Check
Drives the gathering of medical history and clinical tests so that nothing is missed.	By physician.	Based on optimal treatment options as determined by literature, specialty societies, study groups, etc. (options shared with patient).	A plan is established by the physician in light of the treatment protocol. Must be written and list specific goals and expected outcomes.	Therapy is undertaken by physician and patient. Must be set out in record.	Physician must check to see if goals are met. Review must appear in record. Process is repeated if goals not met.
Drives processing of data so as to facilitate diagnosis.					

problem-oriented medical delivery system hold out a clear prospect for doing that.

REFERENCES

1. J. M. Juran, *Juran on Quality Planning.* Ace Press, New York, 1988, pp. 11–13, 15, and 71.
2. H. M. Tufo, R. E. Bouchard, et al., "Problem Oriented Approach to Practice: I. Economic Impact," *JAMA* **238:** 414–417 (1977).
3. H. M. Tufo, R. E. Bouchard, et al., "Problem Oriented Approach to Practice: II. Development of the System Through Audit and Implication," *JAMA* **238:** 502–505 (1977).
4. L. L. Weed, *Medical Records, Medical Education and Patient Care.* Case Western Reserve University Press, Cleveland, 1971, pp. 1–297.
5. H. M. Tufo et al., "Implementing a Problem Oriented Practice." In H. K. Walker, J. W. Hurst, and M. F. Woody (eds.), *Applying the Problem Oriented System*, Medcom Press, New York, 1973, p. 29.

PART THREE

MANAGEMENT INFORMATION SYSTEMS

CHAPTER EIGHTEEN

Report Focus

PURCHASER-ORIENTED MANAGED CARE REPORTS

PETER BOLAND, Ph.D., President
Boland Healthcare Consultants, Berkeley, California

Intelligent information is the key resource of delivery systems in the 1990s. How it is applied will largely determine to what extent HMOs and PPOs become third-generation managed care systems. It is also the best barometer of a health plan's orientation to customer needs and can be readily understood by payers, employee benefits managers, and trust fund administrators.

Too few delivery systems recognize the strategic importance of client reporting as a marketing tool for positioning themselves as effective managers of healthcare resources.

The number of managed care products on the market is inundating purchasers with a bewildering array of choices. Plain vanilla-type PPOs and traditional HMOs all compete in their respective market niches with remarkably similar products. Market differentiation —through information technology— has not been widely pursued as a managed care strategy to date.

Unless a corporation or trust fund is large enough to have full-time benefit specialists on staff, it becomes increasingly difficult for buyers to make an intelligent decision about which health plan to select and why they are choosing it.

Many purchasers have little to go on other than general reputation of the PPO or HMO, word-of-mouth from employees or other employers, and marketing appeals from the health plan. As a result, buyers need benchmarks or user-friendly "handles" for judging health plans. One of the easiest benchmarks to comprehend is client reporting. If a report is understandable, it enables benefit managers to make better choices about allocating resources. If the data are hard to interpret or too complex to wade through, they are of little use.

A further weakness of managed care information systems has been limited data flexibility and adherence to rudimentary all-encompassing "averages." The latter can be useful as a point of reference, but it too often becomes a "lowest common denominator" type of yardstick for measuring success.

Both purchasers and health plan sponsors are gravitating toward management information systems as one of the most practical indices of what to look for in terms of PPO and HMO capability. Their reasoning is that sophisticated data management capability signifies a commitment to develop the type of resources a health plan needs to be a market leader in the 1990s.

However, claims administration systems have historically generated numerous statistical compilations but relatively little useful information about the relationship between medical care and costs. Thus, management information systems are now being called upon to gather data which highlight both delivery system performance and claims adjudication capability.

What employers will be looking for in terms of data capability includes:

- The capacity to document real cost savings using valid measurement techniques
- The ability to determine patient management options (on a case-by-case basis) in relation to different treatment modes and settings
- Focused management reports which convey information as a decision-support tool

In order to generate relevant cost savings data, managed care plans must move to incorporate information generated from utilization review procedures with claims-based data that are commonly used. One of the prerequisites of focused customer reporting is a flexible database which links different utilization review screens to other internal management controls like case management, quality assurance, and claims adjudication. The impact of each of these factors must be tracked and reported to purchasers and payers.

These basic data elements must be in place and administered according to a common set of management objectives. This will produce accurate data which can then be massaged into constructive client information. The adage about "so much data, but so little information" is certainly the case for most HMOs and PPOs.

One of the shortcomings of managed care has been the lack of meaningful customer reports. Delivery systems which cannot produce credible performance-based data may be squeezed out of the market as the industrywide shakeout intensifies.

Health plans that develop succinct, usable data will quickly establish a reputation as market leaders. This capacity will enable a delivery system to better define "the rules of the game" on a regional basis and gain a tremendous advantage through skillful market positioning.

As a prerequisite for product accountability, certain information features will become more commonplace; for example,

- Predictable cost estimates that can be used as a basis for risk- and gain-sharing mechanisms, such as exclusive provider organizations or other hybrid arrangements which control price and volume
- Utilization trend highlights which profile providers and patients
- Interactive databases which allow for modeling solutions on a client-specific basis

Thus, to become effective third-generation delivery systems, health plans need to develop a broad information systems strategy. Most HMOs and PPOs develop specific data capability on an ad hoc basis in response to crisis situations. They normally address one or two functional areas at a time, and the order of importance is usually as follows:

- Day-to-day housekeeping functions
- Financial data
- Utilization management
- Quality assurance
- Clinical interface
- External client reporting

HMOs, PPOs, and payers need to give client reporting far more importance than is the case currently. For many purchasers, product accountability equals properly focused data from vendors. Accountability, in turn, is related to internal efficiency standards, management reports that highlight utilization levels, cost figures, and cost savings.

These types of reports provide important planning data for benefit design and budget forecasting. Their intent is to enable employers and other purchasers to make better decisions about employee benefits. Good data will enable them to stretch healthcare dollars further and to preserve the value of current healthcare benefits.

These reports will likewise be useful to payers for benefits design and product development activities and to providers for monitoring and controlling how care is given.

CHAPTER NINETEEN

Information Cycle

COLLECTION, CORRECTION, APPLICATION: THE INFORMATION CYCLE IN MANAGED HEALTHCARE

RICHARD H. ESKOW, Vice President
American International Healthcare, Rockville, Maryland

Managed healthcare, across its many areas of application, is in large part an information-driven field. The questions facing professionals in the managed care field who are evaluating their information needs are (1) how should the information-handling process be enhanced for tomorrow's delivery systems and (2) how can currently available information be used effectively in the meantime?

Several significant statements can be made about managed healthcare information.

1. Managed healthcare programs have increased the amount of available healthcare data significantly.
2. The availability of usable data has always lagged significantly behind the marketplace and industry goals.
3. The lag in the availability of usable data is due in part to problems in the collection of valid data and in part to the fact that segments of the industry do not yet understand the usefulness of certain information that is already available.
4. The process of improving data collection and reporting has an inevitable effect on what is being reported (an "uncertainty principle" in healthcare).
5. The integration of multiple managed care products into unified products increases demands for information-based products.

6. The information objective for managed healthcare administrators must therefore be threefold: to use currently available data to maximum effect, to improve the collection and reporting process, and to use information management techniques to enhance services.

7. These objectives require that managed healthcare administrators utilize three areas of data management: improvement in source information (collection), edits and controls on the entry and use of information (correction), and effective plan management based on reporting (application). These areas represent the information "life cycle."

HISTORICAL OVERVIEW   The need to collect data related to health benefits began with the advent of centralized claims payment operations in order to support the claims payment functions. Clearly there was no need for any kind of claims processing ability until a structure was developed to distribute the costs of healthcare experience. Large employers who provided healthcare services to their employees by running clinics and hospitals needed only two basic types of data. They needed to know who their employees were (eligibility demographics), and they needed to know what kind of services they would provide (benefits design).

Employer-Sponsored Healthcare   Healthcare providers were employed by companies in a role that was roughly parallel to today's group-model health plans. Group-model plans, like the employer-sponsored health programs of the past, have less complex administrative data requirements than independent practice associations (IPAs). For example, IPAs need to track a member's primary care physician affiliation and use that affiliation as a check to ensure that specialty or hospital services were appropriately authorized before they were used. Accounting functions are substantially more complex in an IPA, and discerning physicians will demand substantially more sophisticated cost and utilization reporting in situations where their compensation is based in part on cost incentives.

The informational requirements of employer-sponsored healthcare plans were simple, but they already included three of the four basic categories of information required to pay healthcare claims:

- Membership demographics
- Benefit information
- Provider information

Such organizations were not required to pay healthcare claims on a third party basis. Third party payments in healthcare were a product of the rise of Blue Cross and Blue Shield organizations in the post-Depression years and the advent of group health insurance on a large scale.

Group Health Insurance

Payment of these services required that claims be sent to large, central organizations for payment. These claims covered a variety of services that were provided to individuals in a number of separate employer groups over a widely dispersed geographic area.

In order to pay a claim, indemnity carriers needed to know the following kinds of information:

- Membership information (including dates of eligibility and type of coverage).
- Benefit design (the kinds of services and benefits the member's coverage entitle him or her to at the time of service).
- Type of service—the carrier needed to know the type of service being provided in order to know whether it was appropriate for the member's coverage. The carrier did not need to know the specific service provided, for either the appropriate payable amount or the appropriateness of treatment.
- Amount billed for the service.
- Provider information for Blue Cross and Blue Shield and other plans requiring provider membership.
- Member's required contribution and deductible limits.

During the 1930s, all the essential elements used to pay claims until the advent of alternative delivery systems in the 1970s had been defined. Even after these systems came into being, the basic elements remained the same—the enhancements since then have tended more toward increased detail and increased sophistication rather than a change in the basic elements.

Impact of Medicaid and Medicare

The 1965 laws which established the Medicaid and Medicare programs provided for federal cost sharing and the imposition of federal standards on state programs of healthcare for the poor. The unexpectedly high cost of these programs created a political climate, based on taxpayer concerns, that resulted in government investigation and public disclosure of patterns of healthcare delivery.

The discovery of fraud and abuse in the practice of medicine under Medicare changed public perceptions of the medical profession. It added legitimacy to the idea that payers were entitled to question the delivery of medical care and to intervene in certain cases, and it increased the demand for information on costs, utilization patterns, and the professional decisions that affected utilization and costs.

Most states initially contracted with Blue Cross and Blue Shield and insurance companies to carry out the claims adjudication function using existing systems and procedures. These systems and procedures were oriented toward rapid transaction processing rather than assuring appropriateness of provider payment. This orientation is a reflection of the nature of indemnity claims processing, which does not contain the kinds of edits for prior authorization, appropriateness of care, and provider patterns of treatment that are characteristic of closed-panel payment systems.

For many years there has been significant waste because of such basic errors as payment of duplicate claims, payment for services not covered, overpayment, and payment to ineligible persons. As they begin to examine the performance of their carriers and claims administrators, employers are beginning to find many of the same problems found by the government.

The federal government developed explicit standards for management information systems (MIS) to be used in state Medicaid programs in 1971 and ever since has been increasing the stringency of these standards as well as the effectiveness of federal compliance monitoring.

Utilization Review

In the period 1971 to 1972 the federal programs came to include a surveillance and utilization review (S/UR) subsystem which represented a leap forward in the technology of using Medicaid claims processing systems to detect questionable healthcare patterns by providers and recipients. The S/UR system supported comparatively complex statistical and normative analysis.

Automated model treatment profiling systems (comparing service patterns against diagnosis-specific criteria) began appearing at this time. Simultaneously states began using these techniques for prior authorization and concurrent review of hospital inpatient care. Many of these techniques became part of the new cost-containment rhetoric for employer groups.

HMO Claims Payment

The HMO Act encouraged the development and growth of the HMO industry, which needed to store and use all the types of information described above. In addition, a number of new information elements became necessary in order to know how to pay a claim. These included:

- *Predetermined fee schedules for specific types of services*   Under fee-for-service plans, all the claims payer needed to know was whether the member was covered, what type of service was rendered, and what percentage of charges the carrier was required to pay (within "reasonable and customary" limits). With HMOs and PPOs, fees have been agreed to between the provider and the plan based on the precise service rendered. That makes it necessary to store far more specific information about each procedure performed so that each claim can be paid according to the fee schedule, rather than as a percentage of the billed amount.
- *Provider profile*   Early, prototypical HMOs needed to know who their participating providers were. Greater levels of detail are required in today's HMO environment. These include:

> Has the provider agreed to the general fee schedule, or are their special fee agreements on a procedure-by-procedure basis specific to that provider?
>
> In a provider risk-sharing arrangement, how much of the provider's fee is being withheld for risk pooling?
>
> Has a general discount percentage that is less expensive than the regular fee schedule been agreed to?
>
> Are there restrictions on the types of service the provider can perform for the HMO? In other words, is the provider certified to perform only specific procedures for the health plan and restricted from performing others that may often be performed by members of his or her specialty?

- *Gatekeeper concept*   Is the provider a primary care physician (PCP)? Is the provider accepting new patients? How many patients does the PCP have and within what demographic groups? This information is needed in order to know how much to compensate the physician under capitation.

In the membership area, HMOs have a whole new set of informational needs. These include:

- Member's age and sex profile.
- Member's choice of a primary care provider. Since the choice of the PCP is used to determine whether the services rendered were authorized, it is necessary to record all previous PCPs as well as the dates that each physician filled that role in order to determine if services were properly authorized.
- Other coverage code for coordination of benefits.
- Free-form remarks.

When it actually comes time to pay or deny a claim, an HMO or PPO system also needs additional pieces of information:

- Is the service authorized? This is a critical element in HMO processing since controls are imposed through the "gatekeeper." An HMO system has to first check whether the provider of service was the PCP; if not, it has to check a file to make sure that the service was authorized by the PCP. Otherwise, it will deny the claim.
- What was the specific procedure performed? Was it appropriate to the recipient's demographics (age and sex)? What restrictions does the procedure have, for example, once in a lifetime? Has this member violated those restrictions? Is it a procedure that is included in the capitation payment and therefore no additional fee should be charged?
- What was the diagnosis? Does the diagnosis fit the member's profile? Is the procedure rendered appropriate for the diagnosis?
- Where was the service performed? Prepaid health plans normally restrict certain procedures to outpatient or other specific locations. It therefore becomes important to track the location of the service.

Claims Processing: Current Data Needs

When taken as a whole, the claims processing industry and its related activities have created the following types of data processing needs:

Large-scale fee-for-service processing by large, national carriers.

HMO claims processing with its own set of processing, pricing, and claims editing criteria.

HMO internal reporting requirements.

HMO reporting requirements to employers. This area is receiving increasing attention now as a result of changing marketplace conditions.

Federally mandated requirements for reporting, quality review, and appropriateness of payments in the Medicare and Medicaid environment.

PPO reporting requirements.

Triple-option processing and reporting.

Precertification review requirements, including clinical indicators, national norms for types of service, demographic data, and internal data needs which includes efficiency indicators.

Employers' needs for concise and well-organized data to be used in evaluating their healthcare costs in the fee-for-service and managed care areas.

Employer information requirements for supporting the design and implementation of flexible-spending benefit plans.

Information on the projected and actual cost and utilization impact of benefit design changes in a managed fee-for-service environment.

Comparative data on fee-for-service, HMO, and PPO experience.

Clinical data from hospital and physician care management systems.

Quality of Data The quality, quantity, and consistency of data in these systems varies dramatically from location to location. The problem then becomes how best to recognize what is accurate and usable in the data currently available and to see the true significance of the reports produced. Recognizing useful data and interpreting the data correctly requires an understanding of the individuals who produce the data in its raw form (for example, claims form and medical records) and an understanding of how that information can be applied and by whom.

THE INFORMATION CYCLE

Managed Healthcare: A Behavioral Science

Managed healthcare can be seen as a behavioral science, and a number of managed healthcare reporting functions can be seen as applied behavioral science, where the subject under study is the behavior of social groups. Groups of individuals that participate in the managed healthcare process include providers, enrollees, healthcare managers, and purchasers.

Each group enters into the process with specific needs, biases, and motivations that influence the information they provide. Each in turn is affected by the need to report information and modifies its behavior accordingly. Examples of behavior intended to meet informational needs include a physician recording more detailed diagnostic and procedural information, a patient tracking health plan approval of a restricted service, and an employer group collecting more detailed demographic information for premium payment purposes. Changes in behavior that result from these actions might include a physician's changing the diagnosis code provided to a carrier in order to better justify the procedure performed and a patient's use of an emergency room for treatment in an attempt to avoid a plan's preapproval requirements for selected services.

These are negative changes in behavior caused by actions performed as a result of the need for information, but information demands can have positive effects as well. For example, it can discourage the use of unnecessary services by causing providers to reexamine whether specific procedures will be considered appropriate for the diagnosis being reported, or it can discourage employees from giving their health plan card to nonmembers (by requiring that each family member be identified upon enrollment).

Information as a Management Concern

The information life cycle consists of collection of data from the groups of individuals described above; of correction, that is, the computerized process of clarification, error-elimination, and standardization; and of application, that is, the process of generating usable information and acting on it. Each part of the cycle requires the commitment, involvement, and guidance of senior healthcare management. Issues will arise which include:

- Should enrollees be required to provide more detailed personal histories, even if they feel uncomfortable about the plan as a result?
- Should physicians be subject to automatic review of the care they provide? What actions should be taken if they do not "pass" that review?
- How much information should be gathered when providing authorization for restricted services? Should the requirement for detailed information be used to discourage use of such services?

The importance of these questions ensures that the information cycle will be of primary concern to senior management.

COLLECTION, CORRECTION, AND APPLICATION

Collection

ENROLLMENT It is not possible to properly interpret reports on the cost and use of healthcare services without understanding the population that is using those services. The lack of a proper "denominator" (size, age, and sex mix of the covered population) for the cost and frequency reports produced by many claims payers results in the production of healthcare statistics that lack a proper context. If the number of persons a cost represents is not known then, for example, $247,000 in prescription drug costs per year is not a significant number. Maternity costs that are 34 percent of total expenditures may or may not be appropriate; the age and sex mix of the group can help tell that. Medical costs of $2800 per employee per year may be a sign of overuse of services, or it may be an appropriate cost level for an older population concentrated in a city with costly medical services.

Producing meaningful healthcare reports requires denominators on the population for whom services are being rendered. This requires capturing and updating detailed demographic information on the population being covered. HMOs have traditionally led the field in this area since HMO benefits are often contingent on primary care physician relationships, age and sex restrictions, and other policies that require knowing things about each covered individual, for example, whether the patient had a primary care relationship with the physician performing the service, the age and sex of the patient (to verify medical necessity), and the benefit group of the patient (to confirm the nature and extent of coverage). It is therefore useful to begin by collecting the following information on each subscriber:

Name

Address

Other coverage for the coordination of benefits

Employer and division

Hourly rate and salary

Length of service

Employer standard industry classification

Deductible and copayment limits

Knowing each individual's dependents is also critical to healthcare management information. This requires capturing the following information, at a minimum:

Name

Subscriber

Age

Sex

Family status (subscriber, husband, wife, daughter, son)

Primary care physician (if HMO or EPO)

Dates of coverage

Categories of coverage:

- Single, double, or family
- Benefit plan
- Membership class
- Special restrictions

Past history of coverage categories (with effective dates of each)

- Employer group
- Address

PROVIDER   Profiling provider behavior and understanding how to modify it is a key element in managed healthcare. This cannot be done if all services rendered by an individual physician or hospital cannot be linked together for reporting purposes through a common ID number.

Many carriers do not ensure that the same identifier is used each time, particularly when the subscriber is reimbursed for the service. Some hospitals and physicians do business under multiple tax identification numbers, which means that the computer logic used to generate tax forms (1099s) cannot always be adapted for reporting purposes.

Changing claims administration and computer systems to reliably track providers is not easy. Providers need to provide complete information when submitting a claim form. When patients submit bills that they have paid, they may be required to capture information on the providers who treated them, since detailed provider information will increasingly be required by the payer before the patients are reimbursed. The ability to identify inappropriate patterns in the delivery of care make the inconvenience more than worthwhile.

Provider information that needs to be captured includes:

Provider name

Provider ID

Address

Location

Specialty or type of institution

Secondary specialty

Board certification (for physicians)

Tertiary care facilities (for hospitals)

Group and site affiliations (providers with whom a physician has formed a group practice and separate addresses where a physician may have offices)

Provider's contractual relationship with plan (PPO, HMO, none)

PRIOR AUTHORIZATIONS HMOs and EPOs may require that a primary care physician, or a case manager, provide prior authorization for a range of specialty services. Indemnity plans and PPOs increasingly require preauthorizations for inpatient hospitalizations and a changing spectrum of outpatient services. The prior authorization process represents a means for prospectively gathering data on a case that can be used to provide a number of critical management tasks that are frequently overlooked. These include:

- Identifying potentially catastrophic cases for early case management intervention (referral to tertiary care facilities with special

agreements, home health recommendations, specialist referrals, provision of durable medical goods, and home improvements)
- Identifying inappropriate referral relationships among providers
- Identifying physicians who overrefer (or underrefer)
- Ongoing tracking of incurred but not reported (IBNR) expenses, particularly for higher cost cases with greater potential financial impact
- Capturing initial diagnoses at the inception of a case; this information can be used to profile providers for appropriate diagnoses and to compare the outcome of diagnoses for quality profiling of providers

Authorization data elements include the following:

Authorization ID number

Patient name

Name of authorizing provider

Referred to provider

Date of authorization

Range of dates for services authorized

Type of service authorized

Number of days (or services) authorized

Patient age and sex

Diagnosis (for each authorization and extension of authorization)

Specific procedure(s) authorized

Actual amount paid for service

Actual number of days (or services) used

CLAIMS PROCESSING   The information contained in a claims submission is generally prepared by the provider of service and submitted to the payer directly by the provider or by the subscriber (depending on who is reimbursed by the claims payer). Accurate, complete claims data are critical to information management. Without it, the true picture of healthcare needs (illness) and behavior (services and charges) can never be seen.

The amount of data submitted has historically been driven by the requirements for payment, as discussed above. New needs will drive claims data submission in the 1990s, including ensuring the appropriateness of care, monitoring quality, studying patterns of medical care use in a covered population, and matching delivery systems design to the changing care needs of covered populations.

The applicability of certain key claims data items to retrospective reporting can be questioned by those who have legitimate concerns about the quality of data captured, a concern which can only be addressed by careful consideration of each system and operation. In addition, items used for reporting are often questioned by providers and others who have a financial interest in the outcome of the reports.

For example, providers can question reports which analyze the level of treatment which they provide for certain diagnoses and which purport to demonstrate a pattern of overtreatment by suggesting that the patients they treat are more severely ill and the codes commonly used (International Classification of Diseases, 9th revision, known as ICD-9) lack measurements of the severity of an illness. Conversely, reports that use the procedure codes (such as the standard CPT) submitted by providers can be challenged for the presence of "code creep"; there are many providers who submit claims with procedure codes that describe more detailed and costly procedures than were actually performed or who bill associated procedures (such as multiple activities during a single surgery) as if each were independently performed.

Each concern is legitimate, and each recognizes inherent limitations in current reporting capabilities. However, given the nature of data as they are currently captured, strategies for compensating for these limitations are necessary. With severity of illness, an attempt can be made to compensate for the absence of severity indicators by adjusting provider reports for the age and sex mix of patients. Code creep can be studied through commonsense edits (for example, two initial workups are impossible) and frequency reports on specified procedures.

The key elements that need to be captured during the claims submission process therefore remain:

Patient ID

Subscriber ID

Provider ID

Referring provider ID

Date(s) of service

Type of service

Type of diagnosis (major diagnostic category)

Procedure code

Diagnosis code (primary)

Diagnosis code (secondary)

Other diagnosis codes (up to five may be required for hospital reimbursement under DRGs)

DRG classification

Patient age

Patient sex

Episode of care

Cost center (UB-82) code for hospitalizations

Correction   The entering and updating of data through a computer allows information to be edited automatically. This can happen either on-line, that is, while the information is being entered; batchwise, that is, retrospectively for correction purposes; or both. At the same time, the editing process allows controls that are essential to the true management of healthcare to be placed on the reimbursement process, as they impose changes in the delivery and consumption of covered services.

A set of edits during the entry of enrollment, authorization, and claims information can be instrumental in improving the management of healthcare.

ENROLLMENT DATA ENTRY   The number of useful edits which can be imposed during the entry of enrollment data is minimal. This is because the number of errors is less than, and the nature of the errors is different from, those seen during other stages of the data capture process. The timeliness of enrollment information is critical, however, in ensuring the accuracy of claims payment and the appropriateness of service authorizations. The increasing trend toward the sharing of eligibility information with providers through electronic (computer) media underscores this need.

Verifying a patient's eligibility for a service is only one reason why these data should be captured promptly. Managed healthcare requires timely and detailed information on the age, sex, location, and benefit plan chosen by every covered individual, including all dependents. This information permits accurate interpretation of utilization statistics by allowing comparison to norms. It also allows health plan managers to continue tailoring plan designs toward the specific needs of their population.

These needs are best met by requiring that complete enrollment applications be gotten from every covered individual. The demographic information described above should be provided, together with information on the coordination of benefits (COB) with other carriers (Medicare or spousal coverage) who may share liability for healthcare expenses.

Enrollees should be required to complete and maintain information on COB. Since there is no real motivation for providing this information, membership contracts should invalidate coverage in cases where this information is withheld.

The need for COB information has led to the creation of several databases that pool eligibility information from a number of subscribing carriers. Each carrier can then search for parallel enrollments for its members and seek to recover costs from the other carriers that have been identified. Obviously, the wisdom of participating in this kind of database depends on whether a payer expects to collect more in COB than is collected from it, although this point is often overlooked.

Plans are increasingly restricting their payments as secondary carriers so that the total reimbursement for a service does not exceed the plan's maximum payment. For example, if 75 percent of a service has been paid for by the primary payer and the secondary plan pays 80 percent for that type of care, the secondary plan would traditionally pay the difference in cost up to 100 percent. Under the new designs, the secondary payer would only pay 5 percent, bringing the total up to its own maximum of 80 percent (see the following example).

| | PRIMARY PLAN PAYS | SECONDARY PLAN PAYS | Patient | |
			RECEIVES	PAYS
Nonrestricted	$75	$25	$100	$ 0
Restricted	$75	$ 5	$ 80	$20

One important purpose of the copayment is to provide the patient with an incentive for using medical services selectively. The absence of restrictions on coordination of benefits removes that incentive, as shown above, while restricting the coordinated amount to the limits of the plan retains the incentive.

Other edits that can be applied during the enrollment process include ensuring that the coverage period of the member does not exceed the eligible period of the group, checking that no more dependents are added than is appropriate under the type of contract (single, double, or family), and ensuring that no more employees are enrolled in a group than are signed up for coverage.

AUTHORIZATIONS   The authorization process represents an opportunity to use editing logic on a specific service before that service is rendered. It therefore represents a unique opportunity to use computer logic to impose true management on the healthcare process on a prospective basis.

There are several ways to obtain an authorization. Utilization review services frequently employ a registered nurse or other clinician who can be reached by telephone, each of whom has a computer terminal to support the review process. HMOs tend to use their physicians as case managers. In this model, the primary physician authorizes a service. This authorization is then transmitted to the plan (by telephone, mail, or computer) and verified prior to the delivery of the referred service.

The utilization review process is sometimes controlled by the computer through the use of "logic trees" that dictate the questions to be asked over the phone and that control the interaction based on the answers given to each question. Under these circumstances it is inappropriate to speak of edits, since the computer is controlling, rather than editing, the process. However, these programs have yet to reach widespread acceptance in the utilization review industry because of its reluctance to eliminate the intervention of a trained clinician in a decision about the delivery of medical care.

Computer support for clinician-driven utilization review therefore offers the opportunity to accomplish the following:

- Verify the eligibility of the patient for the services rendered
- Provide supporting information on benefits design which can be given to the patient or provider at the time of authorization and which can influence the rendering of (or the use of) services
- Automatically validate the appropriateness of the proposed treatment to the diagnosis and to the demographics of the patient
- Compare the location of a provider rendering service (if not in a preferred panel) with those of preferred providers, and list nearby preferred providers for patient referral
- Identify requested procedures that require a second opinion
- List reimbursement amounts for requested procedures, which can be reviewed with a provider or patient
- Identify clinical data elements that are needed to determine the medical necessity and support the collection of these data elements

The concurrent review of inpatient hospital stays or of other cases also permits the corrective use of data. Changes in diagnosis for each case can be tracked, as discussed above. Clinical data can be captured and followed over time to yield profiles of provider effectiveness. Indicators of clinical appropriateness that can be followed include:

- Comparison of discharge or final diagnoses to intake diagnoses in order to determine diagnostic accuracy and to identify potential complications
- Determination of the frequency of complicating infections in the hospital setting
- Determination of the presence of extended fevers that may have been inadequately controlled

Sequences and combinations of procedures can be reported and reviewed for appropriateness of medical care.

The authorization process can be used to link a number of discrete services into one episode of care by employing the judgment and inquiries of a clinician during concurrent management of the case. The clinician can assign a single identifying number to the case. This number can link a number of different treatments or diagnoses to a single illness, which is very difficult to do retrospectively. For example, three visits to a physician for bronchial infections in a 6-month period may reflect two or three distinct illnesses, one illness which was difficult to treat, or several illnesses with a single underlying cause, like emphysema.

Episodes of care are very useful in profiling a provider's effectiveness in treating certain conditions and in determining whether the provider may be over- or undertreating patients. This information can be combined with data on a provider's billed charges to get a complete profile. The value that the utilization review (UR) clinician can have during the information-gathering process is highlighted by the difficulty investigators have experienced in the past when they tried to retrospectively link services into a single care episode.

Once the episode of care has been designated and the condition assigned, requested services can be edited against additional appropriateness edits. Other edits, such as the use of the Professional Activities Standards (PAS) approved lengths of stay for hospitalizations, are common.

It should be noted that the editing process need not only be used to restrict services or limit payment. An advanced authorization processing system can identify additional treatments that would be appropriate for a condition and support recommendations for a level of treatment that exceeds that being requested. Such edits not only improve the quality of service delivered when they are properly designed, but they can also prove cost-effective in that timely care is more effective care.

CLAIMS PROCESSING The operation of a sophisticated claims payment process cannot be separated functionally from the authorization process. The same logical edits (for eligibility, provider relationship, and medical appropriateness) that support the authorization process are extended to the payment of claims. The claims payment system need not and should not repeat the edits performed at the authorization stage; rather, if an authorization is required for a service, it is sufficient to check whether one is present and to determine the appropriate payment.

The claims processing function allows the same kind of logic to be extended to services which do not require prior approval. Patients and providers are expected to know whether a policy covers a particular service; the explanation of benefits (EOB) issued with each payment (or nonpayment) is an additional informational tool.

As with authorizations, claims payments can be screened for medical appropriateness: was the treatment applicable to the patient's age and sex, and to his or her medical history? Was the maximum acceptable number of treatments exceeded? Was the treatment appropriate based upon the diagnosis, and was the diagnosis appropriate for the patient? Were the conditions of the coverage met? Is the treatment or diagnosis one that typically involves coordination of benefits (as in traumatic injuries)?

Additional payment edits may be tied to the provider. Was the provider a participant in the plan? Was the physician board certified to perform the service? Were appropriate referrals made? Has there been a history of abuse with that provider (leading the payer to pend future claims for medical review)?

Other edits are primarily financial: what was charged for the service, and (more importantly) what is the reimbursable amount? Was there an agreed-upon fee schedule? Has a discount been agreed to? Has an amount been withheld for provider risk sharing? Is the copayment or deductible dependent on patient behavior (such as acquiring prior approval or seeing a specific provider), and have any such requirements been met?

Still other edits require assigning (or estimating) an episode of care which, as with authorizations, associates a group of treatments with a single condition. Edits can then be applied against a predefined range of treatments (for example, x number of diagnostic procedures, or no more than or no less than y number of procedures within a given date range).

The extent to which the appropriate information has been gathered and edited prior to claims entry (on enrollment, providers, and authorizations) determines the extent to which the claims entry process can be streamlined and automated. That, in turn, is the extent to which claims entry edits (and data entry in general) can be used to support the goal of managed healthcare.

Application   Reporting and making use of the information that has been collected and edited is the last, and most critical, part of the information cycle. Making the best use of the available information requires an intimate understanding of what has been accumulated: who provided the source information, how it was edited, and what were the limitations in every step of the process. The reporting process will be, in the short term, a set of tools for using what is available to compensate for tools that are not yet available, such as standardized measurements of severity and tracking mechanisms for clinical indicators. The tools currently available can be designed to meet selected key objectives.

What are those objectives? Profiling the behavior of providers for the quality, appropriateness, and cost-effectiveness of the care they render is a key goal. Identifying illness patterns in a population that may call for changes in the medical delivery process is another. Intelligent financial planning and reserving, based on observed and predictable cost factors, is another. Understanding how patient behavior is influencing cost and service use and how to design benefits to meet patient needs more effectively are other key goals.

Implicit in all of these goals is the need to use information to create cost savings and quality enhancement and to report the resulting accomplishments in a meaningful way. The first step is to have a set of experiential norms and performance standards with which to compare the results.

NORMS VERSUS STANDARDS It is important at this point to make the distinction between norms and standards in the evaluation of healthcare data, since each have their role. Norms can be defined as the typical patterns of cost, treatment, and other characteristics of medical care delivery. In other words, norms are what the provider community as a whole is doing in a given region. Standards can be thought of as the appropriate patterns of medical care delivery. Unlike norms, standards should not be specific to any region of the country or to changes in overall practice habits (other than changes in medical technology or knowledge).

A number of projects have been undertaken which seek to establish a commonly acceptable standard for practice. The *Patterns of Treatment* product, which was initially developed in California using state Medicaid data, classifies diagnoses into groups and assigns parameters for appropriate treatment for each based on the judgments of the medical college faculty from several universities.

Other research projects address "tracer diagnoses," which are considered indicative of the quality of care, and use them as sample conditions for the evaluation of the care a provider is rendering. Several commercial carriers have experimented with applying the tracer approach in the field as a provider measurement tool. Other vendors are developing related products, including one whose "core sample" product is under development; the product resembles tracer diagnoses but concentrates on diagnosis and procedure patterns that are commonly available in commercial settings.

Certain limitations in the ability to report and analyze data exist in the fee-for-service field that do not exist in the HMO and overall managed healthcare field. For example, HMOs are more likely to store full enrollment and provider data, as noted above, including claims information by provider specialty, that are instrumental in addressing issues of the delivery of care. The available full enrollment data also permit an epidemiological approach to the establishment of norms in which utilization patterns and costs can more easily be expressed in a per person per month basis by age, sex, and geographic groupings.

In the absence of a comprehensive set of standards based on indemnity care data, experiential data from an HMO setting can be used selectively in the analysis of nonmanaged care data. In addition, creation of a comprehensive normative database of managed care experience from non-HMO data is a necessary industry objective for the next decade. Certain groups have experimented with forming consortiums of employers or insurance carriers to pool data, but the logistical difficulties of linking very different databases into a common set, where data elements have common meanings, has been greatly underestimated. In the meantime, use of HMO-based norms with adjustment factors for the type of coverage used and the geographic region may result in the most comprehensive set of population-based norms currently available.

DEMOGRAPHIC REPORTS Having established baseline norms, the next step in analyzing healthcare experience for a group is to produce a set of reports on the population under examination, whether it is health plan enrollees, employees, union members, trust participants, or any subgroup. Healthcare experience should be reported by the appropriate population cohorts and compared to norms only for comparable populations.

Critical reporting elements include:

- Age and sex groups (number in each)
- Geographic location
- Industry classification
- Dependent status (insured, spouse, child)
- Type of coverage
- Benefit plan type
- Employer division

Each of these elements is a determining factor in the use of healthcare services, and each should be considered in developing a set of norms and standards for comparison. This demographic information can be used to create an expected cost and frequency profile for the overall group and for each subgroup within it that provides a first indicator of problems. For indemnity-based plans that are implementing managed care techniques, these demographic reports may also describe, for the first time, the population for whom the payers are providing coverage.

PAYMENT DATES VERSUS SERVICE DATES A traditional characteristic of nonmanaged care reporting is that figures for cost and volume of services are based on the dates that claims were paid, rather than the date the services were rendered. This can be acceptable in a nonmanaged environment, where reports serve as a kind of "check-balancing" function.

Effective management of healthcare requires information that is independent of payment cycles, which are influenced by external factors like cashflow and administrative problems. Trend analyses should give an accurate picture of behavior and how it has changed over time. This permits analysts to examine the relationship between factors that may have caused the change, such as benefits design changes, economic forces, and the actions of providers and patients.

It is becoming increasingly common for misperceptions to develop as reports which were developed for accounting functions get misapplied to the managed care environment. One of the most common types of error is to confuse claims *payment* data with claims *incurred* data. Accounting reports provide claims payment data, that is, when funds were dispersed, while healthcare trend analyses provide claims incurred data, that is, when services were performed. If administrative changes or other factors changed the speed with which claims were paid, the amount paid may vary independently from any true changes in cost or use of healthcare services.

SIGNIFICANCE OF CATASTROPHIC COSTS The issue of catastrophic costs, why they need to be reported, and how to use catastrophic reports for prediction and control is best understood in the light of the following statements:

1. A small number of individuals will incur very disproportionate amounts of medical expense during any period.
2. That cost can be predicted with a fair degree of accuracy for extended periods.
3. Significant fluctuations in that cost can be expected in shorter periods. The shorter the period under study, the more it is likely that fluctuations in these costs will occur.
4. Health plan fund reserves should be able to meet cost fluctuations resulting from catastrophic expenses. The plan should have sufficient capital available to "ride out" the variable nature of catastrophic expense.
5. Plan funding cannot be determined from 1 or 2 years of experience. The variable nature of healthcare costs, and particularly catastrophic costs, means that there is an inherent risk when a plan's funds are based on a "good year," and therefore funding could easily be inadequate.
6. A significant number of high-cost enrollees remain in the high-cost category over a number of years. These are individuals with costly, chronic conditions. These conditions can be iso-

lated in the reporting process and future catastrophic costs can be projected.

7. Coordinated intervention in catastrophic cases has a proportional savings effect of great magnitude (for example, a 5 percent reduction in the most expensive case may equal a 50 percent reduction in 1000 less expensive cases).

8. The impact of catastrophic cases can distort trend analyses. Recent high-cost cases can make cost inflation or use of services appear to increase at a far more rapid rate than they truly are; conversely, an escalation in costs and utilization can be underestimated if there were excessive high-cost cases in an earlier period. Failure to report catastrophic and noncatastrophic experience separately can result in a misunderstanding of changes in a population's healthcare experience.

Costs for catastrophic cases are subject to three general factors:

1. Number of incidents of catastrophic cases which occur
2. Increases in unit costs (inflation)
3. Level of case management applied to each incident

Mathematicians and analysts in a number of different disciplines have long recognized the concept of the "vital few and the trivial many." This concept simply means that in any group a small number of individuals can have a disproportionate influence on a factor that is being measured.

It is a basic statistical principle that prediction becomes less reliable as the number of items being evaluated becomes smaller. The "vital few" are a small group by definition. This means that the behavior of the vital few being measured is far less predictable. The only remedy to this problem is time. Time can be a substitute for volume in restoring statistical balance; the behavior of the vital few conforms more closely to predictions as the length of time that is being studied increases.

The lesson of these statistical principles is clear:

- The cost of catastrophic cases to a medical plan is likely to vary over short periods but tends to become more predictable for longer periods.
- Small changes in the nature of a catastrophic case are as important as great changes in the number of noncatastrophic cases.
- Care has to be taken to ensure that funding projections are not based on costs incurred during periods in which the costs of catastrophic cases were lower than the amount that can be predicted over the long term.
- Catastrophic cases should be closely monitored and controlled.

The availability of norms on catastrophic costs is limited, in part due to the statistical principles described above. Long-term studies of this phenomenon are currently being conducted by a number of organizations.

One commonly made statement concerning catastrophic expense is that 1 percent of all employees can be responsible for 25 percent or more of the total medical costs in a corporate medical plan (when the medical expenses of their families are included). Producing reports of this nature requires the ability to link cases by family, using a social security number or other employee identifier. A more significant indicator, cost per covered life, can be produced provided that there is a unique patient identifier for each covered family member.

In one study performed by American International Healthcare (AIH), 92 families out of 9427 families, equivalent to 1 percent of the employee and retiree enrollment population, accounted for 24 percent of claims payments in the period February 1986 through July 1987. This study showed that 40 individuals in a plan with an expected total covered population of approximately 23,000 used 21 percent of the plan's total medical claims expense.

In another AIH study, 0.1 percent of the individuals incurred 20 percent of all inpatient hospital costs in 1986, which dropped to 5.6 percent in 1987. This led to an overall drop in inpatient costs of 2.7 percent, which could have led to a false impression as to cost trends. In fact, when catastrophic cases (over $50,000) were excluded from the reporting process, the cost increase was over 15 percent for that inpatient service in 1987.

The issue of identifying and controlling catastrophic costs is better understood by recognizing that catastrophic cases fall into two distinct categories. The first category includes all cases where the catastrophic expense occurred as a result of a sudden, unanticipated event: heart attack, auto accident, stroke, and cancers with a rapid onset. The second category involves chronic, long-term medical and psychiatric conditions requiring extensive care over long periods of time. These can include schizophrenia, multiple sclerosis, severe brain damage, and quadriplegia. These cases may cause frequent, brief hospitalizations or extended stays, as well as repeated invasive procedures such as surgery.

It is clear that the second category of catastrophic care is likely to result in greater medical cost, particularly over the long term. Those individuals who are likely to be the "vital few" in terms of cost can frequently be predicted from year to year. In-depth studies of catastrophic cases usually enable analysts to identify the specific individuals who will be the primary consumers of catastrophic expenses in the following year.

The principle of adverse selection is most pronounced with these individuals. Because they are receiving extensive ongoing care, they are highly unlikely to leave the indemnity plan and change providers. Because of that ongoing care, they are among the most costly individuals in the plan in any given year.

Funding projections can be performed in a more sophisticated manner if catastrophic cases of an ongoing nature are accounted for. Funding calculations are based on expected future costs for the population as a whole. Costs for these individuals, however, can be fixed more precisely if specific clinical information on their conditions is gathered whenever a case is identified as costly and potentially long term in nature. More accurate predictions on the future impact of these cases on cost can then be combined with cost projections for the rest of the population as a whole. The result would be a funding projection that more accurately accounted for the existence of ongoing catastrophic cases.

The goals of catastrophic reporting are therefore:

1. To determine the influence of catastrophic expenses on total costs
2. To observe the cost and usage trends that are independent of the effects of catastrophic cases
3. To identify and support the case management process

MONITORING PROVIDER BEHAVIOR   The general goal of monitoring provider reporting is to monitor provider behavior so that it can be changed when necessary. The problem is that current data extracted from claims payment systems do not permit the generation of computer-based reports that accurately describe a provider's behavior, that is, is the provider overtreating or providing inappropriate service? For the foreseeable future, the monitoring process will have to include a dialog (usually over the telephone) between a clinician representing the payer and the provider, which includes a review of clinical information not typically present in the claims payment environment.

The starting point for the clinician-reviewer is a report which evaluates the service histories of providers and identifies those providers that are potential "outliers," rendering services for specific population groups or diagnoses at a higher or lower level than the norm. The goal for these reports in the interim should be to increase the efficiency of clinician-reviewers by providing them with a list of providers who are more *likely* to be providing treatment that varies unacceptably from that of their peers or from other norms or standards. The process must support the following activities:

- Monitor the effectiveness of preferred provider arrangements
- Target higher quality, lower cost providers for PPO recruitment
- Identify abusive providers for corrective action

Claims experience can be used to model the potential impact of benefits design changes on costs, and benefits modeling reports are increasingly requested from claims processing computer systems. A different approach needs to be taken because of several errors which are commonly made. These errors are:

The offset error Reductions in one benefit are normally offset by increases elsewhere. The most obvious example of this is when a reduction of x dollars in inpatient hospital costs is predicted by a utilization review service, leading to a statement of savings that equates to $x - c$, where c equals the cost of employing the utilization review service. However, additional, hidden costs may not be known to the utilization review service, for example, services rendered on an outpatient basis that would have been denied for inpatient stay. A true estimate of savings would therefore be equal to

$$S = x - (c + a)$$

where S = estimated savings
      x = estimated value of denied inpatient services
      c = cost of employing UR firm
      a = cost of alternate services rendered on outpatient basis

Unexpected complexity Analysis may suggest that raising a copayment amount for hospitalizations from \$250 to \$500 may save \$250 times the total expected number of hospitalizations. However, if this increase in costs is applied against deductible limits, the increase in the number of services paid for by the plan must also be considered when estimating the savings.

Cross-purposes Sometimes multiple managed care programs are put into place in a single setting without coordination. The net result can be that while each program projects a savings, cumulatively they cause an increase in costs. For example, a UR firm may deny a 1- or 2-day stay for a surgery and report it as a savings. Meanwhile a PPO may have negotiated a discount with the hospital where the admission was requested and may have projected its savings by multiplying last year's hospital days by the discount amount. In this case, the savings is not realized this year because UR denied the stay. To add to the confusion, it is possible that the cost of performing this surgery in the hospital for an agreed-upon fee may actually be less than the cost on an outpatient basis if the per diem agreement had been put into effect.

Such are the dangers of benefits modeling. The key to producing accurate benefits reports is correct interpretation. Numbers generated from claims payers, utilization review firms, and PPOs need to be cross-checked, reviewed to ensure that the same periods and populations are being used, and analyzed to study the impact of each managed care intervention on the others. It is only in this way that the effect of each intervention can be reported in a meaningful way.

NEXT-GENERATION DATA ISSUES

Information that has been collected through administrative data processing systems has been acquired according to established needs for handling claims payment, for verifying the appropriateness of the service, and for confirming that the requirements of the benefits program have been met.

Significant trends are likely to change the type of information that will be collected, and these trends also must be considered. There are new demands for health plan information management, specifically regarding the collection of clinical information that can support the management of medical care in a detailed manner.

Improvements in data collection and reporting will be required so that employers can target employee health education to specific problem areas, administrators can concentrate provider training on problem areas in medical practice, and planners can have detailed utilization data to design and finance healthcare.

New information technologies will also change the nature of medical information. Improved clinical information systems for provider offices will capture more detailed medical history in a machine-readable format than is currently the case; this could dramatically improve the ability of analysts to interpret and analyze the entire process of medical care. Expert systems (also known as "artificial intelligence") will become a common decision support tool for providers and conceivably for patients as well.

Understanding the developments currently underway in certain critical areas is essential when speculating on the future of healthcare information. These critical areas include quality management, reimbursement and incentive models, enhancements in reporting design, expert systems, early intervention systems, health information networks, large volume databases, and applied social science.

Quality Management

Three major issues need to be addressed regarding the reporting of quality of care in the current environment:

1. There are significant limitations in the ability of a managed care organization to track and report on current quality of care since key clinical indicators of disease severity are not routinely captured.
2. It is critical that strategies be developed which will permit the use of the available limited data in an effective fashion.

3. The use of currently available claims data for quality assurance purposes requires a clear understanding of their proper application. For example, a review of claims data for medical practice anomalies may indicate that one physician is more cost-intensive than another for a given illness, but that physician may be able to legitimately argue that her or his patients are more seriously ill. Claims data without clinical data can be misused.

The limitations which managed care organizations face are substantial. Utilization review firms are in the best position to capture the clinical data that relate to provider quality, but the firms suffer from two primary limitations. First, in many cases there are insufficient norms available against which the data may be judged since the collection of this information is a new practice and there are no commonly accessible databases to draw from. Second, they collect data only for those cases on which they intervene; this may give a skewed picture of quality.

Claims processing (or preprocessing) organizations have a broader range of historical experience, but they have insufficient depth. Diagnosis codes are imperfectly applied. Frequently there are financial incentives for overstating the complexity of the procedure used since more complex procedures are usually paid at a higher rate. (Similar incentives for overstatement exist for reporting diagnoses under DRG reimbursement methodology.) There are few other clinical indicators available, and there are insufficient safeguards, such as selected medical audits, to ensure they are properly used when submitted on a claim form.

Measuring the severity of illness is also impossible under current diagnostic coding conventions since no common convention is used for measuring severity. Should a common convention be adopted, financial incentives for overstating severity would remain. Several computerized techniques for automatically calculating severity have been developed but have yet to attain general acceptance. It is hoped that such a system, when used, will not be manipulated or "gamed" for financial reasons.

A number of alternate strategies have been proposed or developed for managed care organizations. Some adopt information, such as perinatal mortality analysis, that is collected from third party sources as a quality indicator, on the argument that studies which profile a single set of services in detail can be a valid indicator of overall quality. Other studies review a broader range of treatments using statewide hospital data to offset the limitations inherent in observing one procedure independently as a measurement of quality.

Such studies are generally performed on institutions (notably in California), rather than physicians, and are labor-intensive. Applying these approaches to non-Calfornia institutions would require a massive data collection project to survey institutions on a state-by-state basis.

The profiling of physician care in the outpatient setting remains the most difficult area for quality monitoring. Ambulatory services rarely are subject to utilization review, detailed research on tens of thousands of physicians is impractical, and the subjectivity of the coding process for diagnoses and procedures is at its most extreme and can be distorted by financial motivations.

A number of healthcare organizations have developed medical management reports of varying kinds which are intended to analyze and compare the performance of providers in a healthcare system. Reports can be produced which use certain key assumptions:

1. It is not possible to analyze the quality of care rendered by a provider in a claims processing environment under current conditions.
2. A trained clinician (such as a UR nurse or a medical director) will need to make a trained judgment before a managed care organization can take action based on quality of care.
3. The role of computerized reports is therefore to support these clinicians by allowing more efficient use of their time. This role will not change until the data-gathering process becomes more effective and may never change completely.

In order to proceed with the creation of quality-related reports, it is necessary to examine the options open to a managed care plan for intervening when quality of care is found questionable. Options for intervention with physicians include the following:

1. A reduction of reimbursement under an incentive-based program, such as risk-withholding, that is tied to mutually acceptable definitions of quality can be implemented. It is difficult, however, to find mutually acceptable definitions that are objective enough to be easily implemented. Efforts to date have concentrated on the hospital environment, where the most cost-intensive services are performed and clinical data are more accessible, and one of the currently available products may become a standard.
2. An "educational" approach can be used. Some managed care organizations may opt to begin with an approach that is merely informational in tone: "Dear Doctor, Our research indicates that (treatment 1) is appropriate and effective for (diagnosis type), while reports suggest that you tend to use (treatment 2) with an average cost of ($)." A variant of this approach would be to say that: "Physicians in your area and specialty used (number of

services) at a total cost of ($), while you varied from these norms by (x) for similar age and sex groups." The closing statement may be: "If you wish to discuss our information on treatment of (diagnosis), please call the Medical Director at. . . ." This "reach out and touch someone" approach is nonconfrontational, while employing the "sentinel effect" to alert physicians that outlier behavior is tracked and observed.

3. Physicians can be warned that the quality and appropriateness of the care they render is under question and that further actions (including suspension from the plan) are under consideration.

4. Sanctions are clearly the strongest option available for intervening in a case where the quality of care provided is strongly unacceptable.

Physicians may have evidence with which to contradict any possible set of quality reports, including the clinical specifics of the cases they treated and the possibility that they are known for treating particularly difficult cases in certain areas. Such arguments may be perfectly valid.

The difficulties involved in monitoring the quality of care from claims data alone suggest that quality-oriented reports from claims systems will remain, at least in the near future, a support tool to be used by payer-employed clinicians for judging the quality of care delivery. However, these reports are not used as a sole basis for judging the quality of the delivery of care. The clinician-reviewer will use the reports produced by a quality assurance reporting system to identify providers which have a greater likelihood of being problematic (thereby improving their own efficiency) and to provide supporting information for the review of each instance of questionable care. The only other alternative to this application of a quality-reporting model would be one in which the computer serves as "judge, jury, and executioner" in the as-yet incomplete field of quality measurement.

Most locally based medical staffs for managed care organizations will, if staffed properly, have a strong sense of who the problem providers are in their communities. The computer reports provide the information they need to take actions against individuals that they are already aware of; the methodology, however, remains the same.

The role of quality-based reports then becomes a dual one: first, identifying providers that are more likely to be outliers in terms of quality. The payer-employed medical staff are more likely to discover and correct problems by reviewing these providers than they would be auditing providers at random. Second, the reports provide information which the medical staff can use in provider discussions.

Providers can be analyzed using an approach similar to tracer diagnosis, a variant of which is being developed under the general heading of "core samples." Another approach for determining outlier providers (in terms of cost and level of treatment) is to develop a structure of report tiers which is used to zero in on outlier providers (primarily in terms of cost) and to provide claim-specific documentation on each.

An example of the logical sequence for profiling physicians with a tier-based reporting approach is as follows:

1. Profile all physicians by specialty and region for cost; identify tier 1 outliers. In this example, Chicago gastroenterologists appear costlier than predicted by norms.

2. Profile Chicago gastroenterologists by age and sex composition of patients; that is, identify tier 2 outliers by age- and sex-adjusted cost and frequency of services (with age and sex providing a simplified means of adjusting for the principal factors behind case mix and severity factors).

3. Profile tier 2 outliers on a treatment- and diagnosis-specific basis, and identify tier 3 outliers as those who appear to be cost-intensive for certain diagnoses. In this example, five physicians appear to conduct a greater number of diagnostic procedures (for example, sigmoidoscopy) than the age and sex composition of the patients and their diagnoses appear to warrant.

4. Provide a listing of tier 3 outliers, together with complete claims history data, to the clinical staff for review and physician contact. This case review may either confirm or deny the inference drawn from the report, which is that five "tier 3 outliers" are overusing diagnostic procedures.

Under this scenario it would be the responsibility of the managed care organization's clinical staff to take whatever actions seem appropriate after a review of the clinical records and discussions with the practicing physicians.

There is a role for both the diagnosis-based tracer or core approach and the tier-structure approach in the identification of providers for medical review. Until such time as quality of care can be a more fully automated process, each can support the review function.

Reimbursement and Incentive Models

Intervention by clinical staff cannot take place each time reimbursements need to be made under incentive-based programs. Reimbursements under capitation which require an adjustment for case-mix severity can be handled one of several ways:

1. *Age and sex mix*   Although this remains the standard for capitation variation, many health plans have age and sex capitation

models that are imprecise in their ability to predict costs. Age and sex composition remains the accepted basis for predicting costs under capitation.

2. *Severity adjustments* Various formal and informal measures exist for adjusting capitation reimbursements for severity of illness. These include "severity multipliers" to capitation payments, which are generally developed and applied after discussion between a provider and the plan and which may include as much subjectivity as objectivity in their application. These severity multipliers may be applied when physicians take the position that their patients are, on average, 10 percent "sicker" than those of their peers. The average capitation payment may be multiplied by 1.1 if the argument is accepted by the payer.

3. *Severity-of-illness measurements (SOI)* Computer systems which measure the severity of illness based on clinical data captured by the provider can be used to adjust reimbursement in either a fee-for-service or capitated model. Considerable problems remain, however, in a managed plan's ability to place the same SOI measuring system in every provider's office. The alternative, to receive clinical indicators in paper form and to process them at the plan, requires substantial staff and computing capabilities on the plan's part.

Other incentive programs for providers, such as the withholding of risk funds and their distribution based on cost and quality parameters, are in use. The quality issues associated with these plans will not become critical to plan management, however, until market forces dictate a stronger emphasis on them.

Patient incentives provide an additional area for further cost controls. They include premium incentives for lifestyle factors (for example, nonsmoking rates) and rates based on patient health profiles. One such program is provided by Blue Cross of Virginia, which discounts premium rates to enrollees who meet lifestyle-based risk criteria. Certain employers have even initiated forms of risk pooling for employee groups. In these cases, a group of employees is given a target for their healthcare expenses. If exceeded, the payer assumes all responsibility; however, if costs are below expectations, the surplus is distributed to employees in the form of cash or additional benefits.

Enhancements in Report Design

There must be a number of enhancements in report production if reports are to fill their full role in the information cycle. First, norms and standards must come into fuller use if figures on cost and frequency are to be interpreted in proper context. Second, the intelligent application of reports will require a tier-based reporting structure in partnership with an intelligent information management function. Third, the quality of individual report items (such as procedure codes) must be assessed prior to report generation to ensure that reports mean what they appear to mean and that they have been corrected for errors in data collection, data entry, or interpretation.

The next generation of advancements in healthcare information will not end with enhancements to report design, however. As the type of information being collected changes and as information techniques alter the delivery of medical care, the healthcare industry will need to adapt and advance in new ways.

Expert Systems

Expert systems (often referred to as artificial intelligence) represent the use of logical theory and mechanical models of human thought to develop new computer programming techniques. Medical decision making represented an early area of expert system development, and efforts in this area continue to progress. One of the earliest successful expert system programs was MYCIN, developed at Stanford University, which was designed to aid in the diagnosis of infectious diseases. The design concept was later generalized and used to develop other expert systems under the name EMYCIN.

Expert systems will pose several challenges for managed healthcare information. First, the effectiveness of the systems will need to be monitored. Are these systems more or less effective in the diagnosis process than human clinicians? What are the implications of having one clinician's judgment (the "expert" in the expert system) affecting a large number of decisions? Even if the system improves overall accuracy of diagnosis, are there "blind spots" that are consistently missed?

Expert systems require the capture of clinical data. Are there ways these data can be accessed for reporting purposes? Lastly, are these systems being used appropriately as decision support tools, or are they being used improperly as a substitute for professional judgment? Answering these questions will place new demands on healthcare managers.

Early Intervention Systems

The study of catastrophic cases is likely to lead to an improved understanding of when to intervene early in the delivery of medical care for certain conditions. It will become imperative to identify certain conditions as early as possible in the treatment process. This early identification will require the application of clinical, informational, and systems communication knowledge in order to search for these conditions in hospital records, physician office management systems, utilization review support computers, and claims processing systems.

Health Information Networks

Early intervention is not the only area where disparate information systems need to be integrated into one reporting system. Healthcare organizations will need to organize all their information into one centralized system, a health information network, that can make full use of the information being captured. Hospitals, physician offices, utilization review departments, claims processing offices, and financial analysts all capture and use information which represents aspects of the covered population's health.

New healthcare products which emphasize point-of-service decisions on the type of coverage to be used (for example, "open-ended" HMOs) will be best served by networks that can transmit information in real time and share information on prior authorizations for services, the status of deductibles and copayments, and eligibility for services. Advances in "smart cards," communications technology, computer connectivity, and data storage techniques will all contribute to the conversion of independently functioning computer systems into health information networks.

Large-Volume Databases

The ability to understand and measure the use of healthcare will require advances in the collection and interpretation of normative databases. Norms that are currently available are divided between large-volume databases from insurance company sources, which tend to be incomplete and lack population data, and specialized databases that may have complete population data (for example, those used by HMOs) but lack volume and contain only one organization's data. Clinical information is hard to come by and rarely, if ever, resides in the same database as claims payment information.

Healthcare organizations will need to develop new initiatives for cooperation in the collection and integration of claims payment data, clinical records, and population data on an intercompany basis. This will require a change in the traditional reluctance of payer organizations to share data with their competitors.

It will also require new initiatives to protect the privacy of individuals. Centralized databases must be carefully handled because they are likely to raise concerns about privacy. One physician analyzed the individuals having access to his patients' medical records and estimated that between 25 and 100 professionals and administrators "had access to the patients' records and that all of them had . . . a professional responsibility to open and use the chart." However, despite the legitimate concerns of privacy, these databases must be created to learn more about how to identify and encourage the appropriate use of medical services.

Applied Social Science

This article began with the assertion that managed healthcare is, in effect, an applied social science. There is controversy about the degree to which the rigors of scientific discipline have been adapted to the social sciences, but it can also be argued that managed healthcare will need to adapt social science tools if it is to understand the behavior of individuals in a health plan.

The dynamics of group behavior are undergoing study in a number of disciplines. One intriguing if controversial area of study involves the application of cybernetic or systems theory to social sciences. Anecdotal experience in the field of managed healthcare suggests the presence of social forces at work. Why will providers in one city adapt to managed healthcare programs while others organize political opposition? Why do some groups of healthcare recipients reduce their overall use of medical services when copayments are imposed while others increase it? Can such behavior be quantified or predicted?

The healthcare field may prove to be a laboratory for researching some of the general theories of group behavior. Whatever the current limitations of medical information, the administrative and medical requirements of healthcare payment have required the collection of a great deal of data, all of which describes some aspect of human behavior. With luck, managed healthcare's increasing demand for information will provide raw material for research in the social sciences. That research may, in turn, improve our ability to understand and manage healthcare.

CONCLUSION

Managed care organizations will not be able to simply use information in the 1990s. If managers do not have a comprehensive management strategy, they will not be able to control the information cycle. Instead, they will find that in many ways it is controlling them, as an increasingly complex set of data items and an intricate network of reporting relationships result in misinterpreted reports and unintended behavior.

Managed care in the 1990s will include detailed incentive models, expert system programs, clinical data tracking, new government initiatives, computerized payment edits for medical appropriateness, and new demands for quality control and reporting. Information technology will change as health payers change from organizations which distribute risk to organizations that reduce risk. The result will be the creation of new information and new behaviors. A detailed plan for action, one which includes mastery over the information cycle, can permit new breakthroughs in the understanding and management of healthcare.

REFERENCES

1. Mark S. Blumberg, "Measuring Surgical Quality in Maryland: A Model," *Health Affairs* **7:** 62–78 (1988).

2. J. M. Juran, *Quality Control Handbook.* McGraw-Hill, New York, 1951.

3. D. M. Kessner, "Quality Assessment and Assurance: Early Signs of Cognitive Dissonance." *New England Journal of Medicine* **298:** 381–386 (1978).

4. *Maternal and Child Health Data Base, Statistical Appendix.* Community and Organization Research Institute, University of California, Santa Barbara, 1987.

5. "Perinatal Computing in 1987: An Overview," *J. Perinat. Med.* **15**(1): (1987).

6. John E. Wennberg et al. "Use of Claims Data Systems to Evaluate Health Care Outcomes: Mortality and Reoperation Following Prostatectomy," *JAMA* **257:** 933–936 (1987).

CHAPTER TWENTY

Data Systems

THE MANAGED CARE INFORMATION SYSTEM

PHILIP M. LOHMAN, Ph.D., Research Director
JAMES REEP, Chairman
First Consulting Group, Long Beach, California

In the healthcare industry, as in other industries, needs tend to call forth products. Right now, acute care providers have a need for an information system that can guide them in managing the increasingly complex world of contract care. The response has been *managed care information systems*, automated tools for providing detailed analyses of the hospital's financial performance under managed care contracts and for identifying resource utilization patterns. This article provides a detailed analysis of the strategic context in which these systems have arisen, discusses the systems themselves, and sketches out procedures for selecting and implementing them.

MANAGED CARE AND MANAGED CARE INFORMATION

The upheavals caused in the healthcare industry by the federal government's shift to prospective pricing for Medicare have tended to obscure what is potentially an even more momentous change: the accelerating movement away from indemnity coverage for hospitalization and the corresponding shift toward managed care. The swiftness with which this has occurred is astonishing. This year traditional fee-for-service indemnity coverage, which constituted 72 percent of hospital revenues from nongovernmental sources as late as 1985, may decline to only 5 percent, with the rest being made up of some form of managed care. It is not at all uncommon today to find hospitals with 75 percent of their non-Medicare and non-Medicaid revenues already earned through care provided under contracts. Clearly, another of the established foundations of hospital economics is being radically and permanently transformed.

STRATEGIC CONSIDERATIONS FOR THE CARE PROVIDER

For the acute care provider, the shift to managed care has clearly been something of a mixed blessing. In many cases, managed care can smooth out fluctuations in occupancy and keep beds filled. Despite the equally rapid shift to outpatient care, most hospitals are still largely in the business of providing inpatient services, as they should be since there will always be a need for the modern hospital's assembly of skill, science, and organized technology. Moreover, managed care contracts can promise the hospital, through capitation agreements, a significant benefit even in its inpatient care mode: a predictable cashflow. However, the overriding purpose of managed care is to transfer a major portion of risk to the provider; in return for stable patient populations and revenue streams, managed care contracts create substantial business risks for the hospital. There are two principal risks the hospital faces in signing a health maintenance organization (HMO) or preferred provider arrangement (PPA) contract. The most immediate risk, simply stated, is this: The hospital, which must accept specified rates of reimbursement (increasingly capitation), may not have acquired the same degree of control over its costs and utilization that the payer now has over its revenues and will find itself with full beds and an empty bank account. The result is that the hospital contracts itself out of business. The broader, longer-term risk is that the hospital simply will not be able to operate in the managed care marketplace.

To succeed in managed care, the hospital must be able, in addition to maintaining a high level of quality, to do the following:

- Determine what sort of overall strategy it will pursue. Will it, for example, be a "niche" provider, contracting only for a single service line, such as orthopedic surgery? Or will it, on the other hand, provide a full range of services, perhaps even becoming a "vertically integrated" provider, offering skilled nursing and home health, as well as acute care?
- Establish a network of patient and reimbursement sources.
- Select, from among the contracts proposed to the hospital, those that are in its best interests with regard to such strategic factors as patient market, reimbursement, risk, and administrative costs.
- Negotiate the most advantageous terms once suitable contracts have been selected. Many hospitals have signed managed care

agreements only to find too late that they either signed contracts with the wrong payers or did not obtain the best possible terms.

- Manage its provision of services, particularly in the area of utilization, efficiently enough to maximize margins.
- Ensure that it receives all the reimbursement it is entitled to under its contracts.

INFORMATION IMPLICATIONS OF PROVIDER STRATEGIES

The common element to each of these requirements is, of course, *information*. For the hospital to establish an overall strategy, it must know what services there is a market for and what services it is capable of providing at an acceptable cost. For it to select optimal contracts, it must not only have a clear picture of its costs, but must also be able to project how they will be affected by the changes in patient volume that the particular contract may cause and by the need to provide added administrative support. For the hospital to negotiate the best terms, it must know what its own "bottom line" is for each service. For it to manage its services efficiently, the hospital must understand how its resources are used in relation to the reimbursement it receives. Finally, for the hospital to ensure that it receives the correct reimbursement, it must know what the reimbursement is and what it has received.

CURRENT STATE OF THE ART IN HOSPITAL MANAGEMENT INFORMATION SYSTEMS

Since their inception in the early 1960s, hospital information management systems (HMISs) have evolved in a way that made them ill-suited to providing the information support that hospitals participating in managed care require. As in other industries, the first information functions to be automated in the hospital were financial, particularly those functions, such as payroll, that handle large amounts of routine data. By the late 1970s, most hospitals had acquired financial data processing services. However, the rapid improvement in cost-performance that has made computing power steadily cheaper had by then only begun to appear. The dominant computer of the day, the large and costly mainframe, was financially beyond the reach of most hospitals. Consequently, the majority of the country's hospitals that had automated data processing service were served by timesharing companies such as Shared Medical Systems (SMS) and McDonnell Douglas.

While hospital financial systems were generally similar to those already in use in other industries and were, therefore, relatively cheap to develop and simple to implement, patient care systems were an entirely new field for automation. Information handling requirements for patient care systems were, in many ways, different from those for financial systems. The latter tended to support repetitive and relatively routine operations, such as payroll, accounts payable, and general ledger cycles. Patient care systems, on the other hand, were required to support the manifold, irregular, and complex activities that constitute patient care, such as laboratory order management, medication administration, radiology film handling, and medical records abstracting. Consequently, patient care systems evolved into a related, but separate, information system species, often using specialized, clinically oriented languages (such as MUMPS) and mounted on different makes of hardware. The result has been a plethora of medical software architectures and combinations of patient care and financial systems that often coexist in the hospital somewhat uncomfortably.

In the last few years, an increasing number of integrated, database-oriented hospital management information systems have come onto the market. These systems combine financial and patient care functions and have solved at least some of the most pressing problems of traditional hospital information management—redundant files and data entry, slow, difficult communications between systems, multiple hardware platforms, occasionally uncooperative vendors, and choppy, confusing training. However, the time, effort, and expense needed to overcome these problems, combined with the suddenness of developments in healthcare economics, has left even the most advanced HMISs still struggling to catch up to the needs of the market. While today's HMISs are increasingly effective at supporting both patient care operations and routine financial and accounting functions, they still lack the functional sophistication and degree of integration between clinical and financial data needed to address many strategic issues.

Strategic decision making requires the ability to analyze a wide range of relationships between financial and clinical data and to allow ad hoc inquiries, not just to report the data itself. These are abilities that HMISs are only just beginning to acquire.

The difficulty that contemporary HMISs have in providing strategic information is particularly pronounced in the case of managed care. Hospital systems, as a rule, can provide pieces of the data needed to make strategic decisions about managed care arrangements and to administer this care once it has been contracted for, but it cannot provide all of it. Most hospital patient accounting systems can provide only detail and summary reimbursement data by patient, patient financial class, and payer. A few hospital financial systems can also provide cost data, costs per procedure, department, and individual case, and can summarize costs by type of service and financial class versus reimbursement by financial class. What is generally lacking is the ability to relate expected reimbursement to actual reimbursement (at both the case and contract level) and to relate actual reimbursement to costs (again at both the case and contract levels).

For the hospital with a high level of contract-governed reimbursement, there have been three alternatives, none of them attractive.

The first alternative is to pull together as much of the needed data as possible from the medical records, case mix, patient accounting, cost accounting, and other systems, and to manually key it into a general-purpose analysis tool such as Lotus 1-2-3. This is undesirable for several reasons. First, data definitions (such as "patient day") may not be consistent from system to system, and data may be stored at incompatible levels of detail or stored in a format that makes it difficult to break up the data for analysis. Second, relatively sophisticated and expensive financial skills are needed if worthwhile information is be forthcoming. Third, such "freelance" systems tend to have a lot of problems. Complex spreadsheets are difficult to create without hidden flaws. For example, the system may be excessively dependent on a single financial analyst who may become quite possessive of it and is subject to being pulled away for other work, and it is almost impossible to maintain concurrent data. In any case, the typical hospital has so many contracts, with so many different reimbursement rates and other provisions, that even the most diligent analyst or financial manager is eventually overwhelmed.

The second alternative is to rely on HMOs and other payers for information. This practice is widespread and presents obvious risks: payers' systems are themselves often fragmentary or flawed, and the data may be late in arriving and may not be presented in the way most useful to the hospital. In any case, if the hospital deals with a large number of payers, as most hospitals do, assembling and analyzing data from even a dozen providers presents the hospital with a whole new set of administrative problems.

The third alternative, of course, is simply to do without contract-related information and hope that reimbursements are correct, that the hospital has picked the best contracts and is making a profit on the contracts it has signed. This is simply not a viable alternative.

In fact, most hospitals now use a combination of alternatives one and two; they get as much information as possible from their principal payers and their own HMISs, "massage" it on PC-based spreadsheets, measure it against industry standards, and try to muddle through by keeping a tight lid on costs. This approach may keep the hospital out of serious trouble in the short term, but it will not work as a long-term strategy since it is inherently less effective and more costly than obtaining this information from a full-scale managed care information system.

In a competitive market, information is a strategic asset. A hospital that is able to administer its managed care contracts efficiently will have a significant advantage over its competitors, and, significantly, the "arms race" that the healthcare industry has recently experienced in case mix, cost accounting, and resource management systems is now beginning to appear in the area of managed care information systems. The hospital that attempts to administer its managed care contracts by dead reckoning will see itself fall further and further behind its competitors.

MANAGED CARE INFORMATION SYSTEMS: WHAT THEY ARE AND HOW THEY WORK

First, a note on definitions. *Managed care information system* refers to systems that are intended primarily to be used by a hospital to keep track of its managed care contracts, identify contract-covered patients, assess its financial performance under the contracts in which it participates, and project the consequences of strategic decisions concerning managed care. The term *managed care information system, or MCIS,* is thus synonymous with *contracts management system* and *managed care system,* as these other terms are frequently used in the context of acute care delivery. This clarification is necessary because in some other segments of the healthcare industry, such as HMOs, the term "managed care information system" means something quite different—that is, the system that the HMO uses to manage its *own* operations (encounters, membership, claims, and eligibility).

In the broadest sense, the MCIS simply does what the financial analyst with the Lotus 1-2-3 spreadsheet was doing in alternative one above: reading and correlating existing data, but doing it much faster, more accurately and more comprehensively, and creating a far larger range of reports. The MCIS, in other words, is what is sometimes called a "niche" or "piggyback" system. Unlike transaction-oriented systems, such as the hospital's order entry system, which transmits orders for laboratory tests, or the patient accounting system, which posts charges and credits to individual patient accounts, niche systems do not support operational transactions themselves. Rather, they extract data already residing on other, transaction-oriented systems and reformat it at high speed for analysis and reporting purposes. (Cost accounting and budgeting systems are some other members of the niche systems family.)

BUSINESS OBJECTIVES SUPPORTED BY THE MANAGED INFORMATION CARE SYSTEM

A hospital's ability to manage its resources and make strategic business decisions in the managed care environment requires capabilities in three basic areas: operations, reporting and forecasting.

Operations

- Identify contract-covered patients at admission or registration to confirm that contract requirements for service (for example, preauthorization) have been met.

- Obtain concurrent information on costs, and costs versus antici-pated reimbursement, for contract-covered patients while they are in-house in order to ensure that resource utilization is as consistent with contract requirements as possible.
- Audit billings to HMOs, PPOs, and other contract payers to ensure that invoices are correct when they leave the hospital.
- Follow up on bills to contract payers and audit payments to en-sure that the hospital receives the full reimbursement to which it is entitled.

Reporting

- Analyze hospital and physician performance relative to each con-tract to determine which contracts are profitable and which are not.
- Examine utilization patterns to identify those facilities that are most intensely used in providing covered services.
- Examine individual physician behavior to determine what effect each physician has on the utilization of hospital facilities.

Forecasting

- Model the effects of changes in such variables as case mix, physi-cian behavior, services, costs, and contract arrangements in order to guide the hospital in planning for future managed care contracts.
- Model individual proposed contracts to determine if it is in the hospital's interest to sign them.

WHAT HOSPITALS ARE DOING NOW

Hospitals have adopted a number of stratagems in their attempts to run their managed care business efficiently.

- Preadmit patients, cooperate more closely with admitting physi-cians' offices, and perform more detailed admitting interviews in order to identify contract-covered patients and ensure that con-tract requirements are met.
- Conduct concurrent reviews to ensure that limits on acuity, length of stay, and covered services are adhered to as closely as possible. (This is particularly important for patients covered by contracts under which the provider is capitated.)
- Identify and develop cost data for, at least, the highest revenue procedures.
- Adapt the hospital's financial systems as far as possible to provide contract-related information. One common expedient is to use the "financial class" field in the patient accounting system to identify patients by contract. However, this has a major limitation: The

number of financial classes most patient accounting systems allow is far less than the number of contracts that the hospital is involved in. This means that one or more catch-all financial classes must be devised for the contracts that cannot be individually identified.

- Devote additional financial staff to analyzing and reporting the results of managed care. This is an expensive option.

While all these efforts are worthwhile, none is able to compensate for the lack of timely, accurate information on the hospital's managed care performance. As a result, many hospitals are in the position of simply not knowing how well they are performing in the managed care area—not knowing, literally, where their managed care revenues are coming from or how much it is costing the hospital to earn them.

DATA PRESENTATION   MCISs support the hospital's managed care business objectives in two basic ways. The first is by providing reports presenting various types of aggregate data that have been assembled for correlation or comparison. An example of such a report would be one that provides, by payer and for a specific period, the total number of cases, patient days, gross revenue, net revenue, cost, profit, and margin percentage. The second way is by allowing the hospital to inquire on specific contracts and, with some systems, specific patients in order to determine the authorization requirements for a particular patient's coverage, for example, or to obtain a concurrent report on incurred costs to date versus anticipated reimbursement on the patient.

PROCESSING MODES   Consistent with the two reporting modes, MCISs normally operate in one of two processing modes. The first is "batch" mode—that is, by processing groups of files that have been electronically transferred, or downloaded, from the various transaction systems to which the MCIS has been attached, or interfaced. The second way is by on-line inquiry either into its own database (for specific contract provisions, for example) or into the hospital's transaction systems in order to identify specific items of information, such as the case-cost-to-date inquiry above.

STANDARD REPORT TYPES   The functions of the MCISs on the market are arranged into modules that are somewhat different from product to product, and some systems have as many as 300 standard reports. However, it is convenient to break MCIS functions down into three groups, sketching out some of the typical standard reports for each.

Contract Analysis   This module provides information on hospital performance with respect to its contracts and, in some systems, will provide concurrent patient status information. Examples of typical reports are:

- *Executive summary*   Summarizes all activity and financial performance data for a given payer for a given period
- *Activity by cases*   Ranks all payers in order of activity for a given period
- *Performance by contract*   Ranks all payers in order of hospital financial performance for a given period
- *Performance by service*   Details operating results by hospital service (such as medicine and surgery) for a given payer for a given period
- *Activity by DRG*   Ranks 10 or so DRGs in order of activity for a specific period and payer
- *Physician profile by contract*   Reports activity and financial performance for a selected physician
- *Simulations*   Creates comparative operating statements with and without a particular payer contract, variations in rate structures, activity levels, and so on.

Compliance Reporting   This is the MCIS's "audit" module. Its function is to compare anticipated reimbursements to those actually received from the payer. The reimbursement is calculated by applying the payer's contract-specified rate schedules to services provided by the hospital. Examples of typical reports are:

- *Payment audit report*   Reports for selected contract and period amount of expected reimbursement versus amount of actual reimbursement by case.
- *Out of compliance notice*   Informs payer of reimbursement deficit and requests explanation. Actual wording is determined by the user hospital. Generation is timed by days-to-pay provisions of each contract.

Contract Data   This application provides current information on the provisions of each contract. It is most often used by the admitting department to ensure that requirements for admission (for example, second opinion and authorization for elective surgeries) have been met and by the patient accounting department to review the provisions of particular contracts during collection. The principal function is *contract profiling,* which either reports or displays, on-line, the detailed provisions and requirements of selected contracts.

In addition to the stock library of standard reports that are included with MCISs, these systems normally include a "report writer." This is a software tool that allows the user to create special "ad hoc" reports on demand.

DATA SOURCES AND ARCHITECTURE

MCISs obtain their transaction-level data from the hospital's existing information systems. These source systems are:

- *Patient accounting system* Provides patient financial class, case charges, and payments. It is linked to the MCIS by patient account number.
- *Cost accounting system* Provides cost by procedure. Linked to the managed care system by department code, general ledger code, and charge master number. If the hospital does not have a cost accounting system, these data can be loaded manually, although this is a tedious and time-consuming task.
- *Medical records system* Provides patient demographic and clinical case information which is linked to the managed care system by patient account number and medical record number.
- *Physician staff office system* Provides admitting physician identification number.

"Interfaces" (communications pathways between the on-line MCIS and the various transaction "source" systems) need not themselves be on-line. It is not necessary to develop a direct, electronic, machine-to-machine interface in order to get the necessary transaction data into the MCIS. Managed care systems can usually accept data in several input modes, not only on-line, but also by tape or diskette. Flexibility in adapting to the data output capabilities of systems already installed in the hospital is always a key design objective for MCIS vendors.

SOFTWARE ARCHITECTURE

MCISs typically employ a database structure, often using a commercial database product such as Oracle, dBase III+, or Focus. Transaction data are entered into this database by transferring them from the hospital's transaction systems and are the source data which the MCIS's application programs use. These systems are usually built around this single database and are generally modular, allowing the hospital to buy the system one application module at a time. In addition, vendors often provide modules for related applications that can share data with the MCIS. For example, one popular system is composed of five separate modules. They provide contract analysis, reimbursement auditing, financial analysis, and market analysis, and a contracts reference database.

MCIS HARDWARE

The database systems and application languages that are the software elements of most managed care systems are typically "portable." They will operate on more than one type and brand of hardware. One popular language, for example, will operate on IBM and Compaq microcomputers, AT&T, Digital, NCR, Wang, and Unisys minicomputers, and IBM and Unisys mainframes.

The hardware portability of most managed care systems provides a number of advantages to user hospitals. First, the hospital may not need to buy any hardware at all, if there is capacity available on the hardware it already has. Second, even if the hospital has to purchase additional hardware, it need buy only the amount of additional hardware the MCIS requires. Third, if the hospital wishes to revamp its systems in a year or so, there is a good chance that it will be able to move the MCIS onto its new hardware.

MCIS COSTS

Most MCISs are priced by the type of hardware they are to be installed on. The software license fee for an MCIS that combines contract analysis, reimbursement auditing, and contract reference capabilities currently ranges from $2500 for a simple database system that will keep track of contracts, $55,000 for a multifunctional microcomputer-based single-user system, and up to approximately $125,000 for the same system on a mainframe computer. If the system is to be installed on a local area network, the buyer should expect to pay the additional cost of the network software, which is from $1000 to $5000. "Site licensing" (a license that allows a reasonable number of multiple installations so long as these are operated at a single site) is not common, but the buyer may find discounts for multiple connected workstations (for example, paying two license fees for up to five PC workstations). Software license fees may or may not fully cover the cost of installation and training.

The annual costs of operating the system must not be overlooked. The rule of thumb for maintenance costs is 1 to 1.5 percent of installed software license fees per month. (For example, support for a system on which the buyer paid $50,000 in license fees would cost $500 to $750 per month in maintenance.) Maintenance fees usually include "hot line" telephone assistance and updates and enhancements to the software.

The buyer may also have to pay for any manual conversion work, such as loading contracts, if this has to be done either by the MCIS vendor or by a data conversion service.

A final cost item is the fees for any consulting or outside accounting support required, for example, in the development of cost standards or the validation of results from the MCIS during implementation.

MCIS BENEFITS

Historically, computerized information systems have been implemented to obtain operational benefits such as reductions in the size of the staff performing tasks that the computer is designed to replace or an improvement in the effectiveness of relatively routine operations (such as order communications from the nursing unit). MCISs clearly provide operational benefits of the latter sort, in the form of improved admissions screening of contract covered patients and enhanced reimbursement accuracy.

By most estimates, underpayment on managed care claims averages somewhere between 4 and 8 percent, and it is not unheard-of for a hospital to find that it is being underpaid on a contract by 20 percent. Many hospitals have found that MCISs, through their ability to audit payments against reimbursement earned and to flag other payer liabilities, pay for themselves in a very short time. For example, many hospitals have lost money because they have been unable to track days-to-pay performance and enforce days-to-pay clauses. Reporting on payers that have exceeded their days-to-pay limits is a function that contract management systems provide routinely.

However, there is an entirely different order of benefits that managed care systems provide. These are *strategic* benefits—providing information essential to the hospital in achieving its basic business objectives. This is a type of benefits that the MCIS shares with other "strategic" systems, such as cost accounting and flexible budgeting systems. By providing timely input to pricing, contracting, service line offerings, and other key strategic decisions, the MCIS allows the hospital to foresee the consequences of decisions before they are made (or at least before the hospital is irrevocably committed to them). In so doing, it allows the hospital to navigate its way through today's turbulent healthcare economy.

IMPLEMENTATION OF THE MCIS

MCISs are normally implemented by a team composed of the project leader (usually the controller, contracts officer, or a senior financial analyst), the vendor's installer, and a representative from the information systems department. In addition, the hospital may wish to use a consultant, outside accountant or auditor, or a data conversion service. Implementations usually require 3 to 6 months, with the vendor's representative on-site for 4 or 5 days to 2 or 3 weeks.

MCIS PRODUCTS

The rapid transformation of the nation's hospitals from an economy of fee-for-service to managed care has created an enormous market for MCISs, and new vendors and systems are appearing almost weekly. To give some idea of the types of MCIS products that are now available, three typical systems are briefly sketched out here. Because of the variability of pricing schedules, prices have not been included. None of the systems below sells, in the most fully functional version, for more than $60,000, and some are much cheaper.

MCIS A

Vendor A sells a family of related applications that are installed mainly on IBM or IBM-compatible microcomputers. The applications are contract negotiation, contract management, and contract auditing. These three modular managed care information systems are designed to run on any microcomputer, minicomputer, or mainframe that supports the fourth-generation database language in which they are written. In addition, these applications can download data from other computers. The applications were recently completely rewritten; there are about 130 installed sites on the older versions, and 15 on the new.

- *Negotiation system* This system provides specific cost and profitability information by strategic business unit and product line for each managed care contract. It has rate simulation capability with 54 possible rate structures (others can be added at installation), stop-loss and per diem functions. Hospital procedure costs can be either obtained from automated data at the hospital or loaded manually into the negotiation system cost file.
- *Contract management system* This application provides current department-level information on contract-covered patients. For example, the admitting department has available information regarding the preauthorizations that are required, preauthorization and verification contacts, deductibles, copays, and discharge planning.
- *Contract auditing system* This application produces bills per specific contract terms, audits payments against claims to ensure that the claim has not been underpaid, reports on days-to-pay, generates follow-up bills, and has other collection functions.

MCIS B   This product is a dedicated managed care information system using a fourth-generation relational database system (a different one from that used in MCIS A). It was developed in 1987 and is in use in approximately 40 hospitals. At present, it can operate on IBM mainframes (including the 9370), DEC VAX and microVAX, Hewlett-Packard, and Data General minicomputers. Vendor B expects that IBM will support the database language on the AS/400 midrange system shortly. The system is also available on a shared basis under a service agreement. Vendor B's system supports all informational aspects of managed care contracting and can be used in a multiple-hospital environment. Specific functionality includes:

- *Admission screening*   Uses worksheets, task lists, and audit and performance reports.
- *Concurrent tracking and utilization monitoring*   Uses "alert" reports.
- *Payments auditing*   Compares actual payment to expected payment.
- *Billing support*   Automatically produces a detailed calculation worksheet for each patient, based on the specific terms of the applicable contract (per diems, percentages, minimums, maximums, stop loss, pass throughs, and so on). Contractual writeoffs are passed back to the patient accounting system to provide "net" accounts receivable amounts.
- *Followup*   Provides aging reports and automatic follow-up letters.
- *Contract performance analysis*   Monthly and quarterly reports, comparative reports, and others.
- *Renegotiation*   Uses "alert" reports and simulation capabilities.

MCIS C   MCIS C is a PC-based system that can be used stand-alone or interfaced to the hospital's existing HMIS. When operated stand-alone, MCIS C provides the following functional modules:

- *Contracts*   Serves as a contract reference file, providing information such as reimbursement, reference persons, and activity.
- *Third parties*   Provides reports and supports databases relating to third party administrators and negotiators and utilization review organizations.
- *Physicians and medical groups*   Maintains physician profiles and provides a structure and reporting system to associate physicians and medical groups to specific negotiated contracts.
- *Employers*   Maintains reference file on employer groups and their associated carriers and plans.
- *Admissions*   Ties together information contained in the other modules. It provides the admitting department with information

on employer plans, and it allows the department to select negotiated contracts and identify utilization review requirements and
phone numbers to call for benefits determination.

When interfaced to a source of hospital patient data, the following
functional modules are available:

- *Contract performance* Volume, financial performance, and case
  mix information by contract
- *Billing* Provides reimbursement audit reports
- *Physician* Provides management reports on performance and
  volume by physician
- *"What-if" (simulation)* Provides reimbursement scenario profiles

As noted earlier, these systems are merely examples of the types
available. Other systems are arriving on the market almost daily, and
it is probable that both these systems and their competitors will be
steadily improved.

FUTURE DIRECTIONS FOR MCISs

MCISs are in their infancy, and although the direction of information
systems evolution can never be predicted with certainty, it is likely
that MCISs will be enhanced in several ways.

- *Increased internal integration* With most systems now, it is necessary to leave one functional module in order to enter another.
  The increased use of "windowing" environments, which allow
  more than one module to be run simultaneously, will enable the
  user to compare information from more than one function at a
  time. For example, it will likely become possible to inspect individual physician data while scrolling through activity-by-physician
  reports.
- *Increased integration with other strategic systems* Improved pro-
  gram-to-program communications capabilities will make it possible to manipulate increasingly disparate types of data in real time.
  For example, it should become possible to watch the effects of
  variations in the cost components of major procedures on the
  bottom line of a contract simulation by passing cost information
  on-line from the cost accounting system to the MCIS. This will
  allow the user to reach conclusions such as "Given the projected
  level of total hip replacements, we can earn a positive margin in
  orthopedic surgery under the proposed contract with XYZ Care if
  we can reduce the cost of the procedure by 5 percent."
- *Increased integration with marketing information systems* Increase integration with marketing information, to take another

example, would give the hospital the ability to develop economic and demographic profiles of those areas where it is getting patients for a particular service covered under a particular contract. Hospitals can now obtain information similar to this, but only by financial class. This works well for Medicare or Blue Cross patients, but not very well for "other commercial."

- *Increased integration with external systems*   As hospitals assume the role of the acute care nodes in vast healthcare delivery complexes, it is in the hospital's own interest to coordinate information flow with other nodes in the delivery system. This is particularly important in the area of managed care contracts, since these represent an increasing percentage of the hospital's business. For example, although the hospital is at a distinct disadvantage if it has to rely on its HMOs for utilization information, the HMO *is* the natural source for capitation data. A direct interface between the HMO's membership and eligibility systems and the hospital's MCIS will allow quick reconciliation of this data.

Another area where integration will become increasingly important is in quality of care. The ability to bring together financial and quality of care information on a contract-by-contract basis is becoming essential for hospitals in determining whether they are meeting *both* financial and quality requirements simultaneously for a given contract. For example, a particularly high level of readmits for a contracted service that is only modestly profitable might convince the hospital that the service line should be discontinued as soon as the agreement expires.

These evolutionary directions for the MCIS represent enhancements that will bring MCISs up to their present potential. At the same time that these systems are to go through a period of functional enhancement, HMIS vendors will be racing to build managed care capabilities into their financial management systems. Eventually, stand-alone MCISs are likely to go the same way as stand-alone case mix systems: occupying a relatively small corner of the market as entry-level or small-hospital products and competing with more functional systems sold by HMIS vendors.

Should the hospital wait until its current financial system can be upgraded by the HMIS vendor? The answer, in most cases, will be no for several reasons. First, the need for managed care information exists *now*, particularly for those hospitals that have expanded their managed care business up to (and beyond) the ability of their financial staff to manage it. In such a case, adding more financial analysts will not solve the problem, it will merely increase administrative costs.

Second, while many stand-alone MCIS vendors have gone through the time-consuming process of design, programming, and debugging, most HMIS vendors have only begun trying to build genuine managed care functionality into their systems. Consequently, it may be some time before HMIS vendors have the functionality that is available in many stand-alone systems today. (It is almost always easier and faster to design and build a stand-alone system than it is to add functionality to an existing, large-scale system.)

Third, there is likely to be less overall risk in buying a stand-alone system today than there will be in waiting for managed care functionality in an integrated financial system tomorrow. A stand-alone MCIS can be treated as an interim expedient to handle a short-term problem and can be discarded when convenient; an integrated financial system represents a much larger investment of the hospital's time and money.

There is a further consideration, already familiar to hospitals that have been confronted with the issue of buying, for example, a stand-alone pharmacy system versus buying a pharmacy module as part of an integrated patient care system. When purchasing a stand-alone MCIS, the finance department can expect to get relatively close to what it wants in the way of managed care functionality, support, and other desirable features. An integrated HMIS that includes a managed care information application component, however, will likely present the hospital with trade-offs. Will, for example, the finance department accept mediocre managed care functionality in return for an outstanding billing module, or vice versa? It is this dilemma that accounts for the surprisingly large number of stand-alone ancillary system vendors that are still thriving years after major integrated HMIS vendors have duplicated much of the functionality of the stand-alone ancillary products. It also accounts for the increasing number of integration tools on the market, such as the Simborg Systems STATLAN and NCR's CAI-net. These products are specifically intended to integrate high-functionality, but unintegrated, systems into a functional whole.

WHAT TO DO TODAY

It probably makes sense for a hospital with a substantial amount of managed care business to give consideration to implementing a stand-alone MCIS. Certainly, positive indicators in this regard would include the following examples:

- The finance department is unable to identify the managed care components of the hospital's revenues in a way that allows the hospital to assess and manage its contracts. For example, the finance department must lump a dozen or so revenue sources into an "other private pay" category for reporting purposes.
- The finance department is stretched to the limit of its resources and other important financial work is being repeatedly delayed.

- The hospital is contemplating entering into additional contracts or making other strategic moves involving managed care.
- The hospital is having difficulty complying with the provisions of its various contracts as a result of the difficulty of identifying these provisions at admission.
- There is a problem of underpayment on claims, but because of the sheer volume, the patient accounting department cannot keep up with them.

If any of these conditions exist, it is likely that an MCIS would be a worthwhile investment for the hospital. If most of them do (as they do at many hospitals that have a large managed care business), then such a system is more than a sound investment; it may well be a survival tool.

PLANNING FOR THE MCIS

Planning for specialized financial systems, such as MCISs, should begin with the recognition of an important point: The time and effort invested in planning should be proportional to the value of the information provided and the cost and business risk associated with incorrect information—*not* just to the cost of the system itself. As information systems go, MCISs are relatively inexpensive, but the data they provide is unusually valuable, and the related cost of, and business risk associated with, incorrect information are high. Consequently, planning for these systems should be done carefully.

Within reasonable limits, information systems planning is an almost unmixed blessing: Even a little planning is better than none. As hospitals too often find to their sorrow, it is easy to shortcut planning for information systems in the rush to meet pressing information needs. Poor planning accounts for more project failures and user frustration than does any other controllable shortcoming.

A misstep that creates almost as many problems as insufficient planning is *vendor-driven planning*. Often, a hospital will have a chronic operational problem with a large information component but will not focus its thinking clearly on solutions until it is approached by a system vendor. The vendor representative, skilled at uncovering sales opportunities, will offer to assist the hospital in clarifying and solving the problem and will, predictably, formulate a solution that requires the vendor's product. Since the hospital and the vendor have fundamentally different interests—the hospital's interest is in solving its problem while the vendor's is in selling his or her product—the resulting "solution" may or may not be satisfactory. Indeed, the outcome will rest largely on whether the hospital has been lucky enough to have been approached by the right vendor. In any case, the hospital has effectively lost control of the problem-solving process. Even when vendor influence is exercised less forcefully, it can be equally persuasive. The simple availability of a product can easily influence a hospital toward thinking of problems in terms of a product that the hospital knows, rather than defining the problem independently, developing a set of requirements for a solution, and then looking for a solution.

For these reasons, planning should be part of an independent, carefully worked-out process kept firmly under the hospital's control. The process should begin by concentrating on the hospital's managed care *strategy* rather than on any discussion of *systems.* The plan should show a direct and unbroken linkage between the hospital's managed care strategy, the identification of information requirements for implementing the managed care strategy, and, only then, the alternatives for meeting these requirements. Specifically, the plan should address:

- *The hospital's current approach to providing managed care* This should be a brief review of the managed care arrangements in which the hospital now participates. Each entry should include a definition of the basic business relationship involved, economics (for example, reimbursement amounts and the estimated percentage each contract represents of the overall managed care revenues), restriction on care (for example, authorizations for prior-day admission for elective surgeries), and any special problems or opportunities the contract represents. It should also include a review of utilization, administrative costs, and profitability.
- *Plans for the near term (6 months to 3 years)* This should review any changes that the hospital plans in its managed care business: leaving some areas, entering others, and adding or dropping service lines.
- *Present information needs* This should include not only an inventory of the present managed care information needs but also how they are being met (for example, by rekeying data from payer logs into a microbased spreadsheet).
- *Information systems capabilities* This should include all automated information sources used in managing the hospital's managed care business, and it should also include any changes (such as the implementation of a new patient accounting system) that are planned. It will, therefore, require reviewing the hospital's overall information systems strategy. This section should clearly define the HMIS environment into which any new MCIS will have to fit.
- *Projected information needs* This section may take a certain amount of effort to complete, but it is an important component of the plan since it requires the hospital to think through what

information it will require in order to conduct its managed care enterprises.

- *Information strategy for managed care* This section will be a response to the situation posed by the hospital's managed care information needs (present and future) and will, to some extent, mirror its overall information systems strategy at the level of managed care. For example, to what extent will the hospital depend on external sources, such as HMOs, for information? What financial, technical, and organizational resources will the hospital commit to administering its managed care information? How much risk will it accept in its MCIS technology? How much is it willing to spend on this information technology? What is its timetable?

- *Information tactics for managed care* This section will address the implementation of the managed care information strategy itself. Where the information strategy deals with "what," the information tactics deals with "how to." It addresses such issues as "make versus buy," that is, developing MCISs internally rather than purchasing them; general requirements for vendors; use of outside resources, such as accounting, consulting, and data conversion firms; and day-to-day management of managed care information projects.

This process may make planning for MCISs seem somewhat tedious and overly complex. It can be, but need not. What is required to avoid "paralysis by analysis" is to establish a timetable for the plan, create a planning group that will commit itself to meeting the timetable and that has administrative backing, and then simply proceed. The managed care information plan need not be highly detailed, though discussions of managed care information requirements and technical issues must be sufficiently detailed to make informed decisions possible. What is essential is that the issues be addressed *deliberately* rather than be decided by default and that the plan have the *active and unequivocal* support of the hospital's administration.

The planning group need not be large. Although membership will vary somewhat from one hospital to the next, it may be sufficient to begin with the chief financial officer, the contracts administration officer, the hospital's planning or marketing director, the director(s) of admitting and outpatient registration, and a senior representative of the information systems department. Others that may have an interest in this project, particularly if the hospital believes that significant changes in physician behavior may be needed, are the chief of the hospital's medical staff and the manager of the hospital's Independent Practice Association (IPA), if it has one.

MAKE OR BUY?   One issue that must be confronted in every information systems planning project is whether the hospital should develop its information systems or buy them "off the shelf." The experience of the great majority of hospitals over the last 20 years has been that, unless there are truly compelling reasons to develop systems, it is wiser to buy them. Attempts by hospitals to develop their own information systems too often result in systems that do not justify, in terms of features or benefits, the difference between what the hospital spent to develop them and what they would have cost to buy.

As information systems acquire increased flexibility through the use of relational databases, report writers, and fourth-generation languages, they are able to meet the requirements of more hospitals with fewer modifications. This is especially true of specialized financial systems, such as cost accounting, resource management, flexible budgeting, and managed care information systems, since they are designed to interface to a wide variety of transaction systems and to be as adaptable as possible. For these reasons, it is assumed that the hospital will purchase, rather than develop, its MCIS.

SELECTING THE MCIS

Organizing the Selection

As a rule, the group responsible for preparing the hospital's MCIS plan should be the group responsible for selecting the MCIS vendor. Since the MCIS is highly specialized, with relatively few users, it is not necessary to have the sort of large, representative group that is required when selecting a patient care system. However, it is essential that any departmental representatives involved have the authority to commit their departments to a course of action; otherwise there will be a great deal of time lost as selection group members obtain approvals from their department managers.

Applying the MCIS Strategy

The basic requirements that the vendor should meet must be derived from the hospital's managed care information systems plan. A thorough, carefully developed, and fully reviewed managed care information systems plan will greatly simplify vendor selection by allowing the selection group to simply restate key information requirements as selection criteria.

Requests for Information and Requests for Proposals

These are the two most common types of questionnaire submitted to potential vendors. The difference is that the request for information (RFI) is usually shorter and less detailed than the request for proposal (RFP) and, unlike the RFP, does not ask that the vendor propose a specific product at a specific price (if it does, then it *is* an RFP).

RFIs are normally sent out in order to "qualify" vendors—that is, to identify a group of vendors that are plausible candidates for an RFP. The RFI should present the hospital's intentions in obtaining an MCIS, outline the hospital's business and systems environment, list the overall capabilities expected of the system (for example, maintain on-line reference file of contract terms and provisions for all contracts), and, finally, ask if the vendor is interested in receiving an RFP. (The RFI may also ask for a "ballpark" price quotation, though many vendors do not like to discuss price even in general terms without more detailed information than the RFI provides.)

Once the RFI responses have been received, the selection group can weed out vendors who either did not respond, declined to bid, or were not a good fit. The process can then go forward to the RFP. An RFI is not always necessary. Many hospitals, particularly those that are familiar with the type of product being sought or that have done an initial "vendor sweep" and are satisfied that they have a suitable group of vendor candidates, will go directly to the RFP.

Developing Written Requests for Proposals

While preparing an RFP and evaluating proposals can be tedious, the temptation to select a vendor based on presentations, notes from telephone conversations, and a few reference calls must be firmly resisted. First, absence of a written record inhibits, rather than expedites, communications with the vendor. As the selection process proceeds, it becomes necessary to reestablish on every occasion what has and has not been decided before proceeding further with the vendor. This makes misunderstandings inevitable. Second, the RFP is essential in establishing, for the selection group, precisely *what has been proposed.* Third, when a vendor is required to respond to an RFP with a written proposal, the hospital is able to focus the selection process on getting the information it needs, rather than simply accepting whatever information the vendor wishes to give it. Finally, the vendor's written proposal provides the basis of the sales contract with the vendor.

One important caution regarding the RFP: the selection group should work out its evaluation technique *prior* to writing the RFP, rather than wait until the proposals arrive, and should design the RFP to conform to the evaluation technique selected. For example, will an arithmetic scoring technique be used? If so, will the vendor be evaluated on the basis of gross point score? Percentages? Will high-level "critical factors," key requirements that will conclusively disqualify vendors that fail to meet them, be used?

Managing the Process

It is important that the selection process be governed by some simple, but firm, rules.

- *Stay on schedule*   The selection group should decide early in the selection process what information will be needed to make a vendor decision. Once the information is in, the decision should be made, period. The tendency to look for just "one more" item of information is usually a disguised reluctance to make a decision.
- *Maintain control over vendors*   In order to avoid vendor-promoted factionalization, vendors should be required to deal *only* with the *entire* selection group. "Back channel" conversations between individual members and vendors' representatives quickly assume the character of negotiations and are invariably divisive.
- *Be realistic*   It is unlikely that the selection group will find an MCIS that meets all of the member's requirements. Consequently, members must be prepared to make compromises. Deadlocks create not only delays but organizational stresses as well, and steamrolling the opposition usually creates a legacy of ill will that results in problems during system implementation.

MAKING THE SELECTION

The simplest way to score vendor proposals is to begin by reviewing them for "critical factors" in order to eliminate quickly any vendors that are a poor fit at the strategic level. For example, a system that has no production reference sites is, on these grounds alone, a poor choice. The selection group should be aware, however, that it may not find a vendor that does not fail at least one critical factor, and should decide in advance what to do in such a case. Next, the selection group should score the functionality of each vendor's system using a simple arithmetic scale. The functions may be weighted in order of importance; that is, systems that provide good functionality in key areas will score higher. Then, references for the leaders should be checked *thoroughly*, making certain that the site being contacted is a *production* site for the *same version* of the system being proposed, has a similar transaction systems environment, and that (as well as can be determined) the reference institution does not have a concealed business interest in the system. The selection group should bear in mind that the vendor will list as references only those hospitals that will provide a good report; the selection group should make an effort to locate any other users of the system and find out why *they* were not listed as references.

Particular attention should be paid to vendor support, including implementation, software debugging, trouble-shooting, and general willingness to stay in touch and act as a resource to the user. The best system on the market will be extremely difficult to use if the vendor that sells it will not return phone calls.

NEGOTIATING THE CONTRACT

Once the MCIS has been selected, the hospital can negotiate the purchase contract. The purchase of an information system involves certain potential risks for the hospital, and an attorney who is knowledgeable in information systems contracts should be consulted during the contract negotiation on ways of approaching the contract to ensure that the hospital's interests are protected. One area that should be looked at closely is that of support. Many vendors of specialized financial systems are relatively small and have understaffed user support departments or try to cover both sales and user support with the same staff. This can create delays, confusion, and frustration for the hospital both during and after implementation. Performance incentives, forfeitures, and binding problem-resolution procedures should be included in the contract as appropriate.

It is often possible for the hospital to gain leverage in the contract negotiation by bargaining with two vendors at the same time. While this maneuver is understandably disliked by vendors, it is not unethical, any more than is comparison shopping for any other item. It can be quite productive, since it is usually possible to negotiate a vendor down substantially on price if the vendor is aware that the hospital has another suitor waiting.

Throughout the contract negotiation, the hospital should bear in mind that the contract not only binds the parties, it also establishes the basis for their future business relationship. Therefore, it is advisable for the hospital to limit its demands in the contract negotiation to ensuring that it gets the product at a reasonable price and that its legitimate interests are protected. "Squeezing" a vendor, especially a smaller one, may pay off in the short run, but it invariably creates long-term friction and problems for the hospital.

IMPLEMENTING THE MCIS

While implementation of the MCIS is not especially complex, it requires adequate time and staff, and attention to certain key details.

MCISs can typically be implemented in from 3 to 6 months of elapsed time, that is, 3 to 6 months from the beginning of the project until the first set of monthly reports are produced in "production" (rather than test) status. There does not appear to be an appreciable difference in time required between microcomputer-based systems and those resident on minicomputers or mainframes. Microcomputer-based systems are usually implemented on a dedicated microcomputer, while minicomputer- and mainframe-based systems are usually implemented on a machine that is already in place and will be shared with other applications. Since the hospital may need to purchase and install the microcomputer, it is likely that the microcomputer-based system may actually take longer to implement. This is particularly true if the MCIS is to support multiple users via a local area network, since these configurations often require a certain amount of tinkering before they will operate properly.

The implementation team will vary with the type of system being implemented and with the level of support to be obtained from the vendor. A typical implementation team for a highly functional MCIS might require the hospital's contracts manager for 2 days a week and, due to the quantity of data that must be analyzed by hand in order to validate system results, two full-time financial analysts for the duration of the project. Interfaces may require a day or two of on-site work by support technicians from the vendors of the transaction feeder systems; naturally, the hospital will be billed for this time. The MCIS vendor's installation analyst will typically be on-site for several days at the beginning of the project and for a day or two at system conversion. Otherwise, the hospital is on its own unless it has contracted for additional support from the vendor or from an accounting or consulting firm.

Finance departments are not often involved in hospital system implementations and when they are, as in the case of a new general ledger system, they usually have extensive vendor or consultant support. For the finance department to manage an implementation largely on its own, as in the case of an MCIS, may pose novel challenges. However, the implementation can be made easier by observing a few general rules.

First, the finance department should be certain that all concerned agree on the relative priority of the MCIS implementation and that everyone understands that every day a finance department analyst or other key implementation staff member is pulled away for other work is a day lost to the implementation project. Realistically, it is difficult to dedicate *anyone* to such a project without interruption; however, everyone should agree on which interruptions will be allowed, which will not, and what changes to the overall timetable will be acceptable.

Second, if at all possible, the finance department should not schedule any other major projects during the MCIS implementation. This means that the implementation should be timed so that it does not conflict with the annual financial audit, the implementation of a new release of the patient accounting, general ledger, or accounts payable software, or the introduction of major new service lines (opening an outpatient pavilion, for instance).

Third, the finance department should be certain that it fully understands the implementation process and that the vendor's implementation-related documentation is adequate. If there is any question about the finance department's ability to manage the implementation on its own, it should seriously consider contracting for additional vendor or other support, even though this will increase the overall cost of the system somewhat.

Finally, the temptation to cut corners on training in order to save money or speed the implementation must be avoided. A good rule of thumb is to estimate the amount of training required and increase it by a third.

USING THE MCIS Hospitals that have implemented MCISs invariably report that, having once used them, they could not administer their managed care contracts without them. This applies even to hospitals that experienced some difficulty in the implementation of the system. Like all other automated information systems, the MCIS has some limitations.

First, the system, being a combination of database and calculation software, requires a level of maintenance and validation that the finance department might not have experienced before. A control procedure should be set up to ensure that new contracts are entered into the system and existing contracts updated when the provisions are modified. Calculations performed by the system should be audited periodically to ensure that they are correct. Every report run for every contract should be validated when the system is implemented, every report for every new contract should be validated when the contract is added, and each contract should be spot-checked periodically thereafter, particularly when modifications to any of the terms are made. Validation need not be exhaustive, but column totals should be cross-calculated, and information reported out for particularly sensitive categories should be checked against independently available data (such as the patient accounting system's payer logs) and reviewed for reasonableness.

Second, the MCIS, like other automated information systems, is only a tool. It can contribute important information to a managed care strategy and help implement it; it is not a substitute for it.

Using Population-Based Analysis to Manage Care

MANON SPITZER, Director of Marketing and Educational Programs
PHILIP CAPER, M.D., Chairman
Codman Research Group, Inc., Lyme, New Hampshire

The Rutland Regional Medical Center (RRMC) is a pioneer among hospitals because it uses data from population-based analyses of community-use patterns to predict utilization patterns and educate local physicians about how their decision making influences future growth at their hospital. In the process, physicians and hospital administrators were forced to develop a partnership for healthcare management that demands equal attention to clinical decision making and to facility and resource planning.

RRMC was a reluctant pioneer. In December 1985, RRMC submitted a Certificate of Need (CON) application to the state's Department of Health and Health Policy Corporation. As part of a $24.5 million comprehensive redevelopment plan, the hospital sought to replace obsolete physical plant and equipment, introduce new services, realign and consolidate outpatient services, increase access to radiation therapy and CAT services, and develop nonacute patient care space to better serve the elderly. However, the Rutland hospital market area had for several years attracted the scrutiny of state health officials for its pattern of high per capita rates of hospital use by Vermont standards. In fact, since RRMC's patient day rate for the area's residents was 21 percent above average, RRMC became the subject of intense media criticism because of its perceived contribution to the costs of health insurance in the state. Because RRMC accounts for 85 percent of the hospitalizations of area residents, CON reviewers asked the hospital to justify its requests in light of this utilization pattern.

The RRMC responded by undertaking a detailed population-based analysis of the patterns of hospital use in the Rutland area, compared to other communities in Vermont, and an investigation of how severity of illness among RRMC patients influenced utilization.

At the outset, RRMC's medical staff felt the area's relatively high day rates were due largely to a disproportionate number of elderly citizens in the Rutland hospital market area who, as patients, generated both higher admission rates and longer lengths of stay. The staff also feared that the care residents received from non-Rutland providers could be influencing the rates upward. The small area analysis demonstrated that the area's age demographics were only a minor part of the whole story. Moreover, because residents of the service area used RRMC for most of their care in the admission categories which generated the higher than expected rates, with the remainder scattered among several sites, the staff was convinced that the area's utilization patterns reflected its own practice style.

Population-based analyses provided detailed information on every aspect of utilization by clinical cause of service, age group of user, and market area subregion—in some cases individual zip codes. The results were used to establish criteria for conducting chart reviews of RRMC records for the severity analysis.

The results of each analysis were shared systematically with the medical director and staff physicians from the inception of the project, with a comprehensive interpretation of all the findings presented at a full-day retreat. The data analysis was an eye-opener for the physicians. Practicing clinicians think of medical care in terms of individual patients. The population-based perspective gives them the information they need to understand how their clinical decisions compare to those of their colleagues in other parts of the same state and how those decisions affect use rates and per capita costs in their community. The addition of severity data for some of the more common causes of high rates of admission, provided the detail that practitioners needed to understand the clinical decision making that underlies the practice patterns.

The information provided to RRMC by these investigations provided a base for developing consensus among hospital administrators, trustees, and medical staff about their future resource requirements and how they would be met by the building project. The CON application was revised and resubmitted, asking for 10 percent fewer acute care beds and 10 other beds designated for nonacute stays. It placed more emphasis on out patient services, particularly ambulatory surgery facilities, and called for expanded discharge planning activity. Because RRMC had based its revised request on its analysis of actual clinical practice, state regulators were persuaded that the request was justified, using RRMC's revised projections. The state approved approximately 92 percent of RRMC's request.

RRMC had satisfied the immediate need to deal with regulatory authorities, but the attitudes and objectives of RRMC administration and medical staff had changed in the process. The institution voluntarily incorporated both population-based utilization analysis and investigation of severity into a permanent system for continuous monitoring of quality of care and utilization. The hospital's medical director meets periodically with each clinical service to review detailed quarterly reports on utilization, including severity, compare them to historic patterns, and discuss objectives for improvement. Once somewhat reluctant participants, RRMC physicians developed an *esprit de corps* as leaders in the effort to provide high quality cost-efficient healthcare to the residents of Vermont.

During the 4-year period 1984–1987, the age-sex adjusted per capita admission rate dropped by 23 percent, from 139 to 107 per 1000 residents (the rate excludes maternity-related and newborns). While the decreases were broad-based, affecting 19 out of 21 relevant major diagnostic categories (MDCs), reductions of 30 to 50 percent in total patient days were recorded for MDC 8 (musculoskeletal and connective

tissue), MDC 11 (kidney and urinary tract), and MDC 12 (male reproductive)—all the focus of a project study. Whereas medical back admissions (DRG 243) among Rutland residents at RRMC generated 735 more days than expected in 1984, based on the average for the state of Vermont, in 1987 they recorded 2 days *less than expected*. The overall decrease in the per capita patient day rate was 25 percent. Most of the reductions occurred during formal project activity, but the gains have been maintained and the trend is consistent through 1988.

The key element in this success story was development of information that provided a credible—and shared—basis for dialog among all parties involved. No targets were set for reductions, no physicians were singled out for admonition, but the impact of information feedback on the patterns of practice was discernible within months. Changes in the rates of admissions and days were most dramatic for the clinical categories chosen for project scrutiny, although a sentinel effect seems to have influenced the overall utilization.

Major structural changes are occurring in healthcare that place great stress on hospitals and physicians as the most visible symbols of the industry. Population-based information on utilization and costs can be a catalyst for communication between purchasers and providers of care, providing a common language for resolving their diverse and sometimes conflicting objectives.

CHAPTER TWENTY-ONE

Employer Data

EMPLOYER UTILIZATION DATA

JOHN C. ERB, Managing Consultant
A. Foster Higgins & Co., Inc., Princeton, New Jersey

ROBERT F. GRIFFITH, Managing Consultant
A. Foster Higgins & Co., Inc., Los Angeles, California

Health plan management requires access to a wide range of timely, meaningful utilization and cost data. While such data are currently available to most employers, the task of translating raw statistics into useful information remains daunting to many. In this article, currently available data elements are examined along with an assessment of specific barriers to construction of a viable database. A general approach to analyzing case-specific utilization data and the tools required to conduct such an analysis are described as well. Finally, a view of the future trends in utilization data collection and application is presented.

DATA AVAILABILITY, COLLECTION, AND CONSTRAINTS

Steady progress has been made in the past few years to make available the range of data necessary for health plan managers to assess those factors influencing plan utilization and cost. Blue Cross–Blue Shield plans, commercial insurance carriers, third party administrators, and self-administered employers have expanded the range of data to be entered into the claims processing systems files, allowing retrieval of those data elements critical to a meaningful analysis of indemnity plan experience. Improvements have been made in the systems used to capture demographic data on the employees who participate in the various offerings, making possible the prospective development of risk profiles for each of the indemnity or HMO options. The vendors of cost management services, such as preadmission certification, have been motivated by their clients to record key elements of each transaction as a means of measuring the effectiveness of their efforts.

However, a large gap remains in the mosaic representing the total health plan experience of the typical employer. That missing piece is the utilization and cost experience of employees enrolled in HMOs offered by an employer. Because HMOs reimburse providers in a different manner, that is, capitation, than most traditional health plans, the capture of meaningful utilization and cost data is limited. Comparative utilization measures are also difficult to integrate, especially in staff model HMOs, where tracking specific services — notably physician office services — is conducted in a different context than in a fee-for-service environment. This creates problems for plan managers attempting to assess optimum cost-sharing design and provider performance in experience-rated or self-funded HMO arrangements. A number of constraints may be encountered when an employer tries to retrieve data relating to the demographic characteristics of the population at risk, the utilization patterns of plan enrollees, or the cost-effectiveness of specific providers. These include poorly designed standard utilization reports developed by some administrators, the cost of both standard and customized reports, the time necessary to produce such reports, and, more frequently, the lack of clearly defined objectives on the part of the managers requesting reports.

The sections below address issues related to the availability and collection of useful utilization and cost data. Also, the current constraints to the development of a comprehensive health plan database are discussed and a number of alternative approaches to minimize the effect of such constraints on the analysis are offered.

Enrollee Data

In order to maintain a current listing of individuals who are eligible to use a health benefit plan, data files are maintained which include information pertinent to this identification process. Typically, the needed data relate to the employee identifiers, that is, name, social security number, date of hire, type of coverage selected, and the presence or absence of dependents eligible for plan coverage.

However, many employers conduct a more in-depth analysis of the characteristics of these eligibles. For example, in a flexible compensation scheme, developing an actuarial risk profile of the plan eligibles in each of the health plan options makes possible a prediction of the experience in each plan. Financial subsidization of one plan by the enrollees in another plan may then be either eliminated or enhanced, depending on the goals of the employer.

When analyzing risk assumption by HMO alternatives, the employer can utilize such profiling to determine selection patterns and estimated comparative costs. Table 1 demonstrates a simplified approach to such a rating methodology, using standard underwriting techniques.

TABLE 1   Measurement of Risk Factors in Health Plan Underwriting

EMPLOYEE AGE	NUMBER OF EMPLOYEES	RATING FACTOR	WEIGHTING
MALE			
< 19	10	0.630	6.300
20–24	98	0.630	61.740
25–29	119	0.630	74.970
30–34	113	0.680	76.840
35–39	74	0.730	54.020
40–44	57	0.880	50.160
45–49	59	1.000	59.000
50–54	30	1.300	39.000
55–59	29	1.600	46.400
60–64	20	2.100	42.000
65–69	5	2.800	14.000
70–74	0	2.800	0.000
75–79	0	2.800	0.000
80 +	0	2.800	0.000
FEMALE			
< 19	26	0.940	24.440
20–24	299	0.940	281.060
25–29	402	0.940	377.880
30–34	341	1.040	354.640
35–39	199	1.090	216.910
40–44	148	1.190	176.120
45–49	108	1.350	145.800
50–54	73	1.500	109.500
55–59	45	1.600	72.000
60–64	36	1.900	68.400
65–69	7	2.300	16.100
70–74	0	2.300	0.000
75–79	1	2.300	2.300
80 +	0	2.300	0.000
Total	2229		2369.580
Age-sex factor			1.031

This simple underwriting technique when combined with a similar analysis of dependent age-sex factors provides an employer with the ability to quantify the actual risk represented by a group enrolled in an indemnity plan option or an HMO offering and to compare the relative risk that each group represents. When actual claims cost by age and sex cohort is examined in this way, it is possible to adjust employer HMO contributions based on risk assumption by individual HMOs. Newly passed federal legislation allows employers to base their HMO contributions on the actuarial risk that an HMO assumes rather than on the cost of providing indemnity plan benefits. Employers using such "risk transfer" techniques can virtually eliminate the effects of adverse selection on the indemnity plan by reducing contributions to HMOs enrolling younger, healthier employees.

When age- and sex-adjusted norms are available, the plan manager can analyze the data and compare actual experience with the level of utilization expected for a group with similar demographic characteristics. If the employer's experience varies significantly from the predicted level of use, then efforts will be aimed at improving the efficiency of plan design, plan funding methodologies, and/or use of alternative delivery systems such as HMOs and PPOs.

The plan manager can use employee residence (zip code) data to test the feasibility of implementing a specific PPO or HMO network by predicting geographic penetration of current plan participants. When tied to actual utilization information, such residence data enables profiling of current utilization patterns of specific providers within a geographic area.

A thorough analysis of the demographic characteristics of a group of eligibile employees requires that the following minimal data set should be captured by and retrieved from the system:

- Employee identifiers (name, social security number, employee identification number)
- Employee residence (state, county, zip code)
- Employee age (date of birth)
- Employee sex
- Date of hire
- Employment status (full- or part-time, hourly or salary)
- Health plan selected
- Optional coverages selected
- Dependent coverage selected
- Dependent identifiers [name, social security number of spouse; name, social security number of full-time students covered; name(s) of dependent child(ren)]
- Dependent age and sex (for each dependent)

There are a number of other data elements in the file which are crucial for other human resources tasks, but the above data represent the minimum set of information needed to conduct risk-profile analysis. The acquisition of dependent identifiers, ages and sex, offers an important refinement of the current practice of estimating the number and demographic characteristics of dependents covered under the plans. These data elements are not critical, however, to the success of a baseline analysis of risk assumption in an indemnity plan or HMO offering.

Accurate eligible employee counts are necessary to compute "cost per employee" statistics, which are the basis of comparing utilization patterns from one period to the next.

In the absence of an accurate accounting of dependents covered by the plan, estimates of total covered lives may be made by using simple actuarial assumptions of dependent ratios. For example, in a three-tiered contribution scheme, the simple approach shown in Table 2 may be taken.

This simple approach may be refined by using actuarial assumptions of family size by employee age cohort, as found in an underwriting manual. An example of the practical application of dependent eligibility data is the computation of universal utilization measures for comparison with established norms or with the prior years' plan experience. Hospital admission rates, for example, are computed by dividing the number of admissions by the population covered under the plan. Since this population is the aggregate of employees and dependents, it is important to calculate the estimated number of dependents as accurately as possible. Inpatient days per 1000 insured lives is another important yardstick to measure plan experience. Using the population figures calculated above, measures of hospital admission rates and days per 1000 lives can be computed as shown in Table 3.

Similarly, inpatient days per 1000 insured lives can be computed in the same fashion (see Table 4). While the utility of a comprehensive eligibility file is clear, a number of constraints may compromise an employer's ability to make the proper use of these data. Among these constraints is the validity of the data with regard to covered dependents. Frequently, this information is collected at the initial enroll-

TABLE 2   Estimating Covered Lives Enrolled in Health Benefit Plan

CONTRIBUTION TIER	NUMBER OF EMPLOYEES	CONVERSION FACTOR	TOTAL NUMBER OF LIVES
Employee only	645	1.0	645
Employee and spouse	880	2.0	1760
Family	774	3.5	2709
Total	2299		5114

TABLE 3   Calculating Admissions per 1000 Covered Lives

NUMBER OF ADMISSIONS	÷	ESTIMATED LIVES (1000)	=	ADMISSIONS PER 1000 LIVES
498	÷	5.114	=	97.4

ment of an employee into one of the health plan options. If, however, the enrollee makes no change in plans subsequent to that initial choice, no update is made of the eligibility file to reflect changes in the status of dependents covered by the employee. Thus, the information contained in the file quickly becomes dated. This problem can be solved with an annual reenrollment of all health plan participants, but the added value of this costly approach is often perceived as low by plan managers.

Other constraints to the collection of useful data from the eligibility file lie in the flexibility of the software used to capture the data. Many employers use a variety of systems that must interface with each other to fulfill a number of functions such as salary administration, payroll, financial accounting, and cost allocation. These systems were often installed independently, making retrieval of demographic data difficult—especially when such data must be tied to claims data for analytical purposes. One employer recently attempted to analyze its utilization experience and cost patterns for its 60 locations. Eligibility data, however, were maintained solely by the claims administrator from monthly input by each of those 60 locations, many of which had different payroll and human resource systems. In some cases, only paper transmittal of eligibility data was possible. The credibility of the data was so suspect that the employer was advised not to proceed with the analysis. In this case, the installation of a centralized benefit administration system (which was designed to interface with its payroll and human resource software) was the necessary first step in conducting an analysis of its health plan utilization experience.

TABLE 4   Calculating Inpatient Days per 1000 Covered Lives

NUMBER OF INPATIENT DAYS	÷	ESTIMATED LIVES (1000)	=	INPATIENT DAYS PER 1000 LIVES
2938	÷	5.114	=	574.5

The growing popularity of flexible benefits programs has spurred developmental efforts to improve these systems.

Indemnity Plan Experience Data

The demand by senior management for an accounting of health plan expenditures has motivated plan administrators both to capture the critical data elements in the processing procedures and to generate useful report formats arraying those elements. Most Blue Cross–Blue Shield plans, commercial insurance carriers, and third party administrators have developed standard sets of utilization reports which provide their clients with at least a minimal accounting of how claim dollars are spent, who is spending those dollars, and what specific types of medical services are being purchased.

As described above, the employer can apply data acquired from the eligibility file to develop meaningful profiles of plan utilization from period to period and, from these profiles, detect changing or inappropriate patterns of use.

In order to make the best use of such periodic studies, an employer should define the objectives of the study in advance to eliminate unnecessary data acquisition and analysis costs. The following issues must be clarified prior to undertaking a utilization study.

WHAT ARE THE PERIODS TO BE STUDIED? Since utilization data are generally reported on an incurred rather than on a paid basis, a 3-month lag between the date that the claim is incurred and the date on which the claim is paid must be allowed. For example, if claims incurred from January to December are the target of analysis, then data on those claims cannot be collected until the end of March of the following period. It has been found that a 3-month "tail" or lag to allow for payment of an incurred claim generally captures 96 to 97 percent of incurred charges. The wait for payment of 100 percent of incurred claims, however, can take more than 6 months.

The study of plan experience for one period alone is not generally very useful since there is no prior period with which to draw comparisons. Key trends in utilization may be overlooked if prior experience is not used in the analysis of current experience. For example, if inpatient charges are measured at $1200 per employee during a 1-year study period, does this represent an improvement or a deterioration when compared to the prior period? Since there are no normative data for this figure, how can the analyst characterize it?

Since the utilization of healthcare services is somewhat seasonal in nature, it is best to compare like periods in any study. Elective surgery for children, for example, is generally performed in the summer months. Little elective surgical care is sought from late November to early January because of the holidays. Therefore, a July to December experience should be compared to the July to December period of the prior year, rather than to the January to June experience of the same year.

Claims processing systems are routinely purged of data on a periodic basis to prevent massive storage problems. Claims data are often not retained for more than a specified period, that is, 24 months. Retrospective studies for periods prior to the purge date will not always be possible. It is possible for most administrators, however, to download a client's data onto a storage disk for use in the future, even though utilization reports may not be generated immediately. This generally represents a modest expense each year and is suggested for clients who want to perform such analyses every other year or every third year.

WHAT DISCRETE SUBGROUPS OF THE INSURED POPULATION SHOULD BE STUDIED?   The ability of an employer to examine the utilization patterns of specific subgroups of the plan eligibles is, in large part, determined by the account structure used to identify claimants. Individual account suffix numbers may be assigned to groups on the basis of geographic location, employee status (for example, active or retired, salary or hourly) or other forms of organizational identification (for example, manufacturing, sales, and distribution).

Plan managers must determine in advance which of the discrete subgroupings will lend strength to the analysis and which will merely add unnecessary layers of reports. If there is no difference in the plans offered to hourly and salaried workers, for example, the breakouts of experience may not lend any useful insights into controlling costs. Also, if the number of employees in specific geographic areas is too small to be of significance, then a breakout of their experience will add little to the analytic process.

WHAT SPECIFIC MEASURES OF UTILIZATION WILL ASSIST IN ACHIEVING THE OBJECTIVES OF THE STUDY?   In this case, the tendency of an inexperienced analyst is to order data reports whose measures of utilization are irrelevant to the purpose of the study. For example, the reporting of inpatient admissions classified by diagnostic code can be achieved by means of several classification systems — Major Diagnostic Category (MDC), which combines similar diagnoses into 23 categories; Diagnostic Related Groups (DRG), which expands the MDCs to 470; the International Classification of Diseases, 9th Edition (ICD-9), which provides literally thousands of diagnostic categories for analysis; and unique classification schemes developed by individual plan administrators.

The classification of surgical procedures, on the other hand, is most often achieved by use of the CPT-4 coding scheme. Most claims administrators can produce preformatted reports based on the frequency of, and charges and payments for, surgical procedures using the CPT-4 classification system.

The analysis of noninpatient utilization by diagnostic category, however, has a number of constraints. First, much of this coding is performed by nonprofessionals in the medical records field, that is, a physician's office staff, and is frequently incorrect. Also, many noninpatient services, for example, prescription drug claims, are not coded as to diagnosis. Further, there is little incentive for accurate coding for nonsurgical services since reimbursement does not depend on accurate coding. On the claims administration side, such codes are often truncated, recategorized into an administrator-specific coding scheme, or not entered at all.

Each of these classification systems lends itself to particular analytic tasks. For example, DRGs incorporate aspects of other important factors influencing the length or cost of an admission, such as the age of the patient and the presence or absence of coexisting medical conditions or complications. This allows an analysis of the severity of illness and, hence, a more exact comparison of hospital performance. Also, a number of states now require reimbursement to hospitals based on the DRG assignment. Employers with claimants in these states should require their administrators to provide DRG-based utilization reports.

ICD-9 analysis allows a more detailed assessment of the cause of illness but does not factor in the related influences on the admission, as do DRGs. In noninpatient settings, however, some form of ICD-9 groupings must be used since DRGs are not applicable in noninpatient settings.

If one of the objectives of the study is to determine current levels of reimbursement for specific diagnostic categories so that provider negotiations may be initiated, then more specific classification techniques such as DRG or ICD-9 must be used. If, however, the objective of the study is to determine the general effectiveness of plan design, such expensive specificity is unnecessary.

If one of the objectives of the study is to compare the employer's experience to a national or regional norm, careful attention must be given to the techniques used by the reporting system to calculate standard measures of utilization. For example, in some reporting systems, a normal newborn is tabulated as a separate admission, while in others the newborn is considered part of the mother's admission. Obviously, the number of admissions in the former tabulation will be higher than in the latter. These rates may be misleading if the normative data are tabulated in a different manner from the employer's reports.

Also, some reporting systems require full ICD-9 codes (five digits) in order to assign an MDC or DRG. If a three-digit code is assigned by the hospital, the system will assign that admission to "unclassified," thus artificially lowering the admission rate within the specific diagnostic category in which it should have been placed.

ARE THERE SPECIAL PROGRAMS OR CIRCUMSTANCES IN PLACE OR UNDER CONSIDERATION WHICH WILL REQUIRE OTHER THAN STANDARD REPORTING METHODOLOGIES?

Employers who have initiated cost management programs are often frustrated by their apparent inability to measure the impact of those programs on benefit plan use. Many of those frustrations can be eliminated by the prospective design reports. For example, the effectiveness of an incentive to encourage use of generic drugs cannot be measured from most standard utilization reports. A special report that reflects the frequency of generic drug dispensing and the cost of such prescriptions is usually needed. These data may then be compared to the data relating to brand name drugs.

The effectiveness of a PPO must be assessed by the impact of that arrangement on overall plan experience. PPO and non-PPO provider performance must also be compared. When the arrangement is managed by the party administering the employer's claims, it is important to carefully review the reporting formats in advance to assure that no "spin" is applied to the resulting statistics.

Employer-designed formats, reflecting the employer's objectives in the PPO program, will probably provide a more even-handed analysis of the performance of the program.

Table 5 presents example data that demonstrate the need for an objective analysis of overall PPO impact on an employer's total health plan costs. While the PPO hospitals enjoy the majority of admissions in the PPO service area, it appears that a disproportionate share of high-cost cases are treated outside the network. In this case, further analysis by diagnostic category showed that the PPO was not successful in attracting mental health and/or substance abuse admissions because of a lack of participating hospitals and physicians specializing in such treatment. Only 5 of 45 admissions for these disorders were seen at PPO hospitals. The average charges for these

TABLE 5   PPO versus Non-PPO — Inpatient Market Share

UTILIZATION FACTOR	PPO PROVIDERS	NON-PPO PROVIDERS
Admissions in the PPO service area	65%	35%
Inpatient charges in the PPO service area	41%	59%

TABLE 6   PPO versus Non-PPO — Outpatient Market Share

UTILIZATION FACTOR	PPO PROVIDERS	NON-PPO PROVIDERS
Outpatient claims in the PPO service area	45%	55%
Outpatient charges in the PPO service area	47%	53%

admissions was over $21,000. Also, only 10 percent of admissions for circulatory disorders (average charges per admission of $17,000) were seen in the PPO hospitals, which indicates a hole in the network for cardiac surgery.

In the case of outpatient utilization (see Table 6), it appears as though the PPO network is successful in attracting the employer's eligible population when the percentage of outpatient costs is displayed. However, the analysis in Table 7 shows that this is not necessarily so. This information clearly indicates that the PPO physicians are providing significant discounts from their usual fees and charges for in-office diagnostic work. However, when the ratio of laboratory and x-ray services to office visits is computed, the pattern in Table 8 emerges. The PPO providers appear to be much freer in the use of diagnostic services than the non-PPO providers in this example. The result is that the use of a PPO physician is more expensive than the use of a non-PPO physician despite the substantial discounts involved. The average charges associated with a visit to a PPO physician would be $324.54 [$77 + (2.26 × $67) + (0.89 × $108)] as compared to the average charges associated with a visit to a non-PPO physician, measured at $245.50 [$89 + (1.18 × $89) + (0.33 × $156)]. Thus, a visit to a PPO physician is 32.2 percent more costly than a visit to a non-PPO physician. This analysis also demonstrates that figures associated with the noninpatient PPO market share are in-

TABLE 7   PPO versus Non-PPO — Outpatient Average Charge per Service

TYPE OF SERVICE	Average Charge per Service	
	PPO PROVIDERS	NON-PPO PROVIDERS
Physician visit (fee)	$ 77	$ 89
Diagnostic laboratory	67	89
Diagnostic x-ray	108	156

TABLE 8   PPO versus Non-PPO—Number of Diagnostic Services per Office Visit

	Number of Services per Office Visit	
TYPE OF SERVICE	PPO PROVIDERS	NON-PPO PROVIDERS
Diagnostic laboratory	2.26	1.18
Diagnostic x-ray	0.89	0.33

flated by the greater frequency of claims for diagnostic services attributable to PPO providers and the resulting higher charges per visit for use of those providers.

In general, the basic data needed to conduct a comprehensive review of indemnity plan utilization are captured and retained in current claims processing systems. However, retrieval of these data for the purpose of analyzing plan costs and utilization patterns may be complex when certain levels of detail are required. Many of the data elements captured in the claims payment transaction, such as assignment codes, processing date, coverage code, and administrator-specific special codes, are administrative in nature and are extraneous to the analysis of plan experience. It is imperative that standard reporting formats be reviewed in advance to determine their ability to satisfy the needs of the purchaser. Similarly, customized formats necessary for analysis of specific programs must be constructed so that the appropriate variables are defined in advance.

As a minimum data set, the administrators' standard reports should include the following information (although the specific format for reporting such information does not need to follow this outline exactly).

x-AXIS VARIABLES

Inpatient Experience

- Number of admissions
- Number of inpatient days
- Admissions per 1000 insured lives
- Days per 1000 insured lives*
- Average length of stay (days divided by admissions)*
- Total billed charges

*Indicates optional variables. They can be computed by the analyst from the required variables.

- Total eligible charges
- Total paid amount
- Average eligible charges per admission*
- Average eligible charges per day*
- Average paid amount per admission*

Noninpatient Experience

- Number of claims (or services)
- Claims per 1000 insured lives*
- Total billed charges
- Total eligible charges
- Total paid amount
- Average eligible charges per claim*
- Average paid charges per claim*

y-AXIS VARIABLES

Inpatient Experience

- Inpatient experience by employee relationship

  Employee

  Spouse

  Dependent child

  Newborns

- Inpatient experience by patient age
- Inpatient experience by general diagnostic category

  Surgical

  Maternity

  Psychiatric and chemical dependency

  Other

- Inpatient experience by specific diagnostic category

  Major diagnostic category

  DRG within MDC

  ICD-9 grouping

- Inpatient experience by hospital (may be limited to hospitals with 10 or more admissions during the reporting period)†

*Indicates optional variables. They can be computed by the analyst from the required variables.

†Provider-specific analysis should only be sought in standard reports when a concentration of employees within a specific geographic area makes such information meaningful.

- Inpatient experience by diagnostic category within hospital (may be limited to hospitals with 10 or more admissions during the reporting period)
- Inpatient experience by physician (may be limited to physicians with five or more admissions during the reporting period)
- Inpatient experience by diagnostic category by physician (may be limited to physicians with five or more admissions during the reporting period)

Other, more specialized analytic frameworks may be used in the analysis of inpatient experience. Analysis of preoperative lengths of stay and of weekend admissions may be possible using standard report formats from many claims administrators.

OUTPATIENT EXPERIENCE

- Outpatient experience by employee relationship

    Employee

    Spouse

    Dependent child

    Newborns

- Outpatient experience by patient age
- Outpatient experience by type of service (hospital outpatient, emergency room, surgical facility, surgeon charges, physician office charges, diagnostic x-ray, diagnostic laboratory, prescription drugs, physical therapy, nursing care, and any other categories offered by the claims system)
- Outpatient experience by specific diagnostic category (Major Diagnostic Category or ICD-9 grouping)
- Outpatient experience by hospital (may be limited to hospitals with $10,000 or more in billed charges during the reporting period)
- Outpatient experience by physician (may be limited to physicians with $5000 or more in billed charges during the reporting period)

There remain a number of constraints, however, on the collection and analysis of indemnity plan utilization data by employers. In most cases, the employer must rely on the claims administrator not only to collect the data accurately but also to design report formats which display the data in a meaningful way. Standard report formats developed by the administrator are the cheapest and easiest to obtain in a timely manner. In many cases, however, these standard report formats do not meet the analytic needs of the employer, and ad hoc custom reports must then be generated at considerable expense.

The lack of comparable norms also prevents a thorough examination of claims experience. Since there are many different methodologies employed in calculating and reporting utilization statistics by various administrators, it is best to define the statistics against which the norms will be compared. Then the administrator can be requested to provide normative data for those statistics from their "book of business" experience during the same period.

Finally, it is important to remember that many of the analytic questions will be answered only by combining information found in two or more reports. Thus, the use of spreadsheet software which can display calculations across many different strata of data will be an invaluable aid to the analytic process. The most obvious use for such calculations is to compare statistics from one period to the next. Generally, these data will be contained in separate reports and will have to be displayed together so that the percentage increase or decrease for each period's statistics can be calculated.

Preferred Provider Organization Claims Data

Evaluating the impact of a PPO on health plan costs requires the use of specialized reporting formats which focus on both individual provider performance and overall comparisons of PPO versus non-PPO experience. In this case, it is critical that a measure of inpatient case mix be applied to the analysis so that a realistic comparison of unit prices may be made.

Retrieval of PPO data is dependent upon the administrator of the PPO claims. If this administrator also holds a proprietary interest in the PPO, there is a risk that reporting formats are designed to cast the PPO in the best possible light. Conversely, if the administrator is not involved in the PPO management—and wishes to be—there exists the potential that the evaluation data will be presented in the worst possible light.

Thus it is important to develop a reporting methodology prospectively which will fairly and accurately portray the performance of the PPO. The following framework will allow a reasonably comprehensive analysis of the impact of the PPO on the health plan.

- *Assess the market share that the PPO providers command from period to period* Compared to the total expenditures of plan hospitals, what percentage of admissions and claim dollars is represented by each PPO hospital? The PPO physicians? Is this percentage rising or falling as time goes by? Do any participating hospitals provide little or no service to the insureds?
- *Assess the adequacy of the hospital and physician network* Which geographic areas, if any, have non-PPO providers that hold a predominant market share? If so, who are those providers? Are there specific diagnostic categories, for example, mental disorders

or maternity, in which the non-PPO providers capture the majority of admissions? Is there any pattern of erosion to non-PPO providers in either the geographic or the diagnostic categories?

- *Assess the price differential between billed charges and the negotiated reimbursement rate* Is this differential changing over the period of the contract? For example, are hospital and physician price increases passed along in the middle of a contract period, or is the discount rate applied to the original, agreed-upon charge levels? How do negotiated per diem or DRG reimbursement rates compare to billed charges for the same cases?
- *Assess the trends in utilization by service type* What effect does the PPO benefit incentive have on overall plan utilization in each type of service? For example, has the frequency of claims per 1000 employees for physician office visits increased at a more rapid rate than expected? Have overall hospital admission rates increased or decreased over time? What is the ratio of diagnostic laboratory and x-ray services to physician visits in the PPO network? In the non-PPO market?
- *Assess the effectiveness of the PPO management effort* How do total hospital charges for specific diagnostic categories, for example, normal obstetrical delivery, hysterectomy, or appendectomy, compare between individual PPO and non-PPO hospitals? Are there PPO hospitals which appear to be more costly than other network participants for specific diagnostic categories? Are there trends over time which indicate "gaming" of the reimbursement agreement by hospitals or physicians? Are utilization review programs effective?

The most cost-effective means of obtaining the data for this analysis is to use the administrator's standard utilization reporting formats for PPO claims, for non-PPO claims, and for the total claims experience. In most cases, ad hoc report formats will have to be designed to obtain the data necessary for an analysis of geographic incidence of claims activity; for the price comparisons of specific procedural categories, for example, appendectomy or hysterectomy; and for any analysis of the utilization of specific physicians.

In addition to the standard variables—number of claims or admissions, billed charges, plan payments, and the appropriate inpatient utilization measures (for example, average length of stay)—an effort should be made to identify the number of unique claimants in each report. This will allow the measurement utilization rates such as physician office visits on a per claimant basis. When such use rates are compared over time, both within and outside of the network, adjustments to copayment incentives, for example, may be indicated by abnormally high rates of in-network utilization. In the PPO context, "per claimant" measures are more revealing than "per employee" figures might be.

As with any other claim report formats, it will be necessary to combine the information from several reports in some cases and to compute statistics using several different formats. The proper use of spreadsheet techniques can avert the need for expensive, customized reports, which can often produce more paper than information.

Health Maintenance Organization Claims Data

In the 1988 Foster Higgins Health Care Benefits Survey, a disappointing 18 percent of responding employers who offer HMOs received case-specific claims experience data from their HMO vendors. In the past, community-rated HMOs had no real incentive to produce employer-specific reports. However, the relaxation of the experience-rating regulations for federally qualified HMOs is now sending many employers and HMOs scrambling for such data.

In reviewing HMO claims data, it is again imperative to define the objectives of that review. These data may be used to set contribution levels to specific HMOs, to negotiate rates or alternative funding approaches, or to evaluate the comparative cost-effectiveness of specific networks. In each case, pertinent eligibility data must be obtained to match the claims reporting periods.

HMO claims data may be used to help determine the appropriate employer contributions to specific HMOs by providing one view of the historical risk assumed by an HMO as compared to the risk assumed by the employer in the indemnity plan. Comparable indemnity plan claims data must also be used in making this determination. The claims data from both sources must reflect claims paid—rather than claims incurred—during specific periods. Other factors needed to prepare an analysis of an HMO's risk assumption include demographic data on the enrollees of the organization being studied as well as on the indemnity plan enrollees; a quantitative measure of the comparable value of HMO and indemnity plan benefits; geographic area adjustment factors; administrative costs; adjustments for "incurred but not reported" claims; and appropriate trend factors. Clearly, this methodology goes beyond the common plan utilization analysis.

HMO claims data, when used as a measure of aggregate liability, can also be examined for the purpose of negotiating premium rates or a move to experience rating by an employer. This analysis also requires the use of other factors such as trend, administrative charges, and margin to translate raw claims experience into a projected premium.

The use of case-specific claims data to evaluate the effectiveness of an HMO's cost-management efforts is an emerging trend among employers with large concentrations of HMO enrollees. The movement by employers toward consolidation of existing HMO offerings and competitive bidding for new offerings has produced a need for meaningful utilization reporting mechanisms. The ability of an HMO to produce such reports, however, is dependent on the reporting capabilities of the claims payment software in use. Also, the payment of a claim is, in the world of capitated arrangements, an accounting function rather than an actual reimbursement. So some limitations in validity must be anticipated.

With these limitations in mind, a framework for the analysis of HMO plan benefits can be proposed. Keep in mind that the objectives of this type of investigation are similar to those used to evaluate PPO arrangements, with an eye toward both provider performance and plan design.

- *Strive for consistency between the data elements and report formats of the HMO and the indemnity plan*   Clearly define the service and diagnostic categories contained in both sets of reports. For example, does the HMO's "inpatient services" line item include professional fees? Does the indemnity plan's? Similarly, does "number of claims" in the HMO report represent the number of services? The number of claimants? While it is inevitable that some categories will not match, the prospective determination of differences in definitions will go a long way toward explaining discrepencies in utilization rates.
- *Compare use rates and costs for service and diagnostic categories with indemnity plan experience*   Typically, an HMO will demonstrate low inpatient utilization and a high rate of outpatient physician utilization relative to the indemnity plan experience. So comparisons of use rates by service category must be tempered with the knowledge that normative indemnity data will not represent normative HMO utilization. It is possible, for example, to identify excessive use rates within HMO plans and to address such high rates by altering copayment schedules.
- Examination of use rates by diagnostic category can also assist the employer in evaluating HMO utilization patterns. The preponderance of maternity-related hospitalizations in an HMO's inpatient experience, for example, may indicate a selection pattern of younger insureds using HMO benefits. A comparative scarcity of admissions for mental disorders and chemical dependency in the PPO experience may indicate an inadequacy of coverage by the HMO for these conditions. This situation could cause adverse selection against the indemnity plan, where treatment for these disorders would then be provided in an unmanaged setting.
- *Track HMO utilization over time*   Identify those areas of utilization and cost which change over time, and assess the impact of those changing patterns on HMO plan design and plan management.

In order to thoroughly understand the data presented by an HMO, it is best to review the data with its representative. This allows discussion of the implications of the analysis on future relationships with that HMO and offers the opportunity of working with it, rather than merely accepting premiums and benefits offered.

DATA ACCURACY

In these days of sophisticated data processing systems, it is expected that virtually any and all utilization data are available in readily usable formats. The reality is far from this ideal. Merging data from traditional indemnity plans with that from managed care plans compounds the problem. The accuracy and relevance of the combined database are determined by the data collected, the definitions of the data elements, and the specificity of the data. Part of the difficulty stems from the differing agendas of the various healthcare delivery systems. In the typical indemnity plan, payment for fee-for-service procedures and hospital services dictated the need for appropriate and specific types of coding to facilitate payment of scheduled or reasonable and customary allowances. The data had to be in this format to both pay for the service and determine how to cost the plan for rating purposes. In the HMO arena the focus was somewhat different; capitation or discounting arrangements that decreased much of the coding needed for indemnity plan claim payments.

With changes in competitive and legislative environments brought about by alternative HMO pricing options and IRC Section 89, the situation is improving. Greater emphasis is now being placed on data capture. HMOs in particular will need to capture more detailed utilization, demographic, and financial data. Hopefully, they will not fall prey to many of the pitfalls encountered by indemnity plans in this area: inaccurate claim coding, provider up-coding, and administrative cost pressures to limit the level of specificity in coding. All these factors compromise data credibility and therefore complicate meaningful health plan analysis and strategic decision making.

Required Data

What types of data should be collected? At a minimum, group-specific inpatient and ambulatory utilization categorized by age, sex, major diagnostic categories, and "high volume" providers. The Group Health Association of America has developed a Data Collection Form which details the type of information it believes its members should be gathering. To this data, costs must be added so that the risk assumed by the HMO can be compared to that assumed by other plans of the employer. The "risk transfer" study methodology discussed at the beginning of this chapter describes an approach to this problem.

For indemnity plans, information on per insured per claim benefit payment amounts should be collected. In addition, data for inpatient and ambulatory care that include major diagnostic category information by plan, age, sex, numbers, and type of services; lengths of stay (inpatient care), provider, and provider type may be needed. Finally, the plan administrator needs to capture detailed enrollment information on eligibility, age, sex, and other employee classifications important to the plan sponsor.

Accuracy Experience

What has been the experience regarding the accuracy of HMO and indemnity plan claims experience? On the indemnity plan side, results of audits of data capture accuracy reveal that many administrators do perform exceptionally well, have all of the capabilities necessary to provide the data required, *and* are doing so. For the most part, accurate data capture is a realistic expectation. On the other hand, two situations do occur where gross inaccuracies have been found.

1. Diagnosis and procedures codes have been fudged or not researched as a result of administrator production demands. Claims processors are generally rated on the number of claims processed per hour, and since claim payment system adjudication logic is linked to broad benefit categories, high degrees of specificity in service type, provider type, and specific place of service are generally not necessary to adjudicate a claim. There is little incentive then in the claim payment process to delineate specific diagnosis, provider, place, or service codes; general codes will allow payment.

2. Charges and dates of services have been lumped together in the interest of production needs to limit administrative costs. Much of this lumping of services can be attributed to systems limitations such as screen size, number of service lines, and data storage requirements. A significant degree of inaccuracy is still encouraged by high claim processor production demands.

The percentage of each claim dollar spent for the actual benefit payment in most health plans is between 94 to 96 percent, making the accuracy of the actual claim payment amount far more critical than the typical administrative fee of 4 to 6 percent. From an employer's perspective, it seems short-sighted for claims administrators to limit coding specificity or compromise payment and coding accuracy for slight increases in productivity in an effort to lower administrative costs. Effective health plan management demands accurate claim payment and detailed data capture.

Utilization review (UR) program information data capture has also demonstrated varying degrees of success in accurately reflecting the success or failure of the program. In a recent audit of a hospital precertification program, it was discovered that an information system problem was using original lengths of stay to calculate savings estimates instead of updating them when extensions to the original length of stay were requested and granted. This lead to overstated savings estimates. Had this shortcoming not been noticed, it might well have hidden utilization patterns in need of attention.

Insufficient diagnostic data in UR programs can also interfere with early identification of potential, extensive case management problems. The data system software employed by a UR firm must therefore be programmed to require specific diagnostic and procedural information from providers. The system should also lead the intake nurses via system prompts to obtain this information. Careful evaluation of UR firm capabilities in these data areas will ensure more cost-effective utilization of plan services and availability of necessary utilization data.

HMOs have not had as great a need as indemnity carriers to collect specific information on diagnoses, place of service, procedures, and frequency of utilization because of the capitated nature of many HMOs. It is not surprising, then, that the effort to collect the data has not been as great.

In some instances, the data have been collected, but the HMO has been reluctant to divulge it to the employer citing the "insured" nature of the contractual arrangement with the employer. Changes in legislation have allowed community rating by class, and, more recently, experience rating by some HMOs. These changes make experience and utilization data critical to effective plan management and price evaluations. With these options, employers now have additional choices which will foster competition among HMOs and encourage HMOs to provide the data. The instability and bankruptcies in the HMO marketplace will also serve to pressure HMOs to provide data that plan sponsors need to assess plan performance. But with this increased competitive pressure will come the pressure to keep administrative costs low. HMOs will then be tempted to limit data capture and reporting for cost reasons. Plan sponsors will need to be vigilant in monitoring the types and specificity of data their HMOs are capturing and in ensuring that they are accurate.

Controlling Accuracy

What can be done to ensure the accuracy and reporting of the data? First, employers can explicitly indicate to their indemnity administrators and HMOs the minimal acceptable element of data for capture *and* the expected accuracy of the captured data. An effective vehicle for accomplishing this objective is the establishment of a performance agreement whereby minimal levels of payment and coding accuracy are clearly spelled out in a administration contract. Second, the specific data elements detailed above can be mandated for capture. Adherence to data capture requirements and achievement of accuracy levels can be judged through an audit of the administrator's or HMO's results. To put teeth into the agreement, the employer can build in penalties and rewards. Performance agreements have been negotiated with indemnity carriers by employers who self-fund their plans.

These agreements, while gaining in popularity, are still the exception. A 1988 survey of 1600 employers by Foster Higgins indicated that 10 percent of respondents currently have such an arrangement with their administrative services only (ASO) or minimum premium claims administrator. An additional 11 percent said they are considering negotiating guarantees by 1990. Since these agreements are still new, their effectiveness is just being tested. Administrators at risk for performance generally watch plans with such agreements more carefully.

Performance agreements with HMOs do not appear to be available at present. Given the move toward experience rating, however, the application of the concept will undoubtedly be applied in the future.

As with any management information system, the old but somewhat crass adage "Garbage in, garbage out" holds for health plan information systems. To guard against receiving unusable data reports, employers need to carefully assess the type of data being captured by their claims administrators and HMOs and establish the necessary controls to assure the accuracy of that data.

FUTURE TRENDS IN EMPLOYER HEALTH PLAN DATA ANALYSIS

Analyzing the costs, design, and utilization of employer-sponsored health plans is vastly more complex than it used to be. More comprehensive programs, improved technology, and governmental intervention have all contributed to the current situation.

At least six trends suggest that future analyses will be even more complex.

1. The next frontier for data analysis will be quality of care assessment. From the employers' perspective this issue becomes more critical as the adoption of managed care plans influences provider selection by employees. Employers will have several issues to face in this regard.
    a. Human relations issues regarding the restriction of employee choice
    b. Ethical issues regarding influencing care in life and death situations
    c. Legal concerns about liability in situations of questionable care by preferred or HMO providers
    d. Financial concerns regarding paying for substandard or ineffectual care which does not treat the illness

Sophisticated provider profiling and outcomes analysis will aid in analyzing performance in this vital area. This, in conjunction with advances in epidemiological science, will help to define appropriate patterns of care for many diseases and thus establish standards for quality of care. These standards can then be applied to contracted providers, helping employers meet the objectives of addressing quality of care with "due diligence" and limiting the financial consequences of unnecessary or substandard treatment.

2. HMO product offerings have expanded for both federally qualified and nonqualified HMOs. The range of such options is sure to increase over the next few years. Inherent in more options are different levels of benefits and hence differing "values to the employee" of the various choices. The consequence of having plans that are found to discriminate is that the full value of the benefits received will be treated as taxable employee income. An employer may choose to allow this if the financial consequences are not onerous or are desirable for other reasons. Proper valuing of these plans or assessing the desirability of a particular benefit design cannot be accomplished without credible data however. Employers will need both more data and better information from their healthcare program administrators, be they indemnity carriers or managed care program administrators.

3. With HMOs able to rate by experience, renewal actions will require greater experience reporting and analysis. Utilization of services and costs, as well as trends and projected costs, will require more detailed data capture by HMOs. Many HMOs are gearing up to provide this data; some are already able to produce "first-generation" reports. A major insurer recently provided cost experience reports for one employer that detailed costs and utilization by type and place of service and by diagnostic groupings.

4. Current provider reimbursement arrangements are subject to revision as computer technologies allow for more detailed tracking of utilization and comparisons with standard treatment protocols. Use of withholds, incentives, and risk-sharing will be combined in new ways with fee-for-service, per diem, discount, and case fee reimbursement methodologies such as DRGs. Particular attention will be focused on utilization of outpatient services, such as radiology and laboratory testing, to ensure control in this relatively unmanaged area. Competition in the provider community will drive alternative reimbursement methodologies, as will employer intervention.

5. The range of employer health plan options has been described as occurring along a continuum from the totally unmanaged fee-for-service reimbursement model indemnity plan to the totally

regulated closed-panel staff-model HMO. In between, various options combine features of the two extremes in varying degree. With each new version of managed care program has come the desire to incorporate the advantage of a particular program into the employer's overall benefit plan. In many instances the new program may have a different focus from other components of the benefit plan and actually work at "cross-purposes" with them. To guard against this, employers will seek to integrate utilization and financial data in order to see whether benefit plan objectives were achieved.

6. As services shift increasingly from the inpatient setting to the outpatient area, analytical tools similar to DRGs (Diagnostic Related Groups) are being developed to evaluate utilization in this area. A software package, *Patterns of Treatment* developed by Concurrent Review Technology, compares outpatient treatment to a set of protocols in its database. This increased focus on outpatient care UR will require greater specificity in data capture in the future. Increased service type and/or diagnosis coding will be necessary along with place of service and provider identifiers if employers are to be able to monitor utilization and costs in the ambulatory care arena.

A related issue concerning data will be who "owns" or "controls" the information. Employers and providers may have competing agendas in the area of product pricing. It is critical, therefore, that employers demand complete and credible data. This will be easier as HMOs and other managed care plan administrators can no longer hide behind the insured or capitated banner. IPA and other HMO models will need to become more sophisticated in analyzing utilization patterns because this information is a prerequisite for financial forecasting. They will need to analyze how their subscribers are using services and how contract providers are practicing medicine.

Employers, as the purchasers of healthcare services, must be mindful not to lose access to utilization or enrollment information. If they do, they risk becoming overly dependent on the provider of services for decisions on pricing and benefit design. It is also much harder to change vendors when the latter have all the enrollment, pricing, and utilization data. Employers should applaud the growing sophistication of managed care providers in analyzing data but not lose sight of the fact that they must have the data themselves to make the best possible benefit plan decisions.

American Express: A Corporate Strategy for Managed Care

BARBARA D. LEVINE, Assistant Vice President
Health Strategies Group, *The Alexander &*
Alexander Consulting Group, Westport,
Connecticut

Employer selection of appropriate managed care networks has evolved from purely a numbers game to an evaluation of the quality of service provided by the vendor. It is no longer feasible or desirable to choose a network based on price alone. Concerns over liability as well as employee healthcare needs have led many employers to evaluate process and outcomes as well as price. The following case study describes the experience of one major financial services company in the evaluation of its relationships with its providers.

BACKGROUND

American Express Travel Related Services, a division of the American Express Company (AMEX), had established relationships with a vast number of managed care networks across the country. Of their 19,000 employees, 42 percent were enrolled in some form of managed care system, consisting mainly of HMOs. The quality and pricing of each vendor's services varied greatly from location to location. Adverse selection was suspected because of the disproportionate number of younger, healthier individuals enrolled in the HMOs. With new vendors continually entering the marketplace, AMEX needed a way to determine which and how many vendors to offer.

In 1987, AMEX requested the Alexander & Alexander Consulting Group (A&ACG) to undertake an analysis of its HMO and PPO providers. The goal of the analysis was to determine which providers were delivering the most effective care to AMEX employees, as well as to establish the appropriate pricing levels for the delivery of these services. Ineffective providers would be eliminated, and resources would be channeled to more suitable providers.

APPROACH AND SCOPE

A&ACG determined that a strategy was needed which would maximize AMEX's financial contributions while ensuring that employees received necessary care. A four-pronged approach was developed which would accomplish the following:

1. Quantify the financial impact of current HMO enrollment.

2. Survey employees to determine the level of satisfaction with particular vendors.

3. Assess the process, procedures, and quality assurance activities utilized by the providers through a detailed, written evaluation instrument. The written questionnaire would be followed by local on-site visits.

4. Negotiate new contribution levels with vendors selected for quality and appropriateness of service.

The end result of these activities would be a rationalization of both the numbers and pricing of the vendors used, as well as the development of an integrated HMO and PPO strategy.

RESULTS

Because of AMEX's size and multiple locations, the introduction of a single managed care system was initially considered. National networks presented a possible means of achieving this goal. After further evaluation, however, this approach was rejected in favor of a more finely tuned local strategy.

Local healthcare options were constantly changing and expanding. AMEX needed to be in a position to react quickly to a rapidly changing healthcare marketplace. Committing to a single system or vendor locked AMEX and its employees into a relationship that might prove unsatisfactory in the future. Employee relations might also suffer should AMEX need to change vendors. In addition, national vendors did not always offer the best alternative at the local level.

The healthcare strategy that was developed for AMEX included a 3-year, phased-in plan which focused on introducing competition to the marketplace; eliminating unqualified providers; and implementing a structured, yet flexible, healthcare program. Vendors would be selected based on the quality of their service and their willingness to conform to AMEX specifications in terms of plan design, pricing, and accountability. The introduction of new PPO vendors would provide an additional opportunity to expand healthcare options for employees and force HMOs to become more competitive. The end result would be increased employee choice, a coordinated pricing strategy, and the use of the best providers in the local area.

The highlights of the activities conducted during the 3-year period are outlined below.

Year 1

The goal of the first year was to set the groundwork for future changes. The objective was to reduce the number of vendors based on an assessment of their quality and utilization indicators. A written questionnaire was developed and distributed to HMOs and PPOs in AMEX's largest locations. Vendors were evaluated in the following categories:

- Experience and reputation
- Ability to provide utilization data
- Accessibility (number of providers and geographic distribution)
- Quality assurance activities
- Administrative capabilities
- Pricing

Pricing was not AMEX's main concern. Their primary goal was to establish a quality-based long-term relationship with its vendors. With this approach, it was recognized that little financial impact would be felt in the first year as the ground rules were being established and competition was being introduced. Vendors were put on notice that the collection of utilization data specific to AMEX would be required to establish experience rating in the future. Although greater savings could have been achieved in the first year with a short-term philosophy, it was in AMEX's best long-term interests and in the interest of its employees to establish more lasting relationships with its vendors.

Prior to meeting with vendors during this first year, an employee survey was disseminated to approximately 10,000 HMO and PPO enrollees and subscribers to the company-sponsored medical plan. The survey elicited information about the employee's experience with their present plan or vendor, employee satisfaction with the quality and delivery of care received, and employee plans concerning a switch to some other plan at the next open enrollment.

Of the HMO enrollees surveyed, 40 percent completed and returned the questionnaire. The vast ma-

jority of respondents had used the services of their HMO within the past year and did so on a frequent basis; 78 percent of these respondents utilized the HMO more than 4 times a year, and of that number, 36 percent sought HMO services once a month or more. Of particular significance, 36.8 percent of HMO respondents did not feel they were able to complain about poor HMO service. They indicated they did not know how to register a complaint. Many of the written responses also indicated a resignation to the "system," that their complaints would either be ignored or not addressed by the HMO. Of the 480 respondents who had registered a complaint with their HMO, only 40 percent of these complaints were resolved to the respondent's satisfaction.

The results of this survey played an integral part in the negotiating strategy used with each vendor. Vendors eliciting numerous complaints from employees were confronted with this information during the on-site visits and either were given a "cure" period or were eliminated completely.

An interesting finding of the survey was that employee selection of HMOs was heavily influenced by the lack of claims forms, reduced out-of-pocket expenses, and the availability of prescription drug programs. Preventive care and well-baby care were less significant factors in an employee's decision to enroll in a managed care network.

The result at the end of year 1 was that those vendors with immediate and serious quality problems were eliminated based on:

- A lack of access, for example, emergency rooms were open on a rotating basis in inaccessible locations
- A lack of coverage for insulin or AZT although the HMO accepted diabetics and AIDS patients
- The level of substantive complaints from employees regarding physician treatment
- The practice of balance billing of employees

Vendors with uncertain quality were provided with guidelines for modifications and improvements. Some of these guidelines included:

- The development of workable patient grievance procedures or the existence of an ombudsman.
- The development of better communications to employees regarding the HMO's capabilities. Several HMOs did not communicate their abilities in

specialty areas such as neonatology and nephrology.

- The addition of a "hold harmless" clause to protect employees in the event of fiscal insolvency by an HMO.

Immediate cost savings of $1 million were realized as a result of year 1's efforts. These savings were due primarily to redirecting employees away from inappropriately priced vendors by introducing and encouraging enrollment in preferred provider networks, moving away from strict community rating, and changing the way HMOs were presented to employees. Employees were advised to select HMOs based on their healthcare needs rather than on the lack of copayments and deductibles. This new focus also resulted in a decrease in HMO enrollment by new employees.

Year 2

The greatest impact on AMEX's bottom line occurred during the second year of the study. Vendors realized they would be held accountable for quality, pricing, and accessibility. In one instance, a PPO vendor with questionable quality in year 1, with whom AMEX would not contract, returned in year 2 with a greatly improved product. The number of hospital days was reduced through better utilization management, access was improved through an increase in the number and locations of network providers, and quality assurance activities were enhanced whereby providers were monitored for both over- and underutilization. Based on these enhancements, AMEX was able to introduce this vendor to its employees, expand the number of choices available in that market, and force existing vendors to become more competitive in terms of quality and price.

Negotiations were undertaken with vendors based on the collection of AMEX-specific data. By establishing itself as a proactive employer purchasing health care for the long term, AMEX had created an atmosphere conducive to vendor negotiations. Vendors were more inclined to be flexible on price than in year 1. Indeed, year 1's activities set the stage for reaping even greater savings in year 2. In addition, PPO enrollment substantially increased, aided by a plan design change which persuaded employees to use the PPO.

During the second year of the project, vendors were willing to accommodate AMEX's needs since it was understood that AMEX was most concerned with getting a quality service at a fair price. By the end of year 2, a total of $4 million in savings had been achieved.

Year 3 and Beyond

The third year of the project presented further opportunity to fine tune AMEX's healthcare strategies in each of its key geographic locations. AMEX's new managed care approach had not been implemented companywide in the first year of the project, but had been progressively rolled out over the 3-year time frame. Additional vendors were eliminated because of financial problems, which resulted, in some cases, in bankruptcy. During this third year, service was expanded to some of AMEX's smaller locations. Although not every location was included in the managed care network, sites with as few as 15 to 20 employees had access to appropriate managed care providers.

Guidelines were established for the annual reevaluation of AMEX's options. Data would reveal the continued impact of AMEX's programs on its bottom line, allowing the appropriate pricing or program adjustments to be made. Vendors would be reevaluated each year for their quality assurance activities. With an ever changing healthcare marketplace, AMEX would be in a position to reevaluate its options on an annual basis.

LESSONS LEARNED

The flexibility built into AMEX's decision not to contract with a sole vendor gave it the latitude to continually modify and refine its programs on the local level without affecting the delivery of care in all of the locations. As a result of this managed care strategy, HMO and PPO vendors were consolidated along geographic lines and ineffective providers were eliminated. New providers entering the marketplace were subjected to an established protocol that evaluated quality and scope of service. Vendors were forced to compete for AMEX's business based not only on cost but also on quality. The result was that the employee's choice of healthcare provider was based more on quality and convenience than on price. Employee satisfaction coupled with fair and competitive pricing proved to be the optimal means of achieving AMEX's desire for long-lasting relationships with its providers.

Ryder System: Helping Employees Find Medical Care

W. BRYAN LATHAM, M.D., President

MedFacts, Inc., Miami, Florida

JOSEPH G. CHARLES, Group Director, Employee Benefits

Ryder System, Inc., Miami, Florida

Ryder System instituted the MedFacts program in 1986 in order to give employees and dependents "on the spot, up to date" information about local doctors and hospitals.

Ryder offers the program for two reasons. First, it provides a benefit to employees. The information system enables employees and family members to find good physicians and hospitals at the most reasonable price. After an initial flood of inquiries, requests for provider information have leveled off to several per week (employee population is about 2500). About 20 to 30 percent of those who get medical care every month are using the system.

Second, Ryder hopes to help control medical expenses by offering MedFacts to its employees. By using MedFacts, employees reduce out-of-pocket expenses and save about $120 per call. If the call involves a surgical case, the average savings rises to $500 per call.

GATHERING DATA

In order to develop the database for the program, a survey was mailed to 4000 Florida Medical Association members in the south Florida area. The physicians were asked questions about their education and training, board certification status, languages spoken, HMO and PPO affiliations, and fees charged for the most common procedures performed. About 1700 questionnaires were returned and included a valid distribution of physicians representing all specialties. These physicians were then screened to remove any who had been disciplined by the state medical board.

Information on hospital charges was obtained from the state Health Care Cost Containment Board and was included in the database. These data allowed employees to compare local hospitals charges by diagnosis. A computer software program was developed to accommodate and manipulate the information.

SOME RYDER CONCERNS

Liability

Ryder had some initial concerns about employer liability resulting from the service. Ryder attorneys concluded that there was little if any liability because the service does not choose doctors and hospitals, it simply provides information. The user or consumer makes the choices. There have been no instances of users holding the service responsible for such choices.

Information Limitations

Not all practicing physicians in the area contributed to the database. When an employee requests a physician not in the system, the physician is invited to send in information. While the amount of information contained on physicians is extensive, using the system cannot guarantee that the best choice will be made. Choosing medical care is personal, and there are subjective elements used by consumers that cannot be built into a database.

Costs

The service costs about $50,000 to develop. A large portion was software development expense; the remainder included costs for surveys, mailings, and data entry. The yearly maintenance cost is $10,000, including mailing reports and updating information.

Quality of Care

Some physicians have criticized the program for including fees which, in their view, encourages employees to choose the lowest priced doctors and thereby sacrifice quality for cost. An analysis of cost versus qualifications showed the reverse is true; namely, the best-qualified doctors charged less than their less-qualified colleagues (Table 1).

CASE HISTORY

The spouse of an employee needed gall bladder surgery. Her family doctor had already sent her to a

TABLE 1   Fee Comparison for Board Certified versus Nonboard Certified Physician

CPT	PROCEDURE	BOARD FEE	AVERAGE PHYSICIAN	HIGHER CHARGE NON-BOARD CERTIFIED
59400	Total obstetrical care	Yes	$2093	
		No	2140	$ 47.00
59500	Caesarean section	Yes	2652	
		No	2916	264.00
58150	Hysterectomy	Yes	2619	
		No	2685	66.00
47600	Cholecystectomy	Yes	1824	
		No	2162	338.00
49505	Inguinal hernia repair	Yes	1047	
		No	1246	199.00

surgeon who had scheduled surgery at a local hospital. She heard about MedFacts and called for information. After some discussion, a hospital report was sent (Table 2). It turned out that she was scheduled to go to a more expensive hospital (AMI Palmetto General) for gall bladder removal (cholecystectomy). When she learned that the average cost for this procedure at Palmetto was over twice as much as Doctors Hospital, she decided to change hospitals. By changing, she had the opportunity of saving in excess of $800 (her copay was 20 percent of the hospital bill). As a result of the patient choosing a less expensive hospital, the employer saved $3200.

Since her surgeon had no privileges at Doctors Hospital, a change of physicians was required. A physician report (Table 3) was sent, which contained a list of surgeons who worked at Doctors Hospital and their fees. She chose a doctor who was board certified and who charged $2000 for the procedure (Table 4). The original surgeon recommended by her family doctor was not board certified and charged $2500 for the operation. The maximum amount allowed (UCR) for this procedure by her employer was $2200. By using MedFacts, she identified a doctor with better qualifications as well as one who charged less. She saved $300 (the amount in excess of allowable). The employer saved $160 (80 percent of the additional $200 it would have given to the first surgeon).

TABLE 2   MedFacts Hospital Cost Comparison Report

HOSPITAL	NUMBER OF CASES (6 months)	AVERAGE LENGTH OF STAY (days)	AVERAGE CHARGE
DRG: 198 Description: Total Cholecystectomy			
South Miami Hospital	28	5.07	$4718.46
Baptist Hospital of Miami	43	5.14	4635.53
Doctors Hospital of Coral Gables	20	5.42	3510.17
Coral Reef Hospital	10	5.40	6239.60
AMI Palmetto General Hospital	10	5.30	7524.50
Hialeah Hospital	34	5.12	6399.12

TABLE 3   MedFacts Physician Report

Procedure: Cholecystectomy
Area: South Dade County
Specialty: General Surgery
Usual, Customary, & Reasonable (UCR) Fee Allowance: $2200.00

Doctor A	1152 N W 12th	Miami	$1650.00
Doctor B	7826 N Kendall Dr.	Miami	1700.00
Doctor C	6690 S W 90th St.	South Miami	1800.00
Doctor D	2120 N Kendall Dr.	Miami	2000.00
Doctor E	6200 Sunset Dr.	Coral Gables	2000.00
Doctor F	2500 S W 60th Ct.	South Miami	2250.00
Doctor G	4820 N Kendall Dr.	Miami	2400.00
Doctor H	3250 S W 88 St.	Miami	2500.00

TABLE 4   MedFacts Individual Physician Profile

Physician:
John Doe, M.D. (Doctor E)
6200 Sunset Drive
Coral Gables, Fl. 33143   Telephone: 981-4322

Education & Training
Medical School: University of North Carolina. Year Graduated 1963
Residency: Mayo Clinic, Rochester, Minn. Year Completed 1968
Specialty: General Surgery Year Board Certified 1970

Practice Information
Does not make house calls
Does not charge for telephone advice or prescriptions
Will provide a second opinion
Languages spoken in office: English, Spanish

Hospitals
Baptist, South Miami, Doctors-Coral Gables, Mercy

HMO/PPO Affiliations
Blue Cross HMO, Blue Cross PPO

Fee Information
Will discuss fees with employer or employee
Accepts Medicare assignment

CPT	DESCRIPTION	FEE
19120	Excision of breast lesion, benign	$ 500.00
44950	Appendectomy	1400.00
46255	Hemorhoidectomy, internal and external, simple	750.00
47600	Cholecystectomy	2000.00
49505	Repair inguinal hernia	1200.00
90020	Office visit, New patient, comprehensive service	100.00
90620	Hospital consultation, comprehensive	150.00

PART FOUR

NEXT-GENERATION MANAGED CARE

CHAPTER TWENTY-TWO

Third-Generation Managed Care

THIRD-GENERATION DELIVERY SYSTEM FEATURES

PETER BOLAND, Ph.D., President
Boland Healthcare Consultants, Berkeley, California

The appeal of first-generation alternative delivery systems was characterized by premium predictability (HMOs) and freedom of choice with discounts (PPOs). Standards for care were formed through professional consensus and emphasized "average" norms. Reliable program data were scarce and neither purchasers nor providers had an accurate picture of costs, quality, or performance.

As a result, health plans which emphasized wide consumer choice of physicians and hospitals often ended up guaranteeing access to "average" care. This was similiar to traditional fee-for-service indemnity plans, for two reasons: first, most providers in such plans were poorly screened, utilization management controls were weak, and quality assurance procedures were embryonic at best.[1] And second, freedom of choice does not help consumers unless they are also given meaningful information for making an informed choice.

Information management was the weakest link in delivery system performance. HMOs were unable to report full experience data and PPOs did not generate reliable cost-savings information.[2]

The current generation of managed care delivery systems is largely shaped by employer demands for more cost control and provider efforts to maintain control over reimbursement. This is leading second-generation HMOs and PPOs to incorporate managed care features like utilization management rather than just utilization review, alternative treatment settings when appropriate, and multiple benefit design and reimbursement options.[3] Essentially, more choice is being offered to purchasers in terms of available products and how to pay for them.

Utilization management is expanding to cover outpatient care, ambulatory office visits, and numerous ancillary tests and procedures. Reimbursement penalties are being attached for providers who misuse resources, while financial penalties are applied for enrollees who disregard proper utilization guidelines.

Reporting formats originally developed for accounting and claims administration functions no longer suffice for managed care application. There is a growing emphasis on new data collection and information processing techniques as a basis for third-generation capability.[4]

Third-generation HMOs and PPOs will be distinguished principally by their capability to provide cost-effective care and document it to customers. Internal program resources will enable such plans to identify optimal treatment patterns and appropriate treatment resources. Optimizing models and cost-benefit approaches to individual case management will become a standard, as will rigorous utilization review of all major functions and procedures. Provider-profiling techniques will be sufficiently developed for plans to identify and then exclude both overutilizers and underutilizers of care. Third-generation capability will indicate that a delivery system is managing care, not just cost.

The largest breakthroughs will likely be seen in two areas: first, in the application of medical software for quality assurance functions and monitoring performance standards based on industrywide benchmarks, and second, in information technology for internal and external report generation. The increased emphasis on treatment outcomes will underscore the necessity of carefully selecting providers and building in financial incentives that link performance and payment.

HMOs and PPOs will shift their current emphasis on competing with indemnity insurance plans to battling each other for managed care business. The market will no longer demand rapid expansion. Delivery systems will have to fight for selective demand and market share niches in order to grow in the mid-1990s.

Technology — especially information technology — will be used by HMOs and PPOs to differentiate their products and gain a competitive edge as third-generation delivery systems. Information (like quality) will increasingly be recognized as a strategic asset in managed care.

Some of the most important characteristics of third-generation delivery systems are outlined in relation to essential managed care "building blocks" in Table 1. The combined impact of these delivery system dynamics is that a portfolio of integrated managed care prod-

TABLE 1   Third-Generation Delivery System Characteristics

BUILDING BLOCKS	RESOURCES
Management	Track record of financial performance and operational capability Evidence of timely corporate decisions about capital investment, research and development, human resources, and new technology in response to a rapidly changing environment
Capital	Adequate working capital for operations, sufficient resources to meet regulatory requirements, and access to additional capital for investment in new technology and human resources
Services	Complete primary, specialty, and tertiary care services, settings, and personnel Range of allied health services, practitioners, and alternative treatment settings Integration of mental health services and work site employee assistance programs Health education, illness prevention, and health promotion programs Comparative data analysis on cost, utilization, effectiveness, and efficiency factors for providers and patients Benefits consulting on the potential impact of plan design changes and different premium levels
Network selection	Provider profiles on cost, cost-effectiveness, and appropriate use of medical resources as a basis for selection and recredentialing functions Board certified status for physicians Full professional accreditation status for facilities and delivery systems
Benefit design incentives	Integrated multiple-option plans which balance risk among different parties Premium flexibility which reflects plan design value Different degrees in freedom-of-choice and cost-sharing options related to premium level Significant benefit differential between in-network and out-of-network use of providers, and between indemnity and HMO or PPO options Incentives related to management of lifestyle risk factors
Communications	Full array of employer, employee, and dependent information on appropriate health plan use, covered services, and noncompliance penalties Educational material on lifestyle behavior management Regular interaction with participating providers (and support staff) about health plan provisions, changes, and recent clinical advances in medical management
Utilization management	Complete inpatient, outpatient, and ambulatory care review (including allied health services) for primary, tertiary, and specialty treatment Full medical case management Screening for severity of illness, intensity of treatment, medical necessity, and appropriateness Bill and fee review (including fraud and abuse investigation) Capacity to unbundle basic and supplemental services
Quality	Scientifically based appropriateness standards and medical necessity criteria, including frequency and duration Treatment applications based on risk-benefit and cost-benefit models

(continued)

TABLE 1   Third-Generation Delivery System Characteristics *(Continued)*

BUILDING BLOCKS	RESOURCES
	Outcomes management protocols to determine effect of medical resources on clinical condition and functional status
	Quality improvement processes incorporated into delivery system work functions
	Patient satisfaction information used as a management tool
	Integration of customer-defined and provider-based quality indicators
Reimbursement mechanisms	Full range of pricing methods (for providers, payers, and purchasers) based on actuarial analysis which reflects current program operations, including ability to guarantee savings levels
	Risk-sharing and gain-sharing formulas reflecting degrees of partnership for each party
	Incentive-based reimbursement models linking compensation to performance which include clinical, cost, efficiency, and quality factors
Reporting	Understandable client reports with focused summary data on a quarterly basis
	Internal management reports integrating utilization, cost, and quality data
	Claims data fully integrated with utilization review information
	Cost-savings analysis related to specific intervention factors and separate utilization management functions
	Documented cost savings per individual covered life and per capita based on accurate population denominator data, adjusted for case mix and intensity of service factors
	Routine capture of key clinical indicators
	Quality-based reports with indicators on treatment outcomes, summary provider profiles, medical risk management procedures, and patient satisfaction
	Descriptive data on degree of conformance to contract specifications and performance standards
Information systems	Routine integration of inpatient and ambulatory data with performance indicators on quality, efficiency, and cost
	Ad hoc inquiry into relationships between financial, clinical, and utilization data
	On-line modeling of alternative treatment plans
	Multiple software modules run simultaneously to access data from different delivery system functions
Claims administration	Point-of-service benefit options which administer different fees, copayments, and deductibles
	Flexibility of offering multiple benefit and premium variations for an enrolled group
	Eligibility verification on-line from provider offices
	Integrated utilization review and claims management systems
	Automated bill editing
	Increased electronic claims submission, processing, and payment
	Electronic funds transfer

ucts will likely be available within the next few years to healthcare customers seeking one-stop shopping.

The extent to which delivery systems incorporate these features will determine how well care is managed. It will likewise indicate their capacity to assure quality and generate real savings which can be documented.

REFERENCES

1. Peter Boland (ed.), *The New Healthcare Market: A Guide to PPOs for Purchasers, Payors and Providers.* Dow Jones–Irwin Publishing Company, Homewood, Ill., 1985.

2. Peter Boland, "The Illusion of Discounts in the Healthcare Market," *Health Affairs* pp. 93–97 (Summer 1985).

3. Peter Boland, "The Evolving Market for Preferred Provider Contracting," *The Journal of Ambulatory Care Management* pp. 1–7 (May 1987).

4. Peter Boland, "Trends in Second-Generation PPOs," *Health Affairs* pp. 75–81 (Winter 1987).

PART FIVE

FUTURE TRENDS, GOVERNMENT INITIATIVES, AND RESEARCH DIRECTIONS

CHAPTER TWENTY-THREE

Industry Trends

MANAGED CARE PRIORITIES AND INDUSTRY CONSENSUS

PETER BOLAND, Ph.D., President
Boland Healthcare Consultants, Berkeley, California

The lines which once separated indemnity plans, HMOs, and PPOs in the past are now blurred and will become even more so in the early 1990s. The following trends contribute to this phenomena:

- Insurers are developing HMO look-alike products such as EPOs, as well as HMO high-option and low-option plans.
- HMOs are developing indemnity opt-out products to compete with insurers.
- PPOs are developing EPOs to compete with HMOs.
- HMOs are also developing "point-of-service" or "point-of-purchase" products (that is, open-ended HMOs) to compete with PPOs.
- HMOs and PPOs are being offered as local in-network providers while out-of-network benefits are administered by insurers or TPAs.

Thus, it is difficult to tell just how managed a *managed* care delivery system is according to traditional labels like HMO or PPO. Differentiation among competing health plans will require assessing the extent of internal controls such as physician selection criteria, utilization management procedures, quality assurance protocols, and management information systems.

This task is becoming one of the most perplexing challenges facing healthcare purchasers as they decide:

- What to buy
- Who to buy it from
- What is actually being sold under the umbrella term "managed care"

It is too late in the managed care "life cycle" for insurers and provider-based health plans to oversell their products. Purchasers are far more knowledgeable now about the strengths and weaknesses of managed care products and expect more accountability from providers and vendors as a result. As the last few years have clearly demonstrated, cost savings have not materialized as projected. This resulted in a loss of credibility for many HMOs and PPOs and generated tremendous confusion and frustration among employers. A number of insurers left the group health business altogether.

It is up to providers and health plan sponsors to clearly present their products in ways that purchasers understand, that is, in terms of program elements which can be compared across-the-board for different vendors. In other words, if employers and trust funds are faced with marketing jargon which disguises differences among competing product lines, they will make poor choices (which will eventually come back to haunt both sides) or will turn their back on available HMO and PPO options and approach selected providers directly for managed care services.

HMOs, PPOs, and the multitude of delivery system hybrids coming off the drawing boards will also need to "keep close to the customer" in order to succeed — and this means increased product accountability during the coming years.

Evolving market forces — and the looming specter of increased federal and state intervention — are moving healthcare buyers and sellers closer together. Trade-offs must be made and adversarial relationships must mature into strategic business alliances for managed care to succeed in the 1990s.

While a consensus will never be achieved among all the competing priorities in managed care, there is a growing recognition in the industry that agreement must be reached on many of the following issues.

PROVIDERS
1. Price services in relation to actual costs rather than conforming to prevailing market rates.
2. Aggressively monitor and discipline peers where practice patterns are marginal or unacceptable on cost, utilization, and/or quality grounds.
3. Design balanced risk-sharing and gain-sharing reimbursement formulas which are equitable for all parties.

4. Use resources more appropriately and be held accountable in terms of performance standards which are linked to reimbursement levels.

5. Define quality in operational terms and be judged according to how well it is delivered.

6. Form closer hospital-physician relationships for strategic business purposes.

7. Develop and share more meaningful data with purchasers and payers.

PAYERS — INSURERS AND THIRD PARTY ADMINISTRATORS

1. Pass more managed care savings back to purchasers to maintain credibility.

2. Affiliate with health plans that rigorously screen physicians and hospitals as a condition of initial and ongoing network participation.

3. Develop more effective techniques to appropriately manage psychiatric and chemical dependency cases, as well as other allied health services such as prescription drugs, home healthcare, and long-term care.

4. Upgrade management information systems to produce more useful data and focused reports to improve purchaser decision making.

5. Forcefully advocate to purchasers the adoption of financial incentives and disincentives, such as benefit design differentials, which channel enrollees to selected providers.

6. Integrate different administrative aspects of medical insurance and workers compensation (and disability management) in order to apply managed care techniques to both lines of business simultaneously and to overlapping cases.

7. Develop private sector mechanisms for providing necessary medical care to uninsured and underinsured groups.

PURCHASERS **Enrollees**

1. Share more of the financial burden (for example, copayments, deductibles, and coinsurance) for the cost of medical care.

2. Accept greater "controlled access" to providers as a managed care prerequisite.

3. Assume greater responsibility for treatment compliance.

4. Participate in early screening programs for specific diseases and modify (and preferably avoid) lifestyle behaviors associated with high-risk factors (for example, smoking, eating disorders, and substance abuse).

5. Learn to become more knowledgeable consumers of medical care through health education and health promotion programs and improved doctor-patient communication.

Employers and Trust Funds

1. Accept more financial responsibility for (and better management of) employee healthcare costs that are not under the control of the providers.

2. Develop contract specifications for all healthcare vendors and hold them accountable to agreed-upon performance standards.

3. Reduce the number of healthcare plans available to employees and restrict their freedom of choice of providers.

4. Enter into combined risk-sharing and gain-sharing arrangements with selected providers through multiyear partnerships.

5. Commit additional resources to employee (and dependent) communication to increase awareness about the need for managed care and how to use healthcare services more appropriately.

6. Become more involved in day-to-day managed care activities regarding resource allocation, operational guidelines, and utilization management cases.

Managed care is redefining the parameters for doing business among consumers, employers, insurers, providers, and other healthcare vendors. Purchasers and payers will need to meet providers halfway in structuring new types of business relationships which balance risk sharing and gain sharing within a partnership approach to delivering healthcare. What was tried in the past was not very successful when judged by current levels of cost savings (low) and continuing price escalation (high).

As a result, managed care is in a race with the public's growing frustration over current healthcare programs. The industry is running out of time to prove that providers, payers, and purchasers can voluntarily implement effective, workable strategies before regulatory controls are imposed.

The extent to which major players in managed care resolve these issues and demonstrate genuine results by the mid-1990s will largely determine how satisfied American workers and their families are with the cost, quality, and availability of medical care.

If managed care organizations do not make sufficient progress in addressing the healthcare needs of employers and other healthcare payers, then some form of national health insurance may appeal to a majority of the population in the 1990s.

The Time Has Come for Sacrifice

ANGELO M. MASCIANTONIO, Principal

Vantage Health Partners, Inc., Philadelphia, Pennsylvania

Despite the explosion of "solutions" available in the marketplace, the healthcare cost management problem will not get better until fundamental attitudes, expectations, and special interests change. Providers, payers, employers, and consumers each want to minimize the financial risk associated with the costs of health benefits and services. The result is that the financing of healthcare has become a political hot potato. Therefore, part of the solution lies in making tough political and economic decisions.

THE TRADE-OFFS

The problem brings a fundamental complexity of significant magnitude: How is the goal of entitlement to quality health services addressed without contributing to the erosion of the national economy? Balancing major conflicting objectives is no small feat in a growth-addicted $600 billion healthcare economy. Successful healthcare cost management requires three fundamental changes: understanding the major trade-offs to be made, creating new expectations, and accepting a compromise.

The most important trade-offs for each managed care player include:

1. *Providers* must accept more stringent quality and utilization monitoring, accept competitively priced services and/or more unit price controls, expect modest to minimal income gains, and sacrifice professional independence as they know it today.

2. *Consumers* must accept that freedom to choose physicians and hospitals in oversupplied markets must be restricted to assure access to quality health services at an affordable price. Wealthy consumers need to pay more out-of-pocket for healthcare services in order to help subsidize the cost of maintaining a comprehensive healthcare system for all.

3. *Insurance companies, TPAs, and other third party payer organizations* must share responsibility for promoting cost management if they expect to play a future role in managed care. These organizations are increasingly competing on the basis of cost management as well as administrative capabilities. In order to survive, these healthcare intermediaries must play a lead role in encouraging efficient use of services and in contracting with select providers. They must also provide carefully designed benefits products and meaningful health information which facilitate cost management and not just pay claims.

4. *Employers* must realize that keeping healthcare costs in line with other production costs will require much more restrictive health benefits in terms of both access and scope of services. Employers are unable to tolerate the voodoo cost-containment programs of the past. They must be committed to perform more sophisticated analyses of different benefit options, to conduct tough negotiations with healthcare providers and intermediaries, and to be prepared to contract directly with providers if need be. Most important, employers must make their internal benefits management accountable for results. In addition, employers should use their political clout to support state and national initiatives that complement a broader health cost management strategy.

WELL-COORDINATED, COMPREHENSIVE APPROACH

To restrain the forces which drive healthcare costs, most notably healthcare *inflation* and increasing *volume* of services, a well-defined and coordinated set of actions is needed in four areas (Figure 1):

1. More effective payment controls are needed. When and how medically necessary services are paid varies significantly from plan to plan, payer to payer, and program to program, creating an administrative and accounting nightmare. More consistent reasoning for the determination of benefits coverage must be applied and the most advanced technology in the processing, analysis, and adjudication of healthcare information and claims must be employed.

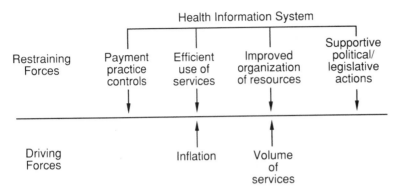

Figure 1 *Healthcare cost dynamics.*

2. Continued efforts to implement more efficient use of expensive health services will reduce unnecessary and inappropriate use of services without jeopardizing quality.

3. New efforts to improve the organization of health resources on a regional basis will better assure that access, supply, demand, quality, and price are reasonably balanced at point of service.

4. A supportive political and legislative environment is a prerequisite for better payment controls and approaches to make efficient use of services. There are too many conflicting and confusing laws and regulations regarding health and benefits policies. This lack of consistency makes it difficult and expensive for multistate companies to impose effective health cost management programs.

Finally, to apply these four restraining forces effectively, a comprehensive and user-oriented health information system is necessary. The dearth of focused healthcare information and relevant analyses remains the nemesis of the American healthcare system.

FACE THE FACTS

There has been a tidal wave of privately initiated managed care ventures, plus several state and federal government sponsored programs such as Medicare's Prospective Payment System. The tendency has been to conceptualize and engineer answers to individual healthcare cost management problems, thereby creating incremental and piecemeal solutions. Unfortunately, this piecemeal approach does not add up to the kind of stability that the healthcare economy so desperately needs.

One of the most important lessons of the last decade is that gaining the necessary consensus among the major healthcare industry players to implement a comprehensive strategy to contain healthcare costs is like trying to brush the teeth of a hungry pitbull terrier. No one private organization or governmental authority seems to possess the insight, courage, resources, clout, and patience to make anything meaningful happen.

The overall failure of this fragmented approach is stunning. More than 38 million Americans lack adequate healthcare coverage. Healthcare costs now exceed 11.5 percent of the United States gross national product versus 9.5 percent in 1980, while major economic competitors, including Japan, West Germany, France, and Canada, currently devote only 7 to 9 percent of their GNP to healthcare.

In addition, as corporations are just beginning to fund retiree health benefits, even greater liabilities for healthcare are accruing. This is not good news since healthcare costs already represent approximately 50 percent of corporate pretax profits. If the healthcare benefits line item of most corporations continues to grow at a multiple of other production line item costs, severe benefits restrictions and/or the deterioration of corporate earnings and viability will result. This is a major problem of national importance given the increasing need to be internationally competitive. The time has come for sacrifice.

Healthcare 2000: Role of Managed Care

RUSSELL C. COILE, Jr., President

Health Forecasting Group, Alameda, California

Managed care will be the dominant scenario for healthcare in the future. In this forecast of the U.S. health system in the year 2000, 90 percent of the American population is covered by managed care plans with extensive cost and utilization controls and with reduced premiums or expanded coverage which would reward enrollees with healthy lifestyles.

The transition to managed care will take 10 years, but it is already beginning in states like California, where nearly 70 percent of the non-Medicare population is already enrolled in a managed care plan. The shift to managed care will be a "quiet revolution." Change will take place gradually, as all parties — government, major employers, insurance, hospitals, physicians, and all health providers — accommodate to the new realities. By the year 2000, managed care will be in full control.

What role would managed care play in such a future? Here is a forecast: Managed care will be the financing mechanism, system controller, and delivery system manager in the healthcare system of the future. More specifically, in a managed care scenario, key components of the U.S. health system would be modified in some important dimensions. Here is a projection of changes ahead.

QUALIFIED HEALTH PLANS

Medicare, Medicaid, and the medically uninsured have been "federalized" by 1995 in one managed care program which covers 25 percent of all Americans. The program has the following features:

- Beneficiaries are enrolled in competing *qualified health plans* (QHP) which are essentially Medicare HMOs with broader provider distribution and which meet federal standards.
- Enrollees are capitated at 100 percent of the former Medicare spending level on a regional basis.

- Hospital and physician participation in QHPs is optional, but 95 percent of all hospitals and 75 percent of all doctors are part of at least one QHP.
- Physicians do not universally support QHPs, but medicine dropped its opposition by 1995 since the alternatives were mandatory assignment or national health insurance.
- There is a limit on hospital days, and organ transplants are not covered to keep costs within the federal budget; however, extended care and home health have been expanded.
- Supplemental coverage to add a "high option" with broader benefits for public beneficiaries is now possible, and more than 50 percent of the QHP enrollees buy the supplemental coverage.

INTEGRATED HEALTH PLANS

Health maintenance organizations (HMOs) and preferred provider organizations (PPOs) in the year 2000 have become *integrated health plans* (IHPs) with 65 percent of the non-Medicare health insurance market and with the following features:

- Distinctions between HMOs and PPOs are blurred, with stronger control features for PPOs and more provider choice in HMOs. This provides a spectrum of options for employers from no-frills to high benefit.
- National IHPs control 50 percent of the market by the turn of the century as indemnity carriers and the Blues reconfigure as managed care plans, and provider-sponsored systems play a niche role in regional and local markets.
- Some IHPs own all of their needed facilities and pay the salaries of their physicians, but most IHPs contract with provider networks on a competitive basis.
- Most IHPs emphasize ambulatory care, use inpatient care sparingly, and have broader coverage of extended care and home health than comparable plans today.
- IHP members with a high-health lifestyle are rewarded with expanded benefits or lower premiums.

INDEMNITY INSURANCE AND THE BLUES

Indemnity insurance plans and the Blues have become IHPs with multiple HMO and PPO options for buyers by the year 2000. The Blue Cross–Blue Shield plan boundaries experienced meltdown under financial pressure in 1989–1992 and collapsed into 15 to 18 multistate "baby Blues" with regional care networks; these "managed indemnity" plans account for another 25 percent of the non-Medicare market by the year 2000.

DISCRETIONARY MEDICINE AND FEE-FOR-SERVICE

Discretionary medicine and fee-for-service has shrunk to 10 percent of the U.S. (non-Medicare) healthcare market. Its enrollees are mostly covered by supplemental health insurance plans, which have become quite popular by the year 2000 as an option in cafeteria-style benefit plans. This is a niche market catering to the wealthy and those frightened of specialized diseases. Many supplemental plans are essentially single-business managed care plans which cover a particular disease such as cancer, stroke, diabetes, or arthritis. Capitation and a provider fee schedule (discounts) are standard in these special-purpose managed care plans, and vision care, dental care, and even plastic surgery are popular options, with services provided by speciality managed care networks.

PLURALISTIC HEALTH SYSTEM

Contrary to some predictions, the United States did not adopt the Canadian health system model in the 1990s. In the year 2000 the American health system is still private and competitive.

Every American — even the poor and the 37 million once "medically uninsured" — are now covered by some type of managed care plan. Providers have organized themselves into competing networks which contract with QHPs and IHPs, and competition within a managed care framework has kept health costs within 3 percent of inflation in the Consumer Price Index.

HUB-AND-SPOKE NETWORKS

All hospitals are part of managed care provider networks, organized like the airlines on a "hub-and-spoke" model with hospitals and physicians channeling patients to the various settings and levels of care. All providers accept discounting as part of the new business environment. Virtually no one pays "retail" prices for hospital or medical services in the year 2000, and health inflation is running only 1 to 2 percent ahead of the overall Consumer Price Index. The volume of healthcare services continues to rise; the aging of the population is the major driving force pushing higher demand for services.

ETHICS AND ECONOMICS

Some call it "rationing." Certainly, managed care plans are very prudent buyers of high technology. Implants and transplants are not covered by many plans, including the federal QHPs, and even supplemental plans require substantial deductibles and copayments. Those over age 75, for example, are not covered for heart or liver transplants by most HMOs or managed indemnity plans.

Managed care plans buy high-technology procedures in volume, driving prices down by 50 percent or more by selectively contracting only with a limited number of regional medical centers which can deliver on both price and quality outcomes.

MARKET SHAKEOUT

Most hospitals survived the transition in the 1990s to managed care as "preferred providers," but 500 small hospitals closed their acute care beds, primarily by down-licensing to subacute or skilled nursing care.

Despite the pervasive influence of managed care in the year 2000, only 15 percent of U.S. hospitals are actually owned by QHPs and IHPs. Managed care plans have not made major capital investments in hospital facilities, but a number of the national managed care firms have bought or built ambulatory care centers.

CORPORATE MEDICINE

The practice of medicine is concentrated in a growing number of medical group practices. These medical corporations are physician-owned and professionally managed. About 40 percent of all doctors are salaried in the year 2000, and many work in ambulatory care centers owned by QHPs and IHPs, or by large group practices which specialize in managed care contracting.

LONG-TERM CARE

The "continuum of care" oriented to chronic illness is still evolving by the year 2000. Nursing home care has been mainstreamed by the year 2000. More than 50 percent of nursing home patients are covered by managed care plans, but stays are half as long as a decade before. Most of the chronically ill are treated at home, and more than 50 percent of the terminally ill die at home.

HEALTHCARE SPENDING

Healthcare's share of the Gross National Product rises to 15 percent in the year 2000 and is still growing. The impact of the "baby boom" on healthcare spending is just beginning to be felt. By the year 2020, health may consume 20 percent of national spending. Health levels are gradually rising as all Americans are now covered by some managed care plan, which are at financial risk for the health of their enrollees.

PUBLIC HEALTH

With a growing consciousness about lifestyle, the United States is increasingly public health oriented. Managed care plans recognize the cost-benefit of public health interventions. For example:

• Managed care plans find that investing in prenatal care of low-income mothers is a business essential as well as sound public policy. Prenatal care reduces the likelihood of a high-cost low-weight birth. By the year 2000, infant mortality has already dropped two percentage points.

• Managed care is collaborating with employers to improve work site safety and health, and supporting research into environmentally linked diseases.

Now we are beginning to see the potential payoff which was always implicit in the term "health maintenance organization."

Looking backward at the 1990s, managed care, while still not an ideal system, has managed a market-driven solution to the nation's needs for healthcare. Americans are willing to spend 12 to 15 percent of their Gross National Product on improving their health and well-being. The nation found a private-sector solution which did not require draconian new regulations or conversion to a national health system like Canada's government-managed model.

Looking forward to the 21st century, the next challenge for managed care will be to respond to the aging of the population. The baby boomers will reach age 65 beginning in the year 2010, as the nation enters into the 21st century. With Americans living longer, can they also lead healthier lives and enjoy a higher quality of life at ages 75, 85, and 100?

Getting there will not be easy, but it is possible. In the coming transition to managed care, the entire health system must be turned on its head. The managed care system must shift the emphasis from acute care to chronic illness and the maintenance of independence. Medicine under a managed care scenario needs a new paradigm—the vision of "health" as a goal. The incentives in a managed care environment will be to keep enrollees healthy (and out of the acute care hospital). Better yet, consumers will take more personal responsibility for their own health. This is the potential of a managed care future.

CHAPTER TWENTY-FOUR

Medicare and Medicaid

MANAGED CARE IN MEDICARE AND MEDICAID

PETER D. FOX, Ph.D., Vice President
Lewin/ICF, Washington, D.C.

EDWARD NEUSCHLER, Director of Policy Studies
Health Insurance Association of America, Washington, D.C.

Managed care, broadly defined from the perspective of the purchaser, can be viewed as any measure that favorably affects the price of services, the site at which they are received, or their utilization. Medicare and Medicaid are the largest purchasers of care in the nation. As such, these programs are almost uniquely situated to negotiate (or as some would argue, unilaterally set prices) because they represent such a large share of the revenues of many providers. Medicare's Prospective Payment System (PPS) for reimbursing hospitals is a case in point; few hospitals could survive without participating in Medicare, and the institutions are not allowed to bill patients for covered services above what Medicare allows. Thus they have little choice but to serve beneficiaries and to accept the program's payment levels.

Physician reimbursement demonstrates both the limits and appeal to providers of Medicare and Medicaid. Physicians are not allowed to balance bill Medicaid patients for the difference between billed charges and the payment received from the agency. In many states, reimbursement is sufficiently low that most physicians limit their Medicaid practice or do not participate at all. In contrast, few physicians refuse to see Medicare patients, particularly as they are permitted to balance bill for amounts over what the program recognizes as reasonable, unless they sign participation agreements. Physicians complain bitterly about Medicare reimbursement levels, yet some 70 percent of bills are assigned, that is, the physician has elected to bill the carrier directly and accept the Medicare allowable as reimbursement in full.[1] Although the average submitted charge is reduced by 27 percent, market behavior as represented by assignment rates seems to indicate that in the current environment Medicare reimbursement is acceptable to many physicians, if not dearly beloved.

Medicare and Medicaid also have adopted various measures to affect the site of care. For example, the Professional Review Organizations (PROs), which are physician-controlled, have been established to review the medical necessity, appropriateness of site, and quality of care provided to Medicare beneficiaries. In practice, the focus has been on retrospective review of inpatient services, although preadmission review is performed on a few services (for example, cataract surgery), and efforts are planned that will address ambulatory care, both surgical and in physicians' offices. Also, the PROs have made a limited effort to review the quality of Medicare-covered nursing home and home health services. Under Medicaid, at least 20 states have specified varying lists of procedures that are not covered if performed on an inpatient basis unless hospitalization has been authorized in advance or the medical necessity for inpatient admission is otherwise justified. A few states pay physicians more if the surgery is performed on an outpatient basis.

Nonetheless, Medicare and many Medicaid programs have not been as forceful in managing care as many private sector programs, which, for example, mandate prior authorization for nonemergency inpatient services, and are beginning to incorporate similar requirements on selected ambulatory services such as surgery and expensive diagnostic interventions.

The rest of this chapter focuses on the programs that have received the most attention, that is, alternative delivery systems (ADSs), which include prepaid health plans or HMOs (terms used interchangeably herein), PPOs, and primary care case management programs. The next section of this chapter summarizes the reasons for public interest in managed care arrangements under Medicare and Medicaid. After that, the major models or decision variables used in structuring government ADS programs are discussed. Then, a statistical profile of Medicare and Medicaid activity is presented, followed by a discussion of some of the major issues. Finally, the prospects and limitations of Medicare and Medicaid efforts are explored.

PUBLIC INTEREST IN MANAGED CARE ARRANGEMENTS

The most obvious reason for public interest in managed care arrangements is budgetary. Between 1980 and 1987, for example, Medicare Part A (which mostly pays for hospital services) outlays rose from $24.3 billion to $50.8 billion, an annual rate of increase of 11.1 percent, and Part B (which mostly pays for physician services) outlays grew from $10.7 billion to $30.8 billion, an annual rate of increase of 16.3 percent. During that period, Medicaid program costs (federal and state combined) rose from $25.8 billion to $49.3 billion, or 9.7 percent annually, while serving essentially the same number of recipients each year. (Despite the recession of the early 1980s and the growth in the number of poor people over the period, the number of Medicaid recipients did not increase significantly because of restrictive federal legislation enacted in 1981 and because most states do not routinely update their income eligibility levels to keep pace with inflation.)

The budget issues are important in their own right. In addition, the changes in public programs needed to address the problems of roughly 37 million uninsured will likely hinge in part on the government being able, first, to demonstrate that the monies are spent efficiently and, second, to achieve better budget predictability, which in turn entails greater and more sophisticated reliance on managed care.

Managed care can improve access to, and continuity of, services. This is principally an issue for Medicaid, and its importance varies by state, reflecting in part state policies regarding reimbursement and benefits. Access can be particularly problematic for physician services. With regard to physician services, Medicaid reimbursement levels vary considerably among states but are low in many. For example, in 1986, payment for a brief office visit rendered by a specialist ranged from $6 in New Hampshire, well below prevailing charges, to $20 in the District of Columbia.[2] In addition to having the potential for improving access to some services, managed care has proven successful in limiting inappropriate use of the emergency room, which is considerably more expensive than a physician visit, and in reducing repeated physician shopping and patient "ping-ponging." Access to physician services for Medicare beneficiaries is much less of a problem, although finding physicians who will accept assignment is difficult in some communities and with some specialists. Inpatient care is generally readily accessible unless the beneficiary has exhausted his or her benefits. This can occur particularly under some state Medicaid programs that impose limits on the number of covered inpatient days. Access to nursing home services is a problem in some communities, especially for Medicaid beneficiaries, but at times this is also true for Medicare recipients; however, most prepaid health plans exclude long-term nursing home care. Another aspiration is that managed care can better meet some of the special needs of the Medicaid population, for example, prenatal and pediatric services.

Finally, but important, managed care can serve as a procompetitive force that exerts a restraining influence on the medical system as a whole rather than fueling increases in medical expenses. Medicare and Medicaid are commonly perceived as the root cause of rising healthcare costs since the initial implementation of the programs in 1966. The reasons include the absence of controls on utilization and payment methods that have generated higher prices, whether through the "usual, customary, and reasonable" (in Medicare parlance: customary, prevailing, and reasonable) payment methods for physician services or the system of cost reimbursement to hospitals that preceded the current Prospective Payment System (PPS). Ascribing the full blame to public programs is unfair because the expenditure increases result from the combined effect of public plans and unmanaged private indemnity plans, not to mention other factors that are beyond the scope of this paper (for example, supply-induced demand due to rising physician supply; changes in technology; the aging of the population; and increasing consumer expectations regarding medical care, leading to greater demand for services). Whatever the distribution of culpability, reliance on managed care entails using the enormous purchasing power of government programs to exert a restraining influence, first, by constraining revenues flowing to the healthcare sector and, second, by inducing physicians and other providers to adopt less resource-intensive practice styles across the board.

MAJOR MODELS OR DECISION VARIABLES

A number of taxonomies of Medicaid managed care efforts have been presented in the literature. These taxonomies are designed to identify key program attributes and to characterize the myriad of programs extant, given the wide variation in approach that states have adopted.[3] They classify both program structure at the government level and organizational structure at the individual plan or ADS level (for example, the nature of physician risk-sharing arrangements and the extent of case management efforts by individual plans). For purposes of this paper, the key concerns are policy decisions faced by the government rather than by individual plans. Among the most critical are (1) whether enrollment in some form of ADS is voluntary or mandatory, (2) who bears the financial risk, (3) which populations and services are included, and (4) the requirements for plan participation.

Voluntary versus Mandatory Participation

Medicare has relied entirely on voluntary programs, although some have proposed a mandatory "voucher" system that would entail each beneficiary selecting among competing private plans and paying for any difference between the value of the Medicare-issued voucher and the plan's total premium. However, the politics of removing the fee-for-service option from Medicare beneficiaries is likely to militate against such a mandatory program for some years to come.

Medicare's major ADS program is one that allows beneficiaries to drop their fee-for-service benefits voluntarily and instead receive care through an HMO or "competitive medical plan (CMP)," which is similar to an HMO except that it does not have to meet all of the requirements to become federally qualified under Title XIII of the Public Health Service Act. In theory, that option has been available since the enactment of the 1972 Social Security Amendments. However, it was not until 1982 that the legislative provisions were changed to make it sufficiently attractive for more than a handful of HMOs to participate and for beneficiaries to join.[4]

Two planned demonstrations are also noteworthy. The first is the "Medicare Insured Group (MIG)," which entails a corporation or union that offers Medicare supplementary benefits accepting risk for both the Medicare and the supplementary benefits. Although the demonstrations are still being planned, three organizations, two large employers and one union-based program, have entered into "cooperative agreements" with the Health Care Financing Administration (HCFA) to develop demonstrations. The expectation is that the risk-bearing organization will receive 95 percent of projected Medicare experience for the group of Medicare enrollees in question. Again, enrollment would be voluntary.

The second is the Medicare PPO. HCFA issued a request for proposal in the summer of 1988 with responses due in October 1988. Five organizations were approved for funding. The expectation is that Medicare beneficiaries who reside within the service area would make a voluntary election to join, in which case benefits would be improved if network providers were used (for example, 10 percent rather than 20 percent coinsurance for Part B services) but would be reduced if nonnetwork providers were used (for example, coinsurance would be increased to 30 percent). Potential applicants were informed that proposals for a "nonenrolled" or mandatory model demonstration in a given geographic area would be entertained; however, for legal and political reasons, Medicare benefits could not be reduced below their current levels if nonnetwork providers were used. One organization (CAPP Care in southern California) did receive approval to test such a model. However, no benefit changes from the current Medicare program are contemplated, and the incentives to use network providers are nonfinancial (for example, assurances that physicians will accept assignment). HCFA's objective in undertaking these demonstrations is to reduce Medicare outlays by constraining utilization rather than through changes from normal Medicare reimbursement practices. Where benefits improvements are introduced as an incentive to use network providers, a key question is whether net savings would result, even given strong utilization management efforts.

Medicaid is another matter when it comes to mandating enrollment in alternative delivery systems. Many states had for some years contracted with prepaid health programs, typically paying them between 90 and 95 percent of estimated fee-for-service, with enrollment being voluntary. However, commonly, enrollment was minimal, in part because in many states the benefit package is sufficiently comprehensive that the plan was limited in its ability to offer additional benefits that would create incentives for the beneficiary to accept being restricted to a limited provider network.

More recently (mostly in the early 1980s), a number of states, either as part of large-scale HCFA-sponsored demonstrations or under the Section 1915(b) authorities that allow the "freedom of choice" provisions in the statute to be waived, have mandated that Medicaid beneficiaries enroll in HMOs or other managed care plans. With the exception of Arizona, the mandate is in selected counties only rather than being statewide, typically in the larger urban areas. Recipient choice among several available prepaid plans is mandated in selected urban areas of Missouri, Minnesota, Oregon, and Wisconsin and is statewide in Arizona. Recipient enrollment in a single managed care plan (sometimes called a "health insuring organization" or "HIO") is required in parts of California (Santa Barbara and San Mateo counties), Minnesota (rural Itasca County), Pennsylvania (part of inner-city Philadelphia), and Washington (Kitsap and two adjacent rural counties). Recent federal legislation, however, limits any future state initiatives that mandate enrollment in a single plan.

Locus of Risk

The second distinction is who bears the risk. By definition, prepaid health plans receive capitation payments and bear the attendant risk, although many state Medicaid programs provide individual (per enrollee) stop-loss protection for very expensive cases. Under the proposed Medicare PPO demonstration, HCFA will retain the risk rather than passing it on to plans or providers, just as employers or insurance carriers do under the typical PPO arrangement.

Medicaid has had greater experience with approaches under which the states retain some or all of the risk. For example, several states capitate small physician groups or clinics for only a limited package of physician and outpatient services while continuing to pay for inpatient hospital and other care on a fee-for-service basis. Recipients enroll in these plans just as they would in an HMO, and the physicians manage all care, including inpatient care, provided to their enrollees. Typically, the state tracks utilization of inpatient and other noncapitated services by plan and pays a bonus if the plan manages such care effectively. California, Michigan, and Oregon have sizable programs.

Under another approach, usually called "primary care case management," the state retains all the risk. Medicaid recipients are required to select and enroll with a primary care physician who has agreed to serve as a case manager and who is required to authorize any referral services. Payment remains on a fee-for-service basis, but services not authorized by the primary physician are not reimbursed, except in a true emergency. In some states, physicians receive a small monthly "case management" fee per enrollee in recognition of the additional responsibilities they have accepted. Programs of this type operate statewide in Colorado, Kentucky, and Utah and in some urban areas of Kansas, Michigan, and Missouri. (Smaller programs operate in Connecticut and Tennessee.) In Colorado, Michigan, Missouri, and Utah, recipients may choose between selecting a physician "sponsor," who serves as case manager, or enrolling in an HMO.

Populations and Services Covered

The Medicare HMO/CMP program encompasses both of its eligibility categories, that is, the aged and the disabled, although it does exempt from the HMO risk-contracting arrangement certain end-stage renal disease patients and those that have elected the hospice program. State Medicaid programs vary considerably. Some are limited to beneficiaries who receive cash welfare payments under the Aid to Families with Dependent Children program (for example, Missouri and Wisconsin). Others (Arizona, California, and New York) also include the aged, blind, and/or disabled eligibility categories. Only a few include the so-called medically needy, those who have incomes above the cash welfare line and who also may qualify by virtue of having particularly large medical expenses (the "spend-down cases").

With regard to services, the Medicare HMO/CMP program places its participating plans at risk for all services covered by Medicare. In contrast, state Medicaid programs commonly exclude certain services and, instead, reimburse them under the regular program. Services that have variously been exempted from prepayment, for substantive or political reasons, include prescription drugs (Missouri), dental care (various states), and most long-term care in nursing homes or mental institutions (all states with prepaid contracts, except for four or five small demonstration projects). It may be noted that most of these excluded services are not covered by Medicare.

Plan Participation Requirements

Both Medicare and most Medicaid programs contract with federally qualified HMOs. However, they rarely limit their contracting to these plans and relax some of the federal requirements (for example, relating to benefit packages and rate setting for private enrollees). Requirements that are usually retained in some form include those related to the adequacy of the provider network, the grievance process for enrollees, the quality assurance system, and financial stability.

ENROLLMENT TRENDS

In April 1985, just after the 1982 Medicare amendments were implemented, some 309,000 Medicare beneficiaries were enrolled in HMOs (or CMPs), almost all under demonstration awards that had been made over the years. In April 1987, only 2 years later, enrollment reached 903,000 and then stabilized. Throughout 1987–1989 enrollment fluctuated around the 1 million level, with a significant number of plans dropping their risk contracts and many others reporting financial losses from the Medicare program. As of March 1990, some 1,124,000 beneficiaries were enrolled in 97 plans, a decline in number of plans with risk contracts from a peak of 161 reached in December 1987. Although most of the plans that terminated their risk contracts had small numbers of Medicare enrollees, and many do continue to serve them under other arrangements, the relationship of HMOs with the Medicare program has been more troubled than either party had envisioned.

The reasons for the financial losses are several. First, in most of the last several years the government underestimated expenses in the fee-for-service system and hence the plan reimbursement levels. Second, some of the plans incurred higher than predicted utilization levels and encountered greater difficulty in controlling costs generally. Third, and related to the second point, most plans did little to reorient their approach to services delivery to meet the specific needs of the Medicare population (particularly the very old and severely disabled), such as more aggressive use of home health or medical-social services. Whether their doing so would have helped the plans' "bottom lines" is conjectural.

Medicaid has also witnessed significant enrollment expansions, reflecting in large measure the increased willingness of the states in recent years to mandate that beneficiaries participate in managed care programs. In June 1981 Medicaid enrollment in prepaid health plans amounted to 282,000 persons in 18 states; in contrast, in December 1987, 28 states contracted with such plans, and enrollment reached 947,000. In addition,

• Five states contracted with health insuring organizations (HIOs), commonly the county-at-risk model described above. These organizations accept risk for a comprehensive service package and also require recipients to select a primary care physician as case manager. Enrollment in December 1987 stood at 145,000.

- Three states (statewide in Texas and Indiana and in three counties in northern California) contracted with HIOs that do not require recipients to select a primary care physician as case manager, accounting for a total enrollment of 1,129,000.

- Six states partially capitate primary care physicians, who serve as gatekeepers for approximately 50,000 enrollees, and another seven states require (usually only in portions of the state) that recipients designate as case manager a primary care physician who authorizes access to nonemergency referral services but is not financially at risk. This requirement affects more than 400,000 individuals.

Many states have adopted more than one approach, and the total number of states that have engaged in one or more of the above-described managed care efforts amounts to 31.

MAJOR ISSUES

This section addresses some of the major issues that Medicare and Medicaid confront, many of which have analogs among private purchasers: (1) rate setting, (2) conditions that plans must meet to participate, (3) problems of monitoring and beneficiary protection, and (4) impact on decision making of public sector due process requirements.

Rate Setting

Issues of rate setting, as might be expected, loom as some of the largest and the most contentious problems between plans and government agencies. Medicare and most Medicaid programs reimburse prepaid health plans a percentage (typically 90 or 95 percent) of prospectively estimated fee-for-service expenditures. A notable exception to the reliance on fee-for-service expenses as the initial benchmark is the Arizona Medicaid program, which mandates enrollment in prepaid health plans statewide and bases reimbursement on a competitive bidding system. The estimate of fee-for-services expenses is commonly referred to as the adjusted average per capita cost, or AAPCC.

The establishment of reimbursement levels can typically be viewed as entailing three major steps. First, per capita expenses in a base year must be determined. Second, these per capita expenses are generally adjusted to reflect factors, for example, enrollee age, that are predictive of the need for medical services and hence resource consumption, and the nature of these adjustments must be determined. Third, the payment level trends must be brought forward from the base year to the current year. (This latter step may occur prior to the application of the adjustments, mentioned above, that reflect the anticipated service needs.)

Determining (or estimating) expenses in the base year is not theoretically difficult, although, complex practical problems do arise. For example, data on benefit payments and eligibility may be on different computer files and so may be difficult to match for purposes of calculating capitation amounts. In addition, estimates for the base year should ideally reflect the services that were *rendered* that year rather than when they were *paid for*, given the propensity of states to delay or accelerate cashflow to meet budget targets. Attributing bills to the correct period and estimating as yet unreported claims (IBNRs, or incurred but not reported claims) can be problematic. However, the more serious issues that arise are those of philosophy and policy rather than of estimating methodologies.

Capitation payment levels are typically county-specific, and per-enrollee fee-for-service expenditures can vary enormously as a result of differences in both *input costs* (for example, costs of supplies, heating and air conditioning expenses, and wages of employees) and *practice styles*. For example, among counties in metropolitan areas, the AAPCC in 1988 for the Medicare elderly population varied from a high of $389 a month in Manhattan to a low of $134 in Pittsylvania, Virginia.[5] Reflecting differences in input cost is generally viewed as appropriate. However, plans in counties that are adjacent to higher-cost (often center-city) counties commonly claim that they face input prices that more nearly approximate those of the more expensive county than their own because of the need to attract personnel. The more critical question is the extent to which variations due to practice styles should be reflected in the HMO payment levels.

Another significant rate-setting problem arises if the bulk of the population enrolls in HMOs, making the base rate within the county meaningless or impossible to calculate. States that have mandated Medicaid enrollment in HMOs have confronted this issue. Some have used the experience of counties within the state that are not subject to the mandate (for example, Minnesota in setting rates for Itasca County); Arizona has adopted a complex bidding system that results in the plans within a given county that have the lower bids benefiting from greater enrollment.

Finally, the percentage of estimated fee-for-service costs that should be paid is controversial. Medicare pays 95 percent of the AAPCC; most state Medicaid programs pay between 90 and 95 percent, and a few pay more. A related issue is whether costs of administration borne by the government should be incorporated in the

AAPCC. Medicare incorporates the costs borne by the fiscal interme-diaries, which process claims under the regular program (and per-form some other functions), on the grounds that the plan assumes these functions. In contrast, most Medicaid programs reflect only medical expenses in determining the AAPCC, in some cases reason-ing that contracting with prepaid health plans *increases* rather than decreases the state's administrative costs.

The second issue relates to the adjustments to the base amount to reflect the likely need for medical resources by individuals who enroll in a particular plan. In addition to county of residence, Medi-care also adjusts the payment level based on enrollee age, sex, wel-fare status (that is, whether the beneficiary is also covered by Medi-caid), and institutional status (for example, whether the beneficiary is a long-term nursing home resident). Many states make similar ad-justments. In contrast the Missouri program, which covers the Aid to Families with Dependent Children welfare category (that is, the el-derly and disabled are excluded), only differentiates whether the enrollee in question is an adult or a child.

Underlying the technical issues of the adjustment factors is the matter of biased selection; that is, within a rate category, enrollees may be, on average, either healthier or sicker than those who do not enroll. The evidence is mixed; although for the Medicare population the preponderance of evidence is that the plans do benefit from favorable selection, at least at the time of initial enrollment. Perhaps the most recent and comprehensive study of adverse selection among the Medicare population specifically is the "National Medi-care Competition Evaluation" performed by a consortium headed by Mathematica Policy Research, Inc. That evaluation focused on dem-onstration projects that preceded the implementation in 1985 of the 1982 TEFRA legislation. One finding, for example, was that HMO enrollees were significantly more likely than beneficiaries who re-mained in the fee-for-service sector to perform basic activities of daily living (for example, bathing and meal preparation) and also had fewer annual bed days prior to enrollment (4.4 versus 9.3 days).[6]

Also, biased selection (favorable or unfavorable) can differ among plans. For example, a study of two group-model HMOs and one IPA that participated in the above-cited demonstrations found that, "the group model HMOs experienced substantial favorable selection but that the IPA attracted enrollees who were representative of the mar-ket area."[7] In addition, whether biased selection persists over time remains a matter of debate. The circumstances under which biased selection occurs, along with its magnitude and direction, remain a highly complex matter for plans and both public and private pur-chasers.

Reflecting this concern, the government and research community is devoting considerable effort to devise ways of adjusting for health status. The leading current effort is that of the Health Care Financing Administration to test a system of "diagnostic cost groups" (DCGs), which incorporates the prior hospitalization experience of individuals at the time of HMO enrollment. Some state programs (for example, Arizona) have partially countered the problems of adverse selection by separately reimbursing for selected high-cost patients, such as neonates and those with AIDS.

The third step relates to the process of bringing trends from the base year forward to the year for which reimbursement is to be made. This in turn entails estimating expenditure changes in the fee-for-service system. Some state Medicaid programs have consciously not passed through the full increase to achieve budgetary savings. In other cases, the problems have been ones of estimation.

Plan Participation Requirements

Both the issue of plan participation requirements and that related to plan monitoring presented in the next subsection address principally the government's responsibility of protecting beneficiaries. Public agencies in electing to contract with plans must make decisions on requirements for participation. The objectives of these requirements include assuring that (1) the delivery network is adequate, (2) the quality of care provided meets acceptable standards, (3) the enrollees understand the plan and how to access services and also have a way of registering complaints, and (4) the plan is financially stable.

Medicare contracts with any plan that is "qualified" under Title XIII of the Public Health Service Act. This qualification process was established in the context of that act's provisions requiring that most employers offer their employees the option of joining an HMO. In the late 1970s, when the Medicare HMO amendments were being debated, the Carter administration proposed limiting Medicare contracting to federally qualified HMOs, in part as a matter of beneficiary protection. However, when the amendments were passed in 1982, they reflected the Reagan administration's perspective that the federal government need not impose the full set of Title XIII requirements, many of which address private-sector benefit and rate-setting practices, and the legislation (which had bipartisan support) authorized Medicare to also contract with so-called competitive medical plans (CMPs). Among the requirements for becoming a CMP are that the plan be financially sound, have an adequate provider network, assume risk for private as well as public enrollees, not discriminate based on health status of enrollees, provide adequate levels of information to enrollees, abide by certain marketing practice limitations, and have acceptable quality assurance and enrollee grievance systems.

In addition, no more than 50 percent of a plan's enrollees may be Medicare and Medicaid combined, if the plan wishes to participate in Medicare. The requirement is more lenient for Medicaid, which allows up to 75 percent of the plan's enrollment to come from the two large public programs, and new plans are given up to 3 years to come into compliance. Philosophically, the intent of the requirement is to protect beneficiaries by assuring that the government contracts only with plans that have proven themselves to be at least minimally acceptable in the competitive private market. Practically, the requirement can be problematic for state Medicaid programs because many mainstream HMOs have little interest in serving the Medicaid population, while plans developed specifically to serve the poor may have great difficulty attracting commercial enrollment.

In establishing their standards for Medicaid participation, many states have taken advantage of the opportunity, made available in 1981, to contract with prepaid plans that do not meet all of the requirements for federal qualification as an HMO under Title XIII. Typically, plans that meet the state's own statutory requirements for operation as a private market HMO can also contract with Medicaid. In a few cases, there is no general state HMO law, and the state Medicaid agency has had to develop detailed standards in its state Medicaid plan in order to contract with non-federally qualified plans. In addition, many states avail themselves of special federal authority permitting capitation contracts with community health centers (CHCs) that receive funds from the U.S. Public Health Service. This approach can be attractive to states because CHCs are, by definition, located in low-income, medically underserved areas where many Medicaid recipients live.

Ongoing Monitoring of Plan Performance

The concerns of government agencies regarding beneficiary protection in establishing qualification requirements remain once a contract has been signed. Problems of performance of major magnitude are not widespread. However, two events that have received considerable public attention highlight the need for ongoing oversight.

The first are the problems that arose in the early- and mid-1970s with the California PHP (prepaid health plan) program. In order to reduce Medicaid expenses, the state aggressively contracted with prepaid health plans without establishing proper mechanisms for qualification or monitoring. While many of the plans delivered adequate, if hardly stellar, levels of service, a number did not or were otherwise engaged in questionable practices. Problems that arose included plans with inadequate provider networks, plans that marketed in areas that were at significant distances from the provider network, access barriers (for example, delays in obtaining appointments), and questionable quality of care. In addition, objectionable marketing practices occurred, including salespeople who wore white physician's coats and told beneficiaries that they would lose their Medicaid coverage if they did not join a particular plan.

A study performed by the U.S. Department of Health and Human Services at the time found quality of care to be roughly equal between the prepaid health plans and those fee-for-service settings where the Medicaid population typically received care. However, wide variability was noted, with the plans that generally performed the worst being those with little or no private enrollment. This finding led to the federal limitations, which have been modified over time, that states only contract with plans that have minimum levels of private enrollees.

In the 1980s, there have been echoes in several states of the early California scandals, for example, complaints of misleading or coercive marketing, allegations of inadequate access or denial of care, and a few documented cases of profiteering. Although nothing has approached the magnitude of the California case, the need for continued vigilance is clear.

The Medicare HMO program has not been free from scandal. Under a Medicare demonstration, the IMC plan in Florida grew rapidly to more than 180,000 enrollees, mostly Medicare. There were allegations of inadequate service delivery and poor quality of care as well as of senior management participating in kickbacks and other illegal activities. In addition, IMC was named in multiple suits by its providers, claiming nonperformance of contract terms, including failure to pay bills. The upshot was that the plan was sold under fire-sale circumstances, and the founder and prior chief executive officer fled the country and is under indictment. Whether earlier and better monitoring could have prevented some of the problems has been debated; their severity has not.

The adequacy of the federal monitoring process has been questioned, and states differ enormously in their processes. Some level of beneficiary protection is needed. Questions arise, however, regarding how far the government should go, and a delicate balance exists between reasonable monitoring and being overly intrusive or imposing requirements that have little bearing on the objectives of the oversight function. In addition, since the oversight process can never be totally mechanical, the skill levels, quality, judgment, and orientation of the staff responsible for monitoring are important.

Impact of the Process Requirements

Medicare and most state Medicaid programs have extensive experience contracting with prepaid health plans. The relevant government bodies are comfortable in doing so because, first, the plans are capitated and bear the risk and, second, they are able to adopt or create conditions for participation that afford a level of protection to the government and enrollees.

PPOs are another matter. Medicare and Medicaid experience has been minimal, despite the significant, if hard to quantify, growth in private purchaser contracting activity. It is not clear whether the lack of Medicare or Medicaid contracting is due to the newness of the PPO phenomenon, which is in considerable flux or, instead, whether government agencies have structural characteristics that limit their ability to engage in PPO efforts. Both factors may be at play, and only time will tell. Nonetheless, the procedural requirements that society places on government will likely limit reliance on PPOs.

PPOs by definition do not accept risk. Rather, risk remains with the payer, thereby necessitating that the payer make decisions regarding which providers or PPO structures practice cost-effective medicine. These decisions can be informed ones if data and analysis are available. However, they are ultimately judgmental, more so with regard to physician selection than with regard to hospitals, where multiple data sources are available (for example, Medicare cost reports and DRG-based claims analyses).

Governmental bodies operate in much more limelight than do private purchasers and in some respects are more accountable (for individual actions, not necessarily end results). One aspect of government accountability is the "due process" requirements, which in the case of PPOs include having clear and, ideally, objective criteria for selecting or terminating those providers that would be designated as preferred. For example, 1981 legislation permits state Medicaid programs (after approval of a waiver) to contract selectively with providers or practitioners that "meet, accept, and comply with" the state's reimbursement, quality, and utilization standards. However, states are specifically prohibited from discriminating "among classes of providers on grounds unrelated to their demonstrated effectiveness and efficiency." Because of these legal restrictions and because quality is so difficult to measure objectively, the few state Medicaid programs that have attempted to contract selectively have focused on inpatient hospital care. Quality, to the extent it is measured at all, is used as a screen, rather than as a basis for competition. California and Illinois are the major medical programs that currently contract for inpatient hospital care on a competitive bid basis. (As noted earlier, Arizona uses a bidding system to select its participating prepaid health plans.) Given the limited and hospital-specific Medicaid experience, the Medicare PPO demonstration, which does break new ground, may prove to be an instructive test of the opportunities of PPO relationships for the two government programs.

PROSPECTS AND LIMITATIONS

In assessing the future of alternative delivery systems, whether from the perspective of the government or of individual plans, a distinction should be made between short- and long-run opportunities.

Under most approaches to contracting, the government typically saves between 5 and 10 percent of expenses, assuming no biased selection, and perhaps a little more if it underestimates fee-for-service expenses. Given the magnitude of the Medicare and Medicaid budgets, such savings, even on a minority of total enrollees, is hardly trivial. However, the greater impact would appear to be long term by using the purchasing power of government to promote a market discipline in the healthcare sector.

Few plans have made significant profits under the Medicare or Medicaid programs; indeed, most have lost money or barely broken even, in part because the opportunities for cost savings are limited. These plans achieve the savings needed for profitability primarily by constraining utilization. However, the savings must be sufficient to offset several advantages that the government enjoys. The first is the 5 to 10 percent of estimated fee-for-services expenses that the government keeps. Second, the plans in some instances reimburse providers at levels that are commonly above those paid by the traditional Medicare and Medicaid programs. Indeed, one of the reasons that physicians, in particular, encourage plans with which they are affiliated to participate in Medicare is to obtain higher payment levels. This phenomenon is particularly true for Medicaid. Third, managed care, regardless of who undertakes it, entails some administrative costs (for example, for utilization review) that the regular program does not incur.

The future of Medicare and Medicaid contracting with alternative delivery systems depends on both the public credibility of the oversight process and the willingness of government agencies to understand and accommodate to the legitimate business and operational concerns of the plans. With regard to oversight, acceptance by the public generally and beneficiaries specifically depends on the programs' operating in an environment that is as scandal-free as possible. The major interests of government are budget control and predictability. Having achieved that objective through capitation, it is tempting for government agencies not to be proactive in assuring that beneficiaries have ready access to care that meets acceptable standards. However, prudent purchasing entails maximizing *value*, not simply minimizing cost. This in turn requires the hiring of a sufficiently large, capable staff, something many government agencies lack.

At the same time, the government should be cognizant that most plans do not participate in Medicare or Medicaid, electing instead to serve only private enrollees. Adequate reimbursement is important; few plans can afford to lose money consistently. Properly functioning administrative processes also matter. For example, many plans have had difficulty with the enrollment systems of Medicaid, and to some extent those of Medicare. Data demands are another issue for government payers, as they are for private ones. While a plea for adequate monitoring was made previously in this chapter, the appropriate level of intrusiveness needs to be considered, including ensuring that data demands are reasonable. Another problem is the fickleness of government, with regard to both payment levels and administration.

In the long term, greater reliance on alternative delivery systems and other forms of managed care seems inevitable. Medicare and Medicaid, like private payers, cannot afford to continue making payments in an unconstrained fee-for-service environment. Furthermore, the Medicare and Medicaid markets are too big for plans to ignore if the contract terms offered are reasonable. However, for the full potential of alternative delivery systems to be realized, the government must not just strive for short-term savings but must also be a good business partner, which it has not always been, and assure that Medicare and Medicaid beneficiaries are protected.

REFERENCES

1. Ira Burney and Julia Paradise, "Medicare Physician Participation," *Health Affairs.* **VI**(2):107–120 (Summer, 1987).

2. Health Care Financing Administration, U.S. Department of Health and Human Services, *Health Care Financing Program Statistics: Analysis of State Medicaid Program Characteristics, 1986,* Baltimore, August 1987, p. 99.

3. See, for example, Robert E. Hurley and Deborah A. Freund, "A Typology of Medicaid Managed Care," *Medical Care.* **XXVI**(8):764–774 (August 1988).

4. The plans that did participate prior to the 1982 amendments did so initially as part of various demonstrations that made the reimbursement system more palatable than the risk arrangements then in law.

5. Susan Jelleg Palsbo, "Analysis of the 1988 AAPCCS in Metropolitan Statistical Areas." Research Brief, No. 3, Group Health Association of America, December 1987.

6. Sheldon M. Retchin and Barbara S. Brown, *National Medicare Competition Evaluation: An Analysis of the Health Status Outcomes and Access to Care for Medicare Beneficiaries in Medicare Risk-Based Plans.* Williamson Institute for Health Studies, Medical College of Virginia, Richmond, VA, July 1988.

7. Louis F. Rossiter and Kathryn Langwell, "Medicare's Two Systems for Paying Providers," *Health Affairs.* **VII**(3):120–132 (Summer, 1988).

Access Issues in Managed Healthcare

JOHN D. GOLENSKI, S.J., Principal

Bioethics Consultation Group, Berkeley, California

While managed healthcare organizations must wrestle with the practical trade-offs between cost containment and access to care, the fundamental *ethical* issue of limiting access will be discussed at the *policy level*. Managed care planners can strive to remain competitive by offering low rates but limiting access to only low-risk clients. As long as all parties — buyers, members, patients, administrators, and providers — understand this reality and enter into a service contract with full consent, no ethical principle is breached. A breech of ethics does occur, however, when managed care organizations limit access to services without adequate planning, negotiation, and consent. This lack of clear policy among affected parties in many managed care organizations today calls out for remedy.

The situation in most state Medicaid programs is directly analogous. Faced with limited resources, most state governments avoid addressing the ethical considerations of limiting access to healthcare services. Instead of making conscious, consensual policy decisions about what services can be funded for particular populations, most state governments respond to the budget crunch by tightening eligibility requirements for coverage and reducing reimbursement rates to providers. Access has been substantially decreased by these actions. The stricter eligibility requirements have squeezed out of the Medicaid program hundreds of thousands of people that are below the poverty level, and cost reimbursement rates, which are often equal to or below the actual costs, have led many physicians to refuse to provide covered services to Medicaid patients.

Private insurers and managed care organizations face the same trade-offs between cutting costs and limiting access and have adopted similar implicit strategies to survive. While managed care plans were once a rational, effective, and efficient alternative to traditional fee-for-service healthcare, many are quickly resorting to the same solution of throwing passengers overboard to keep the boat afloat. Passing off high risks to someone else (frequently the provider of last resort) and limiting access to services needed by members through gatekeepers, bureaucratic hurdles, or deep provider discounts will not enable health plans to survive in the long run. Instead of continuing to struggle to compete on the basis of *cost*, HMOs and PPOs will fare better by offering — and allowing access to — services of *value* to members. In their struggle for economic survival, HMOs and PPOs will benefit by addressing the stark necessity for conscious, comprehensive, consensual decision making about which services they can afford to provide.

In order to develop a capacity for prioritizing benefit offerings, HMOs and other managed care organizations will need at least the following components:

- A credible, open and structured *process* for ranking the *value* of all possible healthcare interventions and benefits according to ethical and cost-effectiveness criteria.

- A mechanism, preferably shared with other provider organizations, for evaluating actual *outcomes* of interventions, procedures, and technologies. Efficacy studies are just beginning to be conducted by researchers and are very useful.

- A capacity for actuarial *costing* of individual interventions, procedures, and technologies within the expected client populations.

The managed care sector will not be able to avoid facing this fundamental ethical dilemma of how to restrict access in order to control costs. The question is no longer whether an inefficient, inappropriate fee-for-service method of providing care should be tolerated. Rather, the question to face is: How can managed care be designed to provide equitable care most effectively and efficiently in light of limited resources?

RATIONING HEALTHCARE TO THE POOR

Oregon Medicaid Priorities

The following priorities scale was considered by the Oregon Medicaid Priority-Setting Executive Group as a means of addressing four areas of medical services covered by Medicaid. The ranking system uses a 10 for the highest priority and a 1 for the lowest priority. In most of the groupings there was more than one 10.

Reproductive Services

- 10 — Family planning services

  - Preconception counseling based on risk
  - Pregnancy testing
  - Reversible and irreversible methods of contraception
  - Genetic counseling and services
  - Termination of pregnancy

- 10 — Prenatal care

  - Prenatal visits
  - Counseling and education
  - Case management, including home visits, child care, regular exams, and outreach programs to achieve equitable access to care
  - Laboratory studies
  - Ultrasound, stress testing, biophysical profile, genetic counseling, amniocentesis and, as appropriate, fetal maturity studies

- 10 — Labor and delivery services in certified birth settings

  - Uncomplicated vaginal and Caesarean-section births
  - Ectopic pregnancy
  - Electronic fetal monitoring
  - Fetal scalp sampling
  - Postpartum care
  - Pap test and pelvic exam

- 10 — High-risk pregnancy services

  - Home care services
  - Antepartum hospitalization only if home care is not possible

- 3 — Infertility counseling and workup services

Health Promotion and Disease Prevention

- 10 — Immunizations
- 10 — Nutritional supplements

  - Providing food to hungry people whose poor nutrition makes them a significant health risk; meant as an addition to federal Women, Infant and Children program and food stamps.

The age priority is: children and the elderly; adults

- 10 — Screenings for infants and children from birth to age 2
- 9 — Periodic focused screening based on risk
- 7 — Periodic screening for other people, e.g., Pap smears, mammograms
- Prevention and education programs in the following order: sexually transmitted diseases and teen parents; quitting smoking; ending alcohol and drug abuse; safety and suicide prevention; physical and sexual abuse prevention; and eating disorders

Chronic Disease Management

- 10 — Procedures, therapies or interventions that can restore patients with chronic diseases or conditions to near-full or manageable levels of function and independence

  - Including cataract surgery, lens implants, or corneal transplants

- 9 — Procedures, therapies, or interventions that would maintain patients in the least restrictive and most appropriate environment

  - Including therapy and clinical case management; education and training for primary caregivers; provision of appropriate support services, for example, respite care, homemaker services, transport, child care, and delivery of medicine

Acute Illnesses and Episodic Treatments

- 10 — Diagnosis and treatment of acute illnesses, conditions, and episodes

  - In-hospital care, including intensive care units
  - Emergency and trauma care
  - Anesthesia and surgery
  - Diagnostic and therapeutic radiology and nuclear medicine
  - Diagnostics, laboratory, and pathology studies
  - Medications
  - Appropriate transport and transfer

- 10—Inpatient admissions for psychiatric emergencies and crises

  - Including incapacitating depression, attempted suicide, or suicidal tendencies or acute psychoses

- 9—Physical therapy with predictable return to acceptable level of function

- 9—Durable medical equipment determined to be necessary

- 9—Preventive dentistry for children

- 9—Restorative dental care for adults where necessary for nutrition

- 9—Occupational therapy and speech therapy with predictable return of functions

- 9—Eye exams and eyeglasses for children and elderly every 2 years

- 9—Hearing exams and aids for children and elderly every 3 years

- 8—Orthopedic procedures for replacement of total hip for intractable pain or because of absence of mobility

- 8—Restorative dentistry for children's permanent teeth

- 8—Restorative dentistry for children's original teeth, only for nutrition

- 8—Routine dental care for the elderly

- 8—Necessary reconstructive surgery

- 7—Rehabilitation for improvement of function

- 6—Therapy for alcohol and drug abuse

- 6—Foot care for elderly

- 5—Eye exams and glasses for others every 2 years

- 5—Hearing exams and aids for others every 3 years

- 4—Routine dental care for adults

- 3—Organ transplantation

  - The authors considered the small number who would benefit, the low probability of benefit in many cases, the poor quality of life afterward, and the high costs in deciding to rank transplantation low.

State of Oregon: Medicaid Healthcare Initiative

JOHN KITZHABER, M.D., Oregon Senate
President
MARK GIBSON, Executive Assistant to the
Senate President
Oregon State Senate, Salem, Oregon

The Oregon Health Care Initiative is an attempt to guarantee access to adequate healthcare to all Oregonians. The centerpiece of the program is Senate Bill 27 which extends insurance for basic medical services to tens of thousands of Oregonians who currently cannot afford it. Furthermore, it establishes a process to achieve social and political consensus on what should be included in an "adequate" package of benefits. Finally, in conjunction with a companion legislation (Senate Bill 935), it will extend at least this basic level of care to all working Oregonians who currently lack access to health insurance through their place of employment. How will it work?

Once the state defines the eligible population, the next step is to determine what each individual within that population should get in terms of healthcare. That means defining the benefit level for adequate care. This is a very critical point. To date, most proposals to achieve universal access to healthcare require insurance coverage for an adequate or basic package of benefits. None of these provides a mechanism to determine what constitutes such a package. Nor do they suggest how to define adequate care. It is fair to say that any package of benefits which does not include a service needed by an individual will not be adequate from the standpoint of that individual. If, however, an agreement can be reached that society cannot afford to pay for everything for everyone who may benefit from it, a consensual and responsible process to determine the level of care to which everyone *should* have access must be developed.

Senate Bill 27 establishes a process to develop social and political consensus on what an adequate or a basic package of benefits should be. It creates a Health Services Commission, made up of consumers and providers, to prioritize healthcare services based on the effect each service has on the entire population being served. The result will be a prioritized list of services which reflects both public values and objective clinical data on the effectiveness and the probable outcomes of various medical services and procedures.

When the process is completed, an independent actuarial firm will be retained to determine the cost of providing each service. The goal is to separate the prioritization process from the legislative and political process. The legislature will use the information to make funding decisions which, by their very nature, are political. No "rationing" decisions will be made by the commission.

To illustrate how the process works, Oregon's Medicaid appropriation for the 1990–1991 fiscal year can be used as an example. By dividing the total appropriation amount by the number of people eligible for the program, a figure of $65 per person per month that can be spent to purchase healthcare services can be obtained. With this number as a budget ceiling, a benefit package can be built by using the list compiled by the Health Services Commission, with its accompanying actuarial data (Table 1).

So far this hypothesized package adds up to about $40 per person, thus leaving an additional $25 worth of benefits to be included in the package. The Health Services Commission will do a far more detailed breakdown of services into subgroupings and individual procedures to produce a final "priority" list.

Since the state has already allocated funds for the additional $25 worth of benefits, a debate will ensue when existing revenue has been exhausted about low priority or additional services. Should further

TABLE 1   Medicaid Appropriation Model

Parental care	$ 0.35
Inpatient hospital	27.00
Well baby	0.36
Nutritional supplement	0.25
Transplants	0.60
Prescription drugs	11.00
Dentures	0.37
Hip replacement	0.07
	$40.00

revenue be committed to the program to buy more services? This is where the charge of rationing care comes in.

The same debate over healthcare occurs during every budget cycle. The difference, however, is that now people will no longer be arbitrarily thrown out of the program because of budgeting expediency. Everyone retains his or her coverage, and the debate centers on the *level* of that coverage and on what the state decides is adequate, that is, the socially acceptable minimum level of care that society is willing to pay for.

If there is a limited amount of money to supplement the program, it will be very clear that adding one service will necessarily be done at the expense of another. If the Health Services Commission has done its job properly, however, a social and clinical consensus will have been reached on relative priorities. This process forces the legislature to make those kinds of trade-offs explicitly, publicly, and honestly.

When this process has been completed, the Adult and Family Services Division will be authorized to enter into managed care contracts with providers to deliver a package of services, at a particular cost, for a 1-year period. Should revenue decline during the budget period, the state can neither redefine the eligible population nor reduce reimbursement below the actuarially determined cost. The only options will be:

- To reduce benefits for the entire population from the bottom of the list of benefits, starting with those that are least important
- To maintain revenue at the expense of other programs (for example, education or corrections)
- To raise taxes

In the first case, everyone is treated the same. Although the benefit level may be slightly reduced, no one is summarily thrown out of the program. Universal access to adequate care is maintained. If the revenue level is maintained, then the state has said that any reduction in benefit level would fall below what is considered adequate.

Senate Bill 935 requires that Oregon employers that are *not* currently providing health insurance to their workers do so at a level that is *equal to or greater than* that provided by the state to people with family incomes below the federal poverty level.

Challenges for Public Hospitals

CAROL B. EMMOTT, Ph.D., Executive Director
California Association of Public Hospitals, San Mateo, California

Public hospitals and government-funded delivery systems have had a predictably schizophrenic relationship with managed care. On the one hand, public facilities play a pivotal role in facilitating negotiated rate arrangements among private providers by absorbing an increasing share of unprofitable patients — much to the public systems' financial detriment. Ironically, public systems themselves may soon be required to offer competitive managed care products in order to serve their traditional patients under a variety of insurance schemes being proposed for the uninsured. Proposals for extending insurance to both the medically uninsurable and the unsponsored population as a whole envision the use of managed care organizations as the principal contractors for providing necessary care.

This approach makes a lot of policy sense, particularly in a competitively oriented market. Public hospitals, however, have spent the last decade responding to an ever-expanding demand for care from the unsponsored population. At the same time, private providers, buffered from such financial demands by public delivery systems, have invested in development of managed care products and technology.

Public facilities now find themselves handicapped by chronic underinvestment in aged, unattractive capital plants and a lack of resources to develop the ability to manage capitated contracts. Nevertheless, these public institutions may be asked to compete with private managed care companies for newly sponsored patients. Whether public facilities are able to withstand the potential loss of revenue and the necessity to compete for newly enfranchised patients with managed healthcare options is yet to be seen.

County systems and other indigent care providers can survive and prosper if they do two things: utilize new Medicaid help for "disproportionate share" hospitals to improve their capital plants and develop management tools that are essential to operate in a capitated environment.

The challenge is a formidable one. Policymakers must be willing to assist in this transition. Without such backing the fiscal infrastructure of the public healthcare safety net will be lost. It will be difficult in the best of circumstances for insurance schemes to accommodate the needs of special population groups (for example, non-English speaking, psychiatrically disabled, drug dependent, and homeless). Some safety net will always be required for these vulnerable groups. In addition, it is likely that a profitability differential will continue to make well-insured employees who are in Cadillac plans more fiscally attractive than government-funded patients. Some public delivery system will in all likelihood be required to ensure access for those patients who are relatively less desirable to private payers and providers.

CHAPTER TWENTY-FIVE

Managed Care Research

THE RESEARCH AGENDA IN MANAGED CARE

LOUIS F. ROSSITER, Director of Williamson Institute
Medical College of Virginia, Richmond, Virginia

The changes in the healthcare system that demand new answers to research questions are examined in this chapter as well as a futuristic view of how the role of managed care will develop and what the new research questions will be. Throughout the chapter there is one recurring theme. The HMO and PPO research agenda of the future will be focused on ways of obtaining, using, and applying information to influence the delivery of healthcare. This must be the research agenda for managed care because information technology is the industry's unique strategic advantage.

Healthcare as a field is notoriously stingy in its research and development efforts in the private sector. Managed care plans may be among the lowest spenders on research, with exceptions such as Kaiser-Permanente, because many plans are new and tend to concentrate initial resources on development and growth. This will change as the priorities for HMOs and PPOs shift from an emphasis on growth and market share to ways to better provide managed care services. The big plans, and perhaps the best plans, will have departments for research and development and a corporate appreciation of the value of reliable, relevant research.

WHAT IS AND WHAT IS NOT KNOWN The literature on HMO and PPO research is only summarized here because it is discussed in more detail elsewhere.[1-3] Briefly, what is known and not known about HMOs and PPOs is as follows.

- HMOs appear to have lower costs than traditional insurance by providing incentives to avoid unnecessary care.
- PPOs appear to have lower costs than traditional insurance by encouraging providers to take a discount from charges or risk losing business to competitors.
- HMOs achieve cost savings primarily by lowering the use of hospital services, including admission rates and length of stay for all types of hospitalizations.
- Group- and staff-model HMOs are more effective at achieving cost savings than traditional independent practice associations (IPAs) or network plans.
- HMOs and PPOs attract enrollees typically by offering more comprehensive coverage and lower out-of-pocket costs for about the same premium as traditional insurance plans.
- Economies of scale are not a major factor in the relative cost effectiveness of HMOs and PPOs, and HMOs and PPOs appear to be no better at reducing general trends in healthcare inflation than traditional insurance.
- HMOs and PPOs engage in shadow pricing in markets where HMO and PPO enrollment is not dominant. Premiums are set at or below prevailing traditional insurer premiums, thus denying expected cost savings to employers.
- Published studies do not indicate that the quality of care provided by HMOs is lower than that provided in the fee-for-service sector. In fact, there is a growing body of studies indicating that the process of care in HMOs may be better than fee-for-service when compared by professional standards.
- HMO enrollees, when compared to fee-for-service enrollees, are more satisfied with their claims processing experience and waiting time to see their physician, but are somewhat less satisfied with their interaction with physicians.

There are a number of areas, however, where conflicting evidence about the results or the methods used in the studies casts doubt on the conclusions. And less is known about PPOs than HMOs. Some of the more important areas of conflicting or nonconclusive research findings are summarized as follows.

- There is some evidence that HMOs may have experienced adverse selection in the 1960s and 1970s, but that has changed; numerous recent studies suggest that HMOs are experiencing favorable selection. The methods for detecting favorable selection are not strong, however, so there is some doubt about whether the results are generalizable and stable.
- There are some findings that suggest that HMOs use more preventive services and achieve their savings by doing so. The results on

the use of preventive services are mixed, and the link to costs is more questionable.

- It would appear that administrative costs in HMOs are higher than they are for traditional insurance. However, some of what is more easily identified as administrative costs in HMOs and PPOs is not as readily observed in fee-for-service plans; thus, the studies may be comparing apples to oranges.
- It would seem that, in principle, the competitive impact of the growth of HMOs would encourage cost consciousness among traditional insurers. Anecdotal evidence and case studies suggest that there is a strong competitive impact from HMOs on the behavior of the fee-for-service market in favor of cost reductions. The empirical results with large data sets on costs and use are very mixed. More studies suggest that geographic areas with high HMO market share have higher overall use and cost than other similar areas.
- It is unclear whether HMOs encourage high-cost users to disenroll, with studies showing both favorable and adverse selection through disenrollment.

There is also growing research evidence on the characteristics and organizational and financial trends in the industry. The leaders in providing this kind of information are Interstudy and the Group Health Association of America; they provide regular and timely profiles of industry growth and performance. Many individual plans, primarily HMOs but not PPOs, are engaging in important research on the technical aspects of managing a plan and providing care.

A FRAME OF REFERENCE FOR THE RESEARCH AGENDA

For years the "uninformed" consumer suspected it, and now research scientists are documenting that much of American healthcare is unnecessary. Studies now suggest that 15 to 40 percent of hip replacements, coronary artery bypass graft surgery, and other major procedures are questionable, if not unnecessary.[4] Evidence abounds that unexplained variation in the use of healthcare exists, even within the same small geographic areas with similar populations.[5] Other findings directly link physician recommendations for follow-up visits, laboratory tests, and x-rays to the number of competing physicians in the area.[6] There can be no doubt that the practice of medicine and the advice of physicians is strongly linked to payment and economic factors.

Despite the link between medical practice and economic factors, the physician has always been expected to do what is best for the patient. After all, the physician has been the health professional with unquestioned authority over the management of patient care. In a sense, managed care questions that authority, challenges the physician's role, and provides new systems of incentives, rewards, and punishment to redefine what is good for the patient.

Physicians permitted their authority to be challenged because they allowed the pervasive influence of economic considerations to inextricably tie them to the fee-for-service system. Physician financial expectations rose sharply in the 1970s and 1980s to the extent that the profession could not think strategically. The profession readily understood what was happening to their incomes, but they could not see what was happening to the tolerance for higher costs and what it would mean if they remained unresponsive. Fee-for-service medicine was no longer competitive with managed care, as indicated by the number of enrollees who were voting with their feet. But the average physician enjoyed the autonomy of fee-for-service and its relative financial rewards so much so that the excesses of fee-for-service were not recognized. Escalating costs and relative inefficiency invited intervention from outside.

But the rising cost of healthcare and the relatively high incomes of physicians alone are not enough to explain the advent of managed care. Costs had risen for many years before Medicare and Medicaid. Even after Medicare and Medicaid and the acceleration of inflation, managed care did not begin to achieve its current level of visibility and dominance in some parts of the country. The growth curve for managed care accelerated when information processing became more accessible, lower in cost, and more easily replicated. Information was required in two ways: to interfere with the central role of the physician in the healthcare system and to manage the care when a physician has ignored cost-consciousness rules of behavior.

With managed care, the effective application and use of information has been turned over not to physicians but to others acting alone or in partnership with physicians. In other words, the growth of managed healthcare is a response to the growth of medical information and its misuse under the fee-for-service system and to the availability of data processing technology to deal with the information. Good management information systems always have a central place in managed care plans. In fact, there are many examples of plans that have failed without an adequate information system. From this view, data processing technology is the new element fueling the growth of managed care. Competition, employer concerns over costs, and government awareness of healthcare budgets are merely bit players in a drama that has information technology as the central character.

WAVES OF CHANGE

A research agenda that is not considered with an eye to the future runs the risk of being outdated before it is implemented. The future for managed care could very well have three waves of development.

First Wave: Focus on Averages

The first wave of change consists of information systems that only begin to challenge the individual physician's central authority. Some of the most sophisticated systems merely compare physicians and their activities to each other so there can at least be a movement toward the average (mediocre) in prescribed service use and cost. Thus, in terms of current utilization review and quality assurance practice, modal patterns of physician behavior are established statistically or by consensus. Physician recommendations may be challenged either through prospective, concurrent, or retrospective review by other physicians or healthcare professionals. Thus, patient care is no longer completely managed by the individual physician, but by others.

Managed care in the first wave puts an emphasis on the average as an objective. For example, IPA-model plans and PPOs need information on relative fees and use it to push excessive charges and reimbursements back to the average. Regular reports on physician inpatient and ambulatory use rates are the cornerstone of utilization review in most plans, and the norm becomes the standard against which to encourage behavior change, deny payments from risk pools, and administer sanctions. A focus on average utilization is the hallmark of the first wave.

Second Wave: Focus on Outcomes

While still serving their current functions, utilization review and quality assurance will evolve into technology transfer systems as the variance in service use for patients with the same conditions diminishes. In other words, the identification of optimal treatment patterns and their implementation will be the emphasis in managed care. Medicine often does not know the optimal treatment, given the available information; this has lead to the new research dealing with outcomes of care. Consequently, the near-term research agenda will address the definition of optimal treatment. It will go far beyond the mere identification and encouragement of average care by discouraging high cost and skimpy care and by seeking the kinds of treatments that produce the best outcomes. The HMOs and PPOs that do well in the second wave will become expert in identifying the right way to do things and then create the working environment or the incentive-reward-punishment systems that get the right things done.

Managed care plans will be required to do four tasks in this regard.

1. Organize themselves and devote the resources necessary to assimilate the flow of research findings on outcomes
2. Disseminate the results to the appropriate people in a way that they will be absorbed despite busy work schedules
3. Ensure that the findings are being used in practice
4. Document their effectiveness in their own settings

This description could be interpreted as merely quality care, but managed care could become synonymous with quality care if the management is extended to the effective application of the results of outcomes research.

Third Wave: Focus on Ethical Dilemmas

The third wave could be one that most will not welcome but will probably accept. Mature managed care systems that have gone beyond simply comparing physician activity among physicians and directing physicians to adopt known optimal treatment patterns will be called upon to apply their resources toward rationing healthcare. Rationing means saying "no." Managed care systems are now saying "no" to physicians more than traditional plans ever did. But their negative pronouncements are characteristics of the first wave, achieving the average. Managed care systems will be the best suited to ration healthcare because of their inherent ability to control (manage) based on the knowledge of appropriate treatments and purposeful cost consciousness. The principal rationing criteria could be the age of the patient, but it will disguise itself in criteria such as the capability for a useful life or medical necessity. Thus, there are ethical dimensions to be researched in the development of managed care.

Ups and Downs

Because of the role of information technology and the managed care industry's leadership in developing practical and effective information systems, the prospects for managed care are bright. Fee-for-service, by its very name, is inherently fragmented and uncoordinated, and the incentives are clearly to do more, not less. Detailed management information is not needed to achieve this behavior. Thus all the incentives are in place for traditional insurers to continue to do poorly in the market.

Based on figures from the mid-1980s, if HMO and PPO enrollment growth continues at its recent levels, the entire country will be enrolled in managed care delivery systems by the late 1990s. It is unlikely that recent enrollment growth rates can be maintained, so occasional stumbles are inevitable. But it is equally inevitable that the prospects for growth favor HMOs and PPOs rather than traditional insurance, because of the comparative advantage enjoyed by HMOs and PPOs in information application. Consequently, research must be focused on the organization and application of information in order for HMOs and PPOs to maintain their advantage.

RESEARCH ISSUES IN MANAGED CARE

In the near term the research conducted on managed care issues will continue to focus on the first wave of information application, identification of the average level of care. The definition of what constitutes a managed care plan will evolve as quasi-managed care systems learn how to better interfere with the hitherto central role of the physician and enforce average patterns of practice. Consequently, near-term research issues will continue to focus on comparisons with fee-for-service. The information that will be used for the study will consist of available administrative data involving claims. For example:

- What types of PPOs are as effective as HMOs in lowering costs? What about PPOs compared to fee-for-service? Do exclusive provider organizations do better or worse in cost containment?
- Is quality and satisfaction for PPOs comparable to those of fee-for-service plans, as HMO enrollee satisfaction apparently is?
- Do discounts under PPOs merely encourage physician unbundling and supplier-induced demand, blunting the cost reductions expected under discounts?
- Is favorable selection for HMOs an inherent and stable phenomena? How do PPOs fare in terms of biased selection?
- What benefit packages and premiums would make HMOs and PPOs competitive with traditional insurance?
- Do the incentives and utilization review systems used by IPA-HMOs and PPOs lead to spillover effects on participating providers and, in turn, even have an impact on cost consciousness in their fee-for-service practice?
- What are the provider incentive-reward-punishment systems that best achieve the objectives of providing cost-conscious and high quality care that attracts and retains enrollees? How important are incentives, rewards, and punishment alone and in combination?

It could very well be that the current diversity in the industry in terms of the relationships of providers to plans and to incentives, rewards, and punishment will diminish as research and experience shows what works best. As a relatively new service in the health care industry, managed care will mature as a service delivery system, especially compared to the very small role played by HMOs only in selected areas of the country for the last 50 years. A uniformity of approaches will emerge. Research will help establish uniformity. When it does, the questions about comparisons to traditional insurance will be answered, by in large, and the field will have already entered the second wave of information application.

The second wave will be known for its improvement in the delivery of care and for the virtual elimination of unnecessary services, even though service use rates will be high. Outcomes of care will become a major consideration in the recommendations of physicians, and an awareness of the importance of outcomes will greatly influence the relationship between physicians and patients. The sources of data for the second wave will shift from the claims files, used in the first wave, to the contents of medical records and the results of interventions under controlled situations.

The second wave is just beginning as the government and private industry now ask for more money to study the effectiveness of treatment patterns. National Institute of Health–funded research into arcane and high technology applications is only one part of the second wave. The real story is with HMOs and PPOs themselves as they develop protocols for treatment and standards for care in their own plans. Many plans have already progressed well beyond simply statistical analysis of outlier physician activity (although many others have trouble tackling this) and are well versed in protocol development and defining physician expectations. For example, the "Kaiser way" for Kaiser-Permanente Health Plans depends to a large extent upon group-model peer review and agreement on acceptable patterns of care. It is not only the development and growth of outcomes-oriented medicine but the discovery of appropriate outcomes that will characterize the second wave. A partial list of research issues would include the following:

- What are the indications for any procedure that are predictive of health outcomes?
- Which procedure, when competing procedures exist, is preferred under what circumstances for optimal health outcomes?
- What are the probabilities associated with achieving a health outcome for a given procedure?
- Can alternative sites of care or providers produce better outcomes or similar outcomes at lower cost?
- How can experience or the clinical research literature that has reached conclusions about optimal treatment patterns be best conveyed to practitioners, and are they using the information?

The managed care industry is being held back from going beyond piecemeal entry into focus on outcomes because of the lack of necessary information, information systems, and sources of data. Current analysis, when it is done at all, is largely focused on processed claims.

In the third wave of information application, research will focus upon the ethical dilemmas posed by the management of care and the limits of spending imposed by payers. Much more of the caregiving will be for those with chronic conditions than it is now, because of the aging of the population. With this in mind some of the upcoming research issues will be:

- When is it appropriate to deny preventive services that are not cost effective?
- When is exclusion of experimental and high-cost procedures ap-

propriate, especially when the funds could otherwise be spent on more cost-effective procedures?

- What is cost effective? Cost-effectiveness studies of almost any kind will be done.
- When is it appropriate to deny services? Heroic or extraordinary healthcare when the quality of life is not helped and death is near will probably be eliminated.
- When should patients that are to be channeled to alternative modes of treatment be screened if the cost effectiveness of their desired procedure is not apparent?

The third wave will be fraught with difficult questions and answers. Most plans will not like the expanded scope of concern for managed care when the role of devising a mechanism for rationing will be thrust upon the managed care industry. But it will be an easy role for payers to require. What better system to ration scarce resources than one that provides a fixed amount of money per person which must be used to provide all the necessary care? If payers are willing to live with some rationing to lower costs, the management advantage offered by HMOs and PPO will be best suited to achieve their goals.

CONCLUSIONS   The marketing methods and actuarial research now used by managed care plans will not necessarily change, but the currency of the results will change, requiring frequent updates as HMO and PPO growth continues. It will become increasingly difficult and costly for plans to identify the next low-cost group for enrollment as enrollment grows. So applied research will be even more important in marketing and financial functions as a prerequisite for efficient HMO and PPO operations.

Likewise, the special needs and care requirements of those covered by public programs is important. This is especially true for the elderly, because their needs are so different from the under-65 population that HMOs and PPOS are accustomed to dealing with. Successful plans in these markets will have clinical people who specialize in caring for publicly supported patients. Much research needs to be done on who are the best specialists and what services they can provide.

Finally, the impact and value of the research will become even more apparent when industry competition turns from pitting HMO and PPO growth against traditional insurance coverage to competition among HMOs and PPOs themselves for managed care business. In some parts of the country such competition is already the norm.

Answers to such research questions will give managed care plans the operational advantage they need to succeed.

REFERENCES

1. H. S. Luft and J. B. Trauner, "The Operations and Performance of Health Maintenance Organizations." Prepared under NCHSR Contract No. 233-79-3016 (1981).

2. K. M. Langwell and S. F. Moore, "A Synthesis of Research on Competition in the Financing and Delivery of Health Services." DHHS Pub. no. (PHS) 83-3327, U.S. Department of Health and Human Services, National Center for Health Services Research (1982).

3. L. F. Rossiter et al. "New Reimbursement Systems for Medical Care for the Elderly" In: (I. Parham and J. Teitleman, eds.), pp. 201–225, Greenwood Press, Westport, Conn., 1989.

4. J. Wennberg and A. Gittelsohn, "Variations in Medical Care Among Small Areas." *Scientific American* **246:**120–134 (1982).

5. C. M. Winslow, "The Appropriateness of Performing Coronary Artery Bypass Surgery," *JAMA* **260**(4):505–509 (July 22/29, 1988).

6. L. F. Rossiter and G. R. Wilensky, "A Reexamination of the Use of Physician Services: The Role of Physician-Initiated Demand," *Inquiry* **20:** 162–172 (1983).

INDEX